# DIAGNOSTIC ANGIOGRAPHY

**Saadoon Kadir, M.D.**

Associate Professor
Division of Cardiovascular and Interventional Radiology
The Johns Hopkins University
School of Medicine
and The Johns Hopkins Hospital
Baltimore, Maryland

*1986*
*W. B. Saunders Company*
Philadelphia — London — Toronto — Mexico City
Rio de Janeiro — Sydney — Tokyo — Hong Kong

W. B. Saunders Company:   West Washington Square
                          Philadelphia, PA 19105

**Library of Congress Cataloging in Publication Data**

Kadir, Saadoon.

Diagnostic angiography.

1. Angiography.     2. Blood-vessels—Diseases—Diagnosis.     I. Title.     [DNLM: 1. Angiography—Methods.     WG 500 K11d]

RC691.6.A53K32        1986        616.1'30757        85–11872

ISBN 0–7216–1055–2

*Editor:*  Dean Manke
*Designer:*  Terri Siegel
*Production Managers:*  Laura Tarves and Bill Preston
*Manuscript Editor:*  Charlotte Fierman
*Illustration Coordinator:*  Walt Verbitski
*Indexer:*  Carol Wolf

Diagnostic Angiography                                    ISBN 0–7216–1055–2

Last digit is the print number:     9    8    7    6    5    4    3    2

*TO MY PARENTS*

*TO MY WIFE SALMA,*
*OUR CHILDREN ADNAN, TARIK,*
*KHALID, and AYESHA*

# Foreword

*Diagnostic Angiography* clearly was written primarily for radiologists. No doubt this text will be of great value to them. However, I think many general surgeons will find much of interest in this outstanding effort. Particularly those surgeons whose chief interests lie in vascular and/or biliary tract work will find a great deal of material in this text that will be of practical use.

Vascular surgeons obviously must have a firm background in diagnostic angiography. This book deals completely but concisely with the indications for angiography and the appropriate studies to be ordered for the various vascular diseases. The chapters are conveniently organized, mostly on the basis of regional anatomy. There is an ample supply of clear angiograms to emphasize points and to demonstrate appropriate pathology. In addition, differential diagnoses are tabulated, and pitfalls of interpretation that can befall radiologists and vascular surgeons alike are contained within each chapter.

There are few areas of surgery in which management has changed, and improved, as dramatically as in the field of biliary tract surgery. This is in large part due to the advances in diagnostic cholangiography and therapeutic intervention championed by the Cardiovascular Radiology Division at Johns Hopkins and other centers throughout the United States. The chapter on the biliary system is outstanding. It reviews indications for percutaneous cholangiography, describes differential diagnoses, and provides many cholangiograms to supply examples of a wide range of pathological processes.

Although *Diagnostic Angiography* will quickly find its way into the libraries of radiologists, it clearly is a text that has much to offer the vascular and biliary surgeons. It is beautifully organized and well written, and the illustrations are superb. I think it is a welcome addition to the consultative-type textbooks that many general surgeons wish to have on their bookshelves.

JOHN L. CAMERON, M.D.
*Professor and Chairman*
*Department of Surgery*
*The Johns Hopkins Medical Institutions*

# Foreword

The advent of interventional radiology and improved surgical techniques has strongly stimulated improvements in diagnostic angiography to provide more detailed information for the benefit of patient management. *Diagnostic Angiography* reflects the remarkable advances in this field over the past few years. This book provides guidelines for the proper utilization of equipment and the choice of support systems to accomplish the important task of diagnostic evaluation of the vascular and biliary tracts. Based on a rich experience in cardiovascular angiography, Dr. Kadir discusses in 23 chapters the proper approach to many relevant clinical questions. He demonstrates that, in many ways, angiography requires different and often unique approaches to the various organs of the body in order to be effective and safe in the conduct of each examination. In addition to demonstrating how one tailors each examination to the patient's individual needs, appropriate attention is called to overall patient care in association with the diagnostic study. Preangiographic patient evaluation and post-procedure follow-up by the radiologist are prerequisites to the success of patient management by interventional radiologists and vascular surgeons alike.

Written primarily for radiologists, this well-illustrated book also offers valuable clinical information and discusses interpretation of angiographic studies and how to avoid pitfalls. It is carefully stipulated that unless good diagnostic information is available, interventional procedures cannot be performed successfully and safely.

Moreover, *Diagnostic Angiography* will also be of considerable value to vascular surgeons in pointing out the potentials of the field as they exist today. Therefore, I feel that this book reflects the state of the art in diagnostic angiography and addresses itself effectively to the needs of all specialists dealing with vascular and biliary tract disorders.

Martin W. Donner, M.D.
*Professor and Chairman*
*Department of Radiology and Radiological Sciences*
*The Johns Hopkins Medical Institutions*

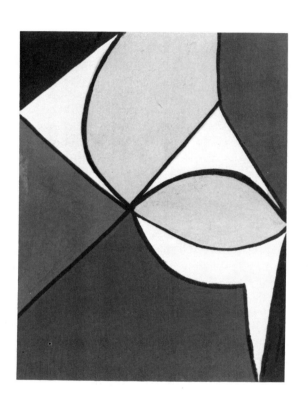

# Preface

The impact of angiography upon patient management is more significant today than it was one or two decades ago. This is primarily due to the increasing applications of transcatheter interventional procedures. Over the past four years we have experienced a 2½-fold increase in the number of such procedures, which has brought with it a concomitant increase in the number of diagnostic studies.

Newer imaging techniques have not replaced diagnostic angiography but have redefined its role in patient management. The introduction of intravenous digital subtraction angiography, predicted to replace much of diagnostic arteriography, has failed to provide an acceptable alternative in all but a small number of cases. On the other hand, intraarterial digital subtraction angiography has become invaluable for both diagnostic studies and transcatheter therapy.

Diagnostic angiography is no longer an independent subspecialty. It is a part of the exciting and sophisticated field of interventional radiology. Interventional angiography is a natural extension of diagnostic angiography, and a meticulously performed diagnostic study provides the very basis for successful transcatheter intervention. In fact, without some of the selective catheterization techniques, many interventional procedures could not be possible.

This book was conceived with a twofold purpose: to serve as a manual of current angiographic techniques and to provide a didactic textbook of angiography. There are many different approaches to the performance of angiography, and this text describes some of the established methods without intending to be dogmatic. It should be of value to the practicing radiologist, cardiovascular and interventional radiology fellows, and radiology residents. Furthermore, it should serve as a source of reference for our colleagues in the medical and surgical subspecialties.

With the exclusion of cerebral and cardiac angiography, this book covers the entire spectrum of diagnostic angiography, including digital subtraction angiography and chol*angiography*. There is a special emphasis upon angiographic technique, with a large chapter (Chapter 3) being devoted entirely to this topic. Each chapter includes pertinent clinical information, radiological findings, and indications and contraindications for angiography. In addition, pertinent techniques and details for performing individual studies, as well as relevant complications, are also discussed. Each chapter also contains a complete description of the angiographic findings and discusses the angiographic pitfalls resulting from interpretive errors or angiographic "look alikes."

SAADOON KADIR, M.D.

# Acknowledgments

The completion of this book would not have been possible without the invaluable help and support of numerous individuals. The list of names is far too long and thus cannot be included here. A significant stimulus for this work came from our residents and fellows in cardiovascular and interventional radiology.

I would like to express my gratitude to Dr. Frederick Eames from the Section of Neuroradiology and Dr. Glenn Robeson, chairman of the Department of Radiology, Albany Medical Center, for writing the chapter on Spinal Angiography. I would also like to thank my department chairman, Dr. Martin W. Donner, and Dr. John L. Cameron, chairman of the Department of Surgery, for reviewing several of the chapters and for writing the forewords.

The literature searches and compilation of the references would not have been possible without the help of Ms. Elaine Pinkney. Most of the artwork was done by Jonathan Dimes and the logo was prepared by Naseer Farooqui. The photographs were prepared in the Photography Laboratories of the Departments of Radiology and Pathology, The Johns Hopkins Medical Institutions.

Many of the illustrations used in this book have been published previously. I would like to thank those authors and the publishers for their permission and for providing me with these invaluable illustrations. In particular, I would like to thank Dr. Christos A. Athanasoulis, my teacher and friend, for permission to use some of the illustrations from the teaching files of the Massachusetts General Hospital. I would also like to thank the manufacturing companies that provided me with equipment photographs used in Chapter 1.

The enthusiastic help and support that I have received from my editor, Mr. Dean Manke, my former editor, Mrs. Lisette Bralow, and all the people at W. B. Saunders Company have contributed significantly toward the preparation and completion of this text.

Finally, the virtuous patience and understanding displayed by my family and friends and their unrelenting support and encouragement throughout the difficult period during which this book was in preparation deserve very special mention.

SAADOON KADIR, M.D.

# Contents

# EQUIPMENT

## Angiography Room, Imaging Systems, Monitors, Life Support and Accessory Equipment

In this chapter, an attempt will be made to identify the basic requirements for an angiographic room and some of the optional equipment and materials that may be helpful in the performance of both diagnostic and therapeutic procedures. For more information regarding angiographic room design and equipment performance and purchase, the reader is referred to references 1 to 4.

### ROOM DESIGN (Fig. 1–1)

When planning an angiographic room, it must be kept in mind that such procedures require a degree of asepsis. Since foreign bodies are introduced into the vascular, uri-nary, or biliary system, inadequate precautions may have serious consequences.

The angiographic room should be large enough to accommodate all the equipment required for angiography and still provide ample space for additional emergency equipment such as emergency carts, respirators, and other anesthesia equipment. The ideal room should be at least 5000 to 6000 sq ft with a minimal width of 20 ft (not including the observation/control room).

The radiographic tubes, image intensifier, and monitors should be ceiling mounted. Together with concealed wiring, these prevent unnecessary congestion and provide for a clear floor space. In addition, the room should be appropriately ventilated and air

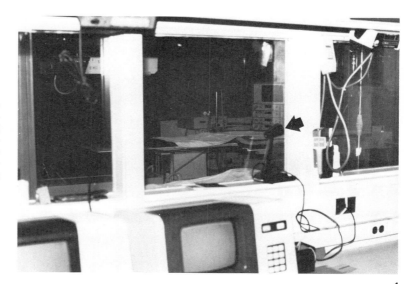

*Figure 1–1.* View of angio-graphic room from the observa-tion/control room. The lead-lined glass window facilitates observa-tion of the patient. Communica-tion between the two rooms is pos-sible via the intercom system (*arrow*) or a split-glass window.

conditioned to prevent equipment and operator breakdown and should not be situated in areas exposed to excessive traffic.

At least two entrances are necessary to the angiographic room. One of these should be to the observation/control room. A large lead-lined glass window between the angiographic and observation/control rooms facilitates observation of the patient during filming. In addition, the observation/control room should have a television monitor to enable visiting physicians and trainees to observe procedures without having to enter the angiographic room. The electrocardiographic monitor should be placed in such a position that it can also be viewed from the observation/control room. Alternatively, an additional electrocardiographic monitor may be placed in this room. The other opening from the angiographic room should be into the hallway. This opening should be large enough to accommodate passage of beds from the hospital's intensive care units.

The angiographic room should be well illuminated and equipped with a dimmer switch (rheostat control). In addition, there should be a high intensity light to enable the vascular radiologist to work with the overhead lights dimmed. This spotlight should have a foot-operated pedal adjacent to the pedal for the fluoroscope to enable the radiologist to operate the light. An adequate number of safety power outlets should be available to operate additional equipment. Ideally, many of these outlets may be located in the base of the radiographic table. These and the power source for the essential radiographic and life support equipment must be connected to the hospital's emergency power supply.

There should also be a countertop work space (minimal size 4 by 2 ft) in close proximity to a sink and closed wall cabinets (over a 10 to 12 ft space) for the storage of frequently used items such as catheters, guide wires, intravenous solutions, and accessories. A sink is required for surgical scrubbing. This may be situated within the angiographic room or immediately outside it. Adjacent to this sink should be a shelf for surgical masks and caps, which should be required for all personnel entering the angiographic room before or during a procedure.

## IMAGING SYSTEMS (Figs. 1–2 and 1–3)

The basic requirements for angiographic equipment are a high capacity generator ca-

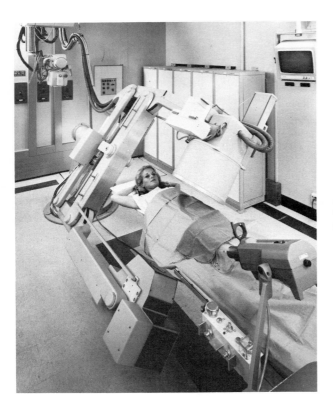

*Figure 1–2.* Versatile C-arm Poly DIAGNOST-A. Complex angulation is possible in all planes. (Photograph courtesy of Philips Medical Systems, Inc., Shelton, Connecticut.)

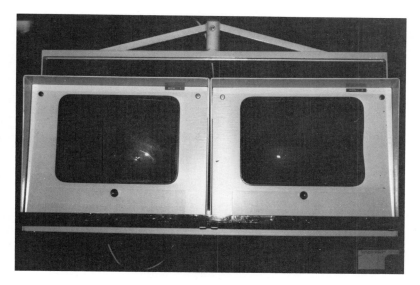

*Figure 1–3.* Dual ceiling-mounted television monitors for interventional and involved diagnostic angiographic procedures.

pable of delivering at least 1000 to 1500 mA with a constant potential. This is necessary to permit short exposure times in order to eliminate motion artefacts and to permit rapid sequence filming in the optimal kVp range. The radiographic tube should have a high speed rotating anode with a 12° target angle and 1.2 or 0.6 mm focal spot to cover a 14 by 14 inch field size. For magnification arteriography, a smaller focal spot (0.3 mm) is necessary in order to obtain high spatial resolution. However, this reduces the field size.

A high resolution image intensifier and a television chain with the capability for magnification fluoroscopy are necessary for small vessel arteriography and interventional procedures. This capability is further enhanced by a 105 mm rapid sequence spot film device and video recording system. A digital subtraction unit can be coupled to it to complete the imaging system.

Digital subtraction angiography is fast becoming an essential part of every diagnostic radiological department. Thus, new equipment purchases should be made with due consideration of this requirement.[5]

The ideal system for fluoroscopy is a C or U arm. This permits fluoroscopy in variable planes without having to move the patient. Alternatively, a cradle can be used for this purpose. Such multiplanar fluoroscopy is often necessary to determine the location of branch vessels in the sagittal plane for selective catheterization. If the control handles for the table top, collimators, and C or U arm either can be sterilized or are covered by sterile drapes, the system could be operated

by the vascular radiologist, which would free the radiological technologist for other work.

For most nonvascular and nonselective vascular procedures, a single television monitor is sufficient. For selective vascular, interventional, and involved diagnostic procedures, dual ceiling-mounted television monitors are of benefit. Images obtained by digital subtraction angiography or recorded on video tape (or disk) may be replayed and "frozen" on one monitor to serve as a guide for selective catheterization or interventional procedures. This is not necessary if a "road-mapping" program is available for the digital subtraction angiography unit.

## ANGIOGRAPHIC TABLE

The table top should be free floating and capable of being elevated in order to adjust to the height of the vascular radiologist and to perform magnification angiography. In combination with a C or U arm, a flat top table is used. For lower extremity arteriography, a flat top stepping table is required, unless long film changers are used. For other ceiling-mounted image intensifying systems, a cradle top is useful. A tilt table is useful, but not essential; for biliary or urinary tract and venous studies.

## FILM CHANGERS (Figs. 1–4 and 1–5)

Both roll and cut film changers are available. The latter offer several advantages such as ease of handling, processing, viewing, and

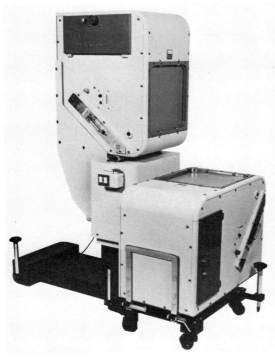

*Figure 1–4.* Biplane AOT-S rapid film changers. (Photograph courtesy of Elema-Schonander, Inc., Elk Grove Village, Illinois.)

The smaller Puck film changers (Elema-Schonander, Inc., Elk Grove Village, Illinois), which hold up to twenty 14 × 14 inch films, fulfill most angiographic requirements. In addition to being small and handy, such changers can be mounted onto the C or U arm. The Puck film changers permit a maximum of four exposures/sec. Alternatively, free-standing rapid film changers that permit 6 exposures/sec and hold up to 30 films (AOT-S, Elema-Schonander, Inc., Elk Grove Village, Illinois) can be used.

For lower extremity arteriography, either a stepping table with a Puck or AOT-S film changer or an extra large field changer using cassettes can be employed. Such large field changers are advantageous for arteriography and venography of the lower extremities, since the entire extremity can be evaluated on each exposure (maximum field size approximately 14 by 51 inches), and calculation of the timing for lower extremity arteriography is less crucial. The disadvantages are the need for an additional ceiling mounted radiographic tube with a tube to floor distance between 87 and 110 inches and a maximal filming speed of 1 film/sec.

storage. In addition, during biplane angiography, roll film is more likely to be affected by scatter radiation, despite the use of cross hatched grids, and may thus lead to degradation of the image. With cut film changers, alternating exposure will circumvent this problem.

## SCREENS AND FILMS

Rare earth screens provide better resolution and decrease patient exposure, especially during magnification arteriography, as a result of a decreased mA requirement. They are usually 2 to 4 times faster than the cal-

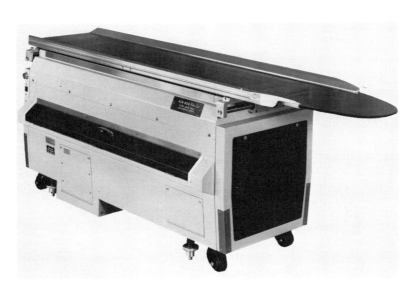

*Figure 1–5.* Long cassette film changer for lower extremity arteriography and venography. (Photograph courtesy of B. C. Medical Manufacturing Ltd., Montreal, Canada.)

cium tungstate screens. With the use of high speed screen–film combinations, the quantum mottle may be disturbing.

## INJECTORS (Fig. 1–6)

Contrast medium injectors are available from several manufacturers. Flow rate–guided mechanical injectors with a pressure-limiting switch are used most commonly. Desirable features of angiographic injectors are (1) a contrast syringe heater (to reduce contrast viscosity), (2) mechanical injection volume limiting capability, (3) flow rates of up to 40 ml/sec, (4) linear acceleration (gradual increase in contrast delivery to prevent catheter recoil), and (5) the capability for injector or film changer delay.

## MONITORS AND LIFE SUPPORT EQUIPMENT (Fig. 1–7)

A three-channel electrocardiographic monitor, cardiac defibrillator, and capability for monitoring and recording intraarterial pressures should be available in every angiographic room. Oxygen (centrally supplied or in portable tanks), suction, and carbon dioxide (for the inflation of flow-directed balloon catheters) should also be available. An emergency cart with instruments and medication for resuscitation should be in the immediate vicinity of the angiographic room.

## MISCELLANEOUS EQUIPMENT

Most patients undergoing a diagnostic or an interventional procedure have some degree of apprehension. In our experience, in addition to a careful explanation of the procedure and the use of sedative medication, soft radio music, according to the patient's request, has helped to decrease this apprehension. A two-way intercom system permitting communication with colleagues and technologists in the observation/control room has also been helpful (see Fig. 1–1).

The cold skin prepping solution is perceived as uncomfortable by most patients. An electric ultrasonic gel warmer (Thermasonic gel warmer, Parker Laboratories, Inc., Orange, New Jersey) provides a simple means for warming the prepping solution.

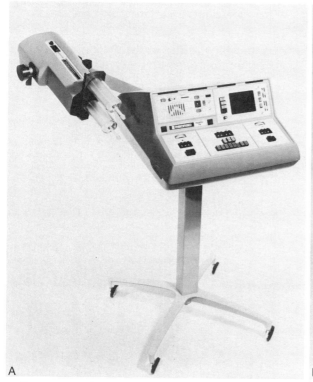
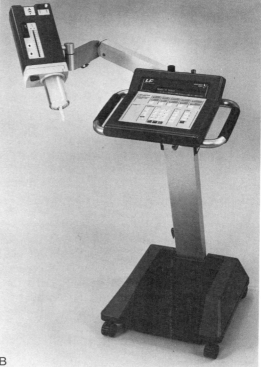

A                                                                      B

*Figure 1–6.* Angiographic injectors. A, Medrad IV. (Photograph courtesy of Medrad, Pittsburgh, Pennsylvania.) B, Angiomat 6000 digital injector. (Photograph courtesy of Liebel-Flarsheim, Cincinnati, Ohio.)

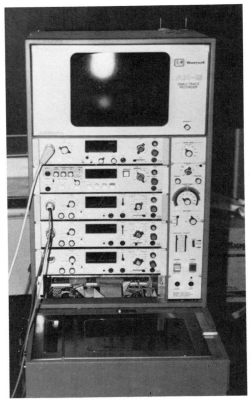

*Figure 1–7.* EKG/arterial pressure monitor and recorder.

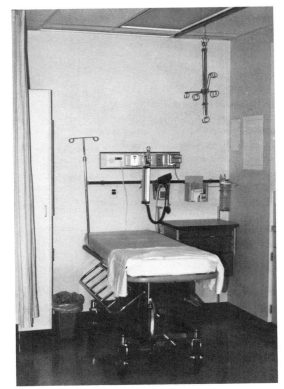

*Figure 1–8.* A cubicle from the post-procedural recovery and observation room for outpatient angiography and interventional radiological procedures.

## POST-PROCEDURE
## RECOVERY/OBSERVATION ROOM
### (Fig. 1–8)

With the availability of 3 to 5 Fr high flow catheters, outpatient arteriography can be performed in selected patients. Currently, some interventional radiological procedures are also being performed routinely on outpatients (eg, varicocele occlusion, percutaneous biliary stone removal). Such outpatient procedures necessitate a facility to permit observation of the patient for recovery from the effects of sedative medication and for the detection of procedure-related complications prior to discharge. This facility should be in close proximity to the angiographic rooms. The observation period for outpatient intraarterial studies is 4 hours, and for venous studies and most other outpatient interventional radiological procedures the period is 2 hours.

## REFERENCES

1. Thompson FT: A Practical Approach to Modern X-Ray Equipment. Boston, Little, Brown & Company, 1978.
2. Fischer HW: Radiology Departments: Planning, Operation, and Management. Ann Arbor, Edwards Brothers, 1982.
3. Christensen EE, Curry TS II, Nunnaly J: An Introduction to the Physics of Diagnostic Radiology. Philadelphia, Lea & Febiger, 1973.
4. Coulam CM, Erickson J, Rollo FD, et al (eds): The Physical Basis of Medical Imaging. New York, Appleton-Century-Crofts, 1981.
5. Levin DC, Dunham L: New equipment considerations for angiographic laboratories. AJR 139:775–780, 1982.

# Materials for Catheterization

The type of materials used for percutaneous catheterization may vary considerably from institution to institution. Among other factors, this reflects the individual philosophy, which is most frequently based upon the experience of the vascular radiologist.

In this chapter, some of the frequently used materials for selective and nonselective angiography will be discussed. Since such materials are available from several manufacturers, only some of the basic types will be described.

## NEEDLES (Fig. 2–1)

The needles used for percutaneous puncture of the femoral, axillary, or brachial arteries or the femoral vein may be of three basic types: (1) with a sharp, beveled outer cannula and matching stylet, or (2) with a squared, blunt outer cannula (this is usually tapered) and a diamond-shaped or pencil point stylet, or (3) with a Teflon outer sheath.

All types function equally well and the choice of needle usually reflects personal preference. A disadvantage of the diamond-shaped or pencil point stylet is the length of the stylet, which protrudes beyond the tip of the cannula. This may also be the case with the beveled needle with the Teflon sheath.

When using a needle with a long stylet protruding beyond the cannula, consideration should be given to the fact that during a shallow puncture the outer cannula or sheath may be only partially within the vascular lumen. In this situation, insertion of the sheath or a guide wire may lead to dissection. This can be avoided by inserting the needle deep, so that it touches the underlying bone. In this case, a two-wall puncture is performed, and as the needle is withdrawn, the true intravascular position of the cannula or sheath is assured.

The needle flange may be funnel shaped (Seldinger type) or may have the proximal end of the outer cannula protruding beyond the hub (Potts-Cournand or Amplatz type). The advantages of the latter type of extension are that pulsatile flow can be recognized easily and that clotting does not occur within the needle hub extension. In addition, the extension permits differentiation between a weak pulsatile flow (partial intramural position of the sheath or outer cannula) and a strong pulsatile flow (true intraluminal position).

Occasionally, the relatively small orifice of the outer cannula extension may give rise to difficulty during insertion of a J guide wire. However, with the aid of guide wire introducers (for straightening the J tip) packaged with all curve-tipped guide wires, this is no longer a problem.

**Amplatz Needle.** This is a 2½ inch long, three-part needle consisting of a beveled cannula, a matching stylet, and an approximately 5 Fr (0.068 inch) fitted radiopaque Teflon outer sheath that is tapered at the tip. The cannula has a Cournand hub extension. The needle is available in 16, 18, and 20 gauge. For adult angiography, the 18 gauge needle is used more frequently. The Teflon sheath from the 18 gauge needle accepts a 0.038 inch or smaller guide wire, whereas the cannula with the Cournand extension will accept only a 0.025 inch or smaller guide wire.

*Application*: The Amplatz needle is used for femoral artery and vein puncture and brachial and axillary artery puncture. In addition, it may be used for puncture of vascular grafts and dialysis access fistulae.

**Angiocath.** This consists of a beveled metal cannula with a Teflon sheath. Such angiocaths are routinely used for venous access by IV teams. Various sizes are used for vascular radiological procedures.

7

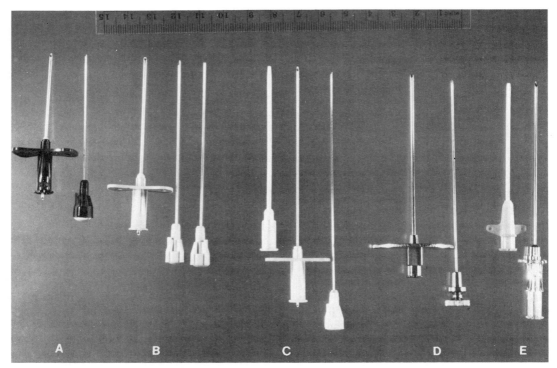

*Figure 2–1.* Needles for arterial and venous puncture. *A*, Pediatric, *B*, Potts-Cournand, *C*, Amplatz, *D*, Seldinger, and *E*, Angiocath.

The Teflon sheath may be advantageous, as it can be advanced into the vessel without the aid of a guide wire. In our own experience, however, this is not always easy and the number of veins lost by attempting this maneuver is high.

**Application:** Either the 16 gauge or the 18 gauge angiocath is employed for cubital vein puncture (digital subtraction angiography), and the 18 gauge angiocath is used for pediatric angiography (arterial or venous puncture). The sheath of the 16 gauge angiocath accepts a 0.035 inch guide wire. The 20 and 22 gauge angiocaths are used for upper or lower extremity venography.

**Butterfly Needle** (Fig. 2–2). Because of its sharp beveled tip, the butterfly needle is ideally suited for obtaining access to small and medium-sized veins. Various sizes are used for vascular radiological procedures. A 19 gauge needle is utilized for cubital vein puncture (for digital subtraction angiography). For this application, the plastic tubing is cut off at the needle hub to permit insertion of a guide wire (0.025 inch). A 23 gauge needle is used for upper or lower extremity venography.

**Potts-Cournand Needle.** This is essentially a two-part needle that is available with or without a rounded, blunt obturator. It is $2\frac{3}{64}$ inches long and has a thin-walled outer cannula that is slightly beveled and a sharp, beveled, hollow inner stylet. Without the obturator, it is available in 16, 17, and 19 gauge. With the 17 gauge needle, a 0.038 inch or smaller guide wire can be used. An 18 gauge, $2\frac{3}{4}$ inch hollow stylet needle with a perforated stylet hub (to identify back bleeding) is also available for single wall

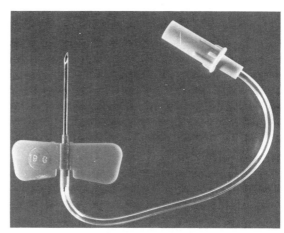

*Figure 2–2.* Butterfly needle with short tubing.

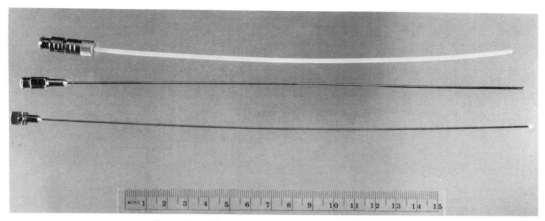

*Figure 2–3.* Needle for translumbar aortography.

arterial puncture (UMI, Ballston Spa, New York).

**Seldinger-type Needle.** This is available as a relatively heavy metal needle or as a lightweight disposable plastic hub needle. It is 2⅞ inches long and has a thin-walled outer cannula, a tapered, squared tip, and a funnel-shaped, open-ended hub. The inner stylet is either diamond shaped or beveled, or it may have a pencil point tip. It is available in 16, 18, and 20 gauge. The 18 gauge needle is used for adult angiography. The outer cannula accepts a 0.038 inch guide wire. The all-metal needle is not used frequently because of the availability of lighter, disposable needles.

*Application:* The Seldinger-type needle is used for arterial and venous puncture. In areas of excessive scarring, eg, after vascular surgery, the metal needle may be advantageous because of its stiffness.

**TLA Needle** (Fig. 2–3). This is a 20 cm long, three-part needle consisting of an 18 gauge (4 Fr) square-tipped metal cannula with a diamond-shaped stylet tip and a fitted outer Teflon sheath (6 Fr). The metal cannula accepts a 0.035 inch or smaller guide wire.

**Percutaneous Transhepatic Cholangiography Needle** (Fig. 2–4). This is a 20 cm long "skinny" needle with a bevel-tipped cannula and matching stylet. Two different sizes are used for cholangiography. The 23 gauge needle (green hub) is very flexible and is easily deflected or bent (by a hard intrahe-

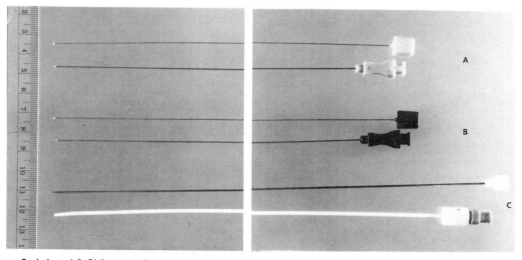

*Figure 2–4. A* and *B,* Chiba needles for percutaneous transhepatic cholangiography: 23 gauge (*A*) and 22 gauge (*B*). *C,* Sheath needle for percutaneous transhepatic biliary drainage, transhepatic portal vein catheterization, and splenoportography.

patic lesion, a rib, or even deep respiration). The larger 22 gauge needle (black hub) is stiffer and thus more easily steerable. The cannula of this needle accepts a 0.018 inch guide wire. Thus, if a suitable radicle has been punctured on the diagnostic cholangiogram, a 0.018 inch "coat hanger" guide wire can be used to gain access to the ductal system for the insertion of a drainage catheter.

Unless a large duct has been entered, intraductal pressures cannot be measured accurately through the cannula of these needles.

*Application*: This needle is used for percutaneous transhepatic cholangiography and percutaneous biopsy of lymph nodes or other masses. Additional applications are the percutaneous rupture of inadvertently migrated silicone mini balloons and splenoportography (22 gauge needle) using digital subtraction techniques.

**Portal Vein/Biliary Drainage Needle** (Fig. 2–4). This consists of a 24 cm long, 19 gauge metal stylet with a diamond-shaped tip and a fitted 16 gauge Teflon sheath (~5½ Fr, tapers down to 18 gauge at the tip). The sheath is radiopaque and accepts a 0.038 inch or smaller guide wire.

*Application*: This needle is used for percutaneous transhepatic portal vein catheterization, percutaneous transhepatic biliary drainage, and percutaneous splenoportography.

**Pediatric Needles.** Most needles are available in pediatric sizes. Such needles are usually shorter (1½ inch), thin walled, and either 19 or 20 gauge. Short bevel–tipped needles are better suited for percutaneous puncture of small vessels and are available as White pediatric needles (Becton-Dickenson, Rutherford, New Jersey). The 19 gauge needles accept 0.028 inch guide wires and the 20 gauge needles accept 0.021 inch guide wires.

**Lymphangiography Needle.** See Chapter 21.

## GUIDE WIRES

Guide wires are required to "guide" the insertion, positioning, repositioning, and exchange of catheters. With the exception of the double flex guide wires (see below), all guide wires have a soft end (either straight or a J-shaped curve) and a stiff end. Only the soft end is designed for intravascular use. However, occasionally the stiff end may be used to carry out certain maneuvers in order to facilitate catheterization (see Chapter 3).

Guide wires consist of two stainless steel inner wires and an outer coil spring. One of the inner wires is rigid and has a core or mandrel that is tapered at the soft end of the wire. The other one is a fine, flexible wire that runs the entire length of the guide wire and is soldered to both ends. The latter wire is a safety feature, which is designed to prevent fracture or separation of the coil spring. The taper of the rigid steel core determines the stiffness or flexibility of the guide wire. Heavy duty guide wires are stiffer because of a thicker or stiffer core wire.

The standard length for adult guide wires is 145 cm. Pediatric guide wires are often 125 cm long. Special guide wires are available in shorter and longer sizes. Most wires for intravascular use are Teflon coated.

### Regular Guide Wires

**Regular Fixed Core Wires.** The inner core of these guide wires is tapered so that the distal 5 cm are flexible. Such wires are available with straight or J tips.

**LT and LLT Wires.** The distal 10 cm of the LT wires are flexible, whereas the distal 15 cm of the LLT (long length tapered) wires are flexible. These wires are available with straight and J tips.

*Application:* The primary use of LT and LLT wires is in selective catheterization for diagnostic and interventional angiography.

**Movable Core Wires** (Fig. 2–5). In the movable core wires, the inner core (mandrel) is stiff (nontapered).* This core can be withdrawn for any distance from the tip of the wire with the aid of a fine handle. The flexibility of the wire tip depends upon the distance over which the core has been withdrawn. Once the core has been withdrawn, the coil spring is extremely floppy and there is an abrupt transition between the floppy coil spring and the rigid core. These wires are available with J or straight tips.

*Application:* Movable core wires are useful for catheterization of tortuous vessels, in which it is difficult to advance wires with a stiffer core. For the most part, however, this task has been taken over by the LT and LLT wires. In addition, other special wires and techniques are available for the catheterization of tortuous and stenotic vessels (see below and Chapter 3). When using these movable core wires for catheterization of se-

---

*Movable core wires with a tapered inner core have also become available from some manufacturers.

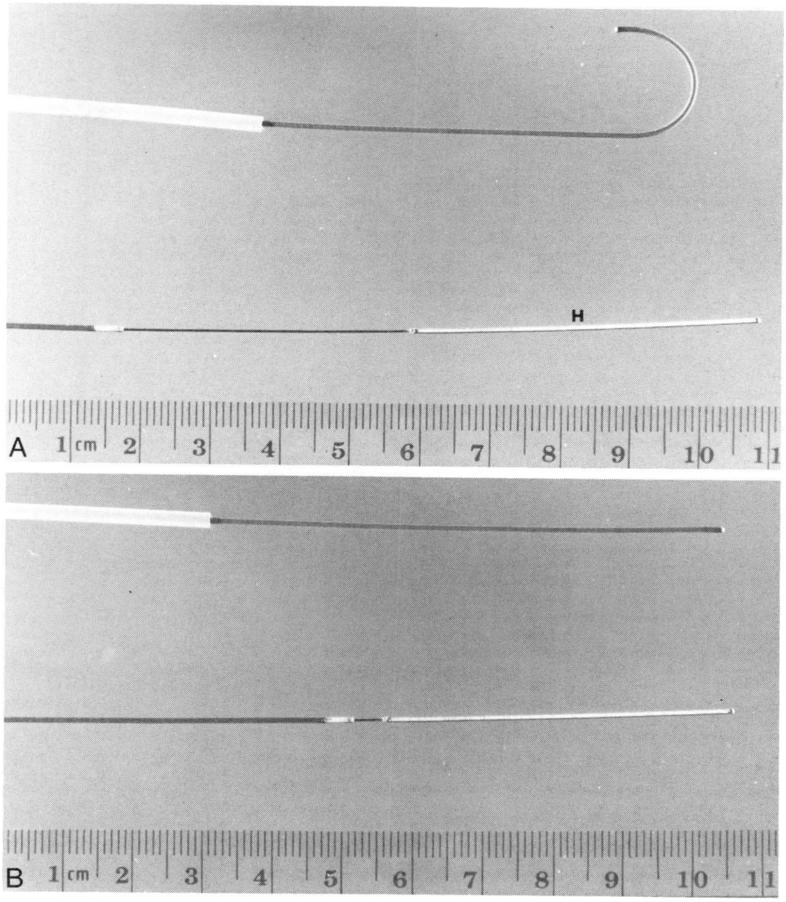

*Figure 2–5.* Movable core J guide wire. *A*, The core has been withdrawn to make the J tip floppy. H = handle for moving core. *B*, The core has been inserted into the wire.

verely tortuous and stenotic iliac arteries, it must be kept in mind that few catheters will follow the floppy coil spring. This is particularly true for the relatively stiff high torque catheters.

**Exchange Wires.** These are usually regular wires with a 5 cm taper and are between 200 and 260 cm in length. The heavy duty exchange wires have a heavier gauge core for added stiffness. In the Rosen-type exchange wire, the floppy segment is shorter in order to provide better anchorage during catheter exchange in shorter vessels, such as the renal arteries. Exchange wires are also available as straight or J-tipped wires.

**Basic Guide Wire Shapes and Sizes** (Fig. 2–6). Guide wires are available in two basic shapes: straight and J. The radius of the J tip may be 1.5, 3.0, 7.5, 10, or 15 mm. In general, straight wires are used for venous catheterization, for narrow vessels (eg, superior mesenteric artery branches), to negotiate stenoses in vessels with a relatively straight

course (eg, percutaneous transluminal angioplasty), and to perform pediatric angiography. In vessels affected by severe atherosclerosis or tortuosity, straight wires (even LLT or movable core wires) can be extremely hazardous.

J-shaped guide wires are the most widely used. They are basically general purpose wires and are used for most vascular catheterizations, in particular to catheterize severely diseased, tortuous, or large vessels (aorta, iliacs), to lead intraarterial catheters, and during percutaneous catheter placement.

Guide wires are available in sizes (diameter) from 0.018 to 0.052 inch. The most frequently used sizes for adult catheterization are 0.035 and 0.038 inch. In pediatric patients, 0.021 and 0.025 inch wires are used most frequently. However, with the introduction of newer, thin-walled, higher flow catheters for pediatric angiography, 0.032 and 0.035 inch guide wires can be used.

**Double Flex Guide Wire** (Kadir 020483

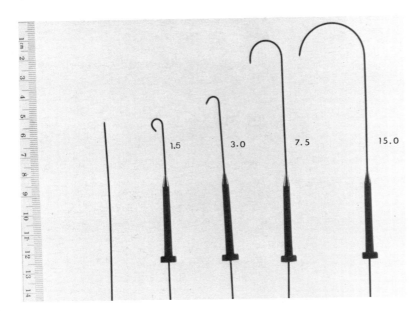

*Figure 2–6.* Basic guide wire shapes. The numbers represent the sizes of the J tip in millimeters (manufacturer's specifications).

TDOC-35-165-0-1.5; Teflon double flex straight and curved, Cook, Inc., Blooming-ton, Indiana). This is a 165 cm. long, 0.035 inch guide wire that is flexible on both ends. The one end has a 1.5 mm J tip and the opposite end is straight, with an LT (10 cm) taper. The double flex guide wire is 20 cm longer than the conventional 145 cm wires in order to compensate for the flexible ends.

*Application:* This combination of frequently used guide wires was designed for percuta-neous cubital vein catheterization for digital subtraction angiography and interventional radiology. It obviates the need for using multiple guide wires, and often the entire procedure can be completed with one guide wire. To facilitate threading a catheter over the J end, a special peel-away introducer (for straightening the J tip) has been developed.

## Special Guide Wires

Several guide wires have been designed for specific applications. With the exception of those guide wires employed for interven-tional procedures in the biliary tract, their use is only occasionally required.

### Biliary Guide Wires

LUNDERQUIST-RING TORQUE WIRE (see Fig. 2–26). This is a 0.038 inch high torque wire that can be shaped into a desired configura-tion. It is not Teflon coated and is not de-signed for use in the vascular system.

*Application:* It is used for selective catheter-ization of the bile ducts, placement of biliary drainage catheters, during percutaneous

stone manipulation, stricture dilatation, or nephrostomy.

LUNDERQUIST EXCHANGE WIRE. Also called the "coat hanger" wire, it is a 112 cm long, 0.038 inch steel wire that has a 7.5 cm flexible spring guide attached to it. Because of its stiffness, it is used for insertion of drainage catheters, for prevention of catheter buckling at the skin or liver capsule.

**Axillary Wire** (Fig. 2–7). This is a regular J-tipped guide wire that has an additional proximal curve with a 22.5 mm radius. The axillary wire is used for catheterization of the descending aorta from the left axillary or brachial artery approach.

**Cope-Eisenberg System.** This is a high torque J wire with a handle at the stiff end. It is used in conjunction with soft nonrein-forced wall catheters for subselective cathe-terization.

**Kadir-Sloan Double Curve Guide Wire** (Fig. 2–8) (Kadir 031082 SCFNA-35-145-1.5; curved Newton 10 cm LT taper, Cook, Inc., Bloomington, Indiana). This is a 0.035 inch guide wire with a 1.5 mm J tip and an LT taper (flexible distal 10 cm). In addition, be-ginning at 10 cm from the wire end, there are two bends at right angles to each other facing in opposite directions. The bends are 10 cm apart and give the wire an S-shaped configuration.

*Application:* This wire is used to negotiate severely tortuous iliac arteries and for place-ment of catheters past eccentric aortic sten-oses and abdominal aortic aneurysms.[1]

**Rosen Wire.** This is a 0.035 or 0.038 inch

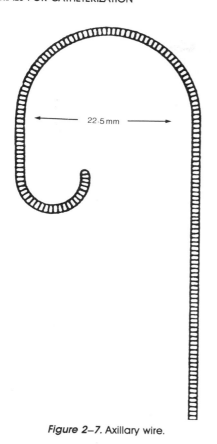

Figure 2–7. Axillary wire.

stiff wire with a heavy duty mandrel and a 2 cm flexible segment (instead of the regular 5 cm). The Rosen wire is available as a regular length or long exchange wire with a straight or J tip.

*Application*: The Rosen wire is used mainly for catheter exchange, especially when work-

ing in short vessels, eg, the renal arteries.[2] Its primary application is for interventional angiography.

**Tip-Deflecting Wire** (Fig. 2–9). The tip-deflecting wire is operated by a special handle, which can be maneuvered by one hand by using the thumb and index and middle fingers. The proximal end of the wire is inserted into the deflecting handle and secured by means of two screws. To operate the system, the fingers and the thumb are adducted toward each other. This puts tension on the core of the wire, thus deflecting the wire tip. If a catheter of matching length is used, a Luer-Lok adapter can be inserted between the handle and catheter hub to prevent the catheter from sliding off the wire. These wires are available with a 3.0, 7.5, and 15 mm radius of deflection.

*Application*: This system is occasionally used in the arterial system for catheterization of vessels arising at an acute angle. Its primary application is in the venous system for the transcardiac placement of a pigtail catheter for pulmonary arteriography, for hepatic venography and pressure measurement, and for renal vein catheterization.

**High Torque J Guide Wire** (Fig. 2–10). This is a 45 cm long, 0.035 inch J-tipped guide wire (Argon Medical Corp., Athens, Texas). The flexible end is 15 cm long and is available in three sizes of J curves: 3, 5, and 10 mm radii. The other end has a short handle to torque the wire. This wire can also be ordered in a 110 cm length and without the handle.

*Application*: The principal applications of this wire are during translumbar aortogra-

Figure 2–8. Kadir-Sloan double curve guide wire. (From Kadir S: Cath Cardiovasc Diagn 9:625–627, 1983. Used with permission.)

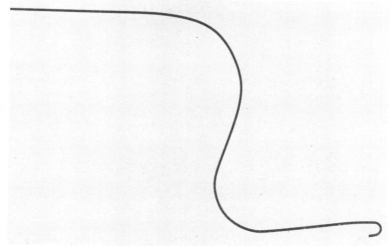

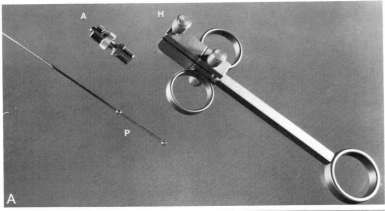

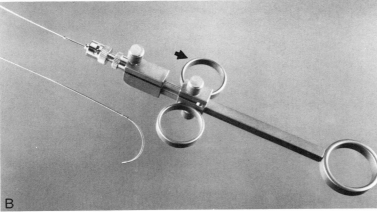

*Figure 2–9.* Tip-deflecting wire with handle (Cook, Inc., Bloomington, Indiana). *A,* Unassembled. P = proximal end of wire, A = adaptor for catheter hub, H = handle. The distal portion (deflectable tip) of the wire is straight. *B,* Assembled. Tension has been applied to the wire by pulling the rings in the direction shown by the arrow. This causes the wire tip to form a J.

phy, percutaneous transhepatic biliary drainage, and nephrostomy placement. We have also used these wires for catheterization of tortuous iliac arteries, for antegrade femoral artery puncture, and for conversion of a retrograde into an antegrade puncture or vice versa.

**Wilson Wire** (Fig. 2–11). This is a 128 cm long, 0.038 inch, straight, movable core guide wire with a plastic handle on the proximal end. It functions in the opposite way to conventional movable core wires, ie, when the handle is withdrawn, the wire tip is stiffened. Catheter exchange is not possible

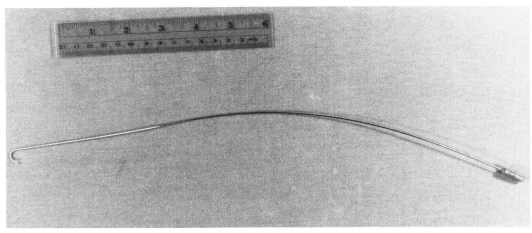

*Figure 2–10.* High torque J guide wire (Argon Medical Corp., Athens, Texas).

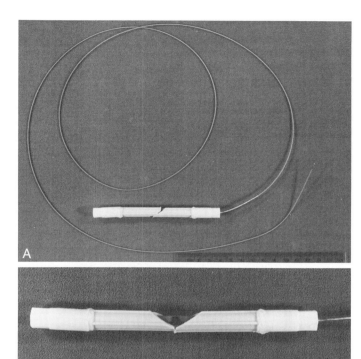

*Figure 2–11.* Wilson wire. *A,* Handle in neutral position. The wire is floppy. *B,* Handle after tension has been applied. The wire tip is stiffened.

over this wire because of the proximal handle but is possible over a modification of this type of wire (Amplatz wire, USCI, Billerica, Massachusetts).

*Application*: The Wilson wire is used for subselective placement of catheters in vessels where the catheter does not follow the conventional floppy tip wires.

**Open-Ended Guide Wire.** The open-ended guide wire (USCI, Billerica, Massachusetts) is a 145 cm-long wire with a removable core and an open-ended spring guide. The wire is available in 0.035 or 0.038 inch diameter and a regular or an LT tapered core. After removal of the core, a Luer-Lok adapter is used for injection or infusion through the end hole of the spring guide.

*Application*: This wire is used for injection of contrast material to verify position for selective catheterization, injection and infusion of diagnostic or therapeutic agents, and measurement of pressure gradients.

## CATHETERS

Catheters are made of polyethylene, Teflon, polyurethane, or nylon. Catheter size is designated by the outer diameter.

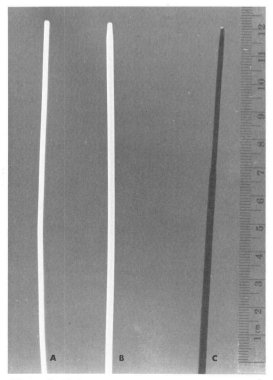

*Figure 2–12.* Straight catheters. A = Nontapered tip (for balloon and other embolizations), B = regular short taper, C = long taper (Staple–van Andel).

Most catheters are tapered at the tip to facilitate atraumatic percutaneous insertion. Nontapered catheters are used for embolotherapy and are inserted through a catheter introducer sheath. They are less suited for diagnostic angiography. The inner lumen (which is determined by French size and the thickness of the catheter wall) and the length determine the maximal flow rate through a catheter. High torque catheters usually have a reinforced wall to permit the catheter to be maneuvered in a desired fashion. Such catheters tend to have smaller lumina than nonreinforced catheters. The thin-walled, high flow catheters do not have braided walls and thus have poorer torque control. Such catheters do have the advantage of a relatively large inner lumen, permitting the use of standard-sized guide wires, and are capable of delivering higher contrast flow rates.

The commercially available preshaped catheters are impregnated with barium, bismuth, lead, or other salts to provide radiopacity. Polyethylene is the most commonly used catheter material. Such catheters are soft and flexible and permit reshaping without much difficulty. Polyurethane and Teflon catheters are stiffer and the former is more difficult to reshape or taper. Polyurethane has a high friction coefficient, which makes it difficult to use unless coated, and requires the use of Teflon-coated guide wires. Some of the newer thin-walled catheters (polyurethane-nylon) are not only softer but permit the use of standard-sized guide wires in 4 and 5 Fr sizes.

Catheters are thrombogenic, ie, deposition of thrombi and fibrin on the catheter surface has been demonstrated by both laboratory studies and angiographic observation. Heparin coating has reduced the affinity for this cellular aggregation and thrombus deposition.[3, 4]

There are four basic catheter shapes: straight, single curve, double or multiple curve, and pigtail. Most catheters used for adult angiography are between 5 and 7 Fr in outer diameter. Since a multitude of catheter variations are available on the market, only a few basic types will be discussed.

**Straight Catheters** (Fig. 2–12 and Table 2–1). The straight catheters most frequently used for diagnostic arteriography are made of polyethylene or Teflon and are available in sizes beginning with 3 Fr. Straight catheters can be ordered with or without side holes.

*Application*: Straight catheters are used for nonselective arteriography (aortography with tip-occluding device, iliac and femoral arte-

**TABLE 2–1. Catheters for Diagnostic Angiography: Straight Catheters**

| Catheter Material (Fr) | Designation | Length (cm) | Guide Wire (inch) | Side Holes | Maximum Flow Rate* (ml/sec) | Application |
|---|---|---|---|---|---|---|
| T (3.0) | T3 | 80–110 | 0.018 | NS | ~4 | Coaxial system for small vessels: adrenal, bronchial, mesenteric, etc; for diagnosis and embolotherapy |
| P (3.6/4.9) | Straight White | 60–100 | 0.021/0.028 | 4/NS | 6/18 | Pediatric angiography |
| N (4.0) | Royal Flush | 65–110 | 0.035 | 6/12 | 15 | Pediatric and femoral angiography |
| N (5.0) | Royal Flush | 65–110 | 0.038 | 6/12 | 27 | Antegrade femoral or pediatric angiography |
| P (6.3/6.7) | Straight | 65–100 | 0.038 | 6/NS | 23/27 | Aortography,† tip-deflecting system for renal and hepatic veins |
| T (5.0/6.3/ 7.0) | Staple–van Andel | 65/80 | 0.035 | 1 | 13–24 | Predilatation, crossover technique, renal exchange |

*Flow rates may vary with catheter length and contrast viscosity. The flow rates shown here are the maximum in vitro rates for the shortest length catheters with side holes.
†For use in conjunction with a tip-occluding device.
N = nylon, P = polyethylene, T = Teflon, NS = no side holes.

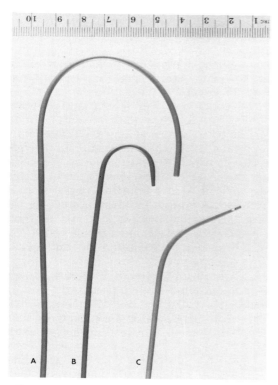

**Figure 2–13.** Single curve catheters. A = Hopkins curve for catheterization of the left gonadal vein, B = hook catheter for visceral angiography, C = A2 multipurpose catheter.

**Single Curve Catheters** (Fig. 2–13 and Table 2–2). Single curve catheters with a 90° or greater gentle or acute angled curve[5] are occasionally used for renal and mesenteric arteriography, for catheterization of the contralateral common iliac artery, and occasionally for directing the guide wire into the descending aorta from the axillary or brachial artery approach. This shape also provides an excellent means for catheterization of gonadal veins from the femoral approach. Such catheters are available commercially or may be shaped at the beginning of the angiographic procedure.

Hockey stick–shaped catheters (45 to 60° curve) are useful for visceral artery catheterization from the axillary artery approach. They are also used for catheterization of head and neck vessels. In addition, they provide an excellent means for hepatic, renal, and gonadal vein catheterization from the cubital vein approach.[6]

**Multiple Curve Catheters** (Figs. 2–14 to 2–16 and Table 2–3). The more commonly used catheters for selective arteriography have multiple curves: cobra, headhunter, sidewinder, Mikaelsson. The Mikaelsson and sidewinder catheters have a preformed loop configuration that provides anchorage (against the aortic wall) during contrast injection in short vessels and prevents catheter dislodgment. In addition, these catheters are ideally suited for catheterization of caudal and craniad directed vessels, eg, inferior mesenteric and left gastric arteries and the adrenal veins.

The cobra catheter is available in three different sizes: C1 for narrow aortas, C2 for most aortas, and the C3 for wide aortas. Similarly, the sidewinder catheter is also

riography) and occasionally for selective angiography. Straight, tapered Teflon catheters with or without side holes (Staple–van Andel catheters) are used for transluminal angioplasty. A modification of the latter catheter with 41 side holes is used for biliary and renal drainage.[4a]

**TABLE 2–2.** Catheters for Diagnostic Angiography: Single Curve Catheters

| Catheter Material (Fr) | Designation | Length (cm) | Guide Wire (inch) | Side Holes | Maximum Flow Rate* (ml/sec) | Application |
|---|---|---|---|---|---|---|
| P (6.5) | Single curve hook | 70 | 0.035 | NS | 25 | Renal, contralateral iliac artery |
| P (6.0–7.0) | N1H type, closed end | 65–100 | | 4 | 11–24 | Renal/hepatic venography from cubital vein approach |
| P/PU (6.0–7.0) | Multipurpose (A1) | 80–125 | 0.035/0.038 | NS | 11–18 | Hepatic wedge pressure measurement, gonadal vein |
| P/PU (6.0–7.0) | Multipurpose (A2) | 80–125 | 0.035/0.038 | 2 | 14–24 | Hepatic and renal veins |

*Flow rates may vary with catheter length and contrast viscosity. The flow rates shown here are the maximum in vitro rates for the shortest length catheters with side holes.

PU = polyurethane, P = polyethylene, NS = no side holes.

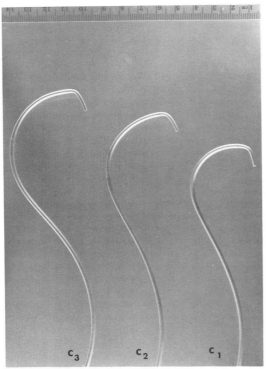

*Figure 2–14.* Cobra-shaped catheters.

available in different sizes: Type 1 with a small loop and a short distal limb for narrow aortas and type 2 with a larger loop and a longer distal limb for wider aortas and the inferior vena cava. Types 3 and 4 are rarely used for visceral angiography.

The cobra and the sidewinder catheters allow visceral artery catheterization to be performed in almost all cases. Of paramount importance is the careful selection of the type of curve, which is determined by the diameter of the aorta. For catheterization of second- or third-order branches of the visceral arteries, soft catheters are required, as the high torque, stiffer catheters may not advance beyond the second or third bends. For this purpose, we have found the thin-walled, polyurethane-nylon, preshaped catheters (Mallinckrodt, St. Louis, Missouri), the 5 Fr polyurethane catheters (Cordis Corp., Miami, Florida), or the 4.9 Fr polyethylene White catheters (Becton-Dickenson, Rutherford, New Jersey) to be invaluable (see Chapter 3).

**Pigtail-type Catheters** (Fig. 2–17 and Table 2–4). Pigtail catheters are usually made of polyethylene and Teflon. Newer high flow,

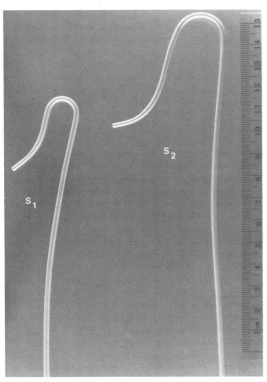

*Figure 2–15.* Sidewinder catheters.

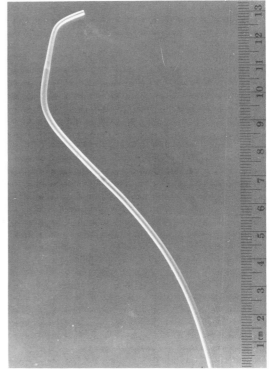

*Figure 2–16.* Headhunter catheter.

**TABLE 2–3.** Catheters for Diagnostic Angiography: Multiple Curve Catheters

| Catheter Material (Fr) | Designation | Length (cm) | Guide Wire (inch) | Side Holes | Maximum Flow Rate* (ml/sec) | Application |
|---|---|---|---|---|---|---|
| P (6.5) | Renal, double curve | 65 | 0.038 | NS | 20 | Renal, spinal, and internal mammary arteries |
| PU†/PU-N‡ (5.0) | Cobra C1–3 | 65 | 0.035 | 2/NS | 14 | Visceral |
| PU†/P§ (6.0–7.0) | Cobra C1–3 | 65/80 | 0.035/0.038 | 2/NS | 17–35 | Visceral |
| PU†/PU-N‡ (5.0) | Sidewinder 1 and 2 | 100 | 0.035 | NS | 14 | Visceral/cerebral |
| PU† (6.0–7.0) | Sidewinder 1 and 2 | 100 | 0.032/0.035 | NS | 14–24 | Visceral/cerebral |
| P§ (6.5) | Sidewinder 1 and 2 | 100 | 0.038 | NS | ~24 | Visceral/cerebral |
| P§ (5.3) | Cerebral H1 | 100 | 0.038 | NS | ~10 | Chemotherapy infusion via left axillary artery |
| P§ (6.5) | Headhunter H1H | 100 | 0.038 | NS | ~20 | Cerebral/brachial |
| P§ (6.5) | Adrenal | 80 | 0.038 | NS | NA | Adrenal vein catheterization |

*Flow rates may vary with catheter length and contrast viscosity. The flow rates shown here are the maximum in vitro rates for the shortest length catheters with side holes.
†Cordis Corp., Miami, Florida.
‡Mallinckrodt, St. Louis, Missouri.
§Cook, Inc., Bloomington, Indiana.
P = polyethylene, PU = polyurethane, N = nylon, NS = no side holes.

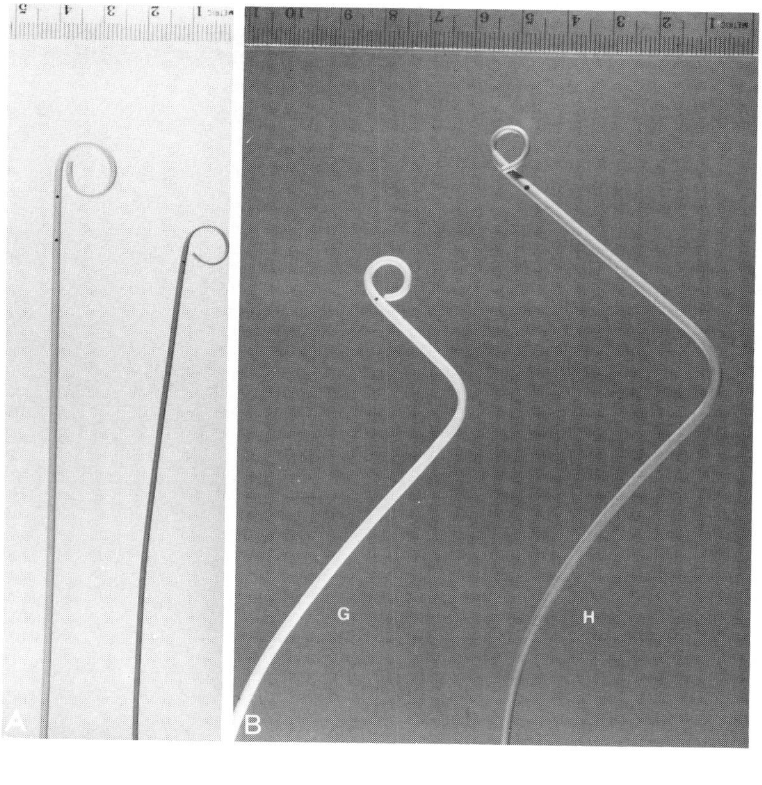

*Figure 2–17.* A, Pigtail catheters. B, Pigtail-shaped catheters for pulmonary arteriography. G = Grollman, H = Hopkins curve for use in patients with large right atria.

**TABLE 2–4.** Catheters for Diagnostic Angiography: Pigtail Catheters

| Catheter Material (Fr) | Designation | Length (cm) | Guide Wire (inch) | Side Holes | Maximum Flow Rate* (ml/sec) | Application |
|---|---|---|---|---|---|---|
| N (4.0) | Royal Flush† | 65–110 | 0.035 | 6 | 15§ | Pediatric angiography, outpatient arteriography |
| PU-N (4.0) | Pigtail‡ | 65/90 | 0.032 | 10 | 18 | Pediatric angiography, DSA |
| N (5.0) | Royal Flush† | 65–110 | 0.038 | 6 | 27§ | Venacavography, IV DSA |
| PU-N (5.0) | Pigtail‡ | 65/90 | 0.032 | 10 | 28 | Abdominal aortography, IV DSA |
| P (6.3) | Pigtail† | 65 | 0.038 | 6/12 | 32 | Abdominal aortography, vena cavography |
| P (7.1) | Pigtail† | 100 | 0.038 | 12 | 37 | Arch aortography, pulmonary arteriography |
| P (6.7) | Grollman (yellow)† | 100 | 0.035 | 4 | 23 | Pulmonary arteriography |
| P (7.2) | Hopkins (green)† | 100 | 0.038 | 4 | 34 | Pulmonary arteriography |

*Flow rates may vary with catheter length and contrast viscosity. The flow rates shown here are the maximum in vitro rates for the shortest length catheters.
†Cook, Inc., Bloomington, Indiana.
‡Mallinckrodt, St. Louis, Missouri.
§When the maximal flow rates are used, the pigtail tends to uncoil.
P = polyethylene, PU = polyurethane, N = nylon, DSA = digital subtraction angiography.

thin-walled pigtail catheters are made of polyurethane and nylon. The pigtail was conceived to permit an even distribution of rapidly injected contrast medium in large vessels, to allow homogeneous opacification, and to prevent an end hole jet. For introduction into a vessel, the pigtail has to be straightened, but resumes its shape as soon as the guide wire is removed. The additional advantages of pigtail catheters are that they can be positioned without the aid of a guide wire and that they can occasionally be used to direct guide wires (for catheterization of the descending aorta from the axillary approach or past abdominal aortic aneurysms or aortic stenoses from the femoral approach). A disadvantage of pigtail catheters is that, when used in the arterial system, they need to be straightened by inserting a guide wire prior to removal.

**Miscellaneous Catheters** (Table 2–5). Many "special" catheters have been described that are designed to facilitate selective visceral arteriography.[7, 8] More often, such catheter designs are products of individual preferences rather than innovations. In the past, before the introduction of high torque catheters, vascular radiologists had to shape their own catheters. Some of the catheter shapes described in the more recent reports are similar to the shapes that were used in the earlier days of vascular radiology. Other than in highly specialized centers, such special catheters are not likely to be used very

**TABLE 2–5.** Catheters for Diagnostic Angiography: Special Catheter Shapes

| Catheter Material (Fr) | Designation | Length (cm) | Guide Wire (inch) | Side Holes | Maximum Flow Rate* (ml/sec) | Application |
|---|---|---|---|---|---|---|
| P (6.0/6.5) | Single curve Visceral RC-1, RC-2 R1M | 65/80 | 0.035/0.038 | NS | 11–20 | Celiac, SMA catheterization, R1M for IMA catheterization |
| P (6.0/6.5) | Right hepatic, Splenic RH, RS | 65/80 | 0.035/0.038 | NS | 11–20 | Hepatic and splenic artery catheterization |

*Flow rates may vary with catheter length and contrast viscosity. The flow rates shown here are the maximum in vitro rates.
P = polyethylene, SMA = superior mesenteric artery, IMA = inferior mesenteric artery, NS = no side holes.

frequently, since the standard selective catheters (cobra and sidewinder) accomplish this task easily. Thus, an inventory of such specially shaped catheters should be unnecessary. If the need should arise, the standard cobra catheter can be steamed into almost any desirable configuration.

**Balloon Catheters** (Fig. 2–18 and Table 2–6). Double lumen balloon catheters are used for cardiac catheterization, but also have application in noncardiac angiography. For introduction of balloon-tipped catheters (other than the angioplasty catheters), catheter introducer sheaths are required. Such sheaths should be either the same size or 1 to 2 Fr sizes larger than the balloon catheter.

FLOW-DIRECTED BALLOON CATHETERS. Flow-directed balloon catheters are available as angiographic catheters with multiple side holes and no end hole or as wedge catheters with an end hole only. The most frequent application for such catheters is in cardiopulmonary angiography and for vascular occlusion in dry field angiography or surgery.

OCCLUSION BALLOON CATHETERS. Large balloon catheters (double and triple lumen) with balloon sizes up to 40 mm are available (Medi-Tech, Watertown, Massachusetts). These can be used for vascular occlusion prior to operation, to provide a dry field for surgery, and for aortic occlusion and embolotherapy.

FOGARTY BALLOON CATHETERS. Small balloon catheters (single lumen) such as the Fogarty embolectomy balloon catheters are occasionally used for occlusion of small vessels (eg, prior to an operation) or for the dislodgment of calculi in the biliary and urinary tracts. They can also be used as an aid for performing cholangiography in patients with Silastic biliary stents.[8a]

HIGH TORQUE, PRESHAPED OCCLUSION BALLOON CATHETERS. High torque visceral angiography catheters are also available as double lumen balloon catheters (7 or 8 Fr cobra 2 or sidewinder 2 catheters in 65 and 80 cm lengths) (Cordis Corp., Miami, Florida). The balloon is located close to the catheter tip.

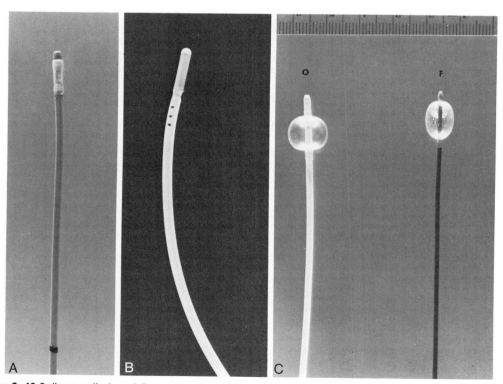

*Figure 2–18.* Balloon catheters. *A,* Berman wedge catheter. Insertion of this catheter requires an introducer sheath at least 1 Fr size larger than the catheter shaft. *B,* Swan-Ganz angiographic catheter. The balloon is recessed, i.e., the balloon segment of the catheter is the same diameter as the remainder of the catheter shaft. This catheter can be introduced through the same size introducer sheath. *C,* Occlusion balloon catheter (O) and Fogarty embolectomy catheters (F).

**TABLE 2–6.** Catheters for Diagnostic and Interventional Angiography: Balloon Catheters

| Catheter (Fr) | Designation | Length (cm) | Guide Wire (inch) | Side Holes | Maximum Flow Rate* (ml/sec) | Application |
|---|---|---|---|---|---|---|
| 5–8 Fr[1] | Balloon wedge | 50–110 | 0.021–5 Fr 0.035–8 Fr | NS | NA | Hepatic, pulmonary wedge pressures, hepatic venography |
| 4–8 Fr[1] | Angiographic balloon catheter | 50–110 | | 6 | 9 (5 Fr) 20 (7 Fr) | Cardiac catheterization Pulmonary arteriography |
| 4–8 Fr[2] | Swan-Ganz flow directed | 60–110 | 0.021–7 Fr. | NS | 8 (5 Fr) 28 (8 Fr) | Pulmonary angiography |
| 5–8 Fr[3] | Occlusion balloons (up to 40 mm) | 65–100 | 0.025–0.035 | NS | NA | Hepatic wedge pressure measurement and venography, embolization, preop occlusion |
| 7–8 Fr[4] | Torque controlled (cobra, sidewinder) | 65/80 | 0.032–0.035 | NS | | Hepatic wedge pressure measurement and venography, embolization, preop occlusion |
| 2–4 Fr | Fogarty embolectomy | 60–100 | | NS | NA | Coaxial occlusion of tumors, bleeding, biliary stone dislodgment, cholangiography |

*Flow rates may vary with catheter length and contrast viscosity. The flow rates shown here are the maximum in vitro rates for the shortest length catheters.
[1]Critikon Inc., Tampa, Florida.
[2]American Edwards Laboratories, Irvine, California.
[3]Medi-Tech, Watertown, Massachusetts.
[4]Cordis Corp., Miami, Florida.
NS = no side holes, NA = not applicable.

*Application*: These catheters can be used for balloon occlusion arteriography and venography, hepatic vein pressure measurement, dry field surgery (tumors, trauma), and chemotherapy or embolotherapy.

**Dilators** (Fig. 2–19). Smoothly tapered, stiff Teflon or polyurethane dilators are often used to dilate the subcutaneous and perivascular tissue in preparation for insertion of catheters. The dilators facilitate insertion of catheters that are not well tapered and therefore prevent damage to the catheter tip. In most individuals, dilatation of the arterial wall is not possible unless a large dilator is used. In patients with atherosclerotic arteries that have lost their elasticity, some mural dilatation may occur. Thus, the size of the dilator should not exceed that of the catheter. Dilators are particularly useful in patients with scars or vascular grafts and before introduction of balloon angioplasty catheters.

**Introducer Sheaths** (Fig. 2–20). Vascular introducer sheaths are available with or without a side arm. The self-sealing sheaths have a rubber valve in the hub, which seals around a smaller-sized catheter and prevents leakage of blood. Tight sealing valves on some sheaths are capable of sealing around guide wires.

*Application*: Introducer sheaths are employed when end hole–occluded (eg, balloon), blunt-tipped, or nontapered catheters are used or when multiple catheter exchanges are anticipated. In addition, they may be used in patients with vascular grafts in order to prevent catheter separation at the time of removal. Such sheaths provide continuous access to the vascular lumen and thus avoid repetitive trauma to the vessel as a result of multiple catheter exchanges. These sheaths also protect the catheter tip. Other applications include removal of clogged cath-

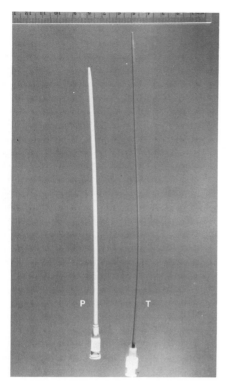

**Figure 2–19.** Vascular dilators. P = polyurethane, T = Teflon.

**TABLE 2–7.** Conversion Table for Outer Dimensions of Catheters

| Fr | mm | Inch |
|----|-----|-------|
| 3 | 1.0 | 0.039 |
| 4 | 1.3 | 0.053 |
| 5 | 1.7 | 0.066 |
| 6 | 2.0 | 0.079 |
| 7 | 2.3 | 0.092 |
| 8 | 2.7 | 0.105 |
| 9 | 3.0 | 0.118 |
| 10 | 3.3 | 0.131 |
| 11 | 3.7 | 0.144 |
| 12 | 4.0 | 0.158 |
| 15 | 5.0 | 0.197 |
| 18 | 6.0 | 0.236 |

A conversion table for catheter sizes is listed in Table 2–7.

## SHAPING AND FLANGING OF CATHETERS AND SHAPING OF GUIDE WIRES

**Catheter Shaping.** Catheter shaping may involve shaping of straight catheters or reshaping of commercially available preshaped catheters. The technique is shown in Figures 2–21 and 2–22.

**Tapering of Catheter Tip and Flanging of Catheter Hub** (Figs. 2–23 to 2–25). The technique for tapering the catheter tip is shown in Figure 2–24*A* and *B*. For flanging of the proximal end of the catheter, a flanging tool and an alcohol burner flame are used. Such

eters and ruptured angioplasty balloon catheters. The side arm is attached to a pressure drip for continuous infusion in order to prevent thrombus from forming within the sheath and around the catheter.

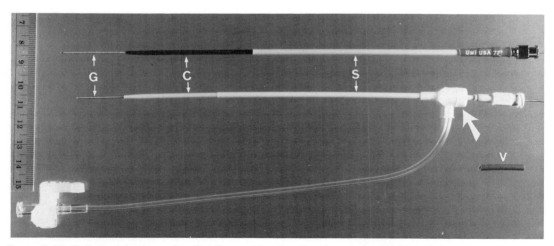

**Figure 2–20.** Catheter introducer sheaths. G = guide wire; C = tapered catheter for introduction of the sheath (S). V = valve made of rubber tubing, which has been slit open on one side. This can be placed around guide wires or small French catheters in order to prevent leakage of blood. Alternatively, the valve in the sheath hub *(arrow)* can be replaced for another tighter, self-sealing valve. Such valves are available separately or as special-order sheaths with tight, self-sealing valves (Cordis Corp., Miami, Florida).

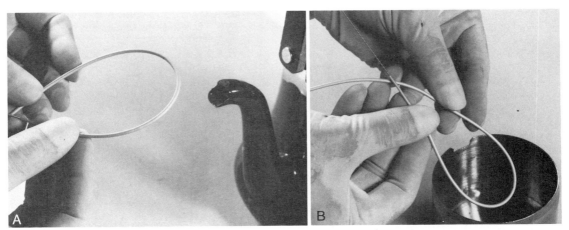

*Figure 2–21.* Steam shaping of catheters. *A,* A guide wire is inserted into the distal segment of the catheter to prevent it from kinking. The catheter is then bent to the desired shape and exposed to steam for 15 to 20 seconds. *B,* Immediately thereafter, the catheter is immersed in cool flushing solution. The guide wire is removed and the catheter shape is assessed.

burners are preferable, since they do not leave soot or other residue. The technique for flanging is shown in Figure 2–24C and *D.* The hot flanging tool often melts the catheter upon contact. To avoid this, saline from a 20 ml syringe is sprayed onto the contact point as soon as the hot flanging tool comes into contact with the catheter.

If a flanging tool is not available, the catheter can be flanged by holding it over the flame. As the polyethylene softens, the catheter is rotated to give it a flange.

**Side Hole Punching** (Fig. 2–25). The presence of side holes in a catheter permits better mixing of the contrast medium with the blood, avoids a strong end hole jet, and thus prevents catheter recoil and dislodgment. In addition, a slightly higher flow rate can be delivered through catheters with side holes.

The side hole punch consists of a sharp

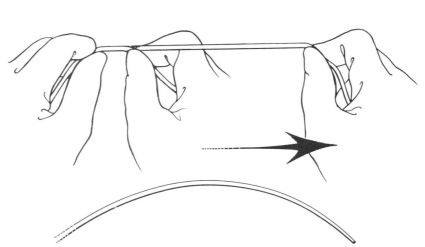

*Figure 2–22.* Hand shaping of catheters. This technique is useful for placement of a curve on Teflon catheters. The distal segment of the catheter is held between the thumb and index finger of both hands. While applying pressure with the thumb, the hand is moved towards the catheter tip. Steam or water immersion is not required unless the catheter is to be reshaped completely. The amount of pressure determines the degree of curvature; ie, slight pressure results in a gentle curve. (From Kadir S et al: Fortschr Roentgenstr 141:378–383, 1984. Used with permission.)

*Figure 2–23. A*, Side hole punch. *B*, Flanging tool.

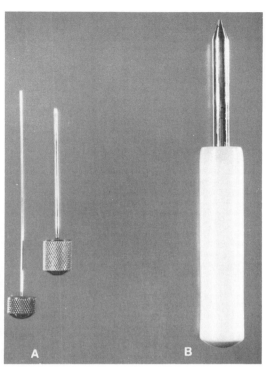

*Figure 2–24. A* and *B*, Technique for forming catheter tip. *A*, The polyethylene catheter is held over an alcohol burner. The catheter is rotated back and forth while maintaining tension in the direction shown by the arrows. As the polyethylene softens, the catheter can be pulled apart, tapering the segment exposed to the heat (*open arrow*). *B*, The tapered segment is cut with a scalpel blade. *C* and *D*, Technique for flanging catheter hub. *C*, The flanging tool is heated over the flame. *D*, The tool is inserted into the catheter. The heat softens the catheter material and molds it to the shape of the tool. Overheating results in melting of the catheter material and makes it adherent to the tool. To prevent this, saline is squirted onto the catheter immediately after the catheter comes into contact with the hot flanging tool.

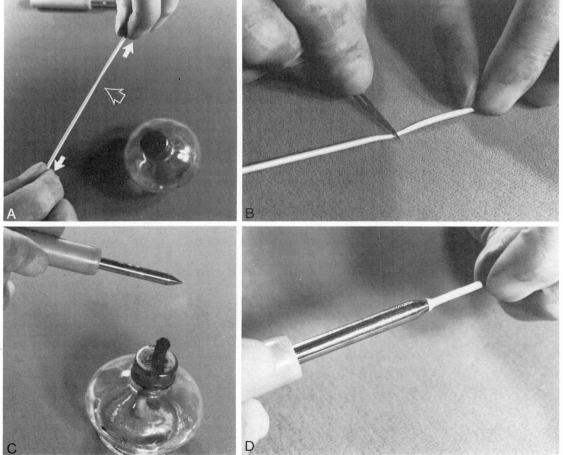

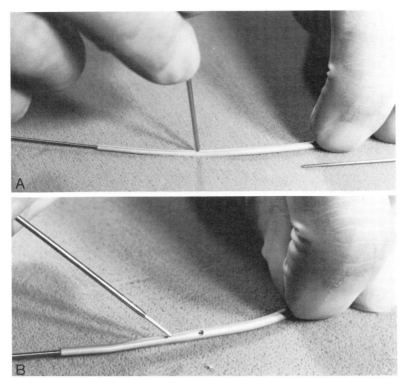

*Figure 2–25.* Punching a side hole. *A,* A guide wire is placed in the segment of the catheter in which a side hole is to be punched. A sharp cannula is placed at the desired spot and is rotated back and forth while applying pressure. *B,* The stylet is used to clear the lumen of the cannula. The catheter must be flushed prior to insertion.

outer cannula with a squared tip and a blunt inner stylet that is used to remove the plug from the cannula (see Fig. 2–23*A*). The sharp cannula is placed on the catheter at the desired spot. Pressure is applied and the cannula is rotated back and forth. A sudden decrease in resistance then occurs as the hole is "punched" through. However, if too much pressure is applied, there is a tendency to damage the opposite wall of the catheter. To avoid this, a guide wire is placed in the lumen while punching side holes.

**Guide Wire Shaping** (Figs. 2–26 and 2–27)

SHAPING HIGH TORQUE WIRES. The most frequent use for manually shaped guide wires is in the biliary system. Here the Lunderquist-Ring torque wire is shaped to facilitate catheterization of the common hepatic/common bile duct or other radicles. For this purpose a hockey stick–shaped curve of approximately 45° is placed 1 to 2 cm from the wire tip. The opposite, nonflexible end of the wire is wrapped into a small coil, which is used as a handle to torque the wire tip. Alternatively, a right angle bend is placed at the nonflexible end and is used as a handle to torque the wire. The latter technique is not preferred, however, because it is often difficult to straighten the bend for insertion of a catheter.

BENDING THE FLEXIBLE END. In general, the floppy end of a guide wire distal to the core cannot be shaped. The flexible segment of the core can be bent manually, and this technique is shown in Figure 2–27. The guide wire is held between the thumb and index finger of both hands, and while applying pressure with the thumb, the hand is moved towards the tip of the guide wire. Depending upon the degree of the pressure applied, this maneuver will result in a gentle curve (mild pressure) or a coiling of the guide wire (heavy pressure).

*Application*: Reshaping of the flexible segment of a guide wire may be used as an aid to facilitate the advancing of a catheter over a bend, eg, across the aortic bifurcation, or into the superior mesenteric artery. For other applications see reference 9.

BENDING THE STIFF END. Bending the stiff end of the guide wire may occasionally become necessary in order to facilitate catheterization. When a 0.038 or 0.035 inch guide wire is used, this technique may be employed as a substitute for a tip-deflecting system. When the curved, stiff end of the guide wire

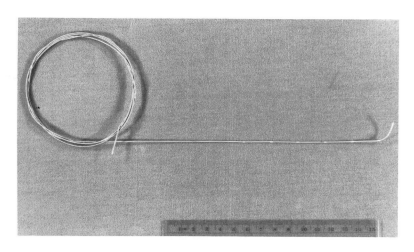

*Figure 2–26.* The Lunderquist-Ring torque wire as used for selective catheterization in the biliary and urinary tracts. A J curve is placed at the wire tip. The proximal end of the wire is rolled up and used as a handle for torquing.

is advanced to approximately 1 to 2 cm of the catheter tip, it will deflect a straight catheter or increase the curvature of a precurved catheter. The technique for bending the stiff end is illustrated in Figure 2–27.

*Application*: This technique can be used to deflect a pigtail catheter for pulmonary arteriography, to increase the curvature of the Grollman curved pigtail catheter for pulmonary arteriography, to re-form the sidewinder curve in the venous system, and to increase the curve of single or multiple curve catheters (eg, for catheterization of renal or hepatic veins and inferiorly directed vessels, such as the gonadal veins and the iliac artery). The stiff end of the guide wire must not be permitted to exit from the catheter tip.

## ANGIOGRAPHIC TRAY (Fig. 2–28)

1. Table on wheels. The table for the angiographic tray should be of steel (so that it can be cleaned). The wheels permit maneuverability. The table size should be at least 2½ by 3½ ft.

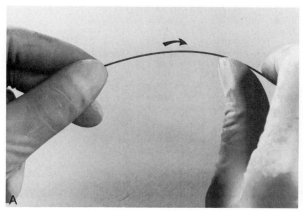

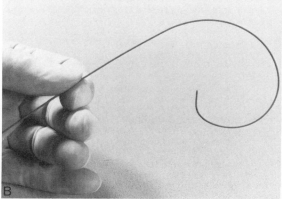

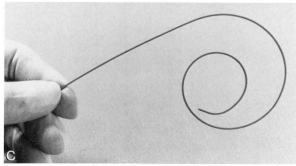

*Figure 2–27.* Shaping guide wires. *A,* The guide wire end that has to be shaped is held between the index fingers and thumbs. While applying pressure with the thumb, the hand is moved towards the guide wire end (*arrow*). *B,* Application of slight pressure results in a gentle curve. *C,* Application of greater pressure results in a more complex curvature.

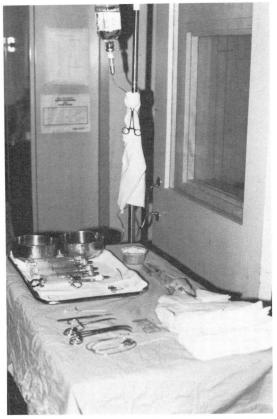

*Figure 2–28.* Angiographic table and infusion stand. A sterile towel is placed around the tubing for the flushing solution to prevent it from contaminating the sterile tray.

2. Infusion stand. Either attached to the table or separate.

3. One small metal tray (approximately 1 by 2 ft). This is used for syringes and other instruments to preserve sterility. The wet unsterile table top would contaminate the materials on the angiographic table. Alternatively, a waterproof table drape may be used to preserve sterility.

4. Two large bowls. One for inflow of the flushing solution and the other for disposal.

5. One small bowl for contrast medium.

6. Syringes: Two 20 ml glass or plastic disposable Luer-Lok syringes. Large syringes are preferable for flushing and, in addition, provide better suction. Smaller syringes must be used in pediatric patients. Two 10 ml plastic disposable Luer-Lok syringes for contrast injection.

7. One 10 ml three-ring plastic syringe for local anesthesia. Plastic syringes are lighter and therefore easier to use.

8. One No. 11 blade.

9. One mosquito clamp to spread subcutaneous tissue.

10. Two Kelly clamps.

11. Six towel clamps.

12. One package of 4 by 4 inch gauze sponges.

13. Three hypodermic needles: 25 gauge for skin anesthesia, 22 gauge for subcutaneous anesthesia, and 18 gauge to draw up local anesthetic.

14. One two-way Luer-Lok metal stopcock.

15. One sterile plastic shower cap for image intensifer.

16. One pack sterile adhesive skin tape, eg, Steri-Strips, to secure catheter.

Optional: a transparent Steri-Drape (3M, Surgical Products Division, St. Paul, Minnesota) with or without a hole.

**Prep Tray.** The contents of the prep tray may be packaged separately or together with the angiographic tray.

1. Two sponge clamps.

2. Eight towels (12 by 24 inches).

3. Four half sheets.

4. Two gowns.

5. One or two small bowls with sponges for prepping.

Alternatively, a one piece absorbent disposable drape may be used (Angiography Drape Pack, Argon Medical Corp., Athens, Texas).

In addition, sterile gloves, disposable masks, and operating room caps should be available. Masks and caps should be required for all persons entering the angiographic room during or immediately preceding the procedure (ie, at any time when the angiographic tray has been prepared).

**Flushing Solution.** Sterile 5% dextrose solution (500 ml bottles) is used; 2000 Units of heparin should be added to each bottle. A closed flushing system is recommended for all procedures lasting longer than 30 minutes.

**Local Anesthesia.** The local anesthetic used is 0.5 or 1% lidocaine without epinephrine. In pediatric patients, 0.5% lidocaine is used.

**Anticoagulation.** If a long arterial catheterization time is anticipated, systemic heparinization is recommended (unless there are contraindications to the heparinization, eg, abnormal clotting parameters, bleeding). The dose for the heparinization is: adults, 40 to 45 Units of heparin/kg or a total of 3000 Units for a 70 kg adult; children, 100 Units/kg.

Reversal of heparinization is rarely necessary. This can be accomplished by administering 10 mg of protamine/1000 Units of heparin remaining in the patient. An overdose of protamine can be hazardous, since protamine itself has an anticoagulant effect.

## PATIENT PREPARATION

**Removal of Hair.** The hair in the region where needle puncture is to be performed should be removed prior to prepping the skin. Hair removal should be generous, so that hair does not come into contact with the sterile field. For preparation of one groin, the pubic hair should be shaved to the midline. If both groins are to be used, *all* pubic hair should be removed. Similarly, all axillary hair should be shaved if the axillary approach is used.

Hair removal can be accomplished with an electric razor or with a razor blade and soap and water. The former is preferable because skin abrasions are infrequent. In addition, reports in the surgical literature indicate a lower incidence of skin infection with an electric razor.[10]

**Skin Prep.** Iodinated prep solutions (eg, Betadine) are used to prep the skin puncture site. The prep solution should remain in contact with the skin for several minutes in order to be effective. In some institutions, alcohol is used to wipe off the iodinated solution. This practice is not to be encouraged because (1) the effectiveness of the prep solution is questionable when applied to the skin for only short periods of time and (2) the use of alcohol is painful if the pubic or axillary hair has been shaved immediately before the application. In patients with skin allergy or sensitivity to such prep solutions, a bactericidal soap solution may be used for skin prepping (Hibiclens, 4% chlorhexidene gluconate and 4% isopropyl alcohol, Stuart Pharmaceuticals, Wilmington, Delaware).

Because of the low temperatures in angiographic rooms, such solutions are usually cold and uncomfortable for the patient. They can be warmed to 37 to 40° C in a water bath prior to use. A convenient apparatus is the gel warmer used for ultrasonic gels. (Thermasonic Gel Warmer, Parker Laboratories Inc., Orange, New Jersey).

## CONTRAST MEDIA

**Fat-soluble Contrast Media.** The only fat-soluble contrast medium utilized in vascular radiology is ethiodized poppy seed oil (Ethiodol), which is used for lymphography. Ethyl iodophenyl-undecanoate (Pantopaque, Alcon Laboratories, Humacao, Puerto Rico) is occasionally used in embolotherapy to prolong the set-up time of cyanoacrylate. In addition, it serves as a radiopaque marker.

**Water-soluble Contrast Media.** The most frequently used contrast media in angiography are triiodinated derivatives of benzoic acid, which are excreted primarily by the kidneys. Important aspects of the composition of contrast media are iodine content, viscosity, osmolality, toxicity, and mode of excretion. For the currently used contrast agents, diatrizoate and iothalamate are the most frequently utilized anions, whereas either sodium or methylglucamine or both (used in different combinations) are the most frequently employed cations.

**Physical Properties of Contrast Agents** (Tables 2–8 and 2–9). The radiopacity of contrast agents depends upon their iodine content. The radiodensity of iodine (4.93 gm/ $cm^3$) is approximately five times that of soft tissue and more than three times that of bone. Thus, the injection of such agents into preformed spaces provides a "contrast" against the surrounding tissues.

In the past, one of the more important considerations in the selection of a contrast agent was its iodine content. With the introduction of digital subtraction angiography, this is more likely to assume a secondary role.

Viscosity is the resistance to the movement of a fluid. The unit for the measurement of viscosity is the centipoise (cP), which compares the viscosity of a given fluid with that of water at 20° C (= 1 centipoise). The dynamic viscosity of blood is 2.5 cP. Kinematic viscosity (measured in centistokes) is used to evaluate the absolute viscosity relative to fluid density.

Osmolarity measures the number of molecules of a substance dissolved in a liter of solution. Osmolarity is measured in mOsm/L. Osmolality is measured in mOsm/kg water. The normal plasma osmolality at body temperature is 291 mOsm/kg. The osmolarity of conventional ionic contrast media is five to nine times that of plasma.

The viscosity of fluids is dependent upon the size of the dissolved molecules—the larger the molecules, the higher the viscosity (eg, methylglucamine). With the use of smaller-sized molecules (eg, sodium), the viscosity of contrast agents can be reduced.

**TABLE 2–8.** Ionic Contrast Media: Chemical and Physical Properties*

| Contrast Agent | Cation/Anion | Iodine (mg/ml) | Sodium (mg/ml) | Osmolarity (mOsm/L) | Viscosity (cP) (25° C/37° C) | pH |
|---|---|---|---|---|---|---|
| Renografin-60 | Meglumine diatrizoate (520 mg/ml), sodium diatrizoate (80 mg/ml) | 292.5 | 3.76 | | 5.6/3.9 | 7.0–7.6 |
| Hypaque, 60% | Meglumine diatrizoate | 282 | 0.02 | 960 | 6.17/4.12 | 6.5–7.7 |
| Conray | Meglumine iothalamate (600 mg/ml) | 282 | 0.03 | 1500 | 6.0/4.0 | |
| Renografin-76 | Meglumine diatrizoate (660 mg/ml), sodium diatrizoate (100 mg/ml) | 370 | 4.48 | | 13.9/9.1 | 7.0–7.6 |
| Hypaque-M, 75% | Meglumine diatrizoate (500 mg/ml), sodium diatrizoate (250 mg/ml) | 385 | 9.0 | 1280 | 13.2/8.3 | 6.5–7.7 |
| Hypaque-76 | Meglumine diatrizoate (660 mg/ml), sodium diatrizoate (100 mg/ml) | 370 | 3.68 | | 15.0/9.0 | 7.0–7.6 |
| Vascoray | Meglumine iothalamate (520 mg/ml), sodium iothalamate (260 mg/ml) | 400 | 9.4 | 2150 | 17.0/9.0 | |

*From ER Squibb & Sons, Inc; Winthrop Laboratories; Mallinckrodt, Inc.

**TABLE 2–9.** Low Osmolality and Nonionic Contrast Media: Chemical and Physical Properties*

| Contrast Agent | Mol/Mol Wt | Iodine (mg/ml) | Osmolality (mOsm/kg) | Viscosity (cP) (25° C/37° C) | pH |
|---|---|---|---|---|---|
| Amipaque | Nonionic monomer 789 | 482 | 484 at 300 mg I/ml at 37° C | 12.7 at 300 mg I/ml at 20° C, 6.2 at 300 mg I/ml at 37° C | 7.4 |
| Hexabrix (ioxaglate meglumine 39.3%, ioxaglate sodium, 19.6%) | Ionic dimer 1269 | 320 | 580 | 15.7/7.5 | |
| Iodecol | Nonionic dimer | 300 | 260 | 7.2 at 37° C | |
| Iopamidol | Nonionic monomer 777 | 280 | 570 | 7.5/3.8 | |
| Iohexol | Nonionic monomer 821 | 280 | 620 | 8.8 at 20° C/4.8 | |

*From Winthrop Laboratories, References 21 and 27.

TABLE 2–10. Hemodynamic Effects of Arterial Injection of Contrast Media

| Site of Injection | Pressure | Vascular Resistance | Cardiac Output | Misc. |
|---|---|---|---|---|
| Heart or Ascending Aorta | Left atrium ↑<br>Left ventricular end-diastolic ↑<br>Aorta ↓<br>Pulmonary artery ↑ | (Systemic)<br>Decreases | Increases | |
| Main Pulmonary Artery | Left atrium ↑<br>Left ventricular end-diastolic ↑<br><br>Aorta ↓<br>Pulmonary artery ↑ | (Pulmonary)<br>Increases, occasionally decreases | Increases | * |
| Abdominal Aorta | (Systemic) ↓ | Decreases | | |

*Injection of hyperosmolar ionic contrast agents may result in an acute but transient pulmonary capillary leak as a result of a transient alteration in the capillary permeability.[28]

However, contrast agents with a high sodium content have a higher toxicity.[11, 12]

According to Poiseuille's law of fluid flow, contrast viscosity, together with the internal diameter and the length of a catheter, determines the maximal flow rate that can be delivered through a catheter:

$$Q = \frac{\Delta P \; r^4 \; \pi}{\eta \; L \; 8}$$

where $Q$ = flow rate, $\Delta P$ = pressure drop along catheter, $r$ = radius of lumen, $\eta$ = viscosity of injected fluid, $L$ = length of catheter, and $\pi/8$ = proportionality constant.

Heating the contrast medium decreases the viscosity and makes it easier to inject (Tables 2–8 and 2–9). However, viscosity plays a minor role for catheters with large lumina.

The most important cause of contrast toxicity is the hypertonicity of the conventional ionic contrast agents. Hypertonicity is responsible for a number of side effects, ie, fluid and electrolyte disturbances, hemodynamic changes, chemical injury to the vascular endothelium, and pain associated with peripheral and mesenteric arteriography. Low osmolality contrast agents such as the nonionic monomeric or dimeric preparations will be better tolerated.[13, 14] The sodium content and the presence of chelating agents in some contrast agents may be responsible for cardiac arrhythmias when these preparations are used for ventriculography or ascending aortography.[15, 16]

**Effects of Contrast Media on Organs or Organ Systems** (Tables 2–10 to 2–12). The cardiovascular effects of contrast agents depend upon the site of contrast injection and the status of the circulatory system, ie, the presence of preexisting anatomical abnormalities.[17] These effects may be electrophysiological (such as alteration in the generation or conduction of impulses and the lowering of the threshold for ventricular fibrillation) or hemodynamic (mechanical or circulatory).[17–19] Both these effects are related to the hyperosmolality of the agents and are possibly due to deficiency in ambient calcium ions.[16, 17, 20] A further review of the subject can be found in reference 21.

The cardiac effects are less pronounced

TABLE 2–11. Systemic Effects of Radiographic Contrast Injection*

| Cardiac Output | Pressure | Peripheral Vascular Resistance | Hematocrit | Intravascular Blood Volume | Blood |
|---|---|---|---|---|---|
| Increases | Decreases | Decreases | ↓ | Increases | Crenation and aggregation of red cells<br>Platelet aggregation ↑ or ↓<br>Complement activation<br>Thrombosis after prolonged contact |

*The systemic effects of nonionic and lower osmolality contrast agents are fewer than those associated with high osmolality ionic contrast agents.

**TABLE 2–12.** Hemodynamic Effects of Contrast Injection into the Renal Artery or Abdominal Aorta*

| Time Following Injection | Renal Blood Flow | Renal Vascular Resistance | PAH Clearance |
|---|---|---|---|
| 30 sec | Increased | Decreased | Decreased |
| 1–5 min | Decreased | Increased | Decreased |
| 30 min | Baseline | Baseline | Baseline |

*Adapted from White RI: Fundamentals of Vascular Radiology. Philadelphia, Lea & Febiger, 1976.
PAH = para-aminohippuric acid.

after contrast injection in the peripheral circulation. Vasodilation with decrease in peripheral vascular resistance occurs, which may lead to hypotension and bradycardia.[22] This is probably due to pooling of blood in the peripheral circulation and is relieved by administration of intravenous fluids, injection of atropine intravenously, and elevation of the legs in an attempt to augment venous return.

The primary mode of excretion of angiographic contrast media is through the kidneys. The injection of angiographic contrast media is associated with a marked increase in plasma volume and subsequent osmotic diuresis. The latter can lead to dehydration and transient renal failure if fluid replacement is not adequate.

Contrast agents exhibit a concentration-related direct toxic effect on the arterial wall.[23] In addition, a dose-dependent anticoagulant effect and impairment of platelet aggregation have been observed.[24, 25] In some patients contrast agents may promote coagulation. In patients with sickle cell anemia, sickling has been observed with the use of the hypertonic ionic contrast agents.[26] This may be avoided by using a nonionic contrast medium. Other patients who are prone to contrast medium–related intravascular complications are those with homocystinuria, proteinuria, multiple myeloma, and diabetes mellitus.

## REFERENCES

1. Kadir S: Double curve wire technique for negotiating tortuous iliac arteries and abdominal aortic aneurysms. Cath Cardiovasc Diagn 9:625–627, 1983.
2. Ring EJ, Mclean GK: Interventional Radiology: Principles and Techniques. Boston, Little, Brown and Company, 1981, p. 214.
3. Kido D, Paulin S, Alenghat JA, et al: Thrombogenicity of heparin and nonheparin coated catheters: clinical trial. Am J Neuroradiol 3:535–539, 1982.
4. Formanek G, Frech RS, Amplatz K: Arterial thrombus formation during clinical percutaneous catheterization. Circulation 41:833–839, 1970.
4a. Kaufman SL: Tapered-tip Teflon catheter for biliary drainage. Radiology 151:251, 1984.
5. Stroem BG, Winberg T: Percutaneous selective angiography of the inferior mesenteric artery. Acta Rad Diag 57:401–410, 1962.
6. Kadir S: Percutaneous antecubital vein approach for hepatic and renal vein catheterization. AJR 139:825–827, 1982.
7. Chuang VP, Soo C-S, Carrasco CH, et al: Superselective catheterization technique in hepatic angiography. AJR 141:803–811, 1983.
8. Levin DC: Catheters for selective arteriography: additional configuration alternatives. Radiology 146:553–555, 1983.
8a. Barth KH: Cholangiography aided by Fogarty balloon catheters after Rodney Smith cholangio-jejunostomy. Radiology 135:517–518, 1980.
9. Heeney D: Shape your guide wire. AJR 141:405–406, 1983.
10. Alexander JW, Fischer JE, Boyajian M, et al.: The influence of hair-removal methods on wound infections. Arch Surg 118:347–352, 1983.
11. Fischer HW: Viscosity, solubility, and toxicity in the choice of an angiographic contrast medium. Angiology 16:759–766, 1965.
12. Fischer HW, Cornell SH: The toxicity of the sodium and methylglucamine salts of diatrizoate, iothalamate and metrizoate. Radiology 85:1013–1021, 1965.
13. Grainger RC: Patient reactions during Hexabrix, Iopamidol and Conray angiography. In Amiel M (ed): Contrast Media in Radiology. New York, Springer Verlag, 1982, pp. 265–268.
14. Senac JP, Prefaut CH, Adda M, et al: Comparative study of the effects of two contrast media of different osmolarity on pulmonary hemodynamics and lung function. In Amiel M (ed): Contrast media in Radiology. New York, Springer Verlag, 1982, pp. 288–290.
15. Snyder C, Cramer R, Amplatz K: Isolation of sodium as a cause of ventricular fibrillation. Invest Radiol 6:245–248, 1971.
16. Violante MR, Thompson KR, Fischer HW, et al: Ventricular fibrillation from diatrizoate with and without chelating agents. Radiology 128:497–498, 1978.
17. Higgins, CB: Considerations of pathogenicity and clinical aspects of contrast media toxicity on the heart in 1981. In Amiel M (ed): Contrast Media in Radiology. New York, Springer Verlag, 1982, pp. 59–69.
18. Higgins, CB: Effects of contrast media on the conducting system of the heart. Radiology 124:599–606, 1977.
19. Higgins CB: Overview and methods used for the study of cardiovascular actions of contrast materials. Invest Radiol Suppl 15:S188–S193, 1980.

20. Thompson KR, Violante MR, Kenyon T, et al: Reduction in ventricular fibrillation using calcium enriched Renografin 76. Invest Radiol 13:238–240, 1978.
21. Amiel M (ed): Contrast Media in Radiology. New York, Springer Verlag, 1982.
22. Roberts PN, Young IP, Windsor CWO: Hypotension after angiography. Lancet 1:985–986, 1967.
23. Guidollette J, Gateau O, Borson F, et al: Iodinated contrast agents: Effect on ATP:creatinine N-phosphotransferase isoenzymes in the arterial wall. *In* Amiel M (ed): Contrast Media in Radiology. New York, Springer Verlag, 1982, pp. 28–30.
24. Belleville J, Cornillon B, Freyria AM, et al: In vivo and in vitro modification of platelet aggregation and release of ATP by ionic and nonionic contrast media used in angiography. *In* Amiel M (ed): Contrast Media in Radiology. New York, Springer Verlag, 1982, pp. 40–43.
25. Schultze B, Beyer HK: The effect of radiographic iodized contrast media on coagulation, fibrinolysis and complement system. *In* Amiel M (ed): Contrast Media in Radiology. New York, Springer Verlag, 1982, pp. 31–39.
26. Rao VM, Rao AK, Steiner RM, et al: The comparative effect of ionic and nonionic contrast media on the sickling phenomenon. Radiology 144:291–293, 1982.
27. Bettmann MA: Angiographic contrast agents: conventional and new media compared. AJR 139:787–794, 1982.
28. Slutsky RA, Hackney DB, Peck WW, et al: Extravascular lung water: effects of ionic and non ionic contrast media. Radiology 149:375–378, 1983.

# Basic Catheterization Techniques

## ARTERIAL PUNCTURE

### Technique

The artery is localized by palpation. In individuals with a weak arterial pulse due to arterial occlusive disease or obesity, localization may be facilitated by Doppler ultrasonography.

Local anesthesia (without epinephrine) is administered through a short 25 gauge needle. Initially, 1 to 2 ml is injected intradermally to produce a wheal. Subsequently, the anesthetic is injected subcutaneously, anterior to and on both sides of the artery, avoiding an intravascular injection. A longer 22 gauge needle may be used for administering deep anesthesia in obese individuals. Arterial puncture with such needles must be avoided because of potential complications, eg, intramural injection of the anesthetic leading to compromise of the arterial lumen and subsequent thrombosis, or arterial spasm due to needle trauma, or dislodgment of a plaque (Fig. 3–1).

With a No. 11 scalpel blade, a 2 to 3 mm stab incision is made through the skin and subcutaneous tissues, approximately 0.5 to 1.0 cm below the anticipated arterial puncture site (ie, below the point at which the needle will enter the artery). In individuals with little or no subcutaneous fat, the skin is lifted between the fingers to avoid trauma to a superficially placed artery (Fig. 3–2).

A mosquito clamp is then used to spread the subcutaneous tissues. The index and middle fingers of one hand are placed above and below the skin incision, so that it lies between the fingers (see Fig. 3–9). Alternatively, the index and middle fingers may be placed above the skin incision. Constant palpation of the arterial pulse serves to guide the direction of the needle. The technique for holding the needle is shown in Figure 3–3.

**Double Wall Arterial Puncture Technique** (Fig. 3–4). The needle tip is inserted through the skin incision, at a 45 to 50° angle from the skin surface. It is advanced slowly until

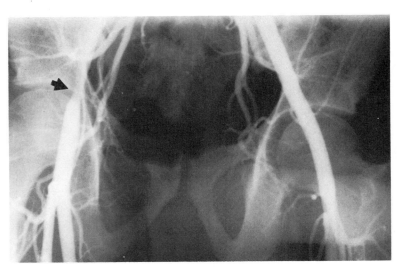

*Figure 3–1.* Focal narrowing of common femoral–external iliac artery due to intramural injection of local anesthetic (*arrow*).

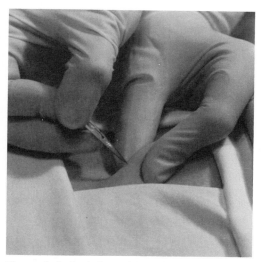

**Figure 3–2.** Technique for making a skin stab in patients with superficially placed arteries. The skin is lifted between the fingers in order to avoid trauma to the artery.

transmitted arterial pulsation is felt. At this point, the needle is advanced through the artery in a single forward thrust. In the groin, the needle tip usually encounters the underlying bone. The stylet is removed, and another 1 to 2 ml of the anesthetic is injected. During axillary or brachial arterial puncture, deep anesthesia is avoided. The needle hub is depressed slightly and the needle is withdrawn slowly. The appearance of a pulsatile jet of blood indicates free intraluminal position of the needle tip. A guide wire is inserted for catheter placement.

If a sheath needle (Amplatz needle) is used for arterial puncture, the stylet is removed and the inner cannula is withdrawn from the sheath by approximately 0.5 cm (rotatory motion must be avoided). This retracts the sharp, beveled cannula into the Teflon sheath. Again the needle hub is depressed slightly and the sheath with the cannula is withdrawn slowly. Once a pulsatile jet of blood is seen, the sheath is slowly advanced into the artery. While this is done, the flow must remain pulsatile.

INDICATIONS. This is the most frequently used arterial puncture technique.

**Single Wall Arterial Puncture Technique** (Fig. 3–5). An arterial needle with a sharp, beveled cannula is used. The stylet is removed and the needle is inserted through the skin incision at an angle of 45 to 50°. It is advanced slowly until a pulsatile jet of blood is observed. At this point the needle hub is depressed slightly and a guide wire is inserted.

INDICATIONS. (1) For a high femoral artery puncture, ie, close to the inguinal ligament (to avoid a retroperitoneal hematoma); (2) during antegrade femoral artery puncture (to avoid entering the profunda femoris artery); (3) occasionally for brachial and axillary artery puncture; (4) in patients with abnormal clotting parameters; and (5) for puncture of synthetic grafts.

**Techniques for Puncture of Arteries with Diminished or Absent Pulses.** In the presence of severe occlusive disease, arterial pulses may not be palpable at the usual

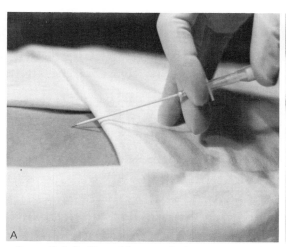

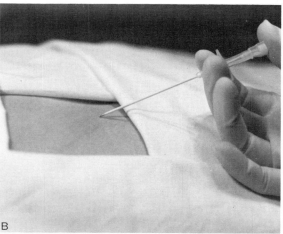

**Figure 3–3.** Position of the needle for arterial or venous puncture. *A,* The angle of puncture is shallow and guide wire and catheter insertion is easier. *B,* With this position, the angle of puncture is steeper and more likely to be perpendicular to the vessel.

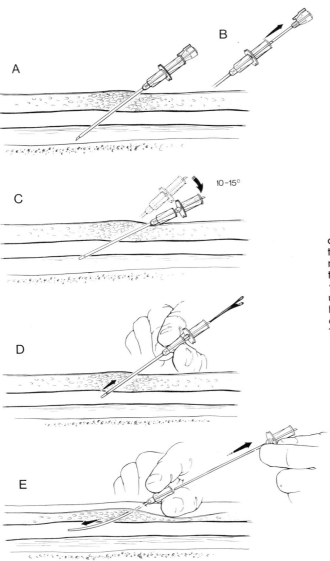

*Figure 3–4.* Double wall arterial puncture with a sheath needle. *A,* The needle is inserted through both walls of the artery. *B,* The stylet is removed. *C,* The inner cannula is withdrawn by 4 to 5 mm. The needle hub is depressed by 10 to 15° and *D,* the cannula and sheath are withdrawn until a jet of blood is observed. *E,* The cannula is held steady with one hand while the sheath is advanced into the artery with the other hand. The cannula is removed subsequently.

arterial puncture site in the groin. Nevertheless, such vessels can be catheterized to provide information about the distal circulation.[1]

When puncturing arteries with a significantly diminished or absent pulse and low intraarterial pressure, it must be remembered that pulsatile flow may be absent and blood return may be in the form of a dribble. In this case, an extension tube is attached to the needle hub for injection of contrast medium to assess the situation by fluoroscopy, spot film, or digital subtraction angiogram (DSA).

1. Doppler technique. The Doppler probe is used to map the course of the artery, which is then marked on the skin surface with indelible ink. After the skin is prepped, the arterial puncture needle is inserted in the direction (along the course of the artery) determined by the Doppler probe.

Alternatively, the Doppler probe can be used after the patient has been prepped. The probe is placed in a sterile rubber glove (with ultrasonic gel at the tip) (Fig. 3–6). The skin surface is moistened with flushing solution or sterile gel.

2. Fluoroscopic technique for femoral artery puncture. With the extremity in a true anterior-posterior position, the course of the normal common femoral artery is over the medial half of the femoral head.[3] This anatomical landmark may be utilized for puncture of a pulseless femoral artery. With the

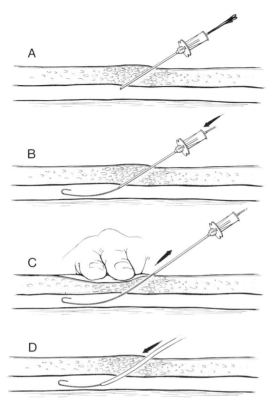

**Figure 3–5.** Single wall arterial puncture. *A*, With the stylet removed, the metal cannula of a Potts-Cournand needle is inserted into the artery. *B*, When a pulsatile jet of blood is observed, a guide wire is inserted. *C*, The needle is removed and *D*, the appropriate catheter is inserted.

aid of fluoroscopy, the arterial puncture needle is inserted over the medial third of the femoral head with the tip inclined medially by about 20°.[3] Any arterial needle may be used; however, long arterial needles are preferable because they permit fluoroscopy during the actual arterial puncture, without exposing the radiologist's hands to radiation. In patients with heavy vascular calcification, the calcification can be used as a fluoroscopic guide for arterial puncture.

3. Palpation technique. A relatively hard cord representing the nonpulsatile artery can often be palpated in nonobese individuals. Such vessels are punctured after their course has been determined by palpation.

4. Venous catheter technique. If the arterial puncture needle enters the femoral vein during an attempt at femoral artery puncture, a short vascular sheath or 5 Fr dilator is inserted. This serves as an anatomical landmark to guide the arterial puncture.

**Common Errors and Problems and Their Solutions**

1. Nonpulsatile jet of blood: A jet of blood coming out of the needle hub that is either nonpulsatile or weak usually indicates a partial intraluminal position of the needle/sheath tip (if the arterial pulse was good by palpation). If a guide wire or the sheath is advanced, this will create a dissection or intramural passage of the guide wire/sheath or may lead to plaque dislodgment.

The needle/sheath is withdrawn slowly until the jet is strong. If this does not occur, the needle/sheath is removed, the groin is compressed for at least 5 minutes, and the arterial puncture is repeated. If the pulse was weak by palpation, a weak jet may be due to the severity of atherosclerotic occlusive disease and not represent a technical problem.

2. Jet of blood diminishes as the sheath

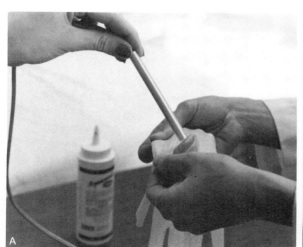

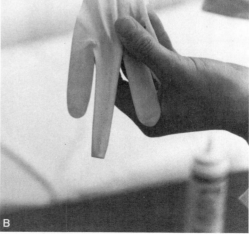

**Figure 3–6.** *A* and *B*, Technique for insertion of the Doppler probe into a glove for localization of artery for percutaneous puncture.

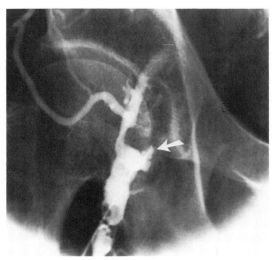

**Figure 3–7.** Importance of contrast opacification to evaluate difficulty associated with arterial puncture. Neither the sheath nor a 0.025 inch guide wire could be advanced into the artery, as the tip of the needle was lying beneath a plaque (*arrow*).

3. Sheath/guide wire does not advance: This indicates either that the tip of the needle or sheath is against the arterial wall or a plaque or that there is an arterial stenosis immediately above the puncture site (Fig. 3–7). The needle or sheath is withdrawn until pulsatile flow is reestablished. The needle is angled in a different direction (either medial or lateral) and the sheath or guide wire is readvanced (Fig. 3–8). Occasionally, a smaller guide wire (0.025 or 0.021 inch) may slip past more easily than a larger wire (0.035 inch). If this is unsuccessful, it usually indicates the presence of an arterial stenosis. Extension tubing is attached to the needle hub and contrast medium is injected and observed fluoroscopically, or a DSA is obtained to document the anatomy. If a stenosis is demonstrated, a 7.5 or 15 mm J or a movable core J guide wire is used to traverse it. If the stenosis is severe, an alternative approach is used.

### Retrograde Femoral Artery Puncture

**Location.** The puncture is made 1 cm or more below the inguinal ligament, in the femoral triangle, at the point where the artery is best palpated. In this location, the course of the femoral artery is medially directed and the artery lies closer to the skin. The location of the inguinal crease may vary considerably with the pannus. Thus, the only safe landmark is the inguinal ligament, which extends from the anterior-superior iliac spine to the pubic tubercle.

**Technique.** The femoral artery is located and the course of the vessel is determined by palpation. For the right femoral artery, the right hand is used for arterial puncture,

(from the Amplatz needle) is advanced: This indicates that the tip is either against the wall or against a plaque. The sheath is withdrawn slightly, until pulsatile blood flow is reestablished. The needle hub is moved either medial or lateral and an attempt is again made to advance the sheath. If the sheath does not advance or the jet diminishes again, a 0.025 inch J guide wire is inserted through the needle cannula and advanced past the obstruction. This soft wire usually advances past the plaques, and the sheath can be advanced over it. Since the 0.025 inch wire is too flimsy to serve as an exchange wire for the insertion of a catheter, it is replaced by a 0.035 inch guide wire for catheter placement.

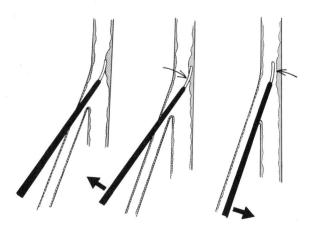

**Figure 3–8.** Angulation of arterial puncture needle to assist guide wire insertion.

with the radiologist standing on the ipsilateral side of the patient. The index and middle fingers of the left hand are placed above and below the anticipated arterial puncture site (Fig. 3–9). The needle is angled medially by 25 to 30° (towards the umbilicus) to correspond to the long axis of the vessel. Similarly, for the left side the left hand is used for arterial puncture, with the radiologist standing on the ipsilateral side of the patient.

**Applications.** This is the most frequently used access for aortography and selective arteriography.

**Contraindications.** (1) Groin infection, (2) recent surgery, and (3) saccular aneurysms (fusiform widening of the femoral arteries, as seen in association with arteriomegaly, is not a contraindication). In severe occlusive disease of the common femoral or iliac arteries, femoral artery catheterization should be undertaken with extreme caution. Similarly, in patients with aorto-bifemoral bypass grafts, graft puncture should be avoided whenever possible.

### Antegrade Femoral Artery Puncture

**Patient Selection.** Only nonobese patients should be considered for antegrade puncture, as this can be extremely difficult in patients with a protuberant abdomen and in obese individuals.

**Technique.** With the leg in neutral posi-

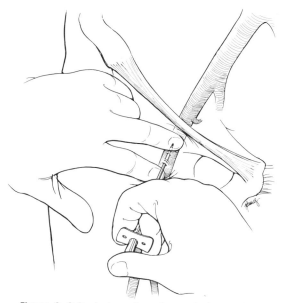

**Figure 3–9.** Technique for retrograde femoral artery puncture.

tion, the femoral artery is punctured from the ipsilateral side. The puncture site should be approximately 1 cm below the inguinal ligament (not the inguinal crease). The needle is held at a 45 to 55° angle from the surface of the skin, since a vertical needle position makes guide wire and catheter insertion difficult. A single wall puncture is preferable because it allows maximal maneuverability. In addition, this permits a high puncture, close to the inguinal ligament.

METAL NEEDLE (POTTS-COURNAND, SELDINGER). With the needle in the common femoral artery, a straight LLT or a 1.5 mm J guide wire is passed into the SFA. If the course of the wire is laterally oriented, it has entered the profunda femoris artery. To catheterize the SFA, the wire is withdrawn, the needle is directed to point laterally, and the wire is readvanced. With this maneuver, the guide wire is deflected off the arterial wall and is directed medially. Similarly, to direct the wire into the profunda femoris artery, the opposite maneuver is used, ie, the needle is directed medially.

If this maneuver is not successful, the wire is removed, and diluted contrast medium (30%) is injected to localize the common femoral artery bifurcation. If the needle tip is in the profunda femoris artery, the skin entry site is marked with a mosquito clamp to permit assessment of the length of the intravascular portion of the needle. The needle is then withdrawn slowly, while injecting contrast medium. Once the needle tip is in the common femoral artery, a straight LLT wire is inserted into the SFA. Alternatively, a 10 mm J high torque wire may be used. Once the wire is in the SFA, a multiple hole straight catheter is inserted. If the torque wire has been used to enter the SFA, the metal cannula is advanced over it and subsequently exchanged for a catheter over a J guide wire.

SHEATH NEEDLE (AMPLATZ NEEDLE). After successful femoral artery puncture, an extension tube is attached to the needle, and diluted contrast medium is injected to locate the common femoral artery bifurcation. A 0.025 inch J wire is inserted, and the needle is used to direct the guide wire into the SFA or profunda femoris artery (similar to the technique described for the metal needle). Once the wire is in the SFA, the sheath is advanced over it. The sheath should not be advanced into the artery without the aid of a guide wire because the flexible Teflon sheath (without the cannula) cannot be used to direct the guide wire if it has to be repositioned, ie, if the sheath does not enter the SFA.

**Applications.** The applications for antegrade femoral arteriography are (1) for better definition of vascular anatomy of the leg, eg, in patients with suspected arterial trauma and in patients undergoing microvascular tissue transfer (intraarterial DSA also provides an excellent delineation of the vascular anatomy from the retrograde femoral approach); (2) transluminal angioplasty and arterial embolization; and (3) catheter placement for intraarterial thrombolysis or catheter thromboembolectomy.

### Axillary Artery Puncture (Fig. 3–10)

**Location.** The location for axillary artery puncture is the lateral axillary fold. Here the artery crosses the humeral head and thus lends itself to compression for hemostasis. In this region, it is also in close relationship to the brachial plexus.

**Patient Selection.** In general, the left axillary artery approach is used. From the right axillary approach, it is difficult to catheterize the descending aorta in older individuals. In addition, this approach is avoided in patients with severe atherosclerosis, because of the potential for thromboembolic cerebrovascular complications as a result of guide wire and catheter manipulation past the cerebral vessels.

A brachial cuff pressure difference of > 20 mm Hg suggests the presence of a hemodynamically significant arterial stenosis of the arm with the lower blood pressure. In this situation, arterial puncture should be undertaken only if other access if difficult.

**Technique.** Axillary artery puncture may be performed with the arm in 90° abduction or with the arm in maximal abduction and the hand tucked under the head. The latter position is preferable, since the artery is stretched maximally and fixed in position (ie, it is less likely to roll).

The artery is punctured at the lateral axillary fold, at the point where it is best palpated. Appropriate sedation and the injection of sufficient local anesthetic are very important, in order to prevent the patient from tensing the arm muscles (contraction of the arm muscles may make the axillary artery pulse unpalpable).

The course of the artery is mapped out by

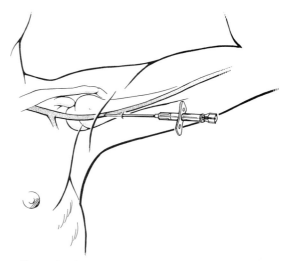

**Figure 3–10.** Technique for retrograde axillary artery puncture.

palpation. The artery is held in place with the index and middle fingers, with the arterial puncture site between the two fingers. The arterial needle is held at an angle of about 45° from the skin surface. After successful arterial puncture with a sheath needle, the sheath can usually be advanced without any problems. A 1.5 or 3 mm J guide wire is used for insertion of the catheter. If another needle is used, a straight LLT guide wire is inserted into the subclavian artery, proximal to the vertebral artery origin (a J guide wire often enters a branch vessel). The needle is removed and a short 5 Fr Teflon dilator is inserted. A J guide wire is then used for catheter placement.

For a description of the techniques for placement of a catheter in the ascending or the descending aorta, see Chapter 8.

**Applications.** (1) Aortography, visceral and lower extremity arteriography in patients with access problems from the femoral approach; (2) interventional procedures (angioplasty of renal and other arteries, embolization, or placement of catheters for chemo- or thrombolytic therapy).

### Brachial Artery Puncture

**Location.** The location for brachial artery puncture is the mid-portion of the humerus in the bicipital groove. In this region, the brachial artery is accompanied by two veins and a nerve.

**Technique.** The technique is described in Chapter 9. For initial catheterization, straight guide wires should be used and large catheters (> 5 Fr) should be avoided.

**Applications.** The indications for retrograde brachial artery catheterization are for (1) an alternative approach for catheterization of the aorta, aortic branches, and lower extremity vessels; and (2) interventional procedures. Applications for antegrade catheterization include (1) interventional angiography, eg, transcatheter embolization of vascular malformations; and (2) evaluation of dialysis access fistulae.

**High Brachial Artery Puncture.** For this approach, the brachial artery is punctured midway between the axillary and brachial artery puncture sites, ie, approximately 5 to 6 cm lateral to the lateral axillary fold. The brachial artery is a relatively small vessel, and in our own experience, catheterization of this vessel is associated with more complications than with the axillary artery. Multiple catheter exchanges, indwelling catheters (eg, for thrombolysis), and large sizes (> 5 Fr) should be avoided.

## Translumbar Aortogram (TLA)

**Location.** With this technique, the abdominal aorta can be punctured at two levels: high TLA, at the lower border of T12; and low TLA, at the lower border of L2.

**Patient Selection**

1. This procedure is difficult to perform in obese individuals because of the short needle.

2. Individuals incapable of maintaining the prone position for at least 1½ to 2 hours owing to obesity, respiratory problems, etc., should not undergo a TLA.

3. Patients on oral platelet aggregation inhibitors, those with abnormal clotting parameters (prothrombin time > 15% over control), and patients with hypertension (systolic > 190 mm Hg and diastolic > 95 mm Hg) should also not be considered for a TLA.

4. A low TLA is not recommended in patients with abdominal aortic aneurysms. In such patients, a high TLA may be performed if another access is not available. Similarly, a high TLA can be performed safely in patients with infrarenal aortic grafts.

**Technique** (Fig. 3–11). The patient is placed in the prone position. A flat sponge or several folded sheets are placed underneath the abdomen to straighten out the lumbar lordosis. The left half of the back (between the lower ribs and the iliac crest) is prepped and draped.

A Kelly clamp is placed at the anticipated aortic puncture site (undersurface of T12 or L2). The spinous processes of the lumbar vertebrae are observed fluoroscopically to insure a true anterior-posterior position (ie, no rotation).

The skin entry site is midway between the lower border of the lowest rib and the iliac crest for the low TLA and approximately 2 cm below the 12th rib for the high TLA. The skin entry site should be approximately 10 cm to the left of the spinous processes of the lumbar vertebrae. Local anesthetic is given initially through a 25 gauge and subsequently through a 22 gauge needle. The skin stab should be 0.5 cm wide and 0.5 to 1 cm deep, and the subcutaneous tissues are spread with a mosquito clamp.

Under fluoroscopic guidance, the TLA needle is inserted at a 60 to 70° angle from the skin surface. As the needle tip reaches the lateral border of the vertebral body, it is advanced slowly until transmitted aortic pulsations are felt through the needle. At this point, a short forward thrust (about 1 cm) advances the needle into the aortic lumen. If no aortic pulsation is felt, the needle is advanced past the midline.

The stylet is removed and the inner cannula and sheath (catheter) are slowly withdrawn as a unit. When pulsatile blood return is observed (the jet of blood is less pulsatile than that seen with puncture needles with a Cournand extension), a high torque J wire is inserted into the upper (for upstream injection) or lower (for downstream injecton) abdominal aorta. Once the wire is in position, with the metal cannula held stationary, the outer sheath is advanced over the wire. Subsequently, the torque wire and inner cannula are removed and the catheter position is confirmed by contrast injection.

If no blood returns as the cannula and sheath are withdrawn past the mid-portion of the transverse process of the vertebral body, the stylet is reinserted and the needle is withdrawn past the tip of the transverse process. The angle is decreased by 5 to 10° after each pass, and the needle is readvanced.

If the needle tip encounters bone, the patient feels a sharp nonradiating pain. The stylet is removed, and 1 to 2 ml of local anesthetic is injected at the periosteum of the vertebral body. The stylet is reinserted and the needle is withdrawn past the tip of the transverse process. The angle of the needle is increased by approximately 5 to 10° after

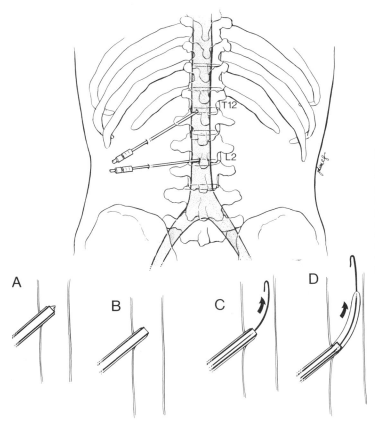

*Figure 3–11.* Technique for translumbar aortography. With the patient in the prone position, the aorta is entered from the left flank (*A*). The obturator is removed (*B*), and a high torque guide wire is inserted. For an upstream catheter placement, the wire is torqued into the descending thoracic aorta (*C*) and for a downstream injection, it is torqued into the infrarenal abdominal aorta. Once the wire is in place, the Teflon catheter is advanced over the wire (*D*).

each pass (ie, the needle tip is directed more anteriorly) and the needle is readvanced.

**Common Errors and Problems and Their Solutions**

1. Absence of transmitted aortic pulsations. This is encountered in patients with heavy mural thrombus deposition or aortic occlusion. In the latter situation, there is also no blood return. In this case a high TLA should be performed.

2. Hard, heavily calcified aorta. In this situation, considerable resistance may be encountered as the needle is advanced through the aortic wall. The mural calcification is usually visible on fluoroscopy, and as the needle is advanced into the aorta, a slight displacement of the calcification is observed.

3. Skin entry site too lateral or too medial. If the skin entry site is too lateral (away from the spine), there is risk of traversing the renal parenchyma. If the skin entry site is too medial (close to the spine), the path of the needle is vertical and a narrow aorta may be missed.

4. The guide wire does not advance. This indicates that the catheter tip is either par-

tially intramural or against the aortic wall. The cannula and sheath are withdrawn a few millimeters and the guide wire is reinserted. If the problem persists, a small contrast injection clarifies the situation.

5. The J tip does not re-form or advances beyond the aortic lumen. This may occur if the needle tip is outside the aorta or if the guide wire has entered a branch vessel. The guide wire is removed and a small volume of contrast medium is injected to clarify the situation (provided there is blood return).

6. The guide wire does not advance downstream. This suggests severe stenosis or occlusion of the lower abdominal aorta. Injection of a small volume of contrast medium clarifies the situation. The guide wire is then positioned for upstream catheter placement.

7. No blood return on a low TLA puncture. No blood return after several attempts suggests complete occlusion of the aorta. In this case a high TLA should be performed.

**Applications.** This procedure is used for (1) arteriography in patients with absent femoral pulses or contraindications to femoral arteriography (eg, infection, recent surgery);

and (2) severe iliofemoral artery disease. It has also been used for catheterization of the thoracic aorta and its branches.[3a]

**Upstream Versus Downstream Catheter Position.** An upstream catheter position is required for abdominal aortography. Downstream positioning of the catheter is used for antegrade arteriography of the pelvis and lower extremity vessels. The latter provides superior opacification of the vessels by virtue of an antegrade contrast injection. Downstream catheter position is used when only the pelvic and lower extremity vessels are to be studied, without the need to evaluate the visceral arteries.

**Conversion of a Downstream to an Upstream Catheter Position or Vice Versa.** Downstream to upstream conversion may be required for evaluation of the abdominal aorta and the visceral arteries upon conclusion of the lower extremity arteriogram. Conversion of an upstream to a downstream catheter position may be necessary for pelvic and lower extremity arteriography following abdominal aortography.

HIGH TORQUE WIRE TECHNIQUE (Fig. 3–12). The Teflon sheath in the aorta is opacified with contrast medium and is withdrawn until it is almost horizontal. A 3 mm J high torque wire is inserted. The tip of the J wire is pointed craniad, and the wire is advanced into the upper abdominal aorta and is followed by the sheath.

Alternatively, the high torque wire is inserted through the sheath and the J tip is allowed to re-form. Both the wire and the sheath are withdrawn until the wire is almost horizontal. The J wire is then torqued into the upper abdominal aorta and is followed by the sheath.

*Note:* It is advisable to measure the length of the guide wire that has to be inserted to re-form the J tip. The proximal end (at the sheath hub) is marked with a sterile tape. This helps in assessing the length of the sheath (which is not very radiopaque) in the aorta and prevents its accidental removal.

TIP DEFLECTING WIRE TECHNIQUE. A sterile tape is placed approximately 8 inches from the tip of a 0.035 inch deflecting wire to mark the length of the sheath. This predetermined length of wire is inserted into the sheath. The wire must not be allowed to protrude beyond the sheath because, upon deflection, the bare wire tip curls up and will not allow the catheter to be advanced over it.

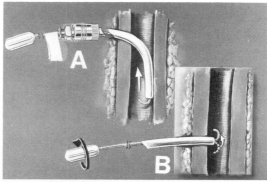

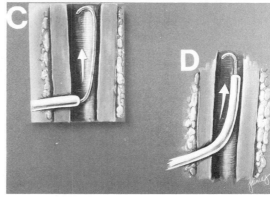

*Figure 3–12.* Technique for conversion of TLA puncture. *A,* A torque wire is inserted into the catheter in the infrarenal aorta and the 3 mm J is permitted to re-form. A piece of sterile adhesive tape is placed on the wire at the catheter hub to mark the length of the wire in the catheter. *B,* The catheter is withdrawn slowly until it is in a horizontal (or nearly horizontal) position. The wire is torqued so that the J points craniad. *C,* The tape is removed and the wire advanced into the suprarenal abdominal aorta and *D,* is followed by the catheter. *Note:* The same technique is used for conversion of an upstream into a downstream puncture.

Both sheath and wire are withdrawn until they are horizontal or almost horizontally oriented. The tip is deflected to point craniad and the sheath is advanced into the upper abdominal aorta.

Both the high torque wire and the tip deflecting wire techniques are also used to convert from an upstream to a downstream catheter position for antegrade arteriography of the pelvis and the lower extremities.

## VENOUS PUNCTURE

### Femoral Vein Puncture

Any arterial puncture needle may be used for femoral vein puncture. The femoral artery is localized in the groin, and a skin incision is made approximately 0.5 cm medial to the artery and 1 to 2 cm below the inguinal ligament. The index, middle, and ring fingers of one hand are placed on the arterial pulse (to guide the needle and prevent an accidental arterial puncture). The puncture needle is inserted through the skin incision at an angle of 45 to 50° from the skin surface, and the patient is asked to take a deep breath and bear down hard (Valsalva maneuver). At this point the needle is inserted swiftly. If the needle touches bone, 1 to 2 ml of local anesthetic is injected.

The stylet is removed, and plastic extension tubing with a 20 ml syringe containing flushing solution is attached to the needle hub. If the Amplatz needle is used, the sheath and inner metal cannula are not separated (unlike the procedure for arterial puncture). The needle hub is depressed slightly and withdrawn slowly while maintaining suction. As soon as venous blood appears in the tubing, the Teflon sheath is advanced into the vein and the cannula is removed. A guide wire is then inserted for placement of the appropriate catheter. If a needle without a sheath has been used, the extension tubing is disconnected as soon as venous blood appears in the tubing, and an appropriate guide wire is inserted for placement of a catheter.

If the vein is not entered on the first puncture, the needle is directed more medially each time it is reinserted. If, however, the initial puncture was at a distance from the arterial pulsation, a more lateral puncture (moving closer to the artery) is attempted.

**Applications.** Femoral vein catheterization is used for (1) evaluation of the inferior vena cava and its branches; (2) pulmonary arteriography and right heart catheterization; (3) venous sampling in patients with hypertension and endocrine abnormalities; (4) gonadal vein catheterization; and (5) intravenous DSA.

### Cubital Vein Puncture (Fig. 3–13)

The arm is placed in 45° abduction, and the antecubital fossa is prepped and draped. A tourniquet is applied over the upper arm, and the median cubital vein is punctured with a 16 gauge angiocath or a 19 gauge butterfly needle.

**Angiocath Technique.** After the vein has been entered, the Teflon sheath is advanced into it. The metal cannula is removed, and a 0.035 inch straight LLT guide wire (or the straight LT end of the double flex guide wire) is inserted into the vein. The tourniquet is released, and 1 to 2 ml of local anesthetic is injected intradermally at the puncture site. The Teflon sheath is withdrawn, the skin puncture site is widened to 1 to 2 mm with a No. 11 blade, and the appropriate catheter is inserted.

Newer sheath needles for cubital venous access (for DSA) have a longer metal cannula protruding beyond a short sheath. Once the vein has been entered with such a cannula, a guide wire is inserted. The tourniquet is released, and the skin incision is made after injection of the local anesthetic. The sheath is then inserted into the vein over the guide wire.

**Butterfly Technique.** The plastic extension tubing of the butterfly needle is cut off close to the needle. Upon entering the vein, a straight 0.025 inch wire is inserted (if a 19 gauge butterfly has been used) and the tourniquet is released. One to 2 ml of local

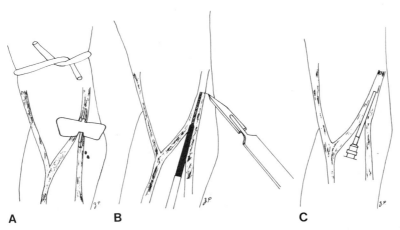

**A**          **B**          **C**

*Figure 3–13.* Percutaneous cubital vein puncture. *A,* The vein is punctured with a butterfly, and a guide wire is inserted. Alternatively, an angiocath may be used. *B,* The butterfly is exchanged for a catheter or introducer sheath. Following injection of local anesthesia, a small skin incision is made. *C,* The catheter or introducer sheath is inserted. (From Kadir S: AJR 139:826, 1982. Reproduced with permission.)

anesthetic is injected intradermally at the puncture site. The needle is withdrawn, and the skin puncture site is widened to 1 to 2 mm with a No. 11 blade. The needle is removed, and a 5 Fr vessel dilator is inserted. The 0.025 inch wire is replaced by a 0.035 inch straight LLT wire. The dilator is removed, and the appropriate catheter is inserted.

If an end hole–occluded catheter is to be used, an appropriate-sized catheter introducer sheath is inserted. If a larger butterfly needle is employed, a 0.035 inch guide wire can be used for placement of a catheter.

**Common Errors and Problems and Their Solutions** (Fig. 3–14)

1. Injection of local anesthetic before venipuncture. This usually obscures the vein and makes the venipuncture difficult. Therefore, local anesthetic should be injected only after access to the vein has been secured.

2. The catheter or guide wire does not advance through the brachial vein. This may be due to venous spasm or extravascular position. One to 2 ml of diluted contrast medium is injected and observed fluoroscopically. If venous spasm is present, a drip infusion is attached to the catheter for several minutes to allow the spasm to resolve. Alternatively, the catheter may be advanced gently while injecting heparinized flushing solution to passively dilate the vein.

3. Use of a laterally oriented vein in the antecubital fossa. This usually leads to the cephalic vein. In the vast majority of cases, this will not pose any difficulties for catheterization of the superior vena cava. The technique for catheterization of the superior vena cava from the cephalic vein is shown in Figure 3–15.

**Applications.** Cubital vein puncture is used for (1) intravenous DSA; (2) catheterization of the superior vena cava and right heart and for pulmonary arteriography; (3) hepatic and renal vein catheterization; and (4) gonadal vein catheterization.[4]

### Internal Jugular Vein Puncture

**Patient Selection.** Percutaneous catheterization of the internal jugular vein provides an alternative route for venous catheterization in patients with abnormal clotting parameters or venous access problems. In patients with massive ascites, this approach may be used for cholangiography or other interventional procedures.

**Location.** The right internal jugular vein is used most frequently, since it provides a straight route to the vena cava. The location of the skin entry site is at the lateral border of the sternocleidomastoid muscle, midway down the neck.

**Technique.** The patient is placed in the supine position and the head is turned to the left. The right side of the neck is prepped and draped and the skin is anesthetized. Initially, a skin wheal is made with a 25 gauge needle. Subsequently, using a 22 gauge needle, deep anesthesia is given along the anticipated track of the puncture needle. The injection of an excessive amount (> 3 ml) of anesthetic is avoided in order to minimize the diffusion of the anesthetic into the recurrent laryngeal and vagus nerves.

A 2 mm skin stab facilitates insertion of the needle (Amplatz needle without the stylet). A 10 ml plastic syringe is attached to the needle hub to provide continuous suction as the needle is inserted at a 45° angle from the

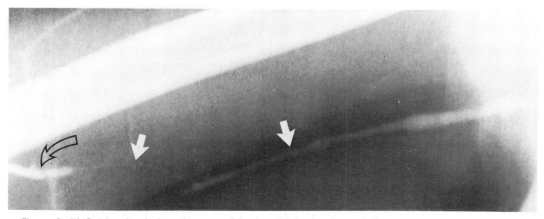

*Figure 3–14.* Guide wire–induced spasm of the brachial veins *(arrows).* Open arrow points to catheter.

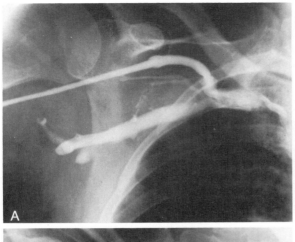
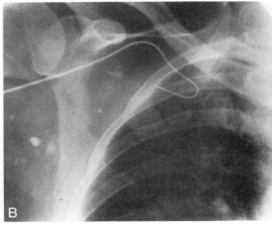
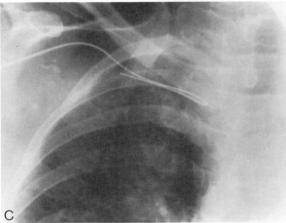

*Figure 3–15.* Technique for catheterization of the superior vena cava from the cephalic vein approach. *A,* Hand injection of contrast medium to delineate anatomy. The cephalic vein joins the axillary vein at a sharp angle. *B,* The tip of the multipurpose catheter is placed several centimeters above the junction of the two veins and a movable core (or LLT) 7.5 mm J guide wire is inserted. The wire tip usually enters the axillary vein. *C,* As the guide wire is advanced, it loops into the subclavian vein. Once it is in the superior vena cava, the catheter is advanced over the wire.

skin surface. The needle tip is directed toward the right breast nipple. The left hand of the radiologist may be used to mark the carotid pulse, which is located 1 to 2 cm medially. To distend the vein, the patient may be asked to perform the Valsalva maneuver.

Once the vein is entered, the Teflon sheath is advanced into it and is subsequently replaced by a catheter introducer sheath. Upon completion of the study, gentle compression is applied for 2 to 3 minutes. A semi-upright position of the patient facilitates hemostasis.

**Applications.** The percutaneous transjugular approach is used for catheterization of the hepatic, renal, and gonadal veins for pulmonary arteriography, portography, and cholangiography. In addition, it can be used for liver biopsy, embolization of gastroesophageal varices, and the creation of portosystemic shunts in patients with portal hypertension (Colapinto, R: personal communication).

## GUIDE WIRE AND CATHETER SELECTION: BASIC CATHETER TECHNIQUES

### Guide Wires

In the adult patient, a J-tipped wire (usually a 1.5 or 3 mm J) is used most frequently for nonselective arterial and venous catheterization (eg, aorta, vena cava, iliac, and proximal extremity vessels). In smaller branches, such as the proximal visceral arteries, a tight J (1.5 mm) can be used. In the distal branches of the visceral arteries (> second-order) or other narrow or stenotic vessels (eg, stenotic subclavian, iliac, or femoral artery), either a large J (7.5 to 15 mm) or a straight LLT wire may be used cautiously.

In the pediatric patient with narrow vessels, either a tight J wire (1.5 mm) or a soft-tipped straight or large J wire (7.5 to 15 mm) is used. Wires with a tapered core (LLT and LT) or movable core wires are ideally suited for getting past multiple bends. However, this distal flexibility often prevents the catheter from following the guide wire past multiple bends. To facilitate catheterization of such vessels, special guide wires are available (Wilson, Amplatz) that are flexible when introduced but can be stiffened once the wire is in the desired location. Alternatively, softer, thin-walled catheters may be used in conjunction with tapered core wires.

An important fact that is often overlooked is that every guide wire, as it makes its exit from the catheter, is extremely stiff and should never be forced out of the catheter against resistance. This is also true for the movable core and LLT wires. For such wires to resume their flexibility, > 2.0 cm length has to be outside the catheter or the J configuration must be resumed. Thus, if a guide wire has to be inserted through a catheter placed in a small diameter vessel or when the catheter tip abuts the arterial wall, the following technique must be used to prevent intimal trauma: As the guide wire comes through the catheter tip, the catheter is withdrawn to allow 1.5 to 2 cm of the wire to exit from the catheter or the J to re-form. This permits the guide wire to be "deposited" in the vessel and prevents the wire tip from penetrating the arterial wall.

A technique for straightening the tip to facilitate insertion of J guide wires into the Cournand extension of needles or into a catheter hub is shown in Figure 3–16. The J can be straightened by simply applying tension to the spring coil.

## Catheters

For the vast majority of diagnostic arteriographic studies, the commercially available preformed catheters are used. The choice of catheter for selective arteriography is dictated by the angle of origin of the particular vessel from the aorta. Similarly, the confluence of the vein with the vena cava determines the choice of catheter for the venous system.

For nonselective angiography of larger vessels (ie, aortography, pelvic arteriography, and vena cavography), a catheter with multiple holes is used to permit rapid delivery of a large volume of contrast medium and to facilitate better mixing of the contrast medium with the blood. For this purpose, the pigtail and multiple hole straight catheters are used. However, the straight catheters should only be used with a tip occluding device to avoid a large end hole jet when using high contrast delivery rates.

Nonselective arteriography is used to evaluate the major arteries and the proximal segments of their branches (eg, orifice of the celiac, superior mesenteric, and renal arteries) for occlusive or other diseases. Because of poor contrast opacification or overlapping of multiple arteries, the distal branches are not adequately demonstrated on such studies and thus the confirmation or exclusion of a diagnosis is often not possible.

Selective arteriography has the advantage that a single vessel is demonstrated in its entirety and thus permits evaluation of a

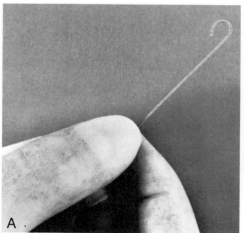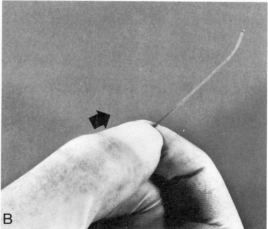

*Figure 3–16.* Technique for straightening J-tipped guide wires. *A,* The guide wire is held between the thumb and index fingers, approximately 3 to 4 cm from the tip. *B,* The outer coil spring is forced towards the wire tip with the thumb and index fingers, while the proximal segment is held by the palm, middle, ring, and little fingers. Arrow points towards the direction in which the force is applied.

specific organ or section of an organ. In addition, venous drainage can often be demonstrated, especially by DSA.

**Catheter Selection.** The choice of catheter for selective arteriography (Fig. 3–17) is determined by:

1. The diameter of the aorta (wide or narrow): In most instances this judgment can be made on the basis of the patient's size and age. That is, older individuals with a large body build and men are more likely to have a wide aorta, whereas small or younger individuals and women are more likely to have a narrow aorta.

For selective catheterization of aortic branches in individuals with a wide aorta, a cobra C3 or a sidewinder 2 curve is used. In individuals with a narrow aorta, a cobra C1 or a sidewinder 1 curve is used. In most other individuals, a cobra C2 or a sidewinder 1 is used. In individuals with severe atherosclerotic occlusive disease of the aorta, the sidewinder catheters should be used with extreme caution.

2. The angle of origin and location of the vessel to be catheterized. While the location of most aortic branches and their variations are well known, the angle of origin of some vessels can vary considerably. Thus, unless the catheter selection is made on the basis of a previous aortogram, a universal catheter is used for selective catheterization (eg, cobra C2). If this curve is found to be unsuitable for catheterization of the desired vessel, the appropriately shaped catheter is inserted after the origin and course of the vessel have been identified by a test injection of contrast medium.

Vessels with an acute, inferiorly directed course require a catheter with an inferiorly directed tip (eg, a sidewinder or a cobra C1 curve). Vessels arising horizontally from the aorta require a catheter with a shallow primary curve (eg, renal, or cobra C2 or C3). Such vessels can also be catheterized with the sidewinder catheters. In the venous system, in addition to the cobra catheter, a straight catheter with a tip deflecting system

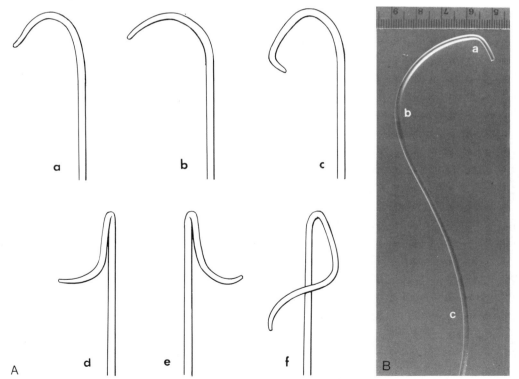

*Figure 3–17. A,* Different catheter shapes for visceral artery catheterization. a = left gastric; b = mesenteric, renal; c = dorsal pancreatic; d = hepatic; e = splenic; f = gastroduodenal artery. *B,* Primary (a), secondary (b), and tertiary (c) curves of a cobra catheter.

may be used for catheterization of larger branches.

Craniad-directed vessels require a catheter that can be inverted to point craniad (eg, sidewinder, shepherd hook, or cobra in the loop configuration).

## TECHNIQUE FOR NONSELECTIVE CATHETERIZATION

### Catheter Insertion Over a Guide Wire

This technique was originally described by Seldinger and has greatly facilitated vascular catheterization.[5]

1. After successful arterial or venous puncture, a J-shaped guide wire is inserted until the flexible segment is well past the puncture site.

2. The needle or sheath is removed and the puncture site is compressed with the 3rd to 5th fingers while the guide wire is held with the thumb and index finger of the same hand. With the other hand, the guide wire is wiped clean using a damp lint-free sponge (eg, Telfa surgical dressing).

3. The desired catheter is threaded over the guide wire. For the insertion of the catheter through the skin and vessel wall, the guide wire must be held taut. Care must be taken not to apply too much tension on the guide wire so as to pull it out.

4. As the catheter is inserted through the skin, it is rotated clockwise (similar to the motion for tightening a screw). If an assistant is not available to help during catheter insertion or exchange, the wire is coiled together and held in the hand used for compressing the puncture site, while the other hand is used for threading the catheter.

5. The catheter is advanced to the desired level, and the wire is removed. After the catheter is flushed, contrast medium is injected to confirm position.

### Catheter Exchange

During catheter exchange, the tip of the guide wire should be observed fluoroscopically. A J guide wire should be used unless the catheter exchange involves a smaller branch.

1. The guide wire is inserted beyond the catheter tip.

2. The catheter is removed in the following manner: The wire is held taut at a distance of about 10 cm from the catheter hub and the catheter is pulled back over it, 5 to 10 cm at a time, without pulling out the wire. If the catheter is in a large vessel, the J guide wire may even be advanced slightly each time the catheter is withdrawn.

3. As the catheter tip exits from the artery/vein, manual pressure is applied at the puncture site with the 3rd to 5th fingers and the guide wire is secured at the skin entry site with the thumb and index finger of the same hand.

4. The wire is wiped clean with a damp lint-free sponge, and the desired catheter is threaded over it.

5. The wire is held taut, and the catheter tip is rotated clockwise as it is inserted into the vessel. Manual pressure at the puncture site should be released as the catheter enters the vessel.

**Common Errors and Problems and Their Solutions** (Fig. 3–18)

1. The catheter is pulled back without holding the wire in place. In this situation the guide wire can be pulled out of the selective position. If long catheters are used (> 100 cm), the standard length guide wire may even be pulled out of the vessel together with the catheter.

2. The length of the guide wire outside the body is shorter than that of the catheter being removed. The proximal portion of the catheter can be cut off with a scalpel blade to expose an additional segment of the wire. Ideally, exchange wires should be used for the exchange of long catheters.

3. The catheter cannot be inserted into the vessel. This can be due to several reasons:

   a. The subcutaneous tissues have not been spread apart adequately. This can be accomplished with a mosquito clamp.

   b. Either the periarterial tissues are fibrotic (eg, postoperative groin, multiple arterial punctures) or the artery is heavily calcified. A dilator should be used to pre-dilate the perivascular tissues and the arterial wall in the latter.

   c. The guide wire has been pulled back so that the flexible segment lies at the puncture site. An attempt should be made to readvance the wire into the vessel. If this is not successful, the sheath (from an Amplatz needle) or a 5 or 6 Fr vessel dilator is inserted and the wire is readvanced. Alternatively,

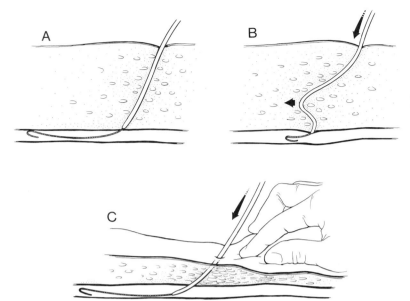

*Figure 3–18.* Technique for insertion of a catheter in patients with excessive subcutaneous tissues or a vertical puncture. *A,* The catheter is inserted at a steep angle. *B,* The catheter buckles in the perivascular tissues resulting in retraction of the guide wire. *C,* Catheter insertion is facilitated by decreasing the angle at which the catheter is being inserted and by compressing the soft tissues adjacent to the puncture site.

the wire is removed, the groin is compressed for 10 to 15 minutes, and the arterial/venous puncture is repeated.

d. The guide wire is not held taut at the time of catheter insertion. This may not only cause the wire to kink at the vascular entry point but may also not provide adequate guidance for the catheter as it is inserted. Thus, the catheter tip may enter the perivascular tissues, causing the wire to retract out of the vessel.

e. The guide wire and catheter do not match (eg, a small guide wire is used to insert a large bore catheter, such as 0.025 inch guide wire for a catheter with a 0.035 inch lumen). In this case it may not be possible to insert the catheter; therefore, a 5 Fr Teflon dilator or short catheter should be inserted and the 0.025 inch wire replaced by a 0.035 inch wire for catheter placement.

f. The angle of vascular puncture is vertical.

4. The wire is not held taut during catheter insertion in narrow vessels and especially when using straight guide wires. If the wire is allowed to advance with the catheter, it may cause intimal damage, spasm, and thrombosis.

5. Excessive tension is placed on the wire. This may lead to accidental removal of the wire.

## Catheter Placement Through a Sheath
(Fig. 3–19)

The following are indications for the use of catheter insertion sheaths:

1. If multiple catheter exchanges are anticipated.

2. If nontapered catheters are used (eg, for embolotherapy).

3. For the introduction of catheters without an end hole (eg, NIH type or multipurpose catheters).

4. For the introduction of balloon-tipped catheters (with the exception of some angioplasty catheters).

5. To facilitate removal of overdistended or accordioned balloon catheters (eg, after angioplasty).

6. To prevent leakage of blood when a large catheter is replaced by a smaller French size (usually > 2 Fr difference).

Once the vessel has been punctured, the short guide wire from the catheter introducer set is inserted. The needle is removed, and the catheter introducer sheath with the coaxially placed dilator is inserted into the vessel. The guide wire and dilator are removed, and a plastic three-way stopcock is attached to the sidearm of the sheath. The sidearm is flushed and attached to a drip infusion (in veins) or a pressure infusion (in arteries) (Fig. 3–20).

Once the sheath is in place, the appropriate

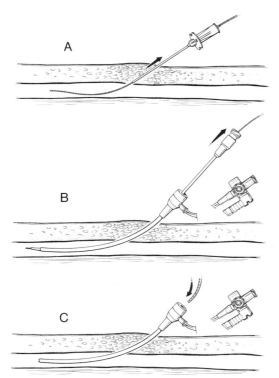

Figure 3–19. Catheter placement through a vascular introducer sheath. A, After arterial or venous puncture, a guide wire is inserted and the needle is removed. B, The catheter introducer sheath is inserted over the guide wire and the dilator and wire are removed. C, The catheter, with a guide wire at the catheter tip, is inserted. The guide wire is advanced out of the catheter and is subsequently followed by the catheter.

catheter is introduced. All catheters with an end hole (with the exception of small, soft-tipped balloon occlusion catheters) are introduced over a guide wire. A J guide wire is placed proximal to the catheter tip. The catheter tip is inserted into the sheath, and the guide wire is advanced into the vessel and is followed by the catheter, or both catheter and wire may be advanced as a unit.

## Catheterization of Tortuous and Stenotic Iliac Arteries

In most patients, a 1.5 mm J LLT wire can be used to get past tortuous and stenotic iliac arteries. If this is not successful, one of the alternatives listed below may be used. However, before proceeding with some of these techniques (ie, high torque wire and curved catheter techniques), the anatomy should be defined with a hand injection of contrast

medium (8 to 10 ml injected during a Valsalva maneuver) or preferably by DSA, both in the anterior-posterior and the oblique projections. The projection that defines the anatomy best should be identified, and when attempting to negotiate severe stenoses, it is very helpful to place either the patient or the image intensifier in the oblique projection that lays out the course of the artery (Fig. 3–21). The following techniques are used:

1. Kadir-Sloan double curve wire technique: This wire has a 10 cm tapered core and has been designed for placement past tortuous iliac arteries. The wire is inserted after femoral artery puncture. If it does not go past all bends in the iliac artery, a straight Teflon catheter (or dilator) is inserted past the first bend in the artery. The wire is then advanced further and is followed by the catheter, until it enters the aorta. If this cannot be done, the catheter (or dilator) is rotated so that the guide wire shape can conform to the bends in the iliac artery and will thus pass through.[6]

2. The 7.5 mm movable core or LLT J wire technique: This is recommended primarily for severely stenotic iliac arteries. This wire

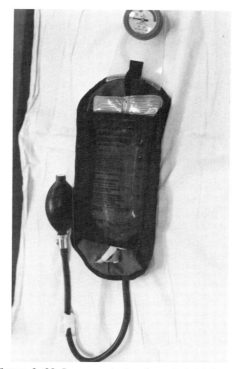

Figure 3–20. Pressure device for arterial infusion of flushing solution.

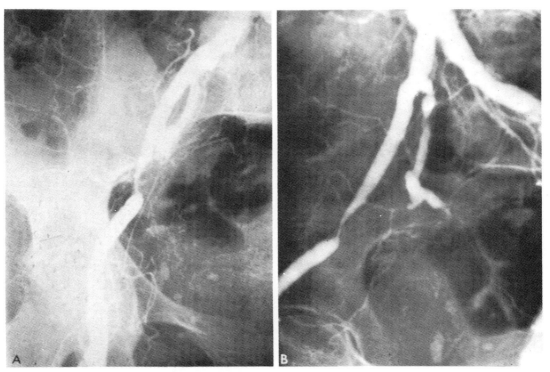

**Figure 3–21.** Importance of oblique arteriography for the evaluation of arterial stenoses. *A,* AP pelvic arteriogram shows a tortuous and stenotic iliac artery. *B,* The right posterior oblique pelvic arteriogram defines the course of the stenotic vessel. (From Kadir S et al: Selected Techniques in Interventional Radiology. Philadelphia, W. B. Saunders, 1982.)

may also be used in combination with a curved tip catheter (see entry 5).

3. The 1.5 or 3 mm movable core J wire technique (Fig. 3–22): When the inner mandrel is withdrawn (by at least 15 cm), the distal portion of the wire becomes extremely floppy. Although the J itself may not advance past a plaque, the floppy wire loops into the artery above the stenosis. When a sufficient length of the wire has been looped above the stenosis (10 to 15 cm), the catheter is advanced over it. Flexible catheters must be used when this technique is employed for arteries that are both tortuous and stenotic. The newer movable core wires that have a variable stiffness mandrel can also be used for this technique.

4. High torque wire technique: This technique is useful for catheterizing both stenoses and tortuous vessels (Fig. 3–23). The arterial needle or the sheath is exchanged for a short catheter or dilator over a 1.5 mm J guide wire. A 10 mm J high torque wire is inserted, and the wire is torqued past the different tortuosities and stenoses and into the proximal common iliac artery or the distal aorta.

Once the wire is past the tortuous and/or stenotic segments and the catheter has been advanced over it, a 0.035 inch J wire is used to exchange for the desired catheter.

5. Curved catheter technique: This technique can also be used for stenoses and tortuous iliac arteries (Fig. 3–24). In addition, it can be employed during catheter placement past abdominal aortic aneurysms. A 45° bend is placed approximately 2 cm from the tip of a straight catheter; alternatively, a preshaped multipurpose or cobra catheter may be used. The catheter tip is placed below the bend or the stenosis. A 7.5 mm movable core J wire (with the core retracted approximately 10 cm) or a 7.5 mm LLT J wire is inserted. As the catheter is torqued, the J tip is used to probe for the stenotic lumen. The wire is advanced as far as it goes, past the stenosis, and is followed by the catheter. If there are several stenoses, the guide wire and catheter can be inched through the vessel in this fashion. Occasionally, the 7.5 mm J wire does not advance past plaques. In this case, a straight LLT wire may be used with extreme caution.

6. If the above techniques are unsuccess-

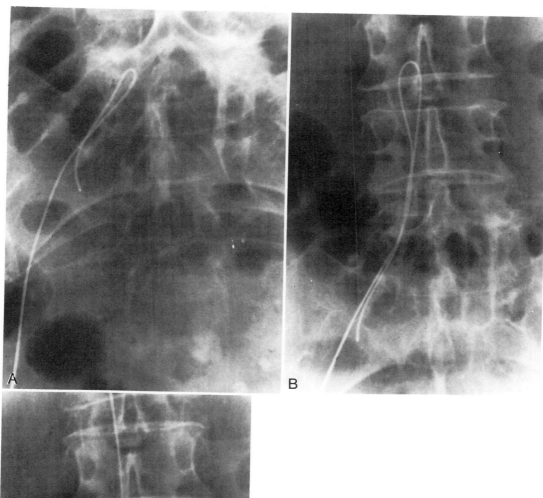

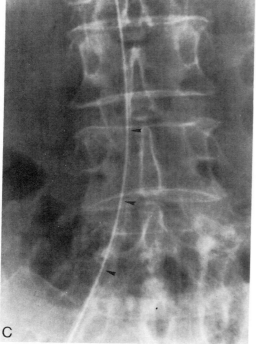

*Figure 3–22.* Movable core wire technique for traversing arterial stenoses. *A,* The J tip of the floppy wire is hooked onto a plaque. *B,* As the guide wire is further advanced, the floppy segment loops into the artery above the stenosis. *C,* Once a long segment of the wire (including the stiff core) has looped into the aorta, the catheter is advanced over it (*arrowheads*).

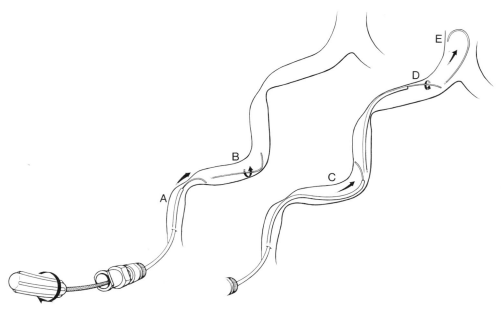

**Figure 3–23.** High torque wire technique for catheterization of tortuous and stenotic iliac arteries. *A,* A short catheter is placed below the area of stenosis/tortuosity and the high torque wire is inserted. The J is torqued past this segment and the catheter is advanced over it. *B* and *C,* The wire is torqued in the opposite direction to negotiate the next area of stenosis/tortuosity and the catheter is subsequently advanced over it. *D* and *E,* This process is repeated until the wire and catheter are advanced into the aorta.

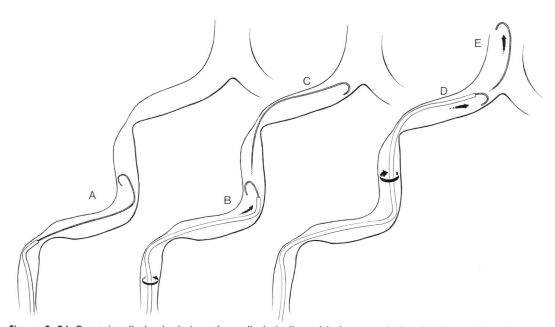

**Figure 3–24.** Curved catheter technique for catheterization of tortuous and stenotic iliac arteries. *A,* A cobra catheter or catheter with a hockey stick–shaped bend is placed below the area of stenosis. With the aid of this catheter a guide wire is torqued past the area of stenosis/tortuosity. *B,* The catheter is advanced over the wire until it can go no farther. *C,* The catheter is again used to torque the guide wire past the next area of stenosis/tortuosity and *D,* it is subsequently advanced over the guide wire. *E,* The guide wire is advanced into the aorta.

ful, the needle or catheter is removed and, if feasible, an attempt is made to catheterize the opposite femoral artery.

**Common Errors and Problems and Their Solutions.** When using any of the techniques just described, force of any kind is never necessary for advancing the guide wire. If a palpable pulse is present (even when severely diminished), this indicates the presence of a patent lumen. Therefore, when force is applied during guide wire manipulation, the course of the wire is usually outside the true lumen. If these techniques are not successful, the indications for arteriography should be reevaluated, and on the basis of that decision either another approach (TLA, axillary) or intravenous DSA may be performed.

If catheterization of such severe stenoses is successful, they may be treated by balloon angioplasty to insure continued patency.

Other problems include:

1. The use of guide wires without a tapered or movable core: The 5 cm flexible segment in these wires will often traverse the most proximal bend. The stiff core prevents the wire from going any farther.

2. The catheter will not advance over the guide wire: This is a relatively frequent problem when high torque, relatively stiff-walled (braided) catheters are used in severely tortuous arteries. When an attempt is made to thread such a catheter over the guide wire placed in the aorta, the guide wire will often retract or the catheter cannot be advanced. This situation may be avoided if thin-walled, flexible, high flow catheters (Mallinckrodt; Cook, Inc.) or heavy duty guide wires (wires with a stiffer core) are used.

## TECHNIQUE FOR SELECTIVE CATHETERIZATION

After the catheter for selective catheterization has been inserted into the aorta, a 12 ml plastic syringe filled with 60% contrast medium is attached to the two-way stopcock at the catheter hub and air bubbles are eliminated from the connection. This makes it possible to inject contrast medium without having to aspirate the air bubbles each time. However, in most instances, contrast medium should be injected only if blood can be aspirated.

The catheter configurations required for catheterization of the different branches are described earlier in this chapter (see Guide Wire and Catheter Selection) and in the specific chapters dealing with those vessels. High torque catheters with good "memory" (ie, that retain the preformed shapes at body temperature) are required for selective catheterization. On the other hand, because of their relative stiffness, such catheters may not be well suited for catheterization of the third- and fourth-order branches.

Some of the prerequisites for selective catheterization are (1) knowledge of the vascular anatomy and its variations, (2) the ability to recognize the vessel selected, and (3) familiarity with alternative methods and techniques.

### Basic Catheter Motions (Fig. 3–25)

The basic seeking motions with a selective catheter are as follows: From the femoral approach, the catheter tip is placed approximately 5 cm above the anticipated origin of the vessel to be catheterized and is pointed

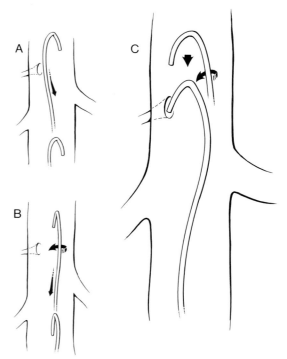

*Figure 3–25.* Basic catheter motions for selective catheterization. *A,* The catheter tip is placed several centimeters above the anticipated location of the orifice of the vessel to be catheterized. The catheter is slowly withdrawn at the groin. *B* and *C,* if the orifice is not found, the catheter is readvanced, the tip is rotated in a slightly different direction, and the maneuver is repeated until the tip engages the desired vessel.

in the direction of that vessel. Under fluoro-scopic observation, the catheter is slowly withdrawn at the groin in a smooth, contin-uous motion. As the catheter enters a branch, the tip either appears to drop forward (larger branches) or gets "hooked" onto a tight ori-fice. If the catheter is withdrawn farther at the groin, the tip tends to straighten out.

Once a catheter has entered a branch, a small volume of contrast medium is injected (approximately 0.5 to 1 ml) in an attempt to identify the vessel. The catheter should not be advanced into any vessel unless the vessel has been identified by contrast injection. This avoids contrast injection in a wedged posi-tion. If a small branch has been catheterized (eg, lumbar, phrenic, or accessory renal ar-tery), the vessel is well opacified by this volume of contrast medium. Injection of con-trast medium into the phrenic and lumbar arteries can be very painful. Thus, if one of these vessels is not the desired artery, the catheter should immediately be withdrawn from the orifice. This permits antegrade blood flow to wash out the contrast medium and alleviate the pain.

If a large vessel (superior mesenteric or renal artery) has been catheterized, such a contrast injection does opacify the vessel suf-ficiently to permit identification. A larger contrast injection then confirms catheter po-sition.

If the catheter does not enter the appro-priate vessel, it is readvanced to above the anticipated location of the vessel. The direc-tion of the catheter tip is turned slightly and the maneuver is repeated.

Once the desired vessel has been entered, the catheter is advanced into it to provide a stable position. The catheter is taped to the skin at the entry site to prevent dislodgment. Subsequently, a small test injection is used to reconfirm the catheter position and/or to check the stability of the catheter in that position (see later section of this chapter on Miscellaneous Techniques).

**Aids for Selective Catheterization**

1. Filling the catheter lumen with contrast medium renders it radiopaque and thus eas-ier to identify fluoroscopically.

2. For the catheterization of laterally ori-ented vessels, the anterior-posterior position (of the patient or the image intensifier) should be used.

3. For catheterization of vessels with an anterior or oblique course, the patient (on the cradle table top or with the aid of a large wedge-shaped sponge if a flat table top is used) or the image intensifier C or U arm is obliqued by 25 to 30°. This facilitates identi-fication of both the direction of the catheter tip (ie, anterior versus posterior) and the vessel orifice.

4. To determine the location of the catheter tip in the anterior-posterior projection, the tip is observed fluoroscopically as the cathe-ter is twisted at the groin in a clockwise direction. If the catheter tip turns to the patient's left, the tip is anteriorly located. If it turns towards the patient's right, the tip points posteriorly.

**Common Errors and Problems and Their Solutions**

1. Attempting to torque the catheter while it is stationary: Unless the catheter is in motion (along its longitudinal axis) at the same time as it is torqued, it may not respond appropriately to the torque. By simply twist-ing the catheter at one level, it will accumu-late torque, and after several twists, it will whip around to uncoil itself. The high torque 7 Fr cobra and sidewinder catheters may be an exception.

2. Cranio-caudad seeking motion too slow: The appropriate seeking speed is approxi-mately 1 cm/sec. If the catheter motion is much slower than this, the aortic pulsations, which also move the catheter back and forth, may make it difficult to identify when the catheter is in a selective position (without the aid of contrast injections).

3. Continuous hand injections of contrast medium into the aorta during selective cath-eterization in an attempt to identify the ori-fice of the aortic branches: This is not rec-ommended as routine practice for the larger branches of the aorta (eg, mesenteric, celiac, or renal arteries). If this technique is em-ployed routinely, large volumes of contrast medium may be used before the filming is begun, which would limit the study or impair renal function. This is acceptable practice only after an attempt at selective catheteri-zation, with the techniques described earlier, has been unsuccessful. This technique may also be used for catheterization of some smaller branches (eg, bronchials, inferior phrenic trunk off the aorta, or subclavian artery branches). It is also helpful during catheterization of the right gonadal vein and during venous sampling.

4. Failure to evaluate the position after the catheter has been taped at the skin entry site: Even a well-seated high torque catheter may

be dislodged from a selective position or may advance into a small branch after it has been secured at the skin entry site. Thus, each time a catheter is handled for any reason, other than flushing, its position should be rechecked.

5. Use of high flow rates for selective arteriography through catheters placed close to the orifice: A catheter placed close to the orifice of an artery should always be checked for stability before injecting a large volume of contrast medium at a high flow rate (see later section of this chapter on Miscellaneous Techniques) (Fig. 3–26).

6. Is an aortogram necessary prior to selective arteriography? An aortogram is rarely indicated to help the vascular radiologist identify the locations of the orifices of the aortic branches. Such a study may prolong the procedure unnecessarily. Other than for the evaluation of vascular diseases or the assessment of arterial blood supply to the kidney (eg, horseshoe kidney, neoplasms), a "survey" aortogram is rarely indicated.

## Catheterization of > Second-order Branches (Subselective or Superselective Catheterization)

**Indications.** Subselective catheterization of > second-order branches may be indicated for interventional radiology (eg, therapeutic embolization), for localization and occasionally characterization of neoplasms and their arterial blood supply (eg, hepatic and endocrine-active tumors), and for preoperative localization of intestinal arteriovenous malformations.

**Technical Considerations.** Most commercially available preformed catheters can be

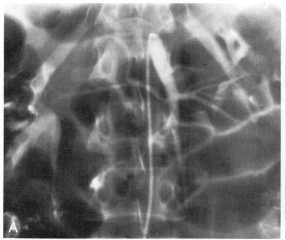
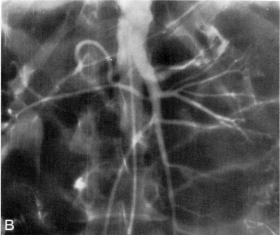
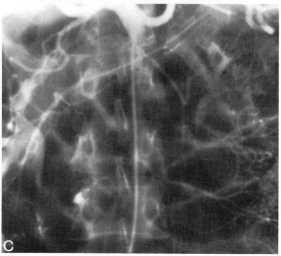

*Figure 3–26.* Catheter dislodgment during contrast injection because of an unstable position. *A,* Early film from a superior mesenteric arteriogram shows the catheter tip close to the orifice. *B,* One second later. The catheter has flipped out of the superior mesenteric artery and lies in the aorta. *C,* Subsequent film shows the catheter in the celiac artery. *Note:* Such inadvertent injection into the renal or lumbar arteries is potentially hazardous.

used for subselective catheterization. For the sidewinder catheter, the length of the inverted limb determines its reach. Sidewinder catheters are well suited for the catheterization of second-order arterial branches (eg, celiac artery branches and occasionally the hepatic arteries arising from the superior mesenteric artery). On the venous side, they can be used for catheterization of the adrenal veins.

The cobra catheters are ideally suited for subselective catheterization. However, the 6 to 7 Fr high torque cobra catheters have reinforced walls, and most of these catheters, irrespective of shape modification, cannot be advanced past several acutely angled bends. This is due to the relative inflexibility of the braided or reinforced segments. The 5 Fr thin-walled cobra catheters are better suited for subselective catheterization. However, these also have inherent problems, ie, poor torque control, especially in tortuous vessels.

The following are some techniques that can be used for subselective catheterization:

CATHETER METHODS. Because of its limited reach, the sidewinder can be used only for catheterization of proximally arising branches. The cobra catheter, with or without modification of the tertiary curve, is best suited for subselective catheterization. In younger individuals, in whom acutely angled bends are less frequent, this catheter can easily be torqued into the distal branches. This is particularly true for the celiac circulation. If the catheter tip hooks onto a branch other than the one desired, a straight LLT guide wire is inserted into the desired vessel and the catheter is advanced over it. Alternatively, the wire is advanced past the catheter tip. The catheter is torqued at the groin to direct the guide wire into the desired branch, and the catheter is then advanced over the wire.

The second- to fourth-order branches are usually of small caliber. Thus, tight J wires are not appropriate, since the diameter of the J is often larger than that of the vessel. The wires that are best suited for catheterization of such branches are the straight LLT and the 7.5 or 15 mm J wires.

CATHETER EXCHANGE METHOD. After the guide wire has been manipulated into the desired vessel, the catheter may not follow. This is usually due to a combination of a flexible guidewire (LLT or movable core) and a relatively inflexible high torque catheter.

As an alternative, once the guide wire is in place, the catheter is replaced by a softer catheter (eg, 5 Fr tapered, cobra or straight catheter or a 4.9 Fr White catheter*). Such catheters can usually be advanced into smaller vessels without difficulty. If a straight catheter is used and has to be advanced past several acute bends, it is advisable to steam a gentle curve several centimeters from the tip.

The commercially available preshaped 5 Fr cobra catheters (Cordis, Mallinckrodt) are very flexible and are thus well suited for subselective catheterization by this method.

LOOP CATHETER METHOD. This method is extremely useful for catheterization of smaller branches of the visceral and pelvic arteries (see following discussion).

GUIDE WIRE METHOD. This method utilizes a flexible guide wire that can be stiffened once it is in the desired position (Wilson or Amplatz wire). The wire is advanced into the desired branch by torquing the catheter. Once it is in place, the wire is stiffened and the catheter is advanced over it. After the catheter is in place, the wire is made flexible and removed.

It may not be possible to advance a 6 to 7 Fr high torque catheter over the wire.

TIP DEFLECTING WIRE METHOD. If the catheter tip cannot be pointed in the direction of the desired branch, a tip deflecting wire may be used. The catheter tip is deflected in the direction of the branch. The wire is held in place while maintaining the deflection, and the catheter is advanced into the branch.

MISCELLANEOUS METHODS. These include the Cope-Eisenberg system, the 0.014 to 0.018 inch platinum alloy steerable guide wire (USCI, Billerica, Massachusetts), and the coaxial catheter techniques using the 3 Fr Teflon catheter or balloon catheters that can be flow directed.

## Loop Catheter Technique

The basic feature of this technique is that it facilitates the catheterization of craniad-directed vessels and second or greater order branches of the visceral, pelvic, and other vessels.

---

*The tapered White catheter does not accept a 0.035 inch wire. To facilitate the use of the tapered catheter over a 0.035 inch wire, approximately a 1 mm piece is cut off the catheter tip with a scalpel blade. If a catheter introducer sheath has been used, a nontapered 4.9 Fr White catheter may be selected.

**Catheter Selection.** The catheter used for this technique is the preshaped 6 to 7 Fr cobra. The thin-walled 5 Fr cobra catheters are not well suited, as they do not retain the loop configuration. The thin-walled polyethylene and polyurethane catheters tend to kink at the apex of the loop. Catheter reshaping is usually not necessary.[7] Occasionally, a single curve catheter can also be used.

**Technique of Loop Formation.**[8] The loop may be formed in the vessel of which a branch is to be catheterized or in a different vessel. In the arterial system, the loop is commonly formed in the iliac, superior mesenteric, or celiac artery branches. Occasionally, a renal artery may be used cautiously. In the venous system, the loop may be formed in iliac or renal veins.

Loop Formation in the Iliac Artery (Fig. 3–27). A cobra catheter is placed over the aortic bifurcation, and a J guide wire is passed into the contralateral common femoral artery. The catheter is advanced over the wire for a distance of approximately 10 to 12 cm, and the wire is pulled back to the aortic bifurcation. The catheter is rotated in a clockwise direction, and at the same time, it is advanced at the groin. Initially, the catheter goes farther into the contralateral iliac artery, but subsequently, as a loop forms in the aorta, the tip begins to retract. The catheter

is further advanced at the groin, and the tip inverts to point craniad.

Loop Formation in the Superior Mesenteric or Celiac Artery Branches (Figs. 3–28 and 3–29). A cobra catheter is placed in the proximal superior mesenteric, splenic, or hepatic artery. A straight LLT or 1.5 mm J wire is advanced into the vessel for a distance of 15 to 20 cm. The catheter is advanced over the wire for about 10 cm, and the wire is pulled back into the aorta. The catheter is now rotated in a clockwise direction, and at the same time, it is advanced at the groin. With the formation of a loop in the aorta, the catheter tip begins to retract and inverts to point craniad.

Occasionally, the catheter will advance into the splenic, hepatic, or mesenteric artery without the guide wire. In this case, the loop is formed without the aid of the guide wire.

If the hepatic or splenic arteries are tortuous, a J guide wire should be used. Movable core guide wires are not suited for this technique because of the extreme flexibility of the wire after the core has been withdrawn.

Loop Formation in the Iliac Vein. The technique for the formation of a loop in the iliac veins is identical to that for the iliac artery. The catheter is placed in the proximal portion of the contralateral common iliac

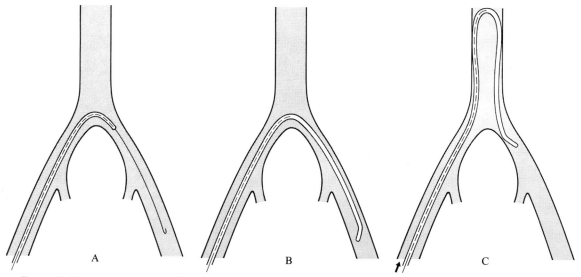

*Figure 3–27.* Loop formation in the iliac artery. *A,* The catheter is placed across the aortic bifurcation and a J guide wire is inserted into the contralateral external iliac or femoral artery. *B,* The catheter is advanced over the wire into the contralateral external iliac artery and the wire is withdrawn to the aortic bifurcation. *C,* The catheter is advanced at the groin in a combined forward and clockwise rotary motion to form the loop in the abdominal aorta. As the loop forms, the tip begins to retract and inverts to point upward. (From Kadir S: Med Radiogr Photogr 57:22, 1981. Used with permission.)

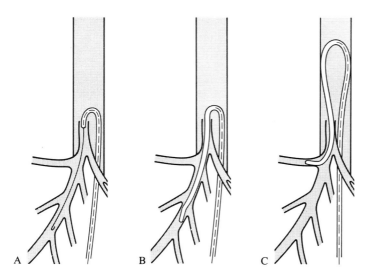

*Figure 3–28.* Loop formation in the superior mesenteric artery. *A,* The catheter is positioned in the proximal superior mesenteric artery and a guide wire is advanced into the vessel. *B,* The catheter is advanced over the guide wire and subsequently the guide wire is withdrawn into the aorta. *C,* The catheter is advanced at the groin in a combined forward and clockwise rotary motion to form the loop in the aorta. (From Kadir S: Med Radiogr Photogr 57:22, 1981. Used with permission.)

vein. A straight LLT or a 1.5 mm J guide wire is advanced into the common femoral vein. The wire is withdrawn to the iliac vein confluence, and the catheter is rotated clockwise and advanced at the groin to form a loop in the inferior vena cava.

LOOP FORMATION IN THE RENAL VEIN (Fig. 3–30). Because of the short length of the right renal vein, this vessel is rarely used for formation of the loop. The catheter is placed in the proximal left renal vein. A J guide wire is advanced to the renal hilum and the catheter is passed over it. The wire is withdrawn to the renal vein orifice. The catheter is rotated clockwise, and at the same time, it is advanced at the groin to form a loop in the vena cava. Initially the catheter tip may advance into a branch of the renal vein, but as the loop forms, the tip begins to retract and inverts to point craniad.

Occasionally, the catheter can be advanced into the renal vein without the guide wire. In this case, the loop may be formed without the aid of the wire.

**Manipulation of the Looped Catheter.** When a catheter in the loop configuration is withdrawn at the groin, the catheter tip goes farther into a vessel. When the catheter is advanced at the groin, the catheter tip comes out of the vessel.

The craniad-directed tip is suited for catheterization of vessels that have a craniad-directed course. Ideally, the loop should be formed in a vessel adjacent to the one that has to be catheterized (eg, in the splenic artery for the catheterization of the left gastric artery or the left gastric–left hepatic artery trunk; in the superior mesenteric artery for catheterization of the inferior pancreaticoduodenal artery or the hepatic artery arising

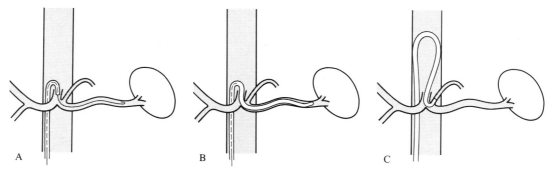

*Figure 3–29.* Loop formation in a celiac artery branch. *A,* With the catheter tip in the celiac artery, a guide wire is inserted into the splenic artery. Alternatively, the guide wire can be inserted into the hepatic artery. *B,* The catheter is advanced over the guide wire and the latter is withdrawn into the aorta. *C,* The catheter is advanced at the groin in a combination of a forward and clockwise rotary motion to form the loop. (From Kadir S: Med Radiogr Photogr 57:22, 1981. Used with permission.)

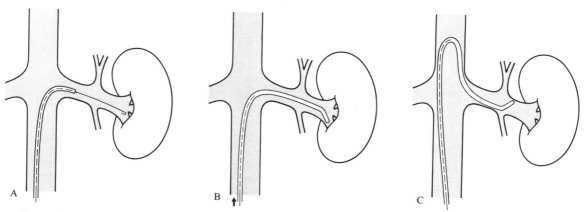

*Figure 3–30.* Loop formation in the left renal vein. *A,* The catheter is placed in the proximal left renal vein and a J guide wire is inserted to the renal hilum. *B,* The guide wire is withdrawn into the vena cava. *C,* The catheter is advanced at the groin, using a combined rotary and forward motion, to form a loop in the inferior vena cava. (From Kadir S: Med Radiogr Photogr 57:22, 1981. Used with permission.)

off this vessel; and in the left renal vein for catheterization of the left adrenal vein).

The upward-directed tip of the looped cobra catheter may lead to difficulty in engaging the orifice of a vessel that has a horizontal or caudad-directed course. To facilitate this, the angle of the catheter tip can be altered by inserting a straight guide wire to about 0.5 to 1.0 cm from the tip (Fig. 3–31). Alternatively, a straight LLT guide wire is advanced to about 1.5 cm beyond the cathe-

ter tip and is used to engage the orifice of the desired vessel.

If the catheter tip cannot be advanced past a branch vessel, a guide wire is placed past the orifice of this vessel, and the catheter is pulled down over it.

**Removal of the Looped Catheter.** From a large vessel (eg, superior mesenteric or iliac artery) the catheter can usually be removed by simply withdrawing it at the groin. However, this must be monitored fluoroscopi-

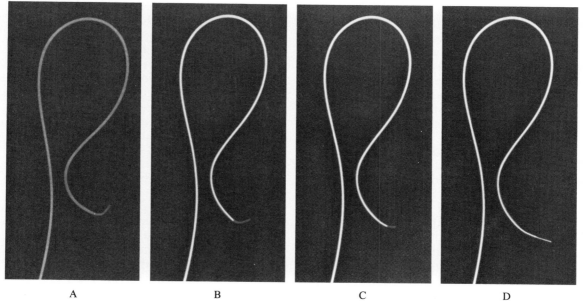

*Figure 3–31.* Use of a guide wire to alter the distal curve of the looped catheter. *A,* Before insertion of the guide wire, the catheter tip points craniad. *B,* The craniad angulation of the catheter tip is decreased by placing the wire approximately 1 cm from the catheter tip. *C,* The angulation is further decreased as the wire is advanced closer to the catheter tip. *D,* The catheter tip points caudad when the guide wire is advanced past it. (From Kadir S: Med Radiogr Photogr 57:22, 1981. Used with permission.)

cally. Any twist in the loop must be undone by rotating the catheter in order to prevent knot formation. As the catheter is pulled out, the tip advances farther into the vessel and may temporarily occlude a small branch. In most circulations with ample collateral blood supply (eg, gastric, hepatic, superior mesenteric, or pelvic branches), this may be without consequence. In smaller vessels (adrenal or intrarenal vessels), this may induce sufficient trauma to cause occlusion.

From small vessels (eg, left adrenal vein) and the renal arteries, the catheter should be disengaged and the loop straightened out in a large vessel, ie, the iliac or superior mesenteric artery or the renal or iliac vein (when working in the venous system). The catheter is advanced at the groin in order to disengage the catheter tip. It is then brought down to contralateral iliac vessel and the loop is straightened out prior to removal.

For removal of the looped catheter from the ipsilateral internal iliac and femoral arteries or external iliac artery branches, the catheter is advanced at the groin and the loop is straightened out in the contralateral iliac artery. Occasionally, a short loop in the ipsilateral internal iliac artery can be removed by simply withdrawing it at the groin. After conversion into an antegrade direction, the catheter is handled like any other catheter that has been placed in an antegrade fashion.

Following the termination of intraarterial chemotherapy for gastrointestinal bleeding or nonocclusive ischemia, the catheter can be removed in the intensive care unit. However, if there is *any* resistance at the time of catheter removal (this is usually due to a twisted loop or the formation of a knot), the patient should be returned to the angiography room for fluoroscopic assessment and removal of the catheter.

### Common Errors and Problems and Their Solutions (Fig. 3–32)

1. The catheter goes into the vessel without forming a loop: The catheter is pulled back to its original position and the guide wire is removed. The stiff end of the guide wire is inserted to lie in the segment of the catheter that is in the aorta or the inferior vena cava, and the loop formation is attempted again. The stiff end of the guide wire straightens the catheter and thus prevents it from advancing into the vessel.

2. The loop is too big: If this happens, the catheter tip may remain within the vessel being used to form the loop. The catheter is withdrawn at the groin, and the length of catheter that was inserted in the vessel for loop formation is shortened to 6 to 7 cm (instead of 10 to 12 cm). The stiff end of the wire is inserted into the aortic (or caval) portion of the catheter, and the loop is re-formed.

3. The loop is too small: If the loop is too short, it tends to straighten out when an attempt is made to engage a vessel. The minimal size of the loop should be about 12 cm (approximately the height of three vertebral bodies).

4. Twisted loop: In this configuration, the catheter cannot be advanced deep into a branch. If the catheter is forced down, it will result in the formation of a knot. The loop can be untwisted by one of the following techniques:
   a. The catheter is pulled down towards the aortic bifurcation. An attempt is made to engage the contralateral iliac artery. If this is successful, the catheter is pulled down slowly, and at the same time it is rotated to untwist the loop.
   b. Alternatively, a J guide wire is advanced past the catheter tip. As the stiffer segment of the core goes through the loop, the catheter is rotated to untwist it.
   c. If the above described techniques are not successful, the catheter is brought down to the aortic bifurcation, and a J guide wire is advanced into the contralateral iliac artery to anchor the tip. The catheter is then withdrawn at the groin, and at the same time it is rotated to untwist the loop.

5. Knotted catheter: This is often the result of pulling down the looped catheter without untwisting it and also occurs when catheter manipulation is not observed fluoroscopically. To undo the knot, the catheter is pushed into the aorta (if it has been pulled into the iliac artery) and a J LLT guide wire is carefully inserted through the knotted segments of the catheter. As the stiffer portion of the wire reaches it, the knot starts to undo itself. As this happens, the catheter is advanced into the proximal abdominal aorta. As the wire is advanced further, the knot becomes undone. Once the knot is undone, the loop is untwisted before removal or any other manipulation. Other techniques for removing catheter knots are described later in this chapter.

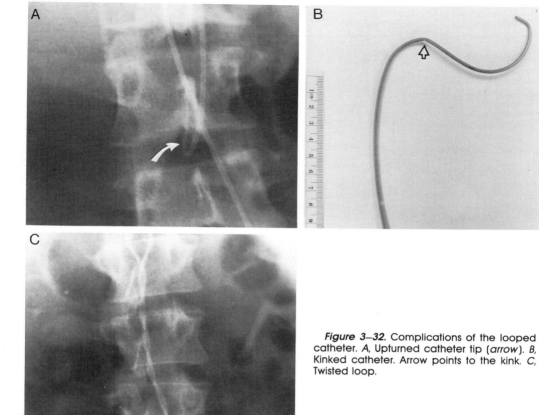

**Figure 3–32.** Complications of the looped catheter. *A,* Upturned catheter tip (*arrow*). *B,* Kinked catheter. Arrow points to the kink. *C,* Twisted loop.

6. Upturned catheter tip: This occurs when an attempt is made to forcibly pull the catheter into a vessel, as well as in individuals with a narrow aorta. To avoid this, a guide wire is inserted into the artery, and the catheter is pulled down over it. To straighten the upturned catheter tip, a J wire is inserted through the catheter. As the stiffer portion of the wire enters the tip, it begins to straighten out. As this happens, the catheter is advanced at the groin to bring the tip into the upper abdominal aorta.

7. Kinked catheter: The apex of the loop is most susceptible to kinking. This is most likely to occur in very narrow vessels (eg, in children, and narrow adult aortas and iliac arteries). A kink is recognized by the inability to inject or aspirate through the catheter. A guide wire does not advance past the apex of the loop. If a wire is advanced forcibly, it is likely to perforate the catheter at the apex of the loop.

Kinking occurs frequently with smaller French sizes and the newer thin-walled polyethylene and polyurethane catheters. For removal, the kinked catheter is brought into the distal aorta and the loop is straightened in the iliac artery. Once this is done, a guide wire can be passed through the kinked segment for replacement of the catheter. Alternatively, the catheter is removed through a sheath.

**Applications of the Loop Technique.** Table 3–1 lists the applications of the loop catheter technique. Details of some of these applications are described next.

LEFT GASTRIC ARTERY AND LEFT GASTRIC– LEFT HEPATIC ARTERY TRUNK (Fig. 3–33). An attempt should be made to form the loop in

**TABLE 3–1.** Applications of
the Loop Catheter Technique

**Arterial**
  Left gastric artery
  Left gastric–left hepatic artery trunk
  Left hepatic artery
  Inferior phrenic arteries
  Renal arteries
  Intrarenal branches
  Superior mesenteric artery:
      Inferior pancreaticoduodenal artery
      Hepatic arteries
      Distal branches
  Contralateral iliac artery
  Ipsilateral internal iliac artery
  Contralateral superior gluteal and iliolumbar arteries
  Ipsi- or contralateral external iliac and common femoral artery branches
  Ipsilateral profunda femoris artery and branches
  Conversion of a retrograde into an antegrade puncture
  Transplant renal arteries off the iliac artery

**Venous**
  Left adrenal vein
  Internal iliac vein branches
  Circumaortic renal vein

**Miscellaneous**
  Stable catheter position for arteriography and intraarterial infusions,

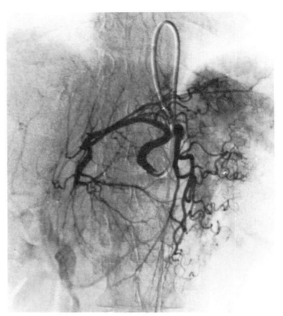

*Figure 3–33.* Catheterization of the left hepatic–left gastric artery trunk, using the loop catheter technique, in a patient with gastritis.

the splenic artery. Once the loop has been formed, the catheter is advanced at the groin to bring the inverted catheter tip into the proximal splenic or the distal celiac artery. A hand injection of contrast medium is used to locate the orifice of the left gastric artery or the left gastric–left hepatic artery trunk. The catheter is withdrawn at the groin to advance the tip into this vessel.

SUPERIOR MESENTERIC ARTERY BRANCHES. The loop is formed in the superior mesenteric artery. As the catheter is advanced at the groin, the catheter tip comes into the proximal superior mesenteric artery. A hand injection of contrast medium is used to identify the orifice of the desired branch, and the catheter is advanced into it by withdrawing at the groin. If the catheter does not enter the desired branch, a straight LLT or 7.5 mm J wire is inserted into the desired branch, and the catheter is pulled down over the wire.

The loop technique is used to catheterize the jejunal, ileal, and colic branches, the inferior pancreaticoduodenal artery, or the hepatic artery arising from the superior mesenteric artery.

IPSILATERAL INTERNAL ILIAC ARTERY (Fig. 3–34). The loop is formed in the contralateral iliac artery, and the catheter is advanced at

the groin to bring the catheter tip into the aorta. The catheter is then rotated so that the tip points towards the ipsilateral common iliac artery. It is withdrawn at the groin to bring the catheter tip into the ipsilateral common iliac artery. Next, it is rotated to point the tip posterior-medially and is pulled down into the internal iliac artery.

The technique for catheterization of the internal iliac artery branches is discussed in Chapter 10.

IPSILATERAL PROFUNDA FEMORIS ARTERY. The technique for catheterization of the ipsilateral profunda femoris artery is similar to that for catheterization of the ipsilateral internal iliac artery. Once the loop has been formed, the catheter tip is brought into the ipsilateral common iliac artery and is pulled down into the common femoral artery. If the catheter does not advance past the internal iliac artery or the loop becomes smaller, a J guide wire is passed into the common femoral artery, and the catheter is pulled down over the wire. Contrast injection is used to locate the profunda orifice, and the catheter is torqued and pulled down into it. Occasionally, a guide wire is needed to guide the catheter into the profunda orifice.

CATHETERIZATION OF THE IPSILATERAL SUPERFICIAL FEMORAL ARTERY OR CONVERSION OF A RETROGRADE INTO AN ANTEGRADE

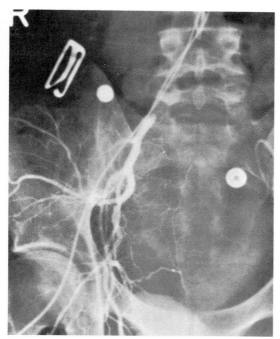

*Figure 3–34.* Catheterization of the ipsilateral internal iliac artery using the loop catheter technique. (From Kadir S: Med Radiogr Photogr 57:22, 1981. Used with permission.)

PUNCTURE[9] (Fig. 3–35). This technique is similar to the one used for catheterization of the ipsilateral profunda femoris artery. Once the catheter tip is brought into the ipsilateral common femoral artery, a 1.5 mm J guide wire is inserted and advanced into the superficial femoral artery. The catheter is pulled down over the wire until the catheter tip has passed the arterial puncture site and lies in the superficial femoral artery.

For the conversion into an antegrade puncture, the catheter is withdrawn until the apex of the loop comes to lie at the arterial puncture site. If further withdrawal of the catheter causes the tip to retract, the conversion is complete. Prior to attempting the conversion, any twist in the loop must be undone to avoid the formation of a knot. In addition, the arterial puncture site must lie immediately beneath the skin incision. This technique should not be used in patients with severe atherosclerosis or narrow iliofemoral arteries.

CATHETERIZATION OF THE CONTRALATERAL COMMON ILIAC ARTERY. It may be difficult to catheterize the contralateral common iliac artery in patients with a steep aortic bifurca-

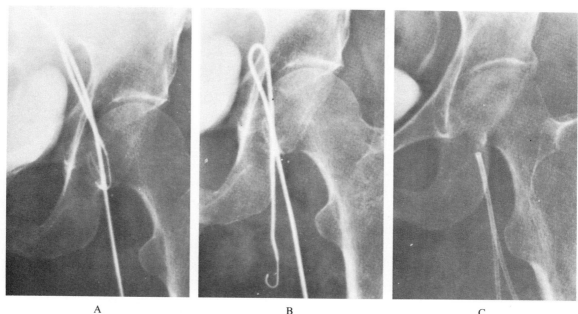

A                                B                                C

*Figure 3–35.* Technique for conversion of a retrograde into an antegrade femoral artery puncture. *A*, The tip of the looped cobra catheter with a leading J guide wire is brought into the ipsilateral common femoral artery. *B*, The catheter is further withdrawn at the groin to bring the catheter tip into the superficial femoral artery. Any twist in the loop must be undone before completing the conversion. *C*, The apex of the loop lies at the arterial puncture site after the conversion has been completed. (From Kadir S: Med Radiogr Photogr 57:22, 1981. Used with permission.)

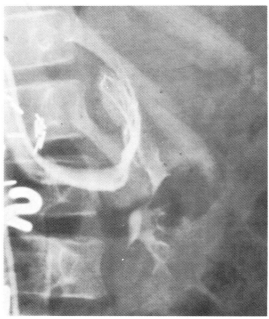

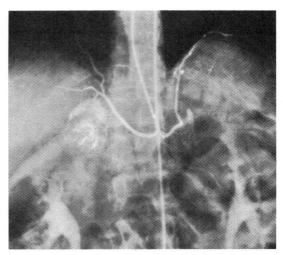

*Figure 3–37.* Stable catheter position for inferior phrenic arteriography using the loop catheter technique. There is a pheochromocytoma of the right adrenal gland. (From Kadir S: Med Radiogr Photogr 57:22, 1981. Used with permission.)

*Figure 3–36.* Loop catheter technique for left adrenal venography. The adrenal venogram is normal. (From Kadir S: Med Radiogr Photogr 57:22, 1981. Used with permission.)

tion. The loop is formed in the superior mesenteric or other aortic branch, and the looped catheter is pulled down into the distal aorta. The catheter tip is rotated to point towards the contralateral common iliac artery and is pulled down into it. If this is not successful, a guide wire is inserted and advanced into the contralateral common iliac artery, and the catheter is pulled down over the wire.

LEFT ADRENAL VEIN[10] (Fig. 3–36). The loop is formed in the left renal vein (or in the contralateral iliac vein). The catheter is advanced at the groin to bring the tip into the proximal renal vein. Contrast injection is used to localize the orifice of the left adrenal vein. The catheter is torqued and pulled down at the groin to advance the catheter tip into the left adrenal vein. If this does not occur easily, a straight LLT wire is inserted into the left adrenal vein for a distance of approximately 2 cm. The catheter is cautiously withdrawn at the groin to advance the catheter tip over the wire. Occasionally, the loop is undone as the catheter tip advances into the adrenal vein. The guide wire must not be allowed to advance with the catheter for fear of causing vascular injury.

MISCELLANEOUS APPLICATIONS. Figures 3–37 and 3–38 show the applications of the loop catheter technique for achieving a stable catheter position for contrast injection in small vessels (Fig. 3–37: inferior phrenic trunk) and for catheterization of craniad-directed branches of the external iliac and common femoral arteries (Fig. 3–38).

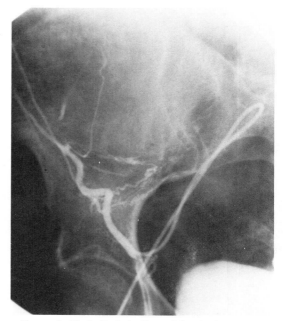

*Figure 3–38.* Catheterization of the ipsilateral deep circumflex iliac artery using the loop catheter technique in a patient with retroperitoneal neoplasm.

## COMPLETION OF THE STUDY

### General Criteria

An angiographic study can be considered as having been completed when (1) the questions that were outlined at the beginning of the study have been answered, and (2) all pertinent information has been obtained. For example, in a patient being evaluated for renovascular hypertension due to atherosclerotic vascular disease, it may not be sufficient to obtain an abdominal aortogram in a single projection. In this case, the study could be considered complete only if the orifices and the entire course of all renal arteries have been defined.

In patients with atherosclerotic peripheral vascular disease, it is frequently not enough to obtain anterior-posterior arteriograms of the pelvis. Oblique views are often required to characterize the lesions and evaluate orifice lesions of the internal iliac and profunda femoris arteries. In addition, hemodynamic data must be obtained in order to permit logical assessment of the situation.

### Compression of the Vascular Puncture Site

After the removal of the catheter, the arterial puncture site should be compressed for at least 15 minutes. A venous puncture site should be compressed for at least 8 minutes. If the clotting parameters are abnormal (eg, after heparin administration), the compression time should be prolonged to approximately 20 to 25 minutes for arterial punctures and to approximately 10 to 15 minutes for venous punctures.

The puncture site should be compressed in the following manner:

1. After the catheter has been removed, a few milliliters of blood are allowed to leak out (approximately 2 to 3 ml).

2. The puncture site is compressed with the gloved hand (without a sponge), using at least three fingers (ie, the index, middle, and ring fingers). The middle finger is used to compress the actual puncture site, while the other two fingers compress above and below the puncture site. Moderate, continuous pressure is applied for at least 10 minutes for arterial puncture and 5 minutes for venipuncture. The pulse must *not* be obliterated during the compression. In patients with excessively hard vessels, the artery may need to be compressed forcibly, with near obliter-

ation of the pulse. However, these are the exception.

3. Subsequently, the pressure is gradually decreased until only the skin puncture site is being gently compressed. Arterial puncture must not be terminated abruptly, as this could induce rebleeding.

4. If rebleeding occurs upon completion of the compression, it is advisable to repeat the entire process.

5. After hemostasis is achieved, the puncture site is cleaned, and antibiotic ointment and a Band-Aid are applied.

Upon completion of the translumbar aortogram, the patient is rolled over onto the stretcher. After the patient is on his or her back, the TLA catheter is removed. A folded towel or sheet may be tucked under the left side to provide some external support. The skin puncture site is cleaned and antibiotic ointment and a Band-Aid are applied.

After translumbar aortography, a 12 hour bed rest is necessary. After femoral arteriography with larger catheters (> 5 Fr) and axillary and brachial artery puncture, an 8 hour bed rest is required. After femoral vein puncture, a 2 to 4 hour bed rest is necessary. The post-angiography orders are shown in Tables 4–5 to 4–7 in Chapter 4. If the clotting parameters are abnormal, prolongation of the period of bed rest may be required. A 4 hour bed rest is sufficient after the use of 4 to 5 Fr catheters for outpatient arteriography.

Pressure dressings utilizing elastic bandages or sandbags should not be used, as these do not offer the focal vascular compression that is required to achieve hemostasis.

### Interpretation

The angiograms, as well as the other pertinent radiographic features demonstrated on the films, should be evaluated. Thus, for example, it is important to evaluate the bones in patients with severe trauma and the bowel gas pattern in patients with mesenteric symptoms and also to assess the urinary system in each patient.

**Flow Artefacts** (Figs. 3–39 and 3–40). Layering of contrast medium in the peripheral arteries may give rise to linear artefacts that may simulate fibrin deposition, clot, or a plaque (Fig. 3–39). Inflow of unopacified blood may also give rise to artefacts in the peripheral vessels and the portal vein (Fig. 3–40). Such artefacts may simulate a thrombus.

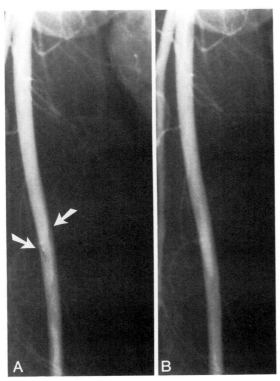

*Figure 3–39.* A, Flow artefacts in the superficial femoral artery (*arrows*). B, A later frame from the same arteriogram. The artefacts are no longer present.

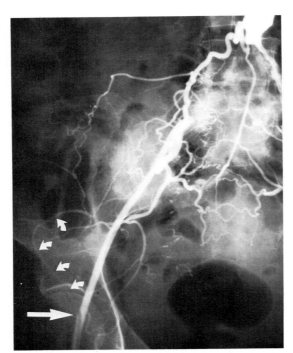

*Figure 3–40.* Artefact caused by inflow of partially opacified blood (*large arrow*) from the deep circumflex iliac artery (*small arrows*) in a patient with occlusion of the ipsilateral common iliac artery.

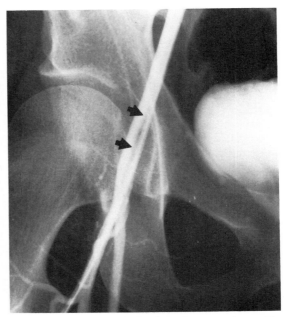

*Figure 3–41.* Focal fibrin deposit on angiographic catheter (*arrows*).

**Fibrin Deposition** (Fig. 3–41). Varying degrees of fibrin deposition occurs on intravascular catheters. This is usually sheared off as the catheter is removed from the vessel and does not bear any clinical consequences. Occasionally (especially in smaller vessels), the catheter wall is outlined by contrast medium and may be mistaken for fibrin deposition, plaque, or a blood clot (Fig. 3–42).

**Standing Waves** (Fig. 3–43). Regular, alternating areas of narrowing may be seen in mesenteric and extremity arteriograms. This is due to focal, circular vasoconstriction[11] and may be related to the flow and pressure changes caused by intraarterial injection of contrast medium.

**Vascular Spasm** (Fig. 3–44). Catheter and guide wire manipulation–induced focal vascular spasm may simulate arterial occlusion or stenosis. Thus, if an area of stenosis is seen in a vessel subjected to guide wire or catheter manipulation, this must be interpreted in light of this consideration.

## Pullout Arteriogram

The use of heparin-coated catheters and systemic heparinization in individuals with severe stenoses and in children has decreased the incidence of post-arteriography thromboembolism. Thus, in the vast majority of patients with relatively atraumatic arterial

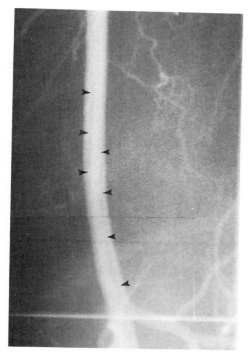

*Figure 3–42.* Catheter wall outlined by contrast material (*arrowheads*).

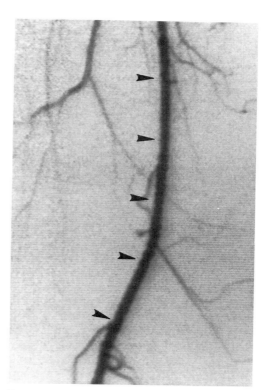

*Figure 3–43.* Intraarterial DSA showing standing waves in the superficial femoral artery (*arrowheads*).

puncture, a pullout arteriogram is not necessary. If, however, symptoms develop after the catheter has been removed, arteriographic reevaluation should be considered. In most cases, this can be accomplished by intravenous DSA.

Small adherent thrombi are occasionally seen close to the arterial puncture site. They are without clinical consequence, as most of these thrombi lyse spontaneously (Fig. 3–45).

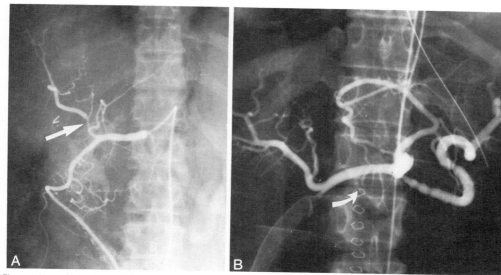

*Figure 3–44.* Focal arterial spasm resulting from guide wire trauma. *A,* Common hepatic arteriogram shows a smooth narrowing of the right hepatic artery (*arrow*). In a patient with suspected hepatic neoplasm, this could be mistaken for arterial encasement. *B,* Beaded appearance of the proximal splenic artery in a patient with an arterioportal fistula (*arrow*) resulting form operative trauma.

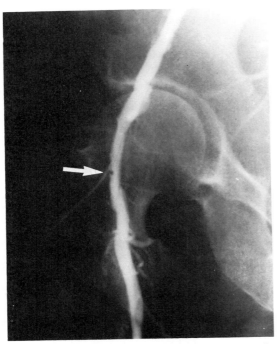

Figure 3–45. Small thrombus at arterial puncture site (*arrow*).

## MISCELLANEOUS TECHNIQUES

### General Guidelines for the Use of Catheters and Guide Wires

1. All catheter and guide wire manipulations should be done under fluoroscopic observation. Similarly, all catheter positions for arteriography must be checked (with a test injection under fluoroscopy) and the catheter secured at the skin puncture site prior to arteriography.

2. When used in arteries, straight catheters should not be advanced without the aid of J guide wires.

3. In patients with atherosclerotic occlusive disease, catheter manipulation should be of limited duration. A J guide wire should be used to readvance the catheter in the aorta. This will prevent unnecessary traumatization of the diseased intimal surface.

4. A straight catheter without an end hole occluding device should not be used for abdominal aortography in adult patients.

5. When a sidewinder catheter is reformed in the aortic arch, a J wire should be used to guide the catheter to and from the arch.

6. During selective arteriography, the sidewinder catheter should not be forcefully pulled down into a vessel. The catheter tip is relatively stiff and is likely to cause a dissection.

7. If there is resistance to advancement of the guide wire or catheter, the manipulation must be stopped and the situation evaluated with a test injection of contrast medium. If an intimal flap has developed, the manipulation should be terminated.

8. Whenever the patient is moved for positioning, the catheter position must be rechecked.

9. The catheter position should be rechecked after each power injection of contrast medium.

10. Before inserting a catheter, the patency of the lumen should be checked. In addition, the guide wire should be checked for compatibility with the catheter. Balloon-tipped catheters should be checked for integrity of the balloons.

11. If a catheter does not advance over the wire, this may be due to the inability of a reinforced wall, high torque catheter to go around bends. A slight twisting motion is applied as the catheter is advanced. In this fashion, the catheter often torques itself into a vessel.

12. Maximal flow rates should not be used in the thin-walled pigtail catheters, since the pigtail may uncoil during the injection (Fig. 3–46). The catheter tip could enter a lumbar

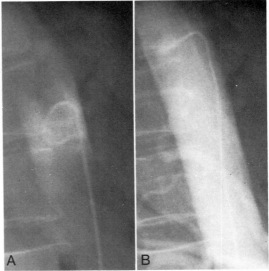

Figure 3–46. Uncoiling of a 5 Fr "high flow" pigtail catheter during aortography using manufacturer's specified flow rate. A, Early frame shows the pigtail catheter in normal configuration. B, Later frame shows the uncoiled pigtail catheter.

or phrenic artery or another aortic branch and deliver a large volume of contrast medium into this vessel.

## Catheter Flushing Technique

To preserve lumen patency, every catheter must be flushed every 2 to 3 minutes with heparinized flushing solution (2000 Units of heparin in 500 ml of 5% dextrose). If the patient is heparinized at the beginning of the procedure, frequent flushing is not required. In patients with fluid restriction, the volume of flushing solution injected each time must be decreased.

**Double Flush.** This technique requires two syringes: one for aspiration and the other for flushing. It is used (1) each time a guide wire has been used in the catheter and (2) in multiple hole (ie, straight and pigtail) catheters. Once the catheter is in place and the guide wire has been removed, a two-way stopcock is attached to the catheter hub. Using one of the syringes, approximately 2 to 3 ml blood is aspirated rapidly and discarded. Thus, if a clot is present at the catheter tip, it will be sucked into the syringe. With the other syringe, 5 to 10 ml of flushing solution is injected over 2 to 3 seconds. While the last portion of the flushing solution is being injected, the stopcock is turned off. In doing so, reentry of the blood into the catheter is prevented.

When flushing multiple hole catheters, the injection of the flushing solution should be rapid, in order to clear the side holes.

**Single Flush.** This technique requires a single syringe containing heparinized flushing solution. It is used for (1) single hole catheters, except after catheter exchange, and (2) patients who are fully heparinized.

Approximately 1 to 2 ml of blood is aspirated rapidly. The aspirated blood settles to the bottom of the syringe, and if it does not contain clots, some of it is reinjected along with 5 to 10 ml of the flushing solution. The stopcock is turned off as the last portion of the flushing solution is being injected. If the syringe is held in a horizontal position, the blood that is aspirated remains at the bottom and does not mix with the flushing solution.

## Test Injection

A test injection serves to (1) check the catheter position, (2) check the stability of the catheter position, and (3) assess the con-

trast flow rate that may be optimal for that particular vessel (judged by the degree of reflux into the aorta). Catheter position is checked by a hand injection of contrast medium and has been described earlier. The methods to check the stability of a catheter position (prior to power injection for filming) are described next. Assessment of optimal flow rate for arteriography can be made by either a hand or a power injection of contrast medium.

**Rapid Hand Injection.** With a 12 ml syringe, a flow rate of between 6 and 8 ml/sec can be easily achieved by a forceful hand injection. The syringe is filled with 30% contrast medium (50:50 mixture of the 60% contrast and flushing solution) or, preferably, with only flushing solution. The contents are injected rapidly through the catheter, and the catheter tip is observed fluoroscopically. Some recoil of the catheter tip may be observed, but if the catheter position is stable, it will not dislodge. If flushing solution has been used for the test, 1 ml of contrast medium is injected to reconfirm position.

**Power Injector Test.** The catheter is attached to the power injector. Contrast medium is injected at the desired flow rate for 1 sec, and the catheter tip is observed fluoroscopically. If the catheter has "kicked out" of the selected position, it is reinserted and one of the following precautions is taken: (1) a better catheter position is selected, (2) a slower contrast injection rate is chosen for the filming, or (3) a different catheter configuration is chosen, ie, instead of the standard cobra, the loop technique or a sidewinder catheter is used.

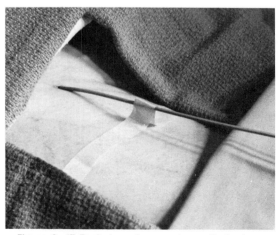

*Figure 3–47.* Technique for securing catheter for angiography.

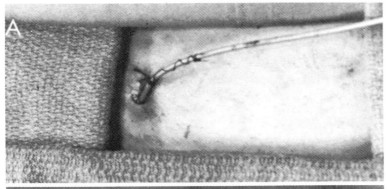

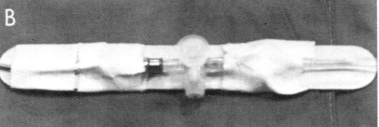

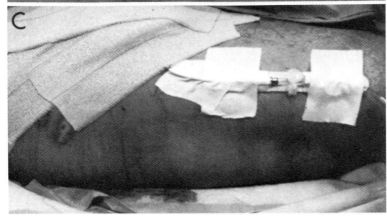

*Figure 3–48.* Technique for securing catheter for intraarterial chemotherapy (eg, vasopressin infusion). *A,* The catheter is sutured to the skin at the groin. *B,* The catheter hub is attached to a K-50 connecting tubing with interposed three-way stopcock. The connections are taped onto a tongue blade to prevent accidental disconnection. *C,* The groin is bandaged with 4 × 4 inch gauze and elastic bandage. (Reproduced with permission from Kadir S and Ernst CB: Current Concepts in Angiographic Management of Gastrointestinal Bleeding. In Ravitch MM et al (eds): CURRENT PROBLEMS IN SURGERY. Copyright © 1983 by Year Book Medical Publishers, Inc., Chicago.)

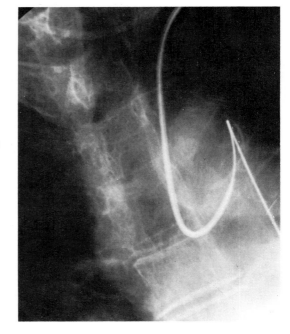

*Figure 3–49.* Formation of a loop in the aortic arch as the selective catheter is inserted.

## Securing a Catheter at the Skin Entry Site (Fig. 3-47)

Once the catheter is in position, it must be secured at the skin entry site to prevent dislodgment. Sterile tape (sterilized adhesive paper tape or Steri-Strip) is used for this purpose. If this is unavailable, a sterile Band-Aid may be used. Figure 3-48 shows the technique for securing a catheter for intraarterial chemotherapy. If a catheter introducer sheath has been used, this must also be secured at the skin entry site (hub and side arm) with sterile adhesive tape to prevent dislodgment during catheter manipulation.

## Prevention of an Aortic Loop During Axillary or Brachial Artery Catheterization

During initial catheterization or catheter exchange from the axillary approach, a loop may form in the aortic arch. This is more likely to occur in patients with an elongated arch and if there is a stenosis in the vessel being catheterized (Fig. 3-49). The formation of such a loop results in retraction of the guide wire tip from the selective position. A loop should be suspected when (1) the wire tip begins to retract as the catheter is advanced, or (2) the catheter tip does not appear at the selected vessel despite its being advanced at the arterial puncture site. To prevent the formation of such a loop, the following measures can be undertaken:

1. The wire is held taut during catheter insertion.
2. The catheter tip is observed fluoroscopically as it passes through the arch.
3. The arm is hyperextended with the hand tucked underneath the head to straighten out the course of the subclavian and axillary arteries.
4. A heavier gauge wire is used.
5. Stiff, high torque catheters are avoided; instead the thin-walled 5 Fr catheters are used.
6. Respiratory mobility is utilized to change the angle at which the catheter is inserted into an aortic branch.

## Re-formation of the Sidewinder Curve

The sidewinder curve can be re-formed in the aortic arch, over the aortic bifurcation or with the aid of a tip deflecting wire. In the venous system, it can be re-formed in the renal, the iliac, or occasionally the hepatic veins. The sidewinder 1 curve can be re-formed rather easily in the ascending aorta. The longer limb of the sidewinder 2 catheter makes it more difficult to re-form the curve in the ascending aorta. Figures 3-50 to 3-52 show the different techniques for the re-formation of the sidewinder curve.

**Applications.** The sidewinder catheter can be used for catheterization of most aortic branches distal to the upper thoracic aorta. The greatest advantage of this catheter is that it provides a stable position for the arteriography. It is also suited for catheterization of the proximal visceral arteries and their craniad-directed branches (eg, left gastric artery and the hepatic artery arising from the superior mesenteric artery). In the venous system, the sidewinder catheter can be used for catheterization of the adrenal and the right gonadal veins.

## Catheterization of the Contralateral Iliac Artery

In individuals with a wide aortic bifurcation, catheterization of the contralateral iliac artery (from the femoral approach) is easily accomplished with a cobra or single curve visceral catheter. In younger individuals with an acute angle of the aortic bifurcation, the cobra catheter may not advance across the bifurcation, but dislodges into the distal aorta. For the catheterization of the contralateral iliac artery in such patients, one of the following techniques may be used: (1) cobra catheter–assisted guide wire technique, (2) sidewinder catheter, or (3) cobra catheter in the loop configuration. Figure 3-53 shows the technique for catheterization of the contralateral iliac artery using a cobra catheter.

## Technique for Replacement of a Clogged Catheter (Fig. 3-54)

Clogging of a catheter may occur as a result of clot formation or during embolotherapy. In the latter case, a coil or an Ivalon plug may occlude the catheter. Occasionally, a kinked catheter cannot be exchanged over a guide wire and may require replacement using this technique.

The hub of the clogged catheter is cut off, and a catheter introducer sheath is inserted over it. The sheath should be selected to fit the outer diameter of the catheter closely (eg, a 7 Fr sheath for a 6.5 Fr catheter). The

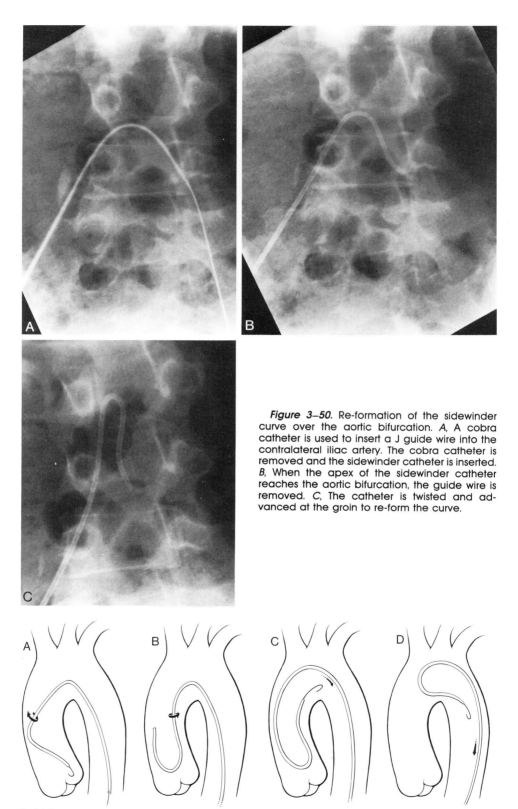

**Figure 3–50.** Re-formation of the sidewinder curve over the aortic bifurcation. *A,* A cobra catheter is used to insert a J guide wire into the contralateral iliac artery. The cobra catheter is removed and the sidewinder catheter is inserted. *B,* When the apex of the sidewinder catheter reaches the aortic bifurcation, the guide wire is removed. *C,* The catheter is twisted and advanced at the groin to re-form the curve.

**Figure 3–51.** Re-formation of the sidewinder curve in the ascending aorta. *A,* The catheter is brought into the ascending aorta over a J guide wire and the guide wire is removed subsequently. A combination of a rotary and forward motion is used to re-form the sidewinder curve. *B,* The re-formed catheter is rotated to bring the catheter tip away from the head and neck vessels. *C,* A leading J guide wire is inserted, and *D,* the catheter is brought into the descending or abdominal aorta.

*Figure 3–52.* Re-formation of the sidewinder curve in the left subclavian artery. *A,* Over a J guide wire, the catheter is advanced into the left subclavian artery. *B,* The guide wire is removed or placed at the apex of the catheter. As it is advanced at the groin, the catheter loops into the aortic arch. *C,* Further advancement of the catheter disengages the tip from the left subclavian artery orifice. A J guide wire is again used to bring the re-formed catheter into the descending or abdominal aorta.

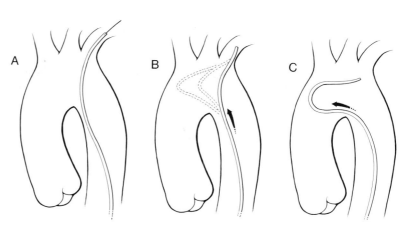

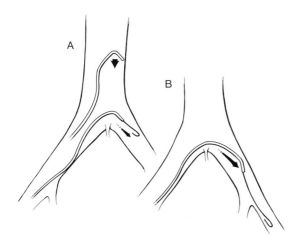

*Figure 3–53.* Catheterization of the contralateral iliac artery with a cobra catheter in patients with an acute-angled aortic bifurcation. *A,* The tip of the cobra catheter is placed across the aortic bifurcation. A J LLT guide wire is inserted into the contralateral iliac artery for a distance of 3 to 4 cm. *B,* The catheter is advanced over it for a short distance. The wire is again advanced for 3 to 4 cm and in this fashion the catheter is inched into the contralateral iliac artery.

*Figure 3–54.* Technique for replacement of a clogged catheter. *A,* The hub of the clogged catheter is cut off. *B,* A catheter introducer sheath is threaded over the catheter and advanced into the vessel. *C,* The clogged catheter is removed. *D,* The new catheter is inserted.

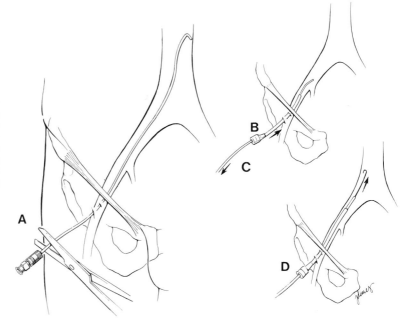

sheath is inserted into the vessel over the clogged catheter, and the latter is removed subsequently. The sheath provides access for the insertion of another catheter.

## Removal of Catheter Knots

Frequent causes of catheter knots are catheter manipulation without careful fluoroscopic observation, during re-formation of the sidewinder curve, and manipulation of the looped cobra catheter. In our own experience, such knots are more likely to occur with softer catheters. Several catheter and guide wire techniques have been described to facilitate nonsurgical reduction of knotted angiographic catheters.[12–16] Figure 3–55 shows some of these techniques.

**Guide Wire Method.** A heavy duty J guide wire (eg, Rosen wire) is inserted into the catheter. As the stiff mandrel enters it, the knot begins to open. At this point, the catheter is advanced into the widest portion of the aorta to facilitate the process of unknotting. Alternatively, the stiff end of a guide wire may be used, provided it passes into the knot easily. The wire tip should *not* be permitted close to the catheter tip. If the stiff end of a guide wire is inserted forcibly, it may perforate the catheter and vessel wall. Once the knot is undone, the catheter is withdrawn over the guide wire and replaced

by a new catheter (if it was kinked or damaged).

**Tip Deflecting Wire Method.** The knotted catheter is brought into the distal abdominal aorta or vena cava. From the contralateral femoral approach, a tip deflecting wire is brought into the distal aorta or vena cava. In the arterial system, this wire should be introduced through a catheter, which is subsequently withdrawn. In the venous system, it may be introduced through a catheter introducer sheath. The wire tip is deflected around the catheter knot. The catheter and wire are pulled down to the bifurcation, and the catheter is anchored with the tip deflecting wire. The catheter is then advanced at the groin in an attempt to loosen the knot. If this is unsuccessful, a heavy duty J-tipped guide wire is inserted as the catheter is readvanced at the groin, to facilitate loosening of the knot.

**Hook Catheter Method.** A tight, hook-shaped, or sidewinder 1 catheter introduced via the contralateral groin may be used to perform the same maneuvers described in the preceding paragraph.

**Catheter Method Using Selective Catheterization.** If a curved catheter (cobra, sidewinder, hook), introduced through the contralateral femoral vessel, can be passed through the knot and into an aortic branch (eg, renal artery), this may be used to anchor

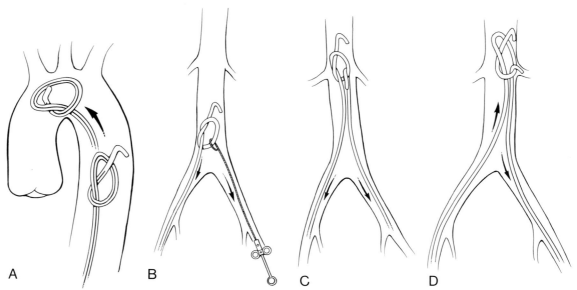

*Figure 3–55.* Techniques for removal of catheter knots. *A,* Guide wire method. *B,* Tip deflecting wire method. *C,* Hook catheter method. *D,* Catheter method using selective catheterization. See text for description of the different techniques.

the knot. The knotted catheter is advanced at the groin in an attempt to loosen the knot. If this is not successful, a heavy duty guide wire is inserted as the catheter is readvanced.

**Straight Catheter Method.** A straight or hockey stick–shaped catheter, introduced via the contralateral groin, is passed through the knot. The knot is pulled down to the aortic bifurcation or the iliac vein confluence. A to and fro motion of the knotted catheter, with or without the aid of a guide wire, is used to loosen the knot.

If knot formation has occurred during catheterization via the axillary artery approach, either the guide wire method is used or, if the knotted catheter can be advanced to the aortic bifurcation and the femoral artery can be catheterized, the tip deflecting wire or hook catheter method can be used.

## REFERENCES

1. Noer I, Praestholm J, Toennesen KH: Supplementary angiography when lumbar angiograms fail to demonstrate the vessels to the leg. Cardiovasc Intervent Radiol 4:77–79, 1981.
2. Kaufman SL: Femoral puncture using Doppler ultrasound guidance: an aid to transluminal angioplasty and other applications. AJR 134:402, 1980.
3. Dotter CT, Roesch J, Robinson M: Fluoroscopic guidance in femoral artery puncture. Radiology 127:266–267, 1978.
3a. Maxwell SL Jr, Kwon OJ, Millan VG: Translumbar carotid arteriography. Radiology 148:851–852, 1983.
4. Kadir S: Percutaneous antecubital vein approach to hepatic and renal vein catheterization. AJR 139:825–827, 1982.
5. Seldinger SI: Catheter replacement of needle in percutaneous arteriography: a new technique. Acta Radiol 39:368–376, 1953.
6. Kadir S: Double curve wire technique for negotiating tortuous iliac arteries and abdominal aortic aneurysms. Cath Cardiovasc Diagn 9:625–627, 1983.
7. Waltman AC, Courey WR, Athanasoulis CA, et al: Technique for left gastric artery catheterization. Radiology 109:732–734, 1973.
8. Kadir S: The loop catheter technic. Med Radiogr Photogr 57:22–30, 1981.
9. Kadir S, Baassiri A, Barth KH: Technique for conversion of a retrograde into an antegrade femoral artery catheterization. AJR 136:430–431, 1981.
10. Kadir S: Loop catheter technique: a simple, rapid method for adrenal vein catheterization. AJR 134:31–33, 1980.
11. Koehler R: Regular alternating changes in arterial width in lower limb angiograms. Acta Radiol Diag 3:529–542, 1965.
12. Young DA, Maurer RM: Successful manipulation of a knotted intravascular catheter allowing nonsurgical removal. Radiology 94:155–156, 1970.
13. Chinichian A, Liebeskind A, Zingesser LH, et al: Knotting of an 8 French headhunter and its successful removal. Radiology 104:282, 1972.
14. Hawkins IF, Tonkin A: Deflector method for nonsurgical removal of knotted catheters. Radiology 106:705, 1973.
15. Stein, HL: Successful nonsurgical removal of a knotted preshaped coronary artery catheter. Radiology 109:469–470, 1973.
16. Holder JC, Cherry JF: The use of a tip deflecting guide in untying a knotted arterial catheter. Radiology 128:808–809, 1978.

# Preangiographic Patient Evaluation

## CHAPTER 4

When a cardiovascular radiologist is asked to perform a procedure or is requested to evaluate a patient, he or she is being asked to serve as a consultant. Therefore, the cardiovascular radiologist must not only perform a diagnostic examination but must also provide an opinion that may have significant therapeutic implications. Thus, it is essential that he or she become familiar with the patient's history and clinical course leading to the need for the diagnostic or therapeutic procedure.

## PRE-PROCEDURAL PATIENT EVALUATION

The establishment of a good patient-physician relationship is an essential part of the vascular radiological consultation. Its importance is twofold. First, it helps to gain the patient's confidence, which in turn helps in the performance of the procedure. Second, if a complication does occur, such a relationship may lessen the likelihood for litigation. Consequently, the patient should be seen by the physician who is to perform the study.

With the exception of an emergency procedure or an urgent "add on" during the day, the pre-angiographic visit should be made the day before the study. This should take place in the patient's room and not in another section of the department where the patient is waiting to undergo another study.

Outpatient examinations such as extremity venograms may be exceptions, since these procedures are often requested on short notice. In such cases, the study can be discussed with the patient after he or she has been brought to the catheterization laboratory.

The pertinent history and laboratory data are reviewed (Table 4–1). The patient is questioned about previous contrast studies and allergic reactions. Pertinent information regarding the past medical and surgical history

(eg, hepatitis) is also recorded. If the hepatitis antigen tests are positive, the catheterization laboratory personnel are notified, so that appropriate isolation and decontamination procedures are used.

Brachial cuff pressure is measured, preferably on both arms. This is of particular importance if an axillary or brachial artery puncture is anticipated.

This is followed by a brief evaluation of the anticipated puncture site. In patients who are to undergo an arteriogram, the distal arterial pulses are also evaluated. The pulse data are recorded in the patient's chart according to the examples given in Table 4–2. This enables comparison of the pulses before and after the procedure and permits the detection of complications.

If the axillary or brachial approach is to be used, the carotid pulses should also be evaluated. In addition, the presence of subclavian and carotid bruits should be noted.

Specifically, the arterial puncture site should be evaluated for the presence of scars, hematoma (from a preceding study), or infection. The quality of the pulse must be determined and recorded, since this may determine the approach to be used.

The anticipated procedure and its indications, alternatives, benefits, and potential risks must be explained to the patient in

**TABLE 4–1. Laboratory Data That Should Be Reviewed Before Angiography or Cholangiography**

Hematocrit
Bleeding parameters: prothrombin time, partial thromboplastin time, platelets
Renal function: BUN, creatinine
*Liver enzymes: serum transaminases, amylase, alkaline phosphatase
*Serum bilirubin
*White blood count and differential

*Required for cholangiography only.

**TABLE 4–2.** Examples of Recording the Extremity Pulses

|       | Axillary | Radial | Ulnar | Femoral | Popliteal | Dorsalis Pedis | Posterior Tibial |
|-------|----------|--------|-------|---------|-----------|----------------|------------------|
| Right | 3+       | 3+     | 3+    | 3+      | 3+        | 3+             | 3+               |
| Left  | 3+       | 3+     | 3+    | 3+      | 3+        | 3+             | 3+               |

simple terms. Written, witnessed informed consent should be obtained. The patient should be advised of the anticipated duration of bed rest that will follow the study.

## PRE-PROCEDURAL ORDERS

1. The patient should not eat any solids for at least 5 to 6 hours before the study. Clear liquids may be allowed in order to prevent dehydration. For elective studies, only clear liquids are allowed after midnight, if the study is to be performed in the morning. If the anticipated time of the study is in the afternoon, breakfast is permitted.

2. In diabetics, the morning insulin dose is withheld. Following the study, the patients are placed on a sliding scale of insulin administration. If the procedure is planned for the afternoon, diabetics are allowed breakfast and should receive half the morning insulin dose. Oral diabetic medication is withheld in either case.

3. For arteriograms and lengthy venous procedures (eg, venous sampling), an intravenous line is placed in the forearm (on the side opposite to the anticipated vascular puncture site). This should be done in the patient's room at least 1 to 2 hours before the study. In patients with proteinuria, diabetics, and others at high risk for contrast-induced renal failure, overnight intravenous hydration is recommended (eg, 5% dextrose and 1/2 normal saline at 100 to 120 ml/hour). The cardiac status must be assessed before embarking upon such a regimen.

4. When the patient is called for the study, he or she should void and is subsequently premedicated and placed on a stretcher (except for severely ill patients from intensive care units, who are transported in their beds). The chart and a completed x-ray requisition should accompany the patient.

5. If a biliary procedure is to be performed, intravenous antibiotics are started approximately 1 hour before the study. A combination of an aminoglycoside and a broad-spectrum cephalosporin is used to cover the most frequently encountered organisms in the biliary tract (Table 4–3). The loading (or initial) dose is determined by the patient's size (estimated lean body mass), and maintenance therapy (dose is determined by renal function) is continued for approximately 24 hours following an uncomplicated procedure. If the procedure was complicated by a fever or sepsis, antibiotic coverage is continued until sepsis clears.

Table 4–4 provides an example of the pre-procedural orders.

## PREMEDICATION

A combination of a sedative and an analgesic is used. Some of the medications and average adult dosages are listed next. In patients with compromised liver function, the dosages must be adjusted accordingly.

**Sedatives**

1. Pentobarbital (eg, Nembutal, IM, 75 to

**TABLE 4–3.** The Most Frequently Encountered Organisms in the Biliary Tract*

| Organism | Gram Stain | Incidence of Occurrence (%) |
|----------|------------|------------------------------|
| *E. coli* | − | 18 |
| *Klebsiella pneumoniae* | − | 16 |
| Enterococci | + | 15 |
| *Pseudomonas* sp. | − | 9 |
| Anaerobes | | 9 |
| *Staphylococcus* sp. | + | 7 |
| *Proteus* sp. | − | 6 |
| Yeast | | 3 |

*From Pitt HA et al: Ann Surg 191:30–34, 1970.

**TABLE 4–4.** Pre-Procedural Orders

1. Only clear liquids after midnight except medication
2. Start IV (L/R) arm at (time) and infuse D5W (or D5W ½ NS) at _____ ml/hr.
3. On call to the cath lab (angiography suite) give: sedative, IM, analgesic, IM*
4. On call to the cath lab (angiography suite) have patient void and send patient down on stretcher with chart and completed x-ray requisition

*PO if IM injections are contraindicated.

100 mg). This is not given to patients with liver disease or emphysema or other airway disease.

2. Hydroxyzine (eg, Vistaril, PO or IM, 25 to 50 mg). This drug is particularly useful in patients who are anxious. It potentiates the effects of narcotic analgesics.

3. Promethazine (eg, Phenergan, PO or IM, 25 to 50 mg). Both hydroxyzine and promethazine also have antihistamine and antiemetic effects.

4. Diphenhydramine (eg, Benadryl, PO or IM, 25 to 50 mg). In addition to being an antihistamine, Benadryl has sedative and anticholinergic side effects. The latter may not be desirable.

### Analgesics

1. Meperidine (Demerol), IM, 75 to 100 mg.

2. Morphine sulfate, IM, 8 to 10 mg.

3. Fentanyl (Sublimaze) IM, 50 to 100 mcg (50 mcg = 0.05 mg or 1 ml). This is a narcotic analgesic. The onset of maximal analgesic effect may require several minutes. Sublimaze must be used cautiously because of its respiratory depressant action. The effects of narcotics can be reversed with naloxone (Narcan).

4. Diazepam (Valium). This drug should not be given intramuscularly because of the variability of absorption. However, intravenous Valium (2.5 mg) followed by Demerol (12.5 mg) can be given as a "cocktail" during the procedure, as the need arises. In several hundred patients, the nausea associated with Demerol alone was not observed when this combination was used. Alternatively, intravenous Sublimaze may be used.

5. Atropine. Premedication with atropine does not fulfill any definable role. Such premedication does not help to prevent a vasovagal episode. On the other hand, atropine can be given intravenously (0.6 to 1.0 mg) should the need arise.

### POST-PROCEDURAL ORDERS AND CARE

Upon completion of the study, the patient is returned to the room with the following orders:

1. Bed rest for 12 hours after translumbar aortography, 8 hours after arterial studies using larger catheters and in adults, 6 hours in older children and adolescents, 4 hours if a 4 to 5 Fr arterial catheter has been used and in younger children, and for 2 to 4 hours after transfemoral venous studies. Bed rest

**TABLE 4–5. Post-Catheterization Orders Following Translumbar Aortography**

1. Complete bed rest until (time); may elevate head end of bed by about 30°
2. Check vital signs:
   q 15 min × 4
   q 30 min × 4
   q 1 hr × 4
3. Resume pre-catheterization orders
4. Encourage PO fluids*
5. Call (telephone number) if any complication should arise

*Unless patient is fluid restricted.

should be longer if the clotting parameters are abnormal, if the patient is placed on systemic anticoagulation, or if rebleeding occurs. Following transhepatic cholangiography, bed rest of approximately 3 to 4 hours should be required. Vital signs should be checked periodically and the patient observed for signs of peritoneal irritation. No bed rest is required after an uncomplicated cubital vein approach.

2. The extremity used for access is immobilized for the duration of the bed rest. For axillary or brachial artery punctures, the arm should be immobilized in a sling.

3. Vital signs are checked periodically.

4. The groin puncture site is checked at the same time as the vital signs to detect hematoma formation or change in quality of the femoral pulse. If a venous puncture was performed, the pulse need not be checked.

**TABLE 4–6. Post-Catheterization Orders Following Femoral, Axillary, and Brachial Arteriography**

1. Flat in bed with (L/R) leg straight until (time); may elevate head end of bed by about 30°
2. Check vital signs:
   q 15 min × 4
   q 30 min × 4
   q 1 hr × 4
3. Check (L/R) femoral pulse(s), (L/R) groin(s) for hematoma, and (L/R) dorsalis pedis and posterior tibial pulse(s) together with the vital signs
4. Resume pre-catheterization orders
5. Encourage PO fluids*
6. Call (telephone number) if any complications should arise

For axillary and brachial artery punctures Steps 1 and 3 are substituted as follows:
1. Complete bed rest until (time) with (L/R) arm in a sling; may elevate head end of bed by about 30°
3. Check (L/R) radial and ulnar pulse(s), sensory and motor function together with the vital signs.

*Unless patient is fluid restricted.

**TABLE 4–7.** Post-Catheterization Orders Following Femoral Vein Puncture

1. Flat in bed with (L/R) leg straight until (time); may elevate head end of bed by about 30°
2. Check vital signs:
   q 15 min × 2
   q 30 min × 2
   q 1 hr × 2
3. Resume pre-catheterization orders
4. Encourage PO fluids*
5. Call (telephone number) if any complications should arise

*Unless patient is fluid restricted.

5. If the distal pulses (dorsalis pedis and posterior tibial) were present before the procedure, these are checked at the same time as the vital signs. If the axillary or brachial artery approach was used, sensory and motor function of the forearm and hand is evaluated in addition to palpation of the radial and ulnar pulses. Frequent examination of the axillary puncture site is usually not necessary if the patient remains asymptomatic and the radial and ulnar pulses remain unchanged.

6. Pre-catheterization orders are resumed and oral fluid intake is encouraged (unless the patient is on fluid restriction).

7. The telephone number of the catheterization laboratory (angiography suite) is recorded to facilitate immediate notification in case a complication should arise.

Tables 4–5 to 4–7 provide examples of the post-procedural orders.

## PRELIMINARY NOTE

Upon completion of the study, the films, pressure data, and other findings should be reviewed and a short note is written to outline:
1. What study was performed.
2. The approach used.
3. What complications (if any) occurred.
4. Pertinent findings, if necessary, supplemented by a diagram.

## POST-PROCEDURAL VISIT

It is recommended that a follow-up visit be made for all inpatients (with the exception of uncomplicated extremity venography). This visit should take place either on the same evening or the following morning (if the procedure was performed in the late afternoon). The appearance of the puncture site, presence of pulses, or other pertinent information should be recorded in the chart.

## REFERENCE

1. Pitt HA, Postier RG, Cameron JL: Postoperative T-tube cholangiography. Is antibiotic coverage necessary? Ann Surg 191:30–34, 1970.

# Pressure Measurements and Hemodynamics

## CHAPTER 5

Knowledge of the physiological principles governing hemodynamics has greatly enhanced our understanding of diseases involving the vascular system. The significance of hemodynamic measurements for the evaluation of peripheral vascular diseases became apparent with advancements in vascular reconstructive surgery and with the introduction of percutaneous transluminal angioplasty. The importance of such physiological measurements for the hepatobiliary and urinary systems is also well established.[1, 2]

## DEFINITIONS

*Systolic pressure*: Peak pressure during ventricular ejection.

*Diastolic pressure*: Lowest pressure during diastole, ie, immediately preceding ejection.

*End-diastolic pressure*: Ventricular pressure immediately before ventricular contraction. It is measured approximately 0.06 second after the Q wave of the electrocardiogram (EKG).

*Mean pressure*: Average pressure in an artery or vein.

*Atrial "a" wave*: Pressure wave due to atrial systole. It occurs between 0.06 and 0.08 second after the beginning of the P wave of the EKG for the right atrium (up to 0.12 second for the left atrium).

*Atrial "c" wave*: Reflects the beginning of the ventricular contraction and closure of the atrioventricular valves. It occurs about 0.08 second after the Q wave of the EKG.

*Atrial "v" wave*: Pressure wave caused by atrial filling during ventricular systole.

*Atrial "x" wave*: Corresponds to atrial relaxation and descent of the atrioventricular valves during ventricular systole.

*Atrial "y" wave*: Lowest point in the atrial pressure pulse before the "a" wave.

The "a," "c," and "v" waves of the atrial pressure tracing are positive waves.

## PRESSURE RECORDING DEVICES

In the venous system and the biliary and urinary tracts, pressures can be measured by using either a saline manometer or a pressure transducer. The measurement of arterial pressure requires a pressure transducer and a recorder. The arterial pressures thus obtained may be recorded upon special recording paper in waveform or as mean pressures and thus may serve as a permanent record.

Systolic limb pressures for the clinical evaluation of peripheral vascular disease are measured by Doppler ultrasound (see section on Hemodynamics of Peripheral Vascular Disease).

## BLOOD FLOW MEASUREMENT

The measurement of blood flow in a nonoperative setting is possible using several methods, including dye dilution, radioisotope diffusion, Doppler ultrasound, and videodensitometry. Using videodensitometry, it is possible to measure blood flow as a fraction of the cardiac output, thus providing an accurate measurement of regional arterial perfusion.[3, 4] Videodensitometry utilizes the video-recorded fluoroscopic image of the arterial contrast injection. Since the images are recorded on video tape, calculations can be made after completion of the arteriogram, avoiding unnecessary prolongation of the duration of arterial catheterization. The regional blood flow in normal individuals, as determined by this method, is shown in Table 5–1.

**TABLE 5–1.** Normal Distribution of Blood Flow*

| Artery | Percent (%) of Cardiac Output |
|---|---|
| Common carotids (left and right) | 17.0 |
| Subclavian (left and right) | 16.2 |
| Celiac | 15.7 |
| Hepatic | 8.8 |
| Splenic | 6.9 |
| Superior mesenteric | 15.4 |
| Inferior mesenteric | 2.0 |
| Renal (left and right) | 17.2 |
| Common iliac (left and right) | 12.0 |

*By videodensitometry. (Adapted from Lantz BMT et al: AJR 137:903–907, 1981.)

## TECHNIQUE FOR PRESSURE MEASUREMENT

The catheter (or catheters) is (are) attached to the female end of a clear plastic tubing through a three-way stopcock (Fig. 5–1). The male end of the tubing is attached to the pressure transducer. The tubing and transducer are flushed with 5% dextrose or normal saline (to remove all air) and the catheter (or catheters) is (are) filled with the same solution. The presence of blood or contrast medium in the catheter may lower the pressure reading. Blood should not be permitted to enter the transducer, since it can damage the sensitive diaphragm.

The stopcock is opened to the pressure transducer, and the pressures transmitted through the column of fluid in the catheter and the plastic tubing are displayed on the oscilloscope of the pressure recorder and/or a digital readout is obtained. For accurate pressure recording, the height of the pressure transducer must be at the level of the right atrium. If the transducer is positioned higher, the pressure reading will be lower

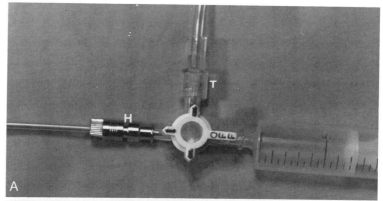

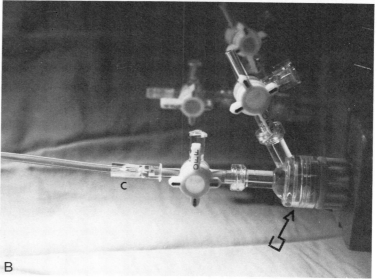

*Figure 5–1.* Setup for measurement of intraarterial pressures. *A,* The catheter hub (H) is attached to the pressure tubing (T) via a three-way stopcock. The syringe is used for flushing the system. *B,* Connection to the pressure transducer. C = to catheter, arrow points to pressure transducer.

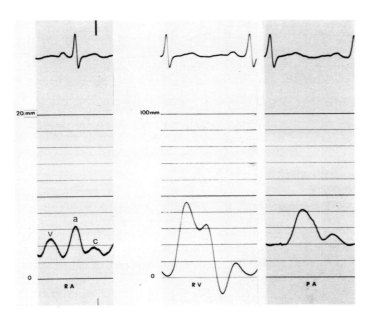

*Figure 5–2.* Venous and arterial pressure tracings. RA = right atrium; RV = right ventricle; PA = pulmonary artery.

and vice versa. Figure 5–2 shows arterial and venous pressure tracings.

## THE PRESSURE GRADIENT

A pressure gradient is defined as the pressure difference across an area of obstruction (stenosis or occlusion). The pressure gradient measured across an area of obstruction depends upon the systolic pressure, the vascular resistance distal to the obstruction and the blood flow velocity. In vessels with multiple, noncritical, sequential stenoses, each stenosis does not contribute equally to the net changes in blood flow. The most proximal lesion has the most significant effect upon flow dynamics, with each subsequent lesion contributing less than the preceding one. Decrease in the peripheral vascular resistance, eg, after exercise or intraarterial injection of a vasodilator, enhances the pressure gradient (Fig. 5–3).

Under normal circumstances, blood flows from an area of higher pressure and fluid energy to an area of lower pressure and fluid energy. Changes in blood flow are an accurate reflection of the presence and severity of a stenosis. The relationship between blood flow, resistance, and pressure gradient is explained by Poiseuille's law:

$$Q = \frac{\Delta P \; r^4 \; \pi}{\eta \; L \; 8}$$

where Q = blood flow, ΔP = pressure gradient, r = inner radius, L = length, and η = viscosity.

The resistance to blood flow is determined by the length of the vessel, severity of the stenosis, and viscosity of the blood:

$$\text{Resistance} \; \alpha \; \frac{L}{r^4} \times \eta$$

Accurate measurement of blood flow is possible with the aid of computer-assisted videodensitometry.[3, 4] However, such methods for the measurement of blood flow have not yet found widespread application. Therefore, pressure gradients are used to assess the hemodynamic significance of arterial stenoses.

Blood flow and arterial pressure gradients do not have a constant linear relationship. Beyond a critical stenosis, there is an exponential decrease in the blood flow and pressure (Fig. 5–4). This critical narrowing corresponds to a 75 to 85% reduction in the cross-sectional area of the vessel. In a stenosis of lesser severity, the blood flow will not be limited at rest (see Fig. 5–3).

Conversely, in vessels with high flow rates, a noncritical stenosis may limit blood flow.[5] Thus, the increase in blood flow through an area of stenosis following decrease in peripheral vascular resistance (after reactive hyperemia or the injection of a vasodilator) enhances the pressure gradient and forms the basis of the stress test used to

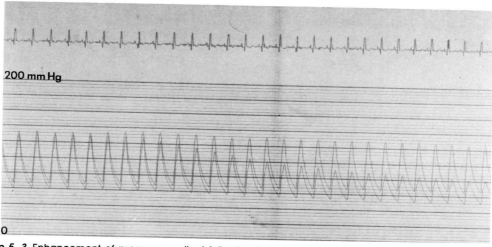

*Figure 5–3.* Enhancement of pressure gradient following injection of vasodilator in a patient with an iliac artery stenosis. Pressures were measured simultaneously in the aorta and the common femoral artery below the stenosis. There is no pressure gradient at rest. Approximately 15 seconds after injection of 10 ml of contrast medium (60% diatrizoate meglumine sodium) in the common femoral artery, the pressure distal to the stenosis falls to a maximal gradient of 48 mm Hg.

assess borderline or insignificant resting pressure gradients. A stenosis is considered hemodynamically significant if the pressure gradient across it is greater than 15 mm Hg at rest or if it is enhanced by at least 10 mm Hg after reactive hyperemia or by greater than 15 mm Hg after intraarterial injection of a vasodilator.

The arteriogram is a two-dimensional representation of the arterial system. Therefore,

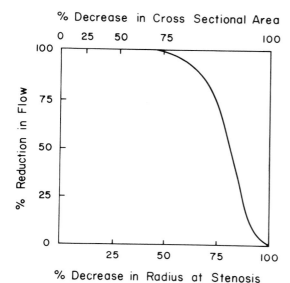

*Figure 5–4.* Relationship of blood flow and severity of vascular stenosis. (After Strandness DE, Sumner DS: Hemodynamics for Surgeons. New York, Grune and Stratton, 1975.)

it does not always permit assessment of the severity of a stenosis or the hemodynamic significance of lesions that do not appear to significantly compromise the arterial lumen. On the other hand, demonstration of a reduction in arterial diameter by more than 66% is indicative of a cross-sectional narrowing of more than 90%, which indicates the presence of a hemodynamically significant lesion. Some hemodynamically significant stenoses may be missed completely on single plane AP arteriography, and are detected only on oblique or lateral arteriograms.

On the other hand, the demonstration of an arterial occlusion by arteriography can be correlated with a predictable pressure drop. For example, in the presence of an occlusion of the infrarenal aorta or iliac arteries, the pressure in the common femoral artery is approximately 40% of the aortic pressure above the occlusion.[6]

## HEMODYNAMICS OF PERIPHERAL VASCULAR DISEASE

Hemodynamic measurements play an important role in the evaluation of peripheral vascular disease, in the prediction of the patency of vascular grafts, and in patients undergoing angioplasty.[7-10] Arterial pressures can be obtained using noninvasive Doppler ultrasound techniques, or intraarterial pressures and gradients can be measured during arteriography. In addition, regional blood flow can be determined by videodensitometry. Other noninvasive methods that may occasionally provide useful physiological information are radionuclide scanning ($^{99m}$technetium-labeled microspheres, $^{201}$thallium, $^{133}$xenon) and thermography.[11-15] The pulse volume recorder permits analysis of the pulse waveform and also helps to evaluate the functional capacity of the collateral circulation.[16]

## Doppler-derived Segmental Arterial Pressures

Segmental limb arterial pressure measurements are obtained by using a Doppler ultrasound velocity detector and blood pressure cuffs placed around the thigh, calf, and ankle (Fig. 5–5). A brachial artery pressure is also measured using the same technique. The pressure index (eg, ankle/arm index = AAI) is calculated by dividing the systolic ankle pressure by the systolic brachial artery pressure. In addition to limb pressures, digital (toes, fingers) and penile pressures can be measured and a toe/brachial or penile/brachial index calculated.

Table 5–2 shows the normal systolic pressures and the pressure indices. Absolute systolic pressures and the pressure indices that can be correlated with the stage of peripheral vascular disease are shown in Table 5–3.

Errors in such pressure measurements can occur if inappropriate-sized blood pressure cuffs are used (narrow cuffs give higher pressure readings and vice versa). The appropriate cuff diameter should be 20% wider than the limb diameter.[7] In general, the following cuff sizes are used: 22 cm for the thigh, 12

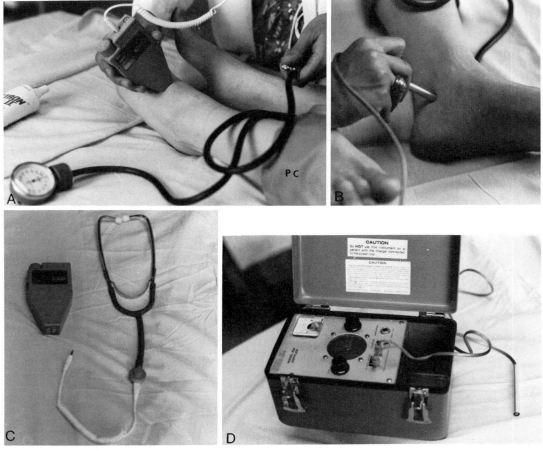

**Figure 5–5.** Doppler ultrasound detectors for obtaining arterial pressures. *A*, Position for the dorsalis pedis artery. PC = blood pressure cuff. *B*, Position for the posterior tibial artery. *C*, Pocket-sized ultrasound detector (Meda Sonics, Mountain View, California). *D*, Portable ultrasound detector (Parks Electronics Laboratory, Beaverton, Oregon).

**TABLE 5–2. Normal Systolic Pressures and Pressure Indices**

| Location | Pressure | Pressure Index |
|---|---|---|
| Thigh | 20–30 mm Hg > brachial pressure | > 1.0 |
| Ankle | ≧ Brachial pressure | 1.0 or greater |
| Toes | < Brachial pressure | 0.7–0.9 |
| Fingers | = Brachial pressure | > 0.95 |
| Penis | < Brachial pressure | 0.75–0.80 |

cm for the ankle, and 2.5 cm for the digits and for penile pressure measurements.

For segmental Doppler-derived pressures, a difference of greater than 30 mm Hg between adjacent segments is considered hemodynamically significant.[7] A temporal change in the pressure index of more than 0.15 is also considered hemodynamically significant.[19]

Absolute pressures are useful in predicting limb viability and amputation stump healing. A systolic pressure of less than 40 mm Hg constitutes limb-threatening ischemia.[20] In diabetics and patients with extensive vascular calcification, the ankle pressures may be elevated, owing to noncompressibility of the arteries, and thus give falsely high readings.

Patients with normal resting ankle pressures or a normal AAI should undergo stress testing. After measured exercise or reactive hyperemia (induced by inflating a blood pressure cuff approximately 50 mm Hg above systolic blood pressure for 3 minutes), the pressures are remeasured. Vascular dilatation following ischemia or exercise leads to a drop in the peripheral vascular resistance,

**TABLE 5–3. Correlation Between Symptoms, Absolute Systolic Pressures, and Pressure Indices\***

| Symptom | Ankle Systolic Pressure | Ankle / Arm Index | Toe Brachial Index |
|---|---|---|---|
| Intermittent claudication | 80–100 mm Hg | 0.5–0.7 | 0.35 ± 0.15 |
| Rest pain: | | 0.4–0.5 | 0.11 ± 0.10 |
| Diabetics | 55–80 mm Hg | | |
| Nondiabetics | 35–55 mm Hg | | |
| Ulcer/gangrene | < 35 mm Hg† | < 0.3 | |
| Impotence | | < 0.6 (penile/brachial index) | |

\*Data from references 7, 17, and 18.
†In diabetics, the absolute systolic pressures are usually higher.

thereby increasing flow and thus enhances the pressure gradient.

## Measurement of Intraarterial Pressure Gradients

Upon completion of the arteriogram, intraarterial pressures are measured in order to quantitate areas of stenosis in the distal aorta and iliac arteries. In general, such pressure measurements do not add more than 15 minutes to the arteriogram. If the intraarterial pressure gradient at rest is less than 15 mm Hg, intraarterial injection of a vasodilator distal to the stenosis is used to simulate exercise. A further fall in the distal intraarterial pressure by greater than 15 mm Hg suggests a significant stenosis. The vasodilatory agents commonly used are (1) tolazoline (Priscoline), 25 mg; (2) 60% contrast medium, 5 to 10 ml; or (3) papaverine 25 mg.

Papaverine produces a dose-dependent fall in distal pressures, and if a large dose is used, a pressure gradient can be produced in even normal arteries.[9] As an alternative to pharmacological reduction of peripheral vascular resistance, reactive hyperemia may be used. A fall in the distal pressure by more than 10 mm Hg following reactive hyperemia indicates hemodynamic significance of an arterial stenosis.[9]

If pharmacological agents are used for simulating exercise, the aortic pressure measurement must be repeated, since the vasodilators also decrease the aortic pressure (Fig. 5–6).

**Femoral Approach: Stenosis on the Side of Femoral Artery Puncture** (Fig. 5–7). If the femoral artery has been punctured on the side of the stenosis, upon completion of the study a pullback pressure is recorded. For accurate pressure recording, a straight catheter, with an end hole only, should be used. The catheter is placed well above the area of stenosis, and intraarterial pressure is recorded. Subsequently, while recording continuously and under fluoroscopic observation, the catheter is slowly pulled back to below the stenotic segment (or segments), and the external iliac/femoral artery pressure is recorded.

**Femoral Approach: Stenosis on the Side Opposite to the Femoral Artery Puncture Site.** Following the arteriogram, the catheter is placed in the aorta, above the stenosis. The contralateral femoral artery is punctured, and the short Teflon sheath of the arterial

# AORTA          FEMORAL

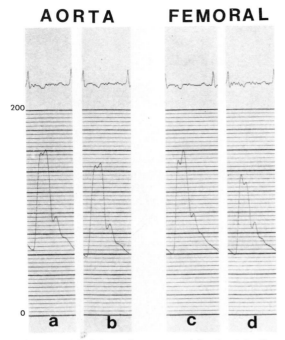

**Figure 5–6.** Fall in aortic pressure following injection of vasodilator (25 mg of tolazoline) in the femoral artery. The resting aortic (a) and femoral artery (c) pressures were equal. After injection of a vasodilator, both the aortic (b) and the femoral artery (d) pressures fell. The actual pressure gradient is 12 mm Hg. If the aortic pressure had not been remeasured, a vasodilator-enhanced gradient of 24 mm Hg would have been implicated. Such a gradient is considered hemodynamically significant.

puncture needle is placed in the external iliac artery distal to the angiographically demonstrated stenosis. Both catheter and sheath are attached to pressure transducers for simultaneous pressure recording.

**Translumbar Aortic (TLA) Approach** (Fig. 5–8). Following the arteriogram via the translumbar approach, the patient is placed in the supine position.[21, 22] The TLA catheter is kept well flushed while the groins are prepped and draped. Femoral artery puncture is performed, and the Teflon sheath of the arterial puncture needle or a short straight catheter is placed below the stenosis and simultaneous pressure recordings are obtained through the femoral artery and TLA catheters.

## PULMONARY HEMODYNAMICS

Pressure measurements should be a part of every angiographic evaluation of the pulmonary arteries. As a matter of routine, the pressures should be monitored constantly as the catheter is passed through the right heart. This is necessary to (1) localize catheter position by means of the pressure (eg, on AP fluoroscopy, the catheter may appear to be in the right ventricle when it is in the coronary sinus); (2) measure right atrial and ventricular pressures; and (3) measure pulmonary artery pressures for the evaluation of

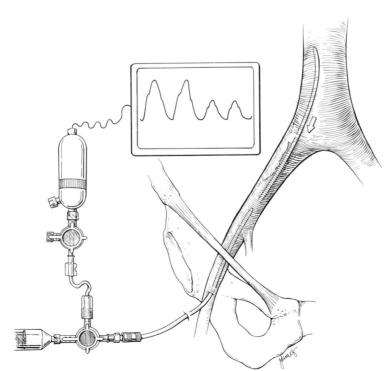

**Figure 5–7.** Technique for measurement of a pullback pressure across a stenosis in the ipsilateral iliac artery. After measurement of the arterial pressure above the stenosis, the catheter tip is pulled down to below the stenotic area while recording continously.

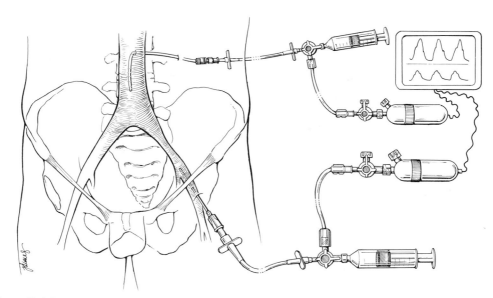

**Figure 5–8.** Technique for measurement of arterial pressure gradients during translumbar aortography.

pulmonary hypertension and prior to the injection of contrast medium.

If the systolic pulmonary artery pressure exceeds 80 mm Hg, a main pulmonary artery injection is avoided, and the total volume of contrast medium injected is reduced in order to prevent ventricular overload. Table 5–4 lists the normal pressures and oxygen saturation.

**Pulmonary Capillary Wedge (PCW) Pressures.** The PCW pressure is equal to the pulmonary vein pressure and thus reflects the left atrial pressure. The diastolic pulmo-

nary artery pressure is also equal to the left atrial pressure in the absence of pulmonary hypertension.

For the measurement of PCW pressure, an end hole catheter is used. This can be inserted over a guide wire or a balloon catheter can be flow directed into the pulmonary arteries. The catheter is wedged into a pulmonary artery branch for recording a pressure. To confirm a true wedged catheter position, a blood sample is drawn to determine oxygen saturation, which should be greater than 95%.

**TABLE 5–4.** Normal Intracardiac and Arterial Pressures and Oxygen Saturation

| Vessel | Pressure | mm Hg | Oxygen Saturation (%) |
|---|---|---|---|
| Inferior vena cava | Mean | < 5 | 65–80 |
| Superior vena cava | Mean | < 5 | 65–80 |
| Right atrium | Mean | < 5 | 65–80 |
| Coronary sinus | Mean | < 5 | 30 |
| Right ventricle | Systolic<br>End-diastolic | 15–30<br>< 5 | 65–80 |
| Pulmonary arteries | Systolic<br>Diastolic<br>Mean | 15–30<br>< 10<br>6–17 | 65–80 |
| Left atrium | Mean | < 10 | > 95 |
| Left ventricle | Systolic<br>End-diastolic | 90–150<br>< 10 | > 95 |
| Aorta | Systolic<br>Diastolic<br>Mean | 90–150<br>60–90<br>70–100 | > 95 |

## HEMODYNAMICS OF THE LIVER

The measurement of hepatic vein wedge pressure (HWP) is an important aspect of the evaluation and classification of liver disease and portal hypertension. The HWP corresponds to the portal vein pressure. It reflects the pressure in the hepatic sinusoids and the intraabdominal pressure.

By subtracting the intraabdominal pressure from the HWP, the actual sinusoidal resistance (corrected sinusoidal pressure = CSP) to portal blood flow caused by liver disease can be determined. Intraabdominal pressure is determined by measuring the inferior vena caval or hepatic vein pressures (also called free hepatic vein pressure).

$$CSP = HWP - \text{free hepatic vein pressure}$$

**Technique for Pressure Measurement.** The inferior vena caval, hepatic venous, and hepatic wedge pressures can be measured with a saline manometer or with the aid of a pressure transducer. An end hole catheter is introduced via the cubital or femoral vein approach and is wedged into a hepatic vein branch. In this position, it is not possible to aspirate blood easily. To insure a true

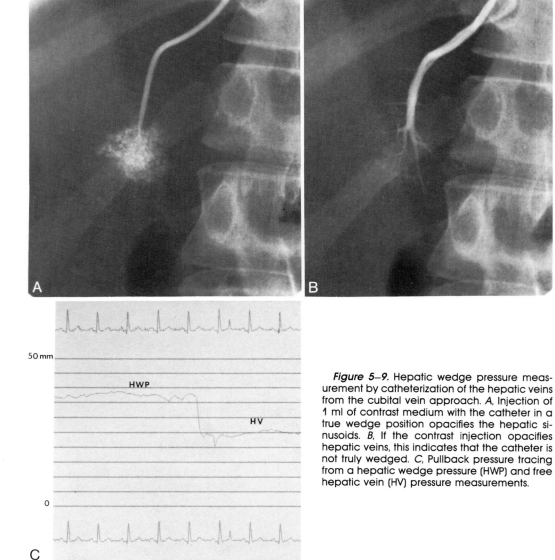

**Figure 5–9.** Hepatic wedge pressure measurement by catheterization of the hepatic veins from the cubital vein approach. *A,* Injection of 1 ml of contrast medium with the catheter in a true wedge position opacifies the hepatic sinusoids. *B,* If the contrast injection opacifies hepatic veins, this indicates that the catheter is not truly wedged. *C,* Pullback pressure tracing from a hepatic wedge pressure (HWP) and free hepatic vein (HV) pressure measurements.

wedged position, a small volume of contrast medium is injected (1 ml). If the catheter is in a true wedged position, a parenchymal stain (sinusoids) is observed (Fig. 5–9). If it is not wedged, a hepatic venule is demonstrated. Prior to pressure recording, contrast medium must be flushed out of the catheter. HWP should be measured in several different right and left hepatic veins. A difference of more than 3 mm Hg between several readings is indicative of technical error but may occasionally occur as a result of segmental differences in the stage of the liver disease.

If it is technically not possible to wedge the catheter, a balloon catheter may be used to obtain balloon occlusion pressures. These correspond closely to hepatic wedge pressures obtained through end hole catheters.[24] However, a wedged position of the catheter is not difficult to achieve from the cubital vein approach. Direct measurement of portal vein pressures is also possible through the umbilical vein or by transhepatic insertion of a skinny needle.[25]

The determination of biliary pressures is useful both for the diagnosis of obstruction and for assessing immediate and long-term success of percutaneous transhepatic balloon dilatation of biliary strictures. The normal pressure in the unobstructed biliary tract is less than 20 cm $H_2O$.

Accurate measurement of biliary pressures through a 22 gauge cholangiography needle inserted into a small biliary duct is possible only occasionally. Pressure measurement through such a needle is accurate if a large duct has been entered. Free intraductal position of the needle tip must be verified after the pressure has been recorded. This is accomplished by injecting 30% contrast medium and observing the needle tip in the AP and oblique projections, using 6 inch mode for fluoroscopy or spot film. The commonly used criteria for confirmation of free intraluminal position (ie, height-induced changes in the saline column) are also observed when the needle tip is partially extraductal or abuts the duct wall. (See Fig. 22–7, Chapter 22.) In this case, elevated pressures may be measured. Injection of a large volume of contrast medium prior to pressure measurement also leads to elevation of intraductal pressures.

**Interpretation of the Pressure Readings.** The normal values are listed in Table 5–5. The CSP has been correlated with the severity of liver disease, as demonstrated by the hepatic venogram and histological studies.[26] (See Chapter 15, Tables 15–3 to 15–5.)

**TABLE 5–5. Normal Hepatic Pressures***

| Pressure | mm Hg | cm Saline |
|---|---|---|
| Hepatic wedge pressure | < 10 | < 14 |
| Free hepatic vein pressure | < 5 | < 7 |
| Corrected sinusoidal pressure | < 5 | < 7 |

*1 mm Hg = 1.36 cm saline.

## REFERENCES

1. Reynolds TB: The role of hemodynamic measurements in portosystemic shunt surgery. Arch Surg 108:276–281, 1974.
2. Barbaric ZL: Interventional uroradiology. Radiol Clin North Am 17:413–433, 1979.
3. Lantz BMT, Foerster JM, Link DP, et al: Regional distribution of cardiac output: Normal values in man determined by video dilution technique. AJR 137:903–907, 1981.
4. Lantz BMT, Foerster JM, Link DP, et al: Determination of relative blood flow in single arteries: new video dilution technique. AJR 134:1161–1168, 1980.
5. Schultz RD, Hokanson DE, Strandness DE: Pressure-flow and stress-strain measurements of normal and diseased aortoiliac segments. Surg Gynecol Obstet 124:1267–1276, 1967.
6. Noer I, Praestholm J, Tonnesen KH: Direct measured systolic pressure gradients across the aorto-iliac segment in multiple level obstruction arteriosclerosis. Cardiovasc Intervent Radiol 4:73–76, 1981.
7. Pearce WH, Yao JST, Bergan JJ: Noninvasive vascular testing. Curr Prob Surg 20:464–537, 1983.
8. Corson JD, Johnson WC, LoGerfo FW, et al: Doppler ankle systolic blood pressure. Prognostic value in vein bypass grafts of the lower extremity. Arch Surg 113:932–935, 1978.
9. Kaufman SL, Fara JW, Udoff EJ, et al: Hemodynamic effects of vasodilators across iliac stenoses in dogs. Invest Radiol 14:471–475, 1979.
10. Kadir S, White RI, Kaufman SL, et al: Long-term results of aorto-iliac angioplasty. Surgery 94:10–14, 1983.
11. Giargiana FA, Siegel ME, James AE, et al: A preliminary report on the complementary roles of arteriography and perfusion scanning in the assessment of peripheral vascular disease. Radiology 108:619–627, 1973.
12. Siegel ME, Giargiana FA Jr, White RI, et al: Peripheral vascular perfusion scanning. Correlation with the arteriogram and clinical assessment in the patient with peripheral vascular disease. AJR 125:628–633, 1975.
13. Siegel ME, Siemsen JK: A new noninvasive approach to peripheral vascular disease: Thallium 201 leg scans. AJR 131:827–830, 1978.
14. Pozderac RV, Miller TA, Lindenauer SM: 133 Xe muscle clearance: A screening test for arterial occlusive disease. Radiology 117:633–635, 1975.
15. Soulen RL, Lapayowker MS, Tyson RR, et al: Angiography, ultrasound, and thermography in the study of peripheral vascular disease. Radiology 105:115–119, 1972.
16. Darling RC, Raines JK, Brener BJ, et al: Quantitative

segmental pulse volume recorder: a clinical tool. Surgery 72:873–887, 1972.

17. Raines JK, Darling RC, Buth J, et al: Vascular laboratory criteria for the management of peripheral vascular disease of the extremities. Surgery 79:21–29, 1976.

18. Carter SA, Lezack JD: Digital systolic pressures in the lower limb in arterial disease. Circulation 43:905–914, 1971.

19. Baker JD, Dix D: Variability of Doppler ankle pressures with arterial occlusive disease: an evaluation of ankle index and brachial ankle pressure gradient. Surgery 89:134–137, 1981.

20. Jamieson C: The definition of critical ischemia of a limb. Editorial. Br J Surg 69(Suppl)S2, 1982.

21. Bardach G: Eine neue Methode zur Direktmessung des aortofemoralen Druckgradienten im Rahmen der translumbalen Aortographie. Fortschr Roentgenstr 128:317–318, 1978.

22. Udoff EJ, Barth KH, Harrington DP, et al: Hemodynamic significance of iliac artery stenosis: pressure measurements during angiography. Radiology 132:289–293, 1979.

23. Criley JM, Ross RS: Cardiovascular physiology. Tampa Tracings, Tarpon Springs, Florida, 1971.

24. Groszmann RJ, Glickman M, Blei AT, et al: Wedged and free hepatic venous pressure measured with a balloon catheter. Gastroenterology 76:253–258, 1979.

25. Boyer TD, Triger DR, Horissawa M, et al: Direct transhepatic measurement of portal vein pressure using a thin needle. Comparison with wedged hepatic vein pressure. Gastroenterology 72:584–589, 1977.

26. Cavaluzzi JA, Sheff R, Harrington DP, et al: Hepatic venography and wedge hepatic vein pressure measurements in diffuse liver disease. AJR 129:441–446, 1977.

## ADDITIONAL READINGS

Bernstein EF (ed): Noninvasive Diagnostic Techniques in Vascular Disease, 2nd Ed. St. Louis, C. V. Mosby Co., 1982.

Levy MN, Berne RM.: Cardiovascular Physiology, 4th Ed. St. Louis, C. V. Mosby Co., 1981.

Strandness DE, Sumner DS: Hemodynamics for Surgeons. New York, Grune and Stratton, 1975.

# Pharmacoangiography

Alterations in blood flow patterns to an organ or an organ system by means of intravascular injection or infusion of vasoactive drugs is used either for improvement of the diagnostic quality of the angiogram or for therapy. In diagnostic angiography, injection or infusion of vasodilators, vasoconstrictors, or other smooth muscle relaxants is used to improve visualization of peripheral small vessels or to differentiate normal from abnormal vasculature (Table 6–1). Of the drugs available for pharmacoangiography, epinephrine, tolazoline, and glucagon are used most frequently.

A basic vascular tone is provided by the sympathetic activity in the form of continuous asynchronous contractions of the vascular smooth musculature. This basic vascular tone is influenced by chemical (medications,

### TABLE 6–1. Applications of Pharmacoangiography

**Vasoconstricting Agents**
1. Differentiation between normal and abnormal blood vessels, especially in hypovascular lesions
2. Redistribution of blood flow to opacify arteries that are difficult to catheterize
3. Retrograde renal venography
4. Treatment of bleeding

**Vasodilatory Agents**
1. Improvement of visualization of the peripheral vascular bed
2. Enhancement of venous opacification
3. Differentiation between organic and functional vascular changes (eg, in Raynaud's disease, vascular trauma)
4. Relief or prevention of arterial spasm (during catheterization, angioplasty, or operation)
5. Provocation of bleeding for diagnosis
6. Management of nonocclusive mesenteric ischemia and other vasospastic disorders

**Agents for Relaxation of Intestinal Peristalsis**
1. Temporary cessation of intestinal peristalsis for digital subtraction angiography (IV glucagon)

hormonal) and physical (temperature) agents.

The response of blood vessels to vasoactive substances can be extremely variable and depends upon (1) the type of vessel (artery or vein: normal artery, neovasculature, or inflammatory vessels), (2) size of the vessel, (3) composition of adrenergic receptors (alpha or beta), (4) dosage of the vasoactive drug used, and (5) route of administration (IV, IA, or IM).

## VASOCONSTRICTING AGENTS
(Table 6–2)

### Epinephrine (Adrenalin)

Epinephrine is a sympathomimetic drug with both alpha (vasoconstriction) and beta (vasodilatation) adrenergic receptor responses. The receptor composition of a given vascular bed and the dose of epinephrine determine the net response. The smaller arterioles and precapillary sphincters are primarily affected, but the larger arteries and veins are also responsive to the drug.[1] Its vasoconstrictive action is most pronounced in the cutaneous, renal, and visceral vessels.[1] Repeat administration does not elicit the same response as the initial dose, suggesting the presence of tachyphylaxis.[2]

**Effects of Epinephrine on Normal Vessels** (Fig. 6–1). Upon administration of 3 to 12 μg of epinephrine, the small and mid-sized arteries respond with constriction. In larger vessels, vasoconstriction is observed when a higher dose is used.[2, 3] The vasoconstrictive response of different normal visceral arteries is quite variable and is listed below in decreasing order of intensity[4]:

1. Splenic artery: extreme constriction of the proximal and distal vessels.

2. Hepatic arteries: constriction of the

**TABLE 6–2.** Pharmacoangiography with Vasoconstricting Agents

| Drug | Dosage | Route of Administration | Half Life | Site of Action |
|---|---|---|---|---|
| Epinephrine (Adrenalin) | 3–6 μg<br>6–8 μg<br>6–8 μg | Renal artery (tumor evaluation)<br>Renal artery (renal venography)<br>Celiac/superior mesenteric artery | | Alpha and beta receptors |
| Angiotensin | 0.5–1 μg<br>1–5 μg<br>5–10 μg | Renal, hepatic mesenteric artery<br>Celiac artery<br>Pelvis, extremity arteries | ~ 20 sec | Vascular smooth muscle; sympathetic innervation |
| Vasopressin | 0.2–0.4 Unit/min<br><br>1 Unit | Intraarterial or intravenous infusion (for gastrointestinal bleeding)<br>Slow intraarterial injection (diagnostic angiography) | ~ 10 min | Vascular and intestinal smooth muscle |

branches. The common and proper hepatic arteries are less responsive.

3. Gastric and gastroepiploic arteries: intense constriction.

4. Renal arteries: constriction of the smaller intrarenal arteries. Focal constriction of the main renal artery.

5. Pancreatic arteries: variable response (from constriction to mild dilatation).

6. Duodenal arteries: mild constriction.

7. Superior mesenteric artery and its branches: mild constriction.

On arteriography, the effects of intraarterial epinephrine are manifested as:

1. A prolongation of the circulation time, ie, increased duration of contrast opacification of the main arteries.

2. Reflux of contrast medium into the aorta.

3. Poor parenchymal stain.

4. Absent or poor venous opacification in the absence of an arteriovenous fistula.

The vasoconstrictive response may be nonhomogeneous, and occasionally an abrupt

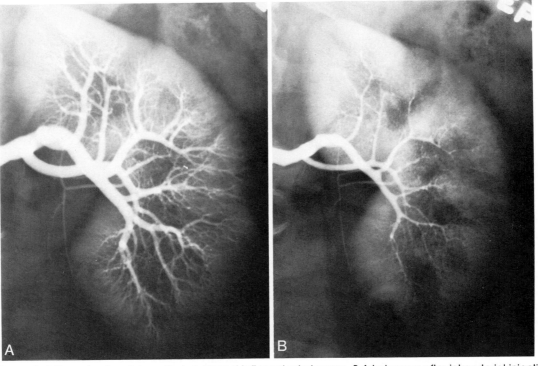

*Figure 6–1.* Normal epinephrine effect. *A,* Normal left renal arteriogram. *B,* Arteriogram after intraarterial injection of epinephrine. There is only minimal construction of the main renal artery. The smaller intrarenal branches show pronounced vasoconstriction.

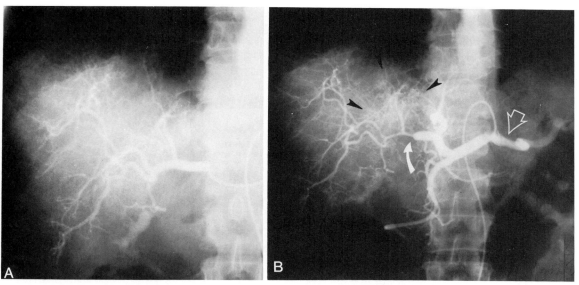

*Figure 6–2.* Abrupt change in caliber of hepatic artery in response to 8 µg of epinephrine. *A,* Hepatic arteriogram before injection of epinephrine in a patient with hepatic cell carcinoma. *B,* Arteriogram after injection of epinephrine. There is an abrupt narrowing of the right hepatic artery (*curved arrow*). Reflux of contrast medium into the splenic (*open arrow*), left hepatic, gastroduodenal, and right gastric arteries is seen. The tumor neovascularity is better demonstrated (*arrowheads*).

change in arterial caliber from normal to severe constriction may be seen (Fig. 6–2). This may simulate dissection or occlusion.

**Effects of Epinephrine on Abnormal Vessels.** In abnormal vessels, the vasoconstrictive response to epinephrine is also variable:

1. Arteries affected by atherosclerosis or fibromuscular dysplasia do not constrict in response to intraarterial epinephrine.[2]

2. In inflammatory diseases of the kidney, the renal arteries may be less responsive to pharmacological stimuli, which may lead to the erroneous diagnosis of malignancy.[4–7] In pancreatitis and inflammatory diseases affecting the intestines, the vasoconstrictive response to epinephrine is maintained.[8]

3. The response of tumor vessels is also variable.[2, 7] Vasoconstriction is seen in only two thirds of cases. This variability of vasoconstrictive response of the tumor is due to the differences in the composition of the vessels supplying tumors. These tumor vessels may be composed of true neovasculature, ie, embryonic, thin-walled, primitive vessels with absent elastic elements, which are not capable of vasoconstriction,[9] or the tumor may be located distal to normal, preformed arteries, which constrict in response to intraarterial epinephrine. In the latter situation the tumor may be obscured (Fig. 6–3).

In the evaluation of primary and metastatic tumors, epinephrine-induced vasoconstriction serves to redistribute the contrast medium into the unresponsive tumor vessels, thereby enhancing tumor opacification. However, such pharmacological tumor enhancement is indicated only in certain cases[9–11]: (1) when the tumor diagnosis is uncertain, ie, when the tumor vessels are obscured by normal vasculature, (2) in hypovascular tumors, (3) in necrotic tumors, and (4) to enhance opacification of abnormal draining veins.

The actions of epinephrine are reversed by ergoloid mesylate (Hydergine), which is an alpha receptor blocker, or sodium nitroprusside.[12]

**Applications**

1. Evaluation of primary tumors: renal, hepatic, pancreatic.

2. Evaluation of metastatic tumors to the liver, eg, carcinoid.

3. Demonstration of abnormal draining veins, ie, arteriovenous shunting in tumors.

4. Retrograde renal venography.[13]

5. Adrenal arteriography—injection of epinephrine into the renal artery to redistribute blood flow into the adrenal arteries: Injection into the celiac artery to demonstrate the inferior phrenic arteries.[4] This technique has

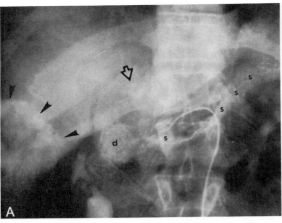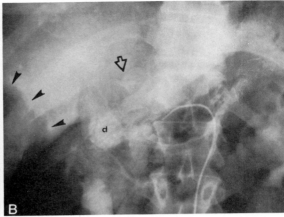

*Figure 6–3.* Differential vasoconstrictive response of tumor vessels to epinephrine in a patient with metastatic colonic adenocarcinoma. *A,* Parenchymal phase of an hepatic arteriogram shows a hypervascular metastasis (*arrowheads*). Another area of abnormal vascularity is seen in the left lobe (*open arrow*). There is hyperemia of the duodenal bulb (d) and stomach (s). *B,* Arteriogram after injection of 8 μg of epinephrine shows absence of the tumor stain in the right lobe of the liver (*arrowheads*). The metastasis in the left lobe is slightly better defined (*open arrow*).

other potential applications for the evaluation of other proximally arising vessels that are difficult to catheterize, eg, injection into the splenic artery to visualize the pancreatic and gastric arteries.

6. Evaluation of primary mesenteric tumors.[14] However, mesenteric arteriography is infrequently used for the evaluation of such tumors, since the diagnosis and extent are easier and better defined by other methods. In patients suspected of having a carcinoid, epinephrine-enhanced arteriography may facilitate establishment of the diagnosis.[15]

7. Resuscitation in cardiac arrest.

8. Relief of respiratory distress due to bronchospasm occurring as a result of a contrast medium reaction.

**Contraindications and Side Effects.** Epinephrine should not be used in patients in shock or those with narrow angle glaucoma. Headache, anxiety, restlessness, tremor, and palpitations have been observed.[1] Occasionally, in susceptible patients, administration of epinephrine may induce an anginal attack. With high doses, tachycardia and flank and abdominal pain (if used in the renal or celiac artery) may be observed. However, in the doses used for pharmacoangiography, side effects are infrequent. The effects of epinephrine may be potentiated by tricyclic antidepressants and certain antihistamines.

**Dosage and Preparation of the Dilution.** The dosage of epinephrine for pharmacoangiography is listed in Table 6–2. Epinephrine, in a dose of 0.5 mg, is added to 500 ml of normal saline. With this dilution 1 ml of the solution contains 1 microgram (μg) of epinephrine. The appropriate concentration is drawn up in a disposable syringe and is injected slowly (over 20 to 30 seconds), and the catheter is flushed with 5 to 10 ml of flushing solution. The syringe is discarded subsequently.

## Angiotensin

Angiotensin is one of the most potent vasoconstricting agents available. Unlike epinephrine, which has both vasoconstrictive and vasodilatory actions, angiotensin is a pure vasoconstrictor. It is effective at the small vessel level (precapillary arterioles and postcapillary venules).[16–18] Contraction of the vascular smooth muscle by angiotensin may be in the form of direct stimulation or indirectly via the sympathetic nervous system.[16, 19] The duration of action is short, with the maximal vasoconstriction lasting for less than 1 minute.[20] Tachyphylaxis occurs after repeated administrations of the drug.[16]

**Applications and Dosage** (Table 6–2). The applications of angiotensin are similar to those of epinephrine. Administration of angiotensin leads to constriction of normal blood vessels, whereas the primitive tumor vessels are unresponsive to this drug. Some of the specific applications are[17, 18, 20–23]:

1. For the evaluation of hypovascular neoplasms of the liver, kidneys, and extremities.

2. For the redistribution of contrast me-

dium into vessels that may be difficult to catheterize, eg, inferior adrenal artery (by injection into the renal artery).

3. For the evaluation of the pancreatic vessels by injection into the hepatic artery. Hepatic vasoconstriction causes reflux of contrast medium into the pancreatico-duodenal vessels.

To utilize the vasoconstrictive effect maximally, injection of contrast medium should be within 30 to 90 seconds of administration of angiotensin.[22] The appropriate dose of angiotensin diluted in saline or dextrose is injected as a slow bolus. The dosage used varies with the circulation (Table 6–2).

**Contraindications and Side Effects.** There are no known contraindications to pharmacological doses of angiotensin. When used in appropriate doses, there is no change in pulse rate or blood pressure.[17] Occasionally, flank pain may be observed.

## Vasopressin

Vasopressin is a short-acting peptide (half life of about 10 minutes) that is produced in the posterior pituitary (neurohypophysis).[24] It causes constriction of the smooth musculature of the arteries and veins and is also an antidiuretic hormone with the site of action in the distal renal tubules.[24] Vasopressin is used primarily in the management of gastrointestinal bleeding.[25, 26] Occasionally, it is also used in diagnostic arteriography to alter blood flow patterns as an alternative to selective arteriography. In response to vasopressin, there is a decrease in blood flow in the splenic, gastric, and mesenteric arteries. Hepatic arterial blood flow is increased.[27, 28]

The duration of action of vasopressin is longer than that of epinephrine. The main indication for the pharmacoangiographic application of vasopressin is vascular redistribution for arteriography of the pancreas. The intense vasoconstrictive response of the splenic, gastric, and gastroepiploic arteries permits redistribution of blood flow into the pancreatic vessels.

**Contraindications and Side Effects.** Vasopressin should not be used in patients with angina. Side effects include abdominal cramps, nausea, and hyperperistalsis of the intestines.

**Dosage.** One unit of aqueous vasopressin is diluted with approximately 20 ml of flushing solution and is injected slowly (over 60 seconds).

## Pitfalls of Vasoconstrictive Pharmacoangiography

Since the vasoconstrictive response is usually dose dependent, a large dose of a vasoconstrictor may obscure small, peripherally located tumors. Thus, for the evaluation of such lesions a small dose (eg, epinephrine, 3 to 6 µg) should be used.[3, 29] In addition, tumors located in the periphery that derive their vascular supply from normal vessels may be obscured after intraarterial injection of vasoconstrictors as a result of constriction of the normal vessels.[30] Finally, hypovascular and also some hypervascular liver metastases may not be demonstrated on epinephrine-enhanced studies.[14]

## VASODILATING AGENTS

The goals of vasodilatory pharmacoangiography are:

1. To allow differentiation between functional and anatomical vascular changes and to assess the reversibility of such changes, eg, in vasospastic disorders.

2. To improve the quality of the arteriogram, eg, opacification of the distal extremity vessels.

3. To enhance venous opacification.

4. To provide a therapeutic intervention for the treatment of nonocclusive mesenteric ischemia or other forms of vasospasm.

## Acetylcholine

Acetylcholine is a short-acting neurohumoral transmitter that is quickly inactivated by circulating and tissue cholinesterases.[31] It is a potent vasodilator that has been used primarily in renal angiography. Infusion of acetylcholine leads to maximal dilatation of renal artery branches and occasionally of the main renal artery. The transit time of contrast medium is accelerated and there is earlier and denser venous opacification. However, the nephrogram is poorer and contrast excretion is delayed.[32]

In normal kidneys, acetylcholine produces a dose-related increase in renal blood flow.[32] Maximal increase in renal blood flow is achieved by infusing < 100 µg/minute. A further increase in the dose may cause a paradoxical decrease in blood flow.[33, 34] The sensitivity of the renal vasculature to acetylcholine is increased in patients who are dehydrated and in essential hypertension and cholinesterase deficiency and is decreased in those with renal failure, parenchymal disease, and arteriolosclerosis.[32, 35, 36] Diphenhydramine and atropine block the actions of acetylcholine by direct action upon the muscarinic receptors.[32] The paradoxical response to higher doses may be mediated by the release of catecholamines[31, 38] or may occur as a result of direct stimulation of the vascular smooth muscle.[34] Tachyphylaxis is not observed in short infusions lasting less than 30 minutes.[32]

### Applications[35–37]

1. For the evaluation of small intrarenal vasculature, eg, in renal transplants.
2. For the evaluation of neoplasms.
3. In renal venography.
4. To differentiate between fixed anatomical changes and vasospasm of intrarenal branches in the evaluation of renovascular hypertension.

**Contraindications and Side Effects.** Acetylcholine is contraindicated in patients with cholinesterase deficiency, bronchial asthma, and hyperthyroidism.[31] Patients with cholinesterase deficiency can be identified by the use of a screening test.[39] Accumulation of acetylcholine leads to hypotension and bradycardia. Serious side effects or unusual sensitivity to the drug can be treated by intravenous atropine, which is a receptor-specific competitive antagonist.

**Pitfalls.** A nonuniform vasodilatory response of the different intrarenal branches may be observed.[36] This may be due to one of several factors: a slow infusion rate, uneven distribution of the drug or selective infusion into a branch vessel, or differential vasodilator response of the branches.

### Nifedipine

Nifedipine is a calcium channel blocker that has been used successfully for the management of coronary artery spasm.[40, 41] Its action is linked to the inhibition of the transmembrane influx of calcium ions into the smooth muscle. In addition to dilation of the coronary arteries and arterioles, nifedipine causes peripheral vasodilatation, which has prompted its use in patients with peripheral vasospastic disorders.

Currently, the drug is available in capsule form for oral intake (Procardia, 10 mg capsules, Pfizer, Inc.). Sublingual application for prompt relief of coronary or peripheral vaso-

spasm is possible by making a hole in the gelatin capsule.

### Nitroglycerin

Nitroglycerin is a short-acting vasodilator that relaxes the smooth musculature of smaller arteries and veins.[42, 43] It is used during coronary arteriography to differentiate between arterial spasm and anatomical lesions and to reverse the spasm induced by ergonovine.[44]

Sublingual nitroglycerin (0.4 mg) has been used successfully to treat renal artery spasm during selective catheterization and angioplasty (unpublished data). Intravenous infusion or bolus injection of nitroglycerin (50 to 100 µg) provides effective vasodilatation and prevents renal or coronary artery spasm due to catheter manipulation.

### Papaverine

Papaverine is a musculotropic smooth muscle relaxant that acts upon arterioles and larger vessels.[43] The precise mechanism of action is not known.

**Applications and Dosage[45, 46]**

1. As a vasodilator in peripheral vascular disease, especially in vasospastic disorders or spasm secondary to trauma or operation.
2. For nonocclusive mesenteric ischemia.

In peripheral vascular diseases 25 mg of papaverine is injected as a slow bolus. In nonocclusive mesenteric ischemia, following a slow bolus injection (25 to 30 mg), papaverine is infused at 1 mg/minute into the superior mesenteric artery for 12 to 24 hours.

**Contraindications and Side Effects.** Accumulation of papaverine or a large bolus may lead to depression of atrioventricular (AV) nodal and intraventricular conduction and may cause arrhythmias.[43] Tachycardia and drowsiness may also occur. In patients with low cardiac output (eg, nonocclusive mesenteric ischemia) a rapid bolus injection of papaverine may cause a fall in systemic blood pressure.

### Prostaglandins

Prostaglandins are highly vasoactive derivatives of the arachidonic acid with an ultrashort half life.[47] Thus, after a single passage through the lungs, 95% of prostaglandin $E_2$ is inactivated.[48]

**Prostaglandin E₁.** Prostaglandin $E_1$ is a potent vasodilator and produces sustained peripheral vasodilatation. It has been used as a vasodilator in peripheral vascular disease,[49] for the evaluation of neoplasms, and for arterial portography.[50] In canine experiments, the superior mesenteric blood flow can be increased by 100% after administration of prostaglandin $E_1$, and the portal vein visualization is enhanced significantly.[51]

**Prostaglandin F₂ₐ.** The vascular effects of this prostaglandin appear to be variable in different species. In humans, it is primarily a vasodilator.[52, 53] In lower doses it may act as a vasoconstrictor.[53] When infused into the superior mesenteric artery of animals, prostaglandin $F_{2\alpha}$ causes vasoconstriction. Injection into the human superior mesenteric artery produces vasodilatation with improved visualization of the portal vein.[52–54]

At recommended dosages, there are no adverse effects on the heart rate and blood pressure.[52] Prostaglandin $F_{2\alpha}$ is contraindicated in patients with bronchial asthma because of its constrictory action on the bronchial smooth muscle.[55]

## Reserpine

The alkaloid reserpine is derived from the shrub *Rauwolfia serpentina*, which is used in the treatment of hypertension. Its pharmacological action is mediated by depletion of catecholamine and 5-hydroxytryptamine (5-HT) stores. Intraarterial injection of reserpine produces sustained peripheral vasodilatation, which makes it an attractive drug for local intraarterial application. At the dosages used for pharmacoangiography, systemic side effects, including hypotension, have not been observed.

**Applications and Dosage**[56, 57] (Table 6–3; see also Fig. 9–23, Chapter 9)

1. For intraarterial bolus injection in the treatment and prophylaxis of peripheral arterial spasm during angioplasty.

2. For evaluation of peripheral vasospastic disorders.

3. For treatment of vasospastic disorders of the extremities.

A dose of 0.5 to 1.0 mg of reserpine is injected as a slow bolus into the appropriate extremity vessel (brachial or femoral artery). The dose may be repeated for the contralateral extremity.

## Tolazoline

Tolazoline (Priscoline, Ciba Pharmaceutical Co.) is one of the most frequently used drugs for vasodilation in diagnostic arteriography. It is an imidazoline derivative and exhibits sympathomimetic, parasympathomimetic, and histamine-like properties. In addition, it stimulates the heart, which can lead to arrhythmias and angina. In the doses used for pharmacoangiography, tolazoline does not exhibit properties of alpha adrenergic block-

**TABLE 6–3.** Pharmacoangiography with Vasodilating Agents

| Drug | Dosage | Route of Administration | Site of Action |
|------|--------|-------------------------|----------------|
| Acetylcholine | 30–100 μg/min | Intraarterial infusion (~ 10 min) | Autonomic effector sites; motor end-plates; autonomic ganglia |
| Nifedipine | 10–30 mg | PO | Calcium channel blocker |
| Nitroglycerin | 0.3–0.4 mg<br>50–100 μg<br>10–100 μg/min | Sublingual<br>Intraarterial bolus<br>Infusion | Vascular smooth muscle |
| Papaverine | 25–30 mg<br>60 mg/min | Intraarterial bolus<br>Intraarterial infusion | ? |
| Phentolamine | 5 mg<br>100 μg/min | Intravenous<br>Intraarterial | Alpha adrenergic blockade; vascular smooth muscle |
| Prostaglandin $E_1$<br>Prostaglandin $F_{2\alpha}$ | 5.0–7.5 μg<br>30–80 μg | Intraarterial bolus<br>Intraarterial bolus | Vascular smooth musle |
| Reserpine | 0.5–1 mg | Intraarterial bolus | Depletion of catecholamine stores |
| Tolazoline | 25 mg | Intraarterial bolus | Vascular smooth muscle |

ade. It produces vasodilatation by direct action upon the vascular smooth muscle.[58]

**Applications and Dosage**[59–62] (Table 6–3; see also Figs. 13–18 and 13–19, Chapter 13)

1. For assessment of the hemodynamic significance of arterial stenoses.

2. For vasodilatation of peripheral vessels during arteriography of the extremities.

3. For evaluation of bone and soft tissue neoplasms.

4. To enhance portal vein opacification during arterial portography.

5. For hepatic or pancreatic arteriography for the evaluation of small vessel abnormalities. The vasodilatory effect of tolazoline on the pancreatic circulation is less than that of glucagon.[63]

6. For the evaluation of hypovascular lesions of the kidney.[64, 65]

A dose of 25 mg of tolazoline is diluted in 10 to 15 ml of flushing solution and injected as a slow bolus over 10 to 15 seconds.

**Contraindications and Side Effects.** Tolazoline should not be used in patients with coronary artery disease, arrhythmias, gastritis, peptic ulcer, or gastrointestinal bleeding.[58] In the dosage used for diagnostic arteriography, serious side effects are uncommon. The safety of intraarterial administration of tolazoline has been established by its widespread clinical usage.[59–62, 64–66]

## Glucagon

Glucagon is a hormone produced by the alpha cells of the pancreatic islets. Secretion of endogenous glucagon is regulated by the serum glucose levels. The biological half life is between 3 and 6 minutes.[67]

**Applications and Dosage.** Because of its actions on many different systems, glucagon has been used in a variety of clinical situations, eg, for the management of congestive heart failure, as a provocative test for pheochromocytoma, for hypotonic duodenography, and for transsphincter expulsion of choledochal calculi.[68, 69] Angiographic applications of glucagon are[70, 71]:

1. For vasodilatation in splanchnic and renal arteriography. The vasodilatory effect is sustained over a long period of time. In animal studies, vasodilatation is observed for up to 2 hours after administration of 0.5 mg of glucagon.[71] This vasodilatory effect is comparable to that of prostaglandin $E_1$ and acetylcholine. The advantages over the latter drug are that glucacon is readily available and can be administered as a bolus.

2. To prevent artefacts caused by bowel peristalsis during digital subtraction angiography.

3. As a physiological stimulant during pancreatic angiography.

For intravenous digital subtraction angiography, glucagon is injected as a slow intravenous bolus. The usual dosage is between 0.5 and 1.0 mg.

**Contraindications and Side Effects.** Glucagon is contraindicated in patients with pheochromocytoma (because of its ability to induce catecholamine release) and in hyperglycemic states. In the dosage used for vascular dilatation, it may cause nausea and vomiting. When used for digital subtraction angiography, reactive hyperperistalsis of the bowel, which occurs after the paretic effect wears off, may degrade the image quality significantly.

## MISCELLANEOUS APPLICATIONS

In addition to pharmacological manipulation of the vascular bed, secretory stimulation of the organ to be studied can be utilized to enhance visualization of smaller vessels (eg, secretin or glucagon stimulation for pancreatic angiography).[8, 72] Newer vasoactive pharmacological substances such as katanserin are also being evaluated and may find clinical application.

## REFERENCES

1. Weiner N: Norepinephrine, epinephrine, and the sympathomimetic amines. *In* Gilman AG, Goodman LS, Gilman A (eds.): The Pharmacological Basis of Therapeutics, 6th Ed. New York, Macmillan Publishing Co., Inc., 1980, pp 138–175.

2. Abrams HL, Obrez I, Hollenberg NK, et al: Pharmacoangiography of the renal vascular bed. Curr Prob Radiol 1:1–37, 1971.

3. Ekelund L, Gerlock AJ, Goncharenco V: The epinephrine effect in renal angiography revisited. Clin Radiol 29:387–392, 1978.

4. Boijsen E, Redman H: Effect of epinephrine on celiac and superior mesenteric angiography. Invest Radiol 2:184–199, 1967.

5. Kahn P, Wise HM: Simulation of renal tumor response to epinephrine by inflammatory disease. Radiology 89:1062–1064, 1967.

6. Caro G, Meisell R, Held B: Epinephrine enhanced arteriography in renal and perirenal abscess. A differential diagnostic problem. Radiology 92:1262–1264, 1969.

7. Rockoff SD, Doppman J, Block JB, et al: Variable response of tumor vessels to intraarterial epinephrine. An angiographic study in man. Invest Radiol 1:205–213, 1966.

8. Uden R: Secretin and epinephrine combined in celiac angiography. Acta Radiol 17:17–40, 1976.

9. Billing L, Lindgren AGH: Die pathologisch-anatomische Unterlage der Geschwulstarteriographie: eine Untersuchung der arteriellen Gefaesse des Hypernephroms und des Magenkarzinoms. Acta Radiol 25:625–640, 1944.

10. Castellino RA: Renal carcinoma demonstrated by postepinephrine arteriography following normal selective arteriograms. Radiology 97:607–608, 1970.

11. Smith JC, Roesch J, Athanasoulis CA, et al: Renal venography in the evaluation of poorly vascularized neoplasms of the kidney. AJR 123:552–556, 1975.

12. Abrams HL, Boijsen E, Borgstroem K-E: Effect of epinephrine on the renal circulation. Angiographic observations. Radiology 79:911–922, 1962.

13. Olin TB, Reuter SR: A pharmacoangiographic method for improving nephrophlebography. Radiology 85:1036–1042, 1965.

14. Kahn PC, Frates WJ, Paul RE: The epinephrine effect in angiography of gastrointestinal tract tumors. Radiology 88:686–690, 1967.

15. Goldstein HM, Miller M: Angiographic evaluation of carcinoid tumors of the small intestine: the value of epinephrine. Radiology 114:23–28, 1975.

16. Bohr DF, Uchida E: Individualities of vascular smooth muscles in response to angiotensin. Circ Res 21(Suppl 2):135–145, 1967.

17. Novak D, Weber J: Pharmakoangiographie mit Angiotensin. Fortschr Roentgenstr 124:301–309, 1976.

18. Ekelund L, Lunderquist A: Pharmacoangiography with angiotensin. Radiology 110:533–540, 1974.

19. Douglas WW: Polypeptides–Angiotensin, plasma kinins, and others. In Gilman AG, Goodman LS, Gilman A (eds.): The Pharmacological Basis of Therapeutics, 6th Ed. New York, Macmillan Publishing Co., Inc., 1980, pp 647–667.

20. Kaplan JH, Bookstein JJ: Abdominal visceral pharmacoangiography with angiotensin. Radiology 103:79–83, 1972.

21. Ekelund L, Laurin S, Lunderquist A: Comparison of a vasoconstrictor and a vasodilator in pharmacoangiography of bone and soft tissue tumors. Radiology 122:95–99, 1977.

22. Jekell K, Sandqvist S, Castenfors J: Angiotensin effect in the human kidney. Acta Radiol 19:329–336, 1978.

23. Weber J, Novak D: Abdominal und periphere Pharmakoangiographie mit Angiotensin und Bradykinin. Radiologe 16:524–536, 1976.

24. Hays RM: Agents affecting the renal conservation of water. In Gilman AG, Goodman LS, Gilman A (eds.): The Pharmacological Basis of Therapeutics, 6th Ed. New York, Macmillan Publishing Co., Inc., 1980, pp 916–928.

25. Baum S, Athanasoulis CA, Waltman AC: Gastrointestinal hemorrhage. II. Angiographic diagnosis and control. Adv Surg 7:149–198, 1973.

26. Kadir S, Ernst CB: Current concepts in angiographic management of gastrointestinal bleeding. Curr Prob Surg 20:287–343, 1983.

27. Simmons JT, Baum S, Sheehan BA, et al: The effect of vasopressin on hepatic arterial blood flow. Radiology 124:637–640, 1977.

28. Kerr JC, Hobson RW, Seelig RF, et al: Vasopressin: Route of administration and effects on canine hepatic and superior mesenteric arterial blood flows. Ann Surg 187:137–142, 1978.

29. Lindvall N: Pharmakoangiographie bei Nierencarcinom und Nierenbeckentumoren. Der Urologe 6:126–133, 1967.

30. Kahn PC: The epinephrine effect in selective renal angiography. Radiology 85:301–305, 1965.

31. Taylor P: Cholinergic agonists. In Gilman AG, Goodman LS, Gilman A (eds.): The Pharmacological Basis of Therapeutics. 6th Ed. New York, Macmillan Publishing Co., Inc., 1980, pp 91–99.

32. Rashid A, Hollenberg NK, Adams DF, et al: Effect of acetylcholine on the renal vasculature in normal man. J Appl Physiol 32:669–674, 1972.

33. Dollery CT, Goldberg LI, Pentecost BL: Effects of intrarenal infusions of bradykinin and acetylcholine on renal blood flow in man. Clin Sci 29:433–441, 1965.

34. Astroem A, Crafoord J, Samelius-Broberg U: Vasoconstrictor action of acetylcholine on kidney blood vessels. Acta Physiol Scand 61:159–164, 1964.

35. Hollenberg NK, Adams DF, Solomon H, et al: Renal vascular tone in essential and secondary hypertension: Hemodynamic and angiographic response to vasodilators. Medicine 54:29–44, 1975.

36. Freed TA, Hager H, Vinik M: Effects of intraarterial acetylcholine on renal arteriography in normal humans. AJR 104:312–318,1968.

37. Chuang VP, Fried AM: High dose renal pharmacoangiography in the assessment of hypovascular renal neoplasms. AJR 131:807–811, 1978.

38. McGiff JC, Burns RBP, Blumenthal MR: Role of acetylcholine in the renal vasoconstrictor response to sympathetic nerve stimulation in the dog. Circ Res 20:616–629, 1967.

39. Swift MR, LaDu BN: A rapid screening test for atypical serum cholinesterase. Lancet 1:513–514, 1966.

40. Antman E, Muller J, Goldberg S, et al: Nifedipine therapy for coronary artery spasm: experience in 127 patients. N Engl J Med 302:1269–1273, 1980.

41. Mueller HS, Chahine RA: Interim report of multicenter double blind, placebo controlled studies of nifedipine in chronic stable angina. Am J Med 71:645–657, 1981.

42. Neurath GB, Duenger M: Blood levels of the metabolites of glyceryl trinitrate and pentaerythritol tetranitrate after administration of a two step preparation. Arzneim Forsch 27:416–419, 1977.

43. Needleman P, Johnson EM, Jr: Vasodilators and the treatment of angina. In Gilman AG, Goodman, LS, Gilman A (eds.): The Pharmacological Basis of Therapeutics, 6th Ed. New York, Macmillan Publishing Co., Inc., 1980, pp 819–833.

44. Chahine RA: The provocation of coronary artery spasm. Cath Cardiovasc Diagn 6:1–5, 1980.

45. Siegelman SS, Sprayregen S, Boley SJ: Angiographic diagnosis of mesenteric arterial vasoconstriction. Radiology 112:533–542, 1974.

46. Athanasoulis CA: Bowel ischemia: Management with intraarterial papaverine infusion and transluminal angioplasty. In Athanasoulis CA, Pfister RC, Greene R et al (eds.): Interventional Radiology. Philadelphia, W. B. Saunders Co., 1982, pp 334–342.

47. Moncada S, Flower RJ, Vane JR: Prostaglandins, prostacyclin, and thromboxane A2. In Gilman AG, Goodman LS, Gilman A (eds.): The Pharmacological Basis of Therapeutics, 6th Ed. New York, Macmillan Publishing Co., Inc., 1980, pp 668–681.

48. Ferreiera SH, Vane JR: Prostaglandins: their disappearance from and release into the circulation. Nature 216:868–873, 1967.

49. Carlson LA, Ericsson M, Erikson U: Prostaglandin E$_1$ in peripheral arteriographies. Acta Radiol 14:583–587, 1973.

50. Jonsson K, Wallace S, Jacobson ED, et al: The use of prostaglandin E$_1$ for enhanced visualization of the splanchnic circulation. Radiology 125:373–378, 1977.

51. Davis LJ, Anderson JH, Wallace S, et al: The use of prostaglandin $E_1$ to enhance the angiographic visualization of the splanchnic circulation. Radiology 114:281–286, 1975.

52. Dencker H, Goethlin J, Hedner P, et al: Superior mesenteric angiography and blood flow following intraarterial injection of prostaglandin $F_{2\alpha}$. AJR 125:111–118, 1975.

53. Robinson BF, Collier JG, Karim SMM, et al: Effect of prostaglandins $A_1$, $A_2$, B, $E_2$, and $F_{2\alpha}$ on forearm arterial bed and superficial hand veins in man. Clin Sci 44:367–376, 1973.

54. Fara JW, Barth KH, White RI, et al: Mesenteric vascular effects of prostaglandin $F_{2\alpha}$ and $B_2$. Radiology 133:317–320, 1979.

55. Mathe AA, Hedqvist P, Holmgren A, et al: Bronchial hyperreactivity to prostaglandin $F_{2\alpha}$ and histamine in patients with asthma. Br Med J 1:193–196, 1973.

56. Kadir S, Athanasoulis CA: Peripheral vasospastic disorders: Management with intraarterial infusion of vasodilatory drugs. In Athanasoulis CA, Pfister RC, Greene R et al (eds.): Interventional Radiology. Philadelphia, W. B. Saunders Co., 1982, pp 343–354.

57. Kadir S, Kaufman SL, Barth KH, et al: Selected Techniques in Interventional Radiology. Philadelphia, W. B. Saunders Co., 1982, pp 142–207.

58. Weiner N: Drugs that inhibit adrenergic nerves and block adrenergic receptors. In Gilman AG, Goodman LS, Gilman A (eds.): The Pharmacological Basis of Therapeutics. 6th Ed. New York, Macmillan Publishing Co., Inc., 1980, pp 176–210.

59. Schreyer H, Schwarz G, Kerl H: Pharmakoangiographie mit Priscol bei progressiver Sklerodermie. Fortschr Roentgenstr 125:232–242, 1976.

60. Hawkins IF, Hudson, TM: Priscoline in bone and soft tissue angiography. Radiology 110:541–546, 1974.

61. Kadir S, Athanasoulis CA, Waltman AC: Tolazoline augmented angiography in the evaluation of bone and soft tissue tumors. Radiology 133:792–795, 1979.

62. Goldstein HM, Thaggard A, Wallace S, et al: Priscoline augmented hepatic angiography. Radiology 119:275–279, 1976.

63. Schmarsow R: Der pankreatographischer Effekt bei der pankreasangiographie nach Verabreichung von Glucagon. Fortschr Roentgenstr 124:310–314, 1976.

64. Smith DC, Faber BE: Priscoline enhancement of renal cyst wall visualization in arteriography. Appl Radiol 134–137:Nov–Dec, 1978.

65. Bron KM, Stilley JW, Shapiro AP: Renal arteriography enhanced by tolazoline. Value in the diagnosis of polyarteritis nodosa complicated by perinephric hematoma. Radiology 99:295–301, 1971.

66. Dahlin PA, Hawkins IF, Doering PL: The safety of tolazoline in renal angiography. AJR 137:381–386, 1981.

67. Alberti KGMM, Nattrass M: Editorial: The physiological function of glucagon. Eur J Clin Invest 7:151–154, 1977.

68. Parmley WM, Glick G, Sonnenblick EH: Cardiovascular effects of glucagon in man. N Engl J Med 279:12–17, 1968.

69. Latshaw RF, Kadir S, Witt WS, et al: Glucagon induced choledochal sphincter relaxation: Aid for expulsion of impacted calculi into the duodenum. AJR 137:614–616, 1981.

70. Danford RO, Davidson AJ: The use of glucagon as a vasodilator in visceral angiography. Radiology 93:173–175, 1969.

71. Danford RO: The effect of glucagon on renal hemodynamics and renal arteriography. AJR 108:665–673, 1970.

72. Taylor DA, Macken KL, Fiore AS: Angiographic visualization of the secretin stimulated pancreas. Radiology 87:525–526, 1966.

# Digital Subtraction Angiography (DSA)

Digital subtraction angiography (DSA) is a method for performing intravenous or intraarterial angiography with the aid of electronic contrast enhancement techniques. It differs from conventional angiography in that it is capable of detecting significantly lower concentrations of contrast medium (1 to 2% iodinated contrast medium) and utilizes electronic data storage and reporting (as opposed to the static recording of the conventional film). DSA and conventional angiography are not mutually exclusive. A combination of conventional angiography and intraarterial or intravenous DSA is often necessary in the evaluation, management, and follow-up of patients with vascular diseases involving multiple organ systems.

Presently, the spatial resolution for DSA is about 2 line pairs/mm, whereas the resolving power for conventional film angiography is greater than 6 line pairs/mm. Although vas-cular structures less than 1 mm can be identified by DSA, they lie below the diagnostic threshhold.

The basic technique involves acquisition of images before and after injection of contrast medium and electronic subtraction of the pre-contrast image from the post-contrast images with subsequent electronic enhancement and manipulation. Figure 7–1 shows a functional block diagram of a typical digital system.

Since a detailed discussion of DSA is beyond the scope of this book, interested readers are referred to references 1 to 5.

## EQUIPMENT AND BASIC PRINCIPLES OF DSA

For maximal utilization, the DSA unit should be integrated with equipment used for conventional angiography and/or inter-

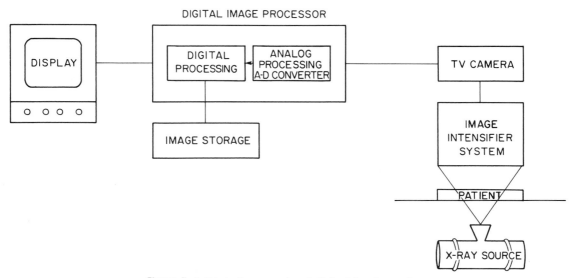

*Figure 7–1.* Block diagram of a digital subtraction system.

ventional radiology. Ideally, this should be a C or U arm in order to facilitate imaging in different projections without having to move the patient. Oblique positioning of the patient is often associated with involuntary patient motion and consequently gives rise to artefacts.

A radiographic tube with a high kV rating and heat dissipation is necessary in order to permit short exposure times. The resolution is best with a large matrix such as $512 \times 512$ pixels, which gives a spatial resolution of 0.7 mm.[6] With a $1024 \times 1024$ matrix, the spatial resolution is improved to 0.35 mm.

**Image Acquisition.** Acquisition of data may be in the form of continuous or pulsed x-ray exposure and the use of interlaced or noninterlaced (progressive) television operations. Pulsed, noninterlaced acquisition provides the best images. The maximal imaging rate for this type of operation is 10 frames/sec. With continuous exposure, dynamic imaging is possible at 30 frames/sec.

The television camera is the single most important factor for image acquisition. A high signal-to-noise ratio (1000:1) is essential for pulsed acquisition. Proper selection of x-ray exposure factors helps to decrease the quantum noise. Large image intensifiers (13 or 14 inch) with a flat field permit examination of larger sections of the body without geometrical distortion.

**Image Processing and Storage.** Images can be processed using either linear or logarithmic amplification. Logarithmic amplification provides a uniform distribution of contrast and may be applicable to body areas with highly contrasting tissue densities, such as the neck. Dual energy subtraction with K-enhancement or hybrid subtraction provides further improvement of the image quality.[7]

Image converters, also called A-D converters, are used to convert an analog into a digital image. This conversion results in a permanent loss of fine detail. The appearance of fine detail on the reprocessed image after digital to analog conversion (for display on a TV monitor or film) is artefactual and represents a creation of the system.[2, 3] Image storage can be in analog or digitized form.

### CATHETERS AND CONTRAST MEDIUM FOR INTRAVENOUS DSA

Contrast medium can be injected into a peripheral vein (brachial) or centrally into the superior vena cava or right atrium. A central injection is preferable, as it provides a better bolus and is associated with fewer complications.

**Catheters.** For a peripheral contrast injection, a short sheath (14 or 16 gauge angiocath) is placed in the brachial vein. For central contrast medium injection, 5 to 7 Fr catheters are used. Pigtail catheters are best suited from both the cubital and the femoral vein approaches. From the cubital vein approach, the catheter is placed in the superior vena cava or right atrium; from the femoral approach, it is placed in the hepatic segment of the inferior vena cava or the right atrium. Straight catheters with an end hole should not be used in the superior vena cava or right atrium. End hole–occluded straight or multipurpose catheters can be used safely in the superior vena cava. If intravenous DSA is combined with renal vein sampling for renin determination, a 6 or 7 Fr multiple hole multipurpose catheter can be used from the cubital vein approach. The catheter tip must be placed below the hepatic segment of the inferior vena cava, and the contrast injection rate should not exceed 18 ml/sec. A more proximally placed catheter or a higher injection rate may cause the catheter to recoil into the right ventricle.

Some of the currently available 5 Fr high flow nylon catheters are not recommended for intravenous DSA if high injection rates (> 17 ml/sec) are used. At high injection rates, uncoiling of the pigtail and catheter recoil have been observed. This may have been responsible for the atrial and caval perforation observed in some cases.

**Contrast Medium.** For intravenous DSA, undiluted 76% iodinated contrast medium is used. The contrast injection rates used in different institutions vary from 12 ml/sec to 35 ml/sec.[8, 9] Higher flow rates reflect the viewpoint that a single bolus of contrast medium provides optimal opacification. However, a bolus effect is possible only in individuals with a normal cardiac output. Moreover, a fast injection rate in the relatively low pressure atrium or vena cava will invariably cause reflux of contrast medium into jugular or hepatic veins and consequently leads to dilution and loss of the bolus effect.

For the peripheral injection into a brachial vein, 30 to 40 ml of contrast medium is injected at 12 to 15 ml/sec as a contrast-saline bolus (approximately 20 ml of 0.45% saline is layered upon the contrast medium in the

**TABLE 7–1.** Catheters and Flow Rates for Intravenous and Intraarterial DSA

| Catheter | | | Flow Rate* (ml/sec) | Guide Wire (inch) | Manufacturer |
|---|---|---|---|---|---|
| Size (Fr) | Type | Length (cm) | | | |
| 4 | Pigtail PU-N | 65 | 18 | 0.032 | Mallinckrodt |
| | | 90 | 15 | 0.032 | |
| 4 | Pigtail | 65 | 15 | 0.035 | Cook, Inc. |
| | Royal flush II | 110 | 11 | | |
| 5 | Pigtail PU-N† | 65 | 28 | 0.032 | Mallinckrodt |
| | | 90 | 25 | 0.032 | |
| 5 | Pigtail | 65 | 27 | 0.035 | Cook, Inc. |
| | Royal flush II | 110 | 19 | 0.035 | |

*Undiluted contrast medium.

†Ultra high flow catheters are also available. These accept 0.035 inch guide wires but do not provide a significantly higher flow rate for the 90 cm length catheter (27 ml/sec).

PU-N = polyurethane-nylon.

injector syringe and serves to drive the contrast medium into the central venous system). However, in our experience 18 to 20 ml/sec for a total of 25 ml injected into the superior vena cava or the right atrium has provided the optimal result. In an occasional patient, a larger volume, ie, 30 to 35 ml of contrast medium, is necessary to provide satisfactory images.

## CATHETERS AND CONTRAST MEDIUM FOR INTRAARTERIAL DSA

**Catheters.** Inpatient intraarterial DSA can be performed with standard angiographic catheters. Outpatient intraarterial DSA is performed with 5 Fr catheters provided the patients can be observed for at least 4 hours following the study. If the 4 Fr catheter system is used for outpatients, the observation period following DSA could be reduced to 3 hours. Bleeding complications can be reduced by a single wall arterial puncture. An 18 gauge, 2¾ inch hollow stylet needle with a perforated stylet hub (for bleeding back) may be used for this purpose (UMI, Ballston Spa, New York). Table 7–1 lists some of the smaller Fr catheters and flow rates for intravenous and intraarterial DSA.

With some 4 Fr catheters, the maximal contrast injection rate is limited to about 15 ml/sec. This is sufficient for the evaluation of the vascular system distal to the aortic arch. In the ascending aorta, the contrast injection rate can usually be increased by approximately 3 to 4 ml over that recommended by the manufacturer. This is possible because the maximal injection rates for catheters are usually determined with undiluted, high viscosity contrast agents. Alternatively, a higher concentration of the contrast medium is used (eg, 30% instead of 15%).

The 5 Fr catheters are ideally suited for outpatient arteriography. The difference in size (in comparison with the 4 Fr catheters) is minimal (1 Fr = 0.33 mm), and the 5 Fr catheters permit a higher contrast delivery rate and provide better torque for selective catheterization.

**Iodinated Contrast Medium.** A 12 to 20% concentration is used for DSA of thoracic and abdominal vessels. The contrast injection rate and volume should be about 75% of that used for standard angiography (eg, 15 ml/sec for a total of 30 ml for abdominal aortography). For pulmonary arteriography with the catheter in the pulmonary artery, a 30% concentration is used. If a right atrial/superior vena caval injection is performed for pulmonary arteriography, undiluted contrast medium is used.

The filming rates for intraarterial DSA are the same as for conventional arteriography. When imaging close to the contrast injection site, the injection must be delayed to provide two or more images without contrast; this is necessary for remasking.

For DSA of the popliteal and distal vessels, a 20 or 30% concentration provides the best images when contrast medium is injected at the aortic bifurcation in a retrograde fashion. A 30% concentration is often necessary for satisfactory demonstration of the vessels distal to the ankles. For antegrade femoral arteriography, a 15 to 20% concentration is used. Between 25 and 35 ml of diluted contrast medium is used for each injection. Tables 7–2 and 7–3 show the different dilution factors for some of the iodinated contrast media for intraarterial DSA.

**TABLE 7–2.** Contrast Dilutions for Intraarterial DSA and Venography Using 60% Diatrizoate Meglumine Sodium

| Contrast Solution | Dilution Factor | Injector Syringe Mixture |
|---|---|---|
| 12% | 4:1 | 20 ml contrast, 80 ml 5% dextrose |
| 15% | 3:1 | 25 ml contrast, 75 ml 5% dextrose |
| 20% | 2:1 | 30 ml contrast, 60 ml 5% dextrose |
| 30% | 1:1 | 50 ml contrast, 50 ml 5% dextrose |

**Carbon Dioxide.** In patients allergic to iodinated contrast agents or in renal failure, intraarterially injected carbon dioxide may be used as an alternative. It is recommended only for use below the diaphragm and in the supine position. The advantages of carbon dioxide as a contrast agent for intraarterial DSA are[10, 11]:

1. It is a vasodilator and therefore provides enhanced visualization of small vessels.

2. There is virtually no limitation to the volume of carbon dioxide that can be used, except in patients with chronic obstructive lung disease.

3. Demonstration of arteriovenous shunting in tumors is enhanced. Early venous opacification is more likely to be detected by carbon dioxide DSA than with iodinated contrast agents. This is most likely due to easier passage of the smaller carbon dioxide molecule through the abnormal arteriovenous communications.

4. Less discomfort is experienced than with conventional iodinated contrast agents. However, approximately one fourth of patients experience a sensation similar to that associated with injection of iodinated contrast agents. The remainder note a "warm, tingling" sensation.

5. There is an absence of allergic reactions.

6. Images obtained by injection of carbon

dioxide are comparable to those obtained by iodinated contrast agents (Fig. 7–2).

The major disadvantage of the use of carbon dioxide as a contrast agent for DSA is the compressibility of the gas, which requires a special delivery system with a variable injection rate. With the development and marketing of a simple delivery system, carbon dioxide may replace iodinated contrast agents for the evaluation of vascular diseases of the extremities.

## PATIENT SELECTION AND PREPARATION FOR DSA

The selection of a patient for DSA should be determined by the status of renal and cardiac function, the type of information desired, and any history of contrast medium–related problems. Not only do these criteria determine whether DSA would provide the information that is sought but they also help decide whether an intravenous or an intraarterial study should be performed.

**Renal Function.** The status of the renal function of many outpatients may not be known. When there is no history of renal problems, diabetes mellitus, or other diseases predisposing to contrast medium–induced renal failure (eg, proteinuria, sickle cell disease), no problems should be anticipated. If an extensive screening is to be performed (eg, for peripheral vascular disease), BUN and creatinine levels should be determined before proceeding with DSA.

Patients with mild renal failure (serum creatinine up to 3.0 mg/dl) should not be considered for intravenous DSA unless a limited study (one or two contrast injections) is to be performed. The risk of further deterioration of renal function, which could occur with contrast administration to such patients, must be weighed against the potential diagnostic benefits of the study. In patients with a serum creatinine > 3.0 mg/dl, intravenous DSA should not be attempted unless for compelling circumstances. Such patients should be studied by intraarterial DSA.

**Cardiac Status.** Patients with congestive heart failure and poor cardiac output are not suited for intravenous DSA because of the fluid load associated with intravenous administration of contrast medium. In addition, the contrast bolus may be diluted significantly, so that the images are of poor quality.

**Type of Information.** Because of the relatively low spatial resolution, DSA may not

**TABLE 7–3.** Contrast Dilutions for Intraarterial DSA and Venography Using 76% Diatrizoate Meglumine Sodium

| Contrast Solution | Dilution Factor | Injector Syringe Mixture |
|---|---|---|
| 15% | 4:1 | 20 ml contrast, 80 ml 5% dextrose |
| 20% | 3:1 | 25 ml contrast, 75 ml 5% dextrose |

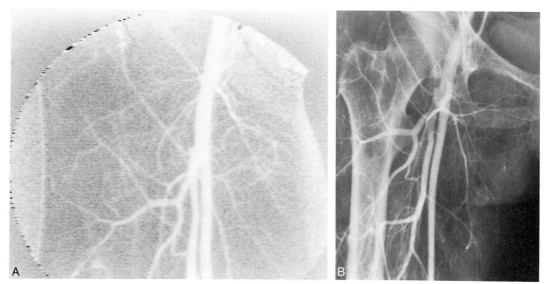

*Figure 7–2. A,* Digital subtraction angiogram using carbon dioxide as a contrast agent. *B,* Conventional cut film arteriogram using iodinated contrast medium for comparison. (Courtesy of Dr. Irwin F. Hawkins.)

be suited for the evaluation of subtle abnormalities or small vessel disease.

**History of Contrast Medium–Related Problems.** Patients with a history of contrast medium reactions, other than a mild skin rash, should not be studied as outpatients. Patients who have developed an urticarial skin rash following a previous contrast study should be premedicated with an antihistamine (eg, Benadryl, 50 mg twice daily for two doses) before the study. At the time of the study, an additional 25 mg of Benadryl is injected intravenously.

Outpatients are hydrated by increasing oral fluid intake. Premedication is usually not necessary. An intravenous sedative, eg, diazepam (Valium), may be given during the study if the need arises. Food intake is withheld for at least 6 hours prior to the study. As with other angiographic procedures, intake of clear fluids is permitted. In patients who are to undergo DSA of the abdominal vessels, a bowel prep (similar to a barium enema prep) is advisable.

During the study, intravenous fluids are administered via the catheter in between contrast injections. Upon completion of the study, the patients are again advised to increase oral fluid intake for several hours to prevent dehydration.

## IMAGING

For intravenous DSA, the time delay between contrast injection and imaging can be estimated by observing the propagation of a small bolus injection of contrast medium after the catheter has been positioned. Considerable individual variations are observed, depending upon myocardial function, pulse rate, venous pressure, injection site, rate of contrast injection, and location of the vessels being imaged. For imaging of the brachiocephalic vessels, the preceding aortic arch study provides an estimate of the time delay. Alternatively, calculation of the circulation time can be used to predict the arrival of contrast medium at the area being imaged.[12]

For larger vessels and those with fast flow (aorta and carotid and pulmonary arteries), images are obtained at 2 to 3/sec for a total of 10 to 15 images and subsequently at 1/sec for an additional 6 to 8 images. In the pelvis and extremities, after an appropriate delay, images are obtained at 1 to 2/sec for a total of 12 to 15 images. In individuals with slow flow, the image acquisition rate may be decreased further. For the evaluation of arteriovenous fistulae, an imaging rate of 3/sec or faster is used. Table 7–4 shows a typical imaging program for the cervicocerebral vessels.

## INTRAARTERIAL DSA

Intraarterial DSA can be used in conjunction with almost any arterial study provided the patient is cooperative. Common applications are:

1. Interventional radiological procedures

**TABLE 7–4.** DSA of the Carotid and
Vertebral Arteries

| | |
|---|---|
| Approach | Cubital or femoral vein |
| Catheter: | 5 or 6 Fr pigtail |
|   Position | Superior vena cava, inferior vena cava, or right atrium |
| Contrast medium: | 76% Diatrizoate meglumine sodium |
|   Injection rate | 18 to 20 ml/sec, total 25 ml |
| Imaging: | |
|   Delay | 4 to 5 sec* |
|   Rate | 2 images/sec for 10 images; 1 image/sec for 8 images |
|   Projections† | a. 55–60° RPO arch aortogram |
| | b. 45–55° LPO neck |
| | c. 45–55° RPO neck |
|   Optional | AP, Townes, lateral, or off-lateral view to evaluate intracranial circulation |
| Image intensifier mode | 9–14 inch for aortic arch |
| | 6 inch for neck and intracranial |

*Varies with cardiac output. Can usually be assessed by the arch study.

†Additional views (steeper oblique or AP neck) may be needed if the carotid bifurcations are not well visualized on two projections.

such as angioplasty and transcatheter embolization.[13] Because of the low contrast load on renal function, diagnostic arteriography and therapeutic embolization can be performed in one sitting.

2. Evaluation of peripheral vascular disease. An additional advantage of this technique is that the arterial catheter can be used to obtain physiological data (intraarterial pressures, blood flow measurements) at the time of the study.

3. Evaluation of patients with suspected renovascular hypertension or transplant renal artery stenosis and potential kidney donors.

4. Other applications. These include arch aortography for the evaluation of carotid and vertebral artery disease (upon completion of a cardiac catheterization or peripheral arteriography),[13] evaluation of arteriovenous malformations, and arterial portography.[14]

The advantages of intraarterial DSA are:

1. Reduction in the total volume of contrast medium needed to complete an arteriogram. This is particularly attractive in patients with compromised renal function.

2. Reduction in arterial catheter time because of the speed of the examination.

3. Significant reduction in contrast medium–related discomfort.

4. Good image quality for both selective

and nonselective arteriography of larger vessels.

5. Smaller catheters (4 and 5 Fr) can be used if necessary. This facilitates outpatient angiography.

6. Carbon dioxide can be used in patients with evidence of an allergy to iodinated contrast medium, in patients with renal failure, or for the evaluation of peripheral vascular disease of the lower extremities.

7. Reduction in cost of the examination (fewer films).

## INTRAVENOUS DSA

The indications for intravenous DSA are derived mainly from its applicability as a relatively less invasive outpatient angiographic procedure. Indications include:

1. Evaluation of the carotid and vertebral arteries in the neck.

2. Screening for diseases of the aorta and its major branches.

3. Screening for vascular diseases of the extremities.

4. Screening for renovascular hypertension. This may be done in conjunction with venous sampling for renin.

5. Evaluation of patients without arterial access for intraarterial DSA or conventional arteriography.

6. Follow-up of patients after vascular reconstruction or interventional vascular radiological procedures.

7. For the detection of venous occlusion.

There are several limitations of intravenous DSA that may compromise its applicability:

1. Susceptibility to artefacts. The most frequent artefacts are due to motion, eg, patient, respiratory, peristalsis, or intrinsic blood vessel motion (systolic/diastolic change in caliber). The single most important factor responsible for poor studies is patient motion. Therefore, such studies can be performed only on patients who can cooperate. Many of the minor artefacts can be eliminated by the use of more advanced methods for subtraction and image manipulation.

2. High contrast volume requirement. This may be the cause of an incomplete study. For example, evaluation of the lower extremities with 9 inch image intensifiers necessitates a second study to complete the evaluation, unless the initial procedure is tailored to the area of interest.[15] In addition, status of

the renal function is often unknown, and the maximal contrast volume used for outpatients should therefore be kept below 180 ml.

3. The overall quality of the images is inferior to that of intraarterial DSA or conventional arteriography because of lower spatial resolution (this may result in a branch vessel abnormality being overlooked), overlapping of vessels, loss of vascular detail (due to overlapping vessels or enhancement of the parenchymal phase), and the variables associated with transportation of the contrast bolus.

4. A higher incidence of contrast reactions has been observed following intravenous administration.[16]

Despite these limitations, when used for the proper indications and with appropriate techniques, intravenous DSA is an excellent procedure for the evaluation of a variety of vascular problems. The results of intravenous DSA are less likely to be disappointing if patient selection is made with due consideration of the capabilities and limitations of DSA.

Although the spatial resolution is lower, DSA does provide higher contrast resolution and is less invasive than arteriography. For the technologist, DSA is faster and easier to perform. In addition, it has a lower procedure cost, thereby providing savings in film and hospitalization costs.

## APPLICATIONS OF DSA

This discussion will focus primarily upon the applications of intravenous DSA. The uses of intraarterial DSA are described in the appropriate chapters.

### Cervicocerebral Vascular Diseases

Intravenous DSA provides an excellent method of screening for extracerebral vascular diseases. In several studies comparing intravenous DSA and conventional arteriography, it is apparent that the diagnostic accuracy depends mainly upon two factors: the quality of the images and the severity of the disease.[8, 17]

With good quality images, the accuracy of intravenous DSA is reported to be 97%.[17, 17a] With poorer quality images this may be as low as 58%, with over- and underestimation of the severity of lesions occurring with greater frequency. Although large ulcerations and plaques are easily recognized, small plaques and shallow ulcers often go undetected by intravenous DSA.[8, 18]

In vertebrobasilar disease, diagnostic quality images of the vertebral arteries have been obtained in 90% of patients, of the basilar artery in 76% of patients, and of the posterior cerebral arteries in only 42% of patients.[18]

However, in our experience and that of some others, intravenous DSA of the neck vessels has been disappointing.[19] The inability to visualize both carotid bifurcations and under- and overestimation of stenosis have been the major problems.

**Applications and Technique** (Fig. 7–3)

1. Screening of symptomatic patients with cerebrovascular ischemia. If a hemodynamically significant abnormality is demonstrated, this finding (with the exception of arterial occlusion) should be confirmed by arteriography (conventional or DSA). However, good quality images can be accepted for preoperative decision making.

2. Evaluation of patients with diminished brachial pulses or upper extremity claudication.

3. Evaluation of asymptomatic patients with a neck bruit or a pulsatile mass.

Evaluation of the neck vessels should include an oblique arch aortogram in a 55 to 60° right posterior oblique (RPO) position. The inaccuracy of single plane arteriography of the cervicocerebral vessels is well known. Therefore, in patients with a supraclavicular bruit or suspected vertebral artery disease, a second projection (55 to 60° left posterior oblique, LPO) should be obtained (see Fig. 9–14, Chapter 9). Similarly, if the carotid bifurcations are not adequately visualized in two projections, significant abnormalities may be overlooked.[19]

Table 7–4 shows a program for intravenous DSA examination of the cervicocerebral vessels. Intracranial views are obtained in patients with vertebrobasilar ischemia, steal syndromes, and occlusion of the cervical portion of a carotid artery. Good quality images can be accepted for preoperative and clinical decision making.[18, 20]

### Thoracic Aorta

Intravenous DSA can be used to evaluate the thoracic aorta in a number of diseases.[21, 22] In one series, a 95% accuracy rate was reported, although comparison was not made with conventional arteriography in all

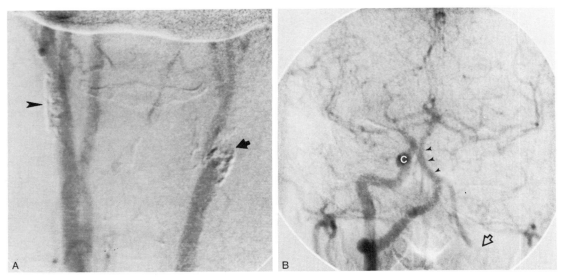

*Figure 7–3.* Intravenous DSA of the neck vessels and intracranial circulation. *A,* AP view of the neck vessels shows a calcified plaque and complete occlusion of the left internal carotid artery (*arrow*). The left vertebral artery is also occluded. A calcified plaque is present at the right common carotid bifurcation (*arrowhead*). *B,* AP view of the intracranial circulation (23 ml of undiluted 76% contrast medium). The intracranial portion of the left internal carotid artery does not opacify. However, there is cross filling of its branches from the right. The basilar artery is nicely demonstrated (*arrowheads*) with retrograde opacification of the left vertebral artery (*open arrow*). C = right carotid artery.

patients studied.[21] Inability to demonstrate the coronary arteries makes this study unsatisfactory for the evaluation of patients with suspected acute dissection of the ascending aorta.[21]

**Applications and Technique** (Figs. 7–4 and 7–5)

1. Screening for aneurysms, atherosclerosis, and other occlusive diseases (eg, aortitis),

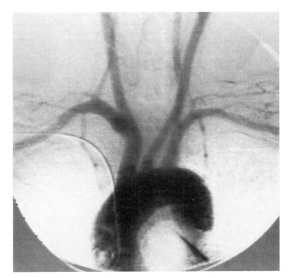

*Figure 7–4.* Normal arch aortogram using intravenous DSA. Pigtail catheter is in the superior vena cava.

type III or B aortic dissection, coarctation of the aorta.

2. Follow-up of patients after surgical repair of aortic dissections[22] and coarctation, vascular bypass surgery of the arch vessels, and follow-up angiography of patients treated by balloon angioplasty for re-stenosis at the surgical repair site of aortic coarctation.

3. Intravenous DSA may provide a satisfactory method for following patients with Marfan's syndrome before and after operation (replacement of the aortic valve and ascending aorta) and in patients with suspected operative complications (eg, false aneurysms).

Conventional aortography is still necessary for the evaluation of subtle abnormalities since image artefacts may seriously limit the accuracy of intravenous DSA of the thoracic aorta. In addition, aortic valve insufficiency cannot be detected by intravenous DSA.

Images are obtained in the standard projections used for conventional aortography. The descending aorta is evaluated in the lateral, LPO and/or steep RPO projections to avoid overlapping of the heart.

### Abdominal Aorta

Intravenous DSA can be used to screen for diseases of the abdominal aorta and its major

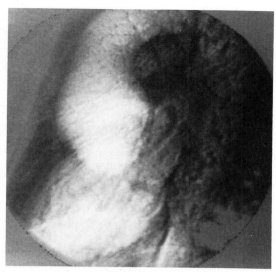

*Figure 7–5.* Ascending aortogram in the RPO projection in a patient with Marfan's syndrome (20 ml/sec; total 25 ml injected into the inferior vena cava). There is a typical "tulip" appearance of the aortic sinuses due to dilation of the sinotubular junction.

branches.[23, 24] One of its major applications is the follow-up and evaluation of a condition previously recognized by contrast aortography, computed tomography, or ultrasonography (eg, asymptomatic abdominal aortic aneurysm, renal artery stenosis, or aortic grafts).

The availability of a method for obtaining measurements of the vascular lumen makes intravenous DSA attractive for the follow-up of patients with asymptomatic aortic aneurysms.[25]

### Applications and Technique

1. Screening for occlusive diseases of the aorta and its major branches.

2. Follow-up of asymptomatic aneurysms.

3. Evaluation of patients with recurrent symptoms after vascular surgery or percutaneous transluminal angioplasty.

Images are obtained in the standard projections used for conventional film arteriography.

### Pulmonary Vessels

Intravenous DSA is a suitable and accurate method of evaluation for patients with suspected large pulmonary emboli, pulmonary arteriovenous malformations, or suspected pulmonary artery aneurysms. However, it requires a cooperative patient capable of suspending respiration for the duration of the imaging. With the catheter in the superior vena cava, diagnostic quality images of the pulmonary arteries can be obtained in 96% of cases.[26] In one study comparing intravenous DSA with conventional arteriography, the accuracy of intravenous DSA for the detection of pulmonary emboli in first- to third-order pulmonary artery branches was 75%.[27] Similar results were obtained in animal studies.[27a]

In addition to the usual angiographic criteria for pulmonary emboli (vascular occlusion, intraluminal defects), evaluation of the parenchymal phase (diminished perfusion) can also be used as an indirect method to aid in establishing a diagnosis and to assess the pattern of pulmonary perfusion.[26, 28] The demonstration of defects in the parenchymal phase images in correlation with an arterial abnormality enhances the accuracy of intravenous DSA.[27a, 28] However, such information may not always be available, as the quality of these images may be compromised by patient motion. The venous phase of the pulmonary angiogram can also be evaluated for anomalies of venous return (see Fig. 19–21, Chapter 19).

One disadvantage of this technique is that pulmonary artery pressures are not measured. In addition, a potential source of error is the right mid-lung window, which normally has diminished perfusion.[29] Suspected embolism to this region must be evaluated carefully to avoid misinterpretation.[28]

### Applications and Technique (Fig. 7–6)

1. Detection of pulmonary emboli.

2. Detection of pulmonary artery aneurysms and arteriovenous malformations.

3. Evaluation of anomalous pulmonary venous return.

4. Assessment of vascular encasement by mediastinal tumor or inflammatory processes (see Fig. 19–36, Chapter 19).

Images are obtained in the standard projections used for pulmonary arteriography.

### Splanchnic Vessels

Intraarterial DSA can be used for the evaluation of some abnormalities of the hepatic, splenic, and mesenteric vessels (eg, occlusive diseases, false aneurysms). It is of invaluable aid for localization of arterioportal fistulae and during transcatheter embolization. We have found it to be particularly useful for arterial portography and the evaluation of shunt patency in patients with portal hypertension (Fig. 7–7).

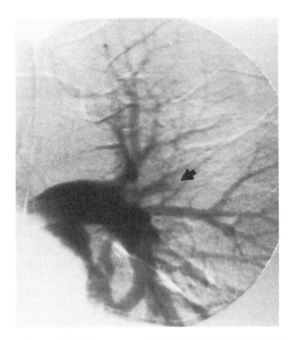

**Figure 7–6.** Intravenous DSA (right atrial injection, 25 ml of undiluted 76% contrast medium) demonstrates an embolus in a second-order pulmonary artery branch (*arrow*).

For the evaluation of the venous phase of superior mesenteric and celiac arteriograms, 15 to 20 ml of undiluted (76%) contrast medium is injected at a rate of 5 to 7 ml/sec. The injection of a vasodilator (25 mg of tolazoline) enhances venous opacification. Images are obtained every other second for a total of 12 to 15 images.

DSA–arterial portography can be used as a substitute for conventional arterial portography. However, in some cases, it provides less information than conventional arterial portography because of the poorer resolution and smaller field size (if a 9 inch image intensifier is used) (Fig. 7–8). In the latter situation, several contrast injections may be required.

Additional applications are percutaneous splenoportography and intravenous DSA for preoperative definition of celiac and mesenteric arterial anatomy (for operative placement of a chemotherapy infusion pump).

## Renal Vessels and Renal Transplants

Intravenous DSA can be used to assess the vascularity and vascular supply of large renal

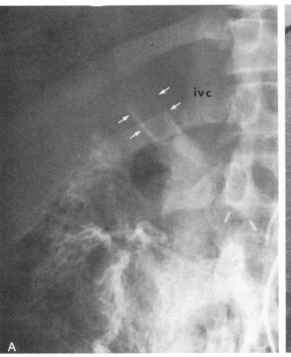

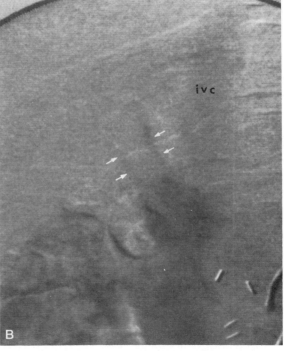

**Figure 7–7.** Digital subtraction arterial portography. Postoperative evaluation of a mesocaval shunt in a patient with sarcoid liver disease. *A,* Venous phase of a conventional cut film superior mesenteric arteriogram shows a thrombus in the portal vein (*arrows*) and opacification of the inferior vena cava (ivc) through the patent mesocaval shunt (60 ml of 76% contrast medium was injected). *B,* Venous phase of a digital subtraction superior mesenteric arteriogram using 18 ml of 76% contrast medium also shows portal vein thrombosis (*arrows*) and vena caval opacification (ivc).

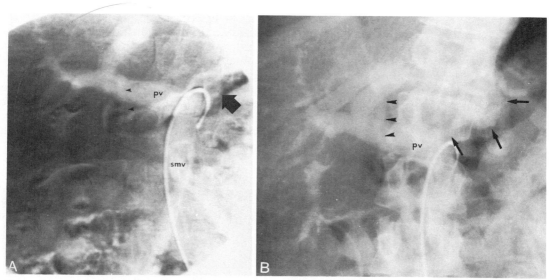

**Figure 7–8.** Digital subtraction arterial portography. Limitations of the technique. *A,* Venous phase of a digital subtraction superior mesenteric arteriogram using 20 ml of 76% contrast medium. The superior mesenteric vein (smv) and the portal vein (pv) are nicely demonstrated. There is only faint opacification of the umbilical vein (*arrowheads*), which could easily be overlooked. Gastric varices are not demonstrated because of small field size (9 inch image intensifier) and gastric air artefact (*arrow*). *B,* Venous phase of a conventional cut film superior mesenteric arteriogram shows the umbilical vein (*arrowheads*) and the gastroesophageal varices (*arrows*).

tumors. Enhancement of the parenchymal phase may obscure some smaller intrarenal lesions. However, with the 6 inch image intensifier mode and careful evaluation of the early images obtained in rapid sequence

(2 to 3 images/sec), some of the smaller lesions can also be detected (Fig. 7–9). The radiologist should personally format the images obtained by DSA so that the appropriate phases are available for evaluation.

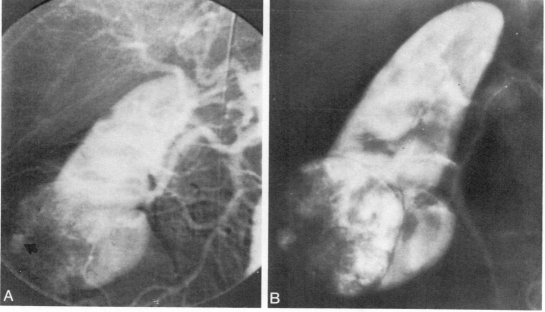

**Figure 7–9.** Digital subtraction renal arteriography for tumor evaluation. *A,* Intravenous DSA (6 inch image intensifier mode) of the right kidney in a patient with renal cell carcinoma. A lower pole mass with a smaller hypervascular nodule (*arrow*) is seen. *B,* Comparative right renal arteriogram using cut film.

In the majority of patients, angiography is no longer necessary for the diagnosis or staging of renal tumors. This is now accomplished noninvasively by computed body tomography. Angiography serves primarily for demonstration of vascularity, vascular supply, and venous involvement (renal vein, inferior vena cava) and occasionally for preoperative embolization of large hypervascular tumors.

Most hypervascular renal tumors are depicted accurately by intravenous DSA. Thus, tumor vascularity and blood supply can be evaluated (Fig. 7–10). If DSA is performed from the femoral vein approach, the inferior vena cava can also be evaluated. This is possible by using diluted contrast medium (digital subtraction venography) or by using a two-phase imaging procedure after a single contrast injection. In the first phase, images

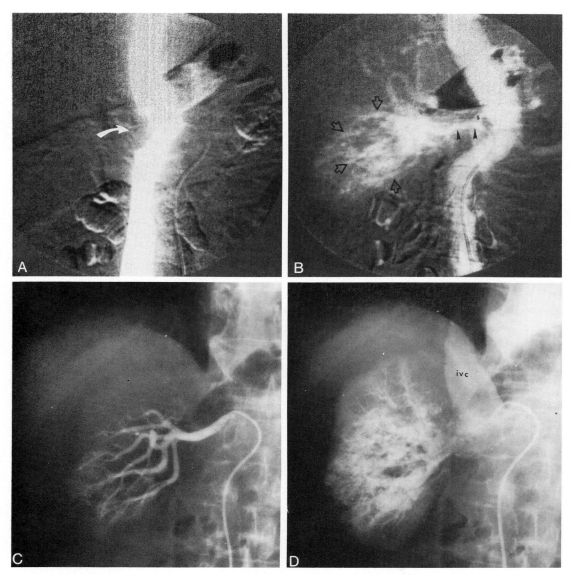

*Figure 7–10.* Digital subtraction renal angiography for tumor staging. *A*, Inferior vena cavagram obtained during contrast injection in the distal inferior vena cava shows tumor protruding into the lumen (*arrow*). *B*, Arterial phase of the DSA shows the right renal artery (*arrowheads*) and a large hypervascular right renal tumor (*open arrows*). S = superior mesenteric artery. *C* and *D*, Early and late arterial phases of the renal arteriogram. There is early opacification of the inferior vena cava (*ivc*). Note that the arteriovenous shunting is not demonstrated on the DSA. (Same patient as in Figures 13–6 and 13–9).

of the inferior vena cava are obtained immediately after injection of undiluted contrast medium. The second (arterial) phase is programmed to begin several seconds later (Fig. 7–10). Computed body tomography together with intravenous DSA may therefore be sufficient for preoperative evaluation of most renal tumors.

The accuracy of intravenous DSA for the assessment of renal artery stenosis is between 71 and 89%.[23, 30, 31] However, stenoses of the intrarenal branches may go undetected. Because of the imaging problems in the abdomen, the incidence of nondiagnostic studies can be as high as 16%.[23] The accuracy of intravenous DSA for the determination of vascular anatomy in potential kidney donors is about 83%.[32] The smaller accessory arteries are most likely to be missed.

Although visualization of the intrarenal branches may be suboptimal in renal transplants, intravenous DSA may provide a method of screening for surgically correctable lesions.[33, 34] However, angiographic assessment of renal transplants is performed only in symptomatic patients. Our experience with intravenous DSA in renal transplants has been disappointing because diagnostic quality images cannot be obtained consistently as a result of bowel artefacts and overlapping vessels. In addition, several injections of contrast medium are frequently required because several projections are necessary to delineate the course of the transplant artery and evaluate the intrarenal branches. Such large volumes of contrast medium are not tolerated well by patients with compromised renal function. Thus, in our experience, renal transplants are best evaluated with intraarterial DSA (Fig. 7–11).

When considering the applications for intravenous DSA of the kidney, the following limitations must be kept in mind:

1. Abnormalities of intrarenal branches may go undetected (Fig. 7–12). This is due to a low spatial resolution and enhancement of the nephrogram, which may then obscure detail.

2. Smaller mass lesions may remain undetected.

3. Accessory renal arteries may be overlooked.

**Applications and Technique** (Figs. 7–9 to 7–13)

1. Screening for renal artery stenosis (main renal arteries or larger branches) in patients with hypertension. The DSA can be combined with venous sampling.

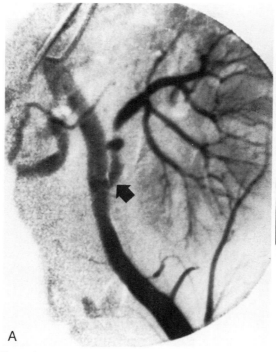

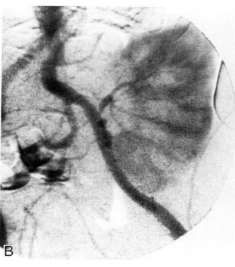

A

B

*Figure 7–11.* Renal transplant evaluation with DSA. *A,* Intraarterial DSA using 12 ml of a 10% contrast solution shows multiple areas of stenosis of the transplant renal artery. Arrow points to the stenosis at the anastomosis with the external iliac artery. *B,* Comparative image from an intravenous DSA. There is overlapping of the main renal and the external iliac arteries. The intrarenal branches are poorly defined.

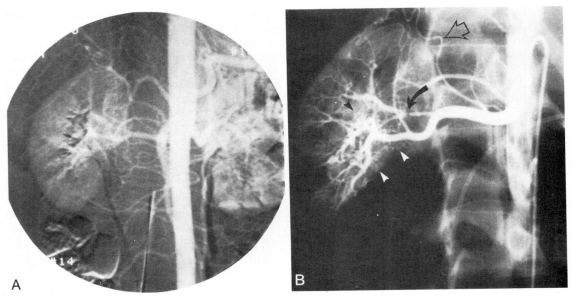

**Figure 7–12.** Limitations of intravenous DSA for the evaluation of small vessel abnormalities. *A*, Intravenous DSA of the right renal artery in an 18 year old hypertensive patient shows no vascular abnormality. *B*, Right renal arteriogram shows a severe stenosis of an extrarenal branch (*arrow*). Numerous intrarenal collaterals are present (*arrowheads*). In addition, the capsular artery is enlarged and also serves as a collateral (*open arrow*).

2. Evaluation of patients after renal artery angioplasty or bypass surgery.

3. Initial evaluation of renal transplants.

4. Evaluation of some cases of renal trauma.

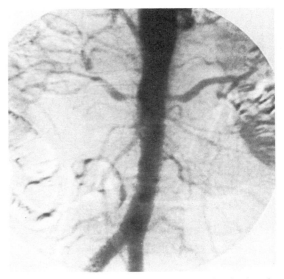

**Figure 7–13.** Intravenous DSA of the abdominal aorta (30 ml of contrast medium injected into the superior vena cava) shows bilateral renal artery stenosis in a patient with hypertension.

5. Preoperative assessment of tumor vascularity and caval extension of renal carcioma.

For evaluation of the renal arteries, the abdominal aorta is imaged in the AP or slight RPO projection or both. For transplant kidneys in the pelvis, an AP or a 25° ipsilateral posterior oblique projection is obtained to evaluate the nephrogram and the proximal branches. The anastomosis often requires imaging in a steep ipsilateral posterior oblique or a lateral projection. In the latter, considerable overlapping of vessels often occurs and significant stenoses can be overlooked. Therefore, renal transplant patients are best evaluated by intraarterial DSA. The added advantage of the intraarterial technique is that the study can be performed with as little as 6 to 10 ml of 76% contrast medium, including test injection for placement of the catheter from the contralateral iliac artery. Similarly, potential kidney donors can also be studied by outpatient intraarterial DSA.

### Extremities

DSA plays an increasingly important role in the management of vascular diseases of the extremities. Presently, intravenous DSA is suited only for a focused evaluation of a given problem, owing to limitations of image intensifier field size and high contrast volume requirements. Comprehensive screening of both extremities for occlusive arterial disease (which may require AP and oblique images) with the widely used 9 inch image intensifiers necessitates two sittings. However, with the 13 and 14 inch image intensifiers, a com-

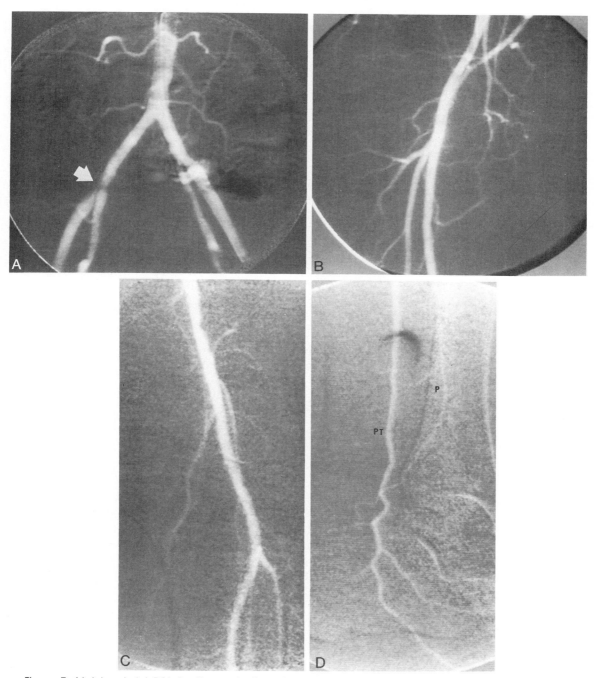

*Figure 7–14.* Intraarterial DSA for the evaluation of peripheral vascular disease (7ml/sec for 12 ml total of approximately 30% contrast medium was injected each time). *A,* AP pelvic arteriogram shows an iliac artery stenosis with a calcified plaque (*arrow*). *B,* Right common femoral arteriogram. *C,* Left popliteal arteriogram. *D,* Lateral view of the distal left lower extremity vessels. The anterior tibial artery is occluded. The peroneal (P) and the posterior tibial (PT) arteries are opacified.

plete examination is possible in one sitting. The development of even larger image intensifiers, the dual field approach, or adaptation to a long leg changer or moving table top will greatly facilitate a complete evaluation in one sitting.[35]

With intravenous DSA, diagnostic quality images of the distal extremity vessels (eg, at the ankle and wrist) can be obtained in patients with normal cardiac function.[36] With intraarterial DSA, images of the distal extremities are not only superior in quality but the entire evaluation can be completed in one examination (Fig. 7–14). The added advantages of intraarterial DSA are the reductions in contrast load, patient discomfort, and in

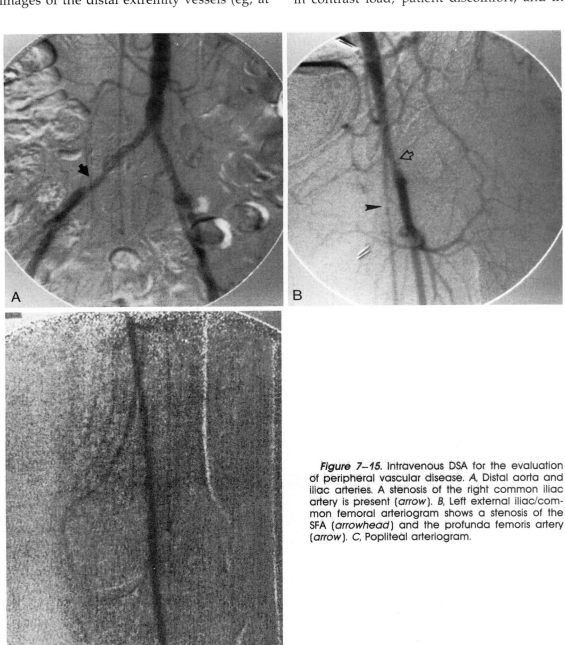

Figure 7–15. Intravenous DSA for the evaluation of peripheral vascular disease. A, Distal aorta and iliac arteries. A stenosis of the right common iliac artery is present (arrow). B, Left external iliac/common femoral arteriogram shows a stenosis of the SFA (arrowhead) and the profunda femoris artery (arrow). C, Popliteal arteriogram.

convenience (ie, no need for a second appointment). Furthermore, hemodynamic data (ie, arterial pressure gradient) can be obtained.

**Applications and Technique** (Figs. 7–14 to 7–16)

1. Screening for occlusive peripheral arterial disease.

2. Follow-up of patients after angioplasty or vascular bypass surgery.[37]

3. Intraarterial DSA can be used for assessment of the patency of distal extremity vessels (distal to the wrist and ankle) or as an aid for selective catheterization.[38]

4. As an aid for interventional procedures (eg, angioplasty) or for the orientation of the surgeon, the bony landmarks can be restored by using the nonsubtracted frame for remasking (Fig. 7–17). Such an image can also be displayed on the TV monitor to guide the catheterization.

For intravenous DSA, images are obtained at 1 image/sec. In patients with slow flow and while imaging distal to the popliteal artery, images may be obtained at every other second. With intraarterial DSA, a more rapid imaging rate is necessary for the proximal extremity vessels. In the pelvis and proximal thigh, both AP and oblique projections are necessary to evaluate the iliac and common femoral bifurcations. Lateral images of the ankle and foot provide the clearest information.

## Venography

Diluted contrast medium (15 to 20%) can also be used to obtain digital subtraction images of the venous system.[39] This is most useful for evaluating the extremity veins in children or when utilizing small gauge needles (when a rapid contrast injection is not possible). We have found digital subtraction venography to be particularly applicable for the upper extremities, the mediastinum and inferior vena cava (Fig. 7–18) (see also Figs. 19–14, 19–42, and 19–44, Chapter 19). In children, the use of diluted contrast medium assures a virtually pain-free study.

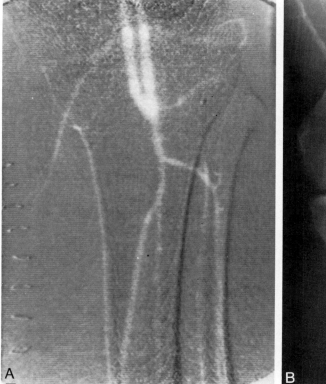 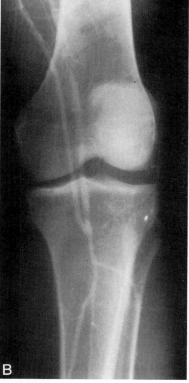

*Figure 7–16.* Intravenous DSA in the evaluation of the postoperative patient. *A,* Intravenous DSA of the left lower extremity demonstrates the patent distal anastomosis of a femoropopliteal bypass graft (20 ml/sec, 25 ml total, 76% contrast medium). The study was performed to determine the cause of recurrent symptoms. *B,* Intraoperative arteriogram obtained at the time of the bypass surgery.

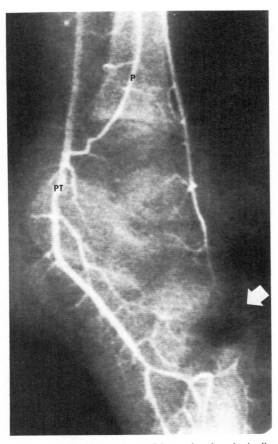

*Figure 7–17.* Restoration of bony landmarks in the DSA image as an aid for the assessment of extent and location of vascular injury. Intraarterial DSA in a 2 year old boy (4 ml of 30% contrast medium injected into the common femoral artery) shows occlusion of the dorsalis pedis artery (*arrow*) at the site of the partial amputation of the foot following a lawn mower accident. P = peroneal; PT = posterior tibial artery.

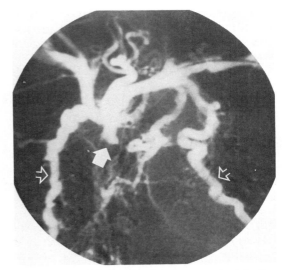

*Figure 7–18.* Digital subtraction venography. Injection of 20% contrast medium into the left brachiocephalic vein demonstrates occlusion of the superior vena cava (*solid arrow*) with collateral flow through markedly enlarged internal mammary veins (*open arrows*).

## IMAGE ARTEFACTS

**Motion Artefacts.** These may be due to patient motion (voluntary or involuntary), respiration, or bowel peristalsis.

PATIENT MOTION. Positive reinforcement and explanation of the sequence of events help to relax most individuals and will prevent many artefacts due to patient motion. In addition, the images can be manipulated electronically (post-processing) to eliminate some artefacts. Motion artefacts over the extremities can often be avoided by using adhesive tape or other devices for immobilization.

RESPIRATORY ARTEFACTS. When imaging in the chest, respiratory motion may be avoided

occasionally by administering oxygen via a nasal cannula.

BOWEL ARTEFACTS. Temporary arrest of bowel peristalsis can be achieved by administration of intravenous glucagon (0.5 to 1.0 mg). Alternatively, a compression band may be applied to the abdomen, or the patient may be imaged in the prone position. A bowel prep eliminates some of the artefacts caused by feces.

**Variations in Contrast Density.** High variations in contrast density (eg, in the chest, neck, or extremities) may also produce image artefacts. These can be corrected by using filtration to reduce the disparity of tissue contrast. In intraarterial DSA, the selection of a different (usually lower) iodine concentration may avoid such artefacts.

**Other Causes of Image Artefacts**

1. Vascular calcifications, especially in the neck vessels, may cause significant imaging artefacts (Fig. 7–19).

2. Systolic/diastolic change in arterial caliber may simulate or obscure a stenosis.

3. Mach effect.

4. Jugular venous reflux. In superior vena caval or right atrial injections, this may be the result of a high injection rate and altered flow dynamics or a manifestation of poor cardiac output (Fig. 7–20). It has also been observed during cerebral radionuclide angiography from the cubital vein approach in patients without a definable underlying abnormality.[40]

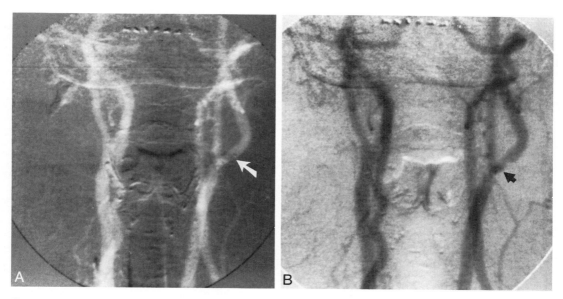

*Figure 7–19.* Subtraction artefact due to calcification and systolic-diastolic change in vascular caliber (20 ml/sec, 25 ml total, 76% contrast medium injected into the superior vena cava). *A,* A calcified plaque obscures an ulcerated left internal carotid artery stenosis (*arrow*). *B,* A subsequent image from the same study shows the lesion (*arrow*).

## COMPLICATIONS

Complications of intravenous DSA are infrequent.[41] Some of the potential complications are (1) phlebitis, (2) transient renal failure due to dehydration of the patient and/or the use of excessive contrast volume, and (3) contrast extravasation due to vein rupture in the arm or to caval or right atrial perforation (Fig. 7–21). Such perforation of the superior vena cava or the right atrium is usually a self-limited complication. Nevertheless, such patients must be hospitalized and observed (cardiac monitoring, hematocrit, and vital signs).

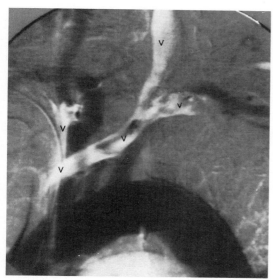

*Figure 7–20.* Jugular venous reflux (20 ml/sec, 25 ml total, contrast medium injected into the right atrium). v = brachiocephalic and jugular venous opacification.

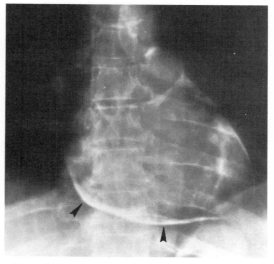

*Figure 7–21.* Complication of intravenous DSA (right atrial injection); 20 ml/sec, 25 ml total, 76% contrast medium injected through a 5 Fr high flow pigtail catheter resulted in right atrial perforation. Arrowheads point to the extravasated contrast medium in the pericardial space.

## FUTURE APPLICATIONS

With continuing emphasis upon the development of improved methods of imaging and physiological evaluation, significant advancements that will enhance the applicability of DSA are to be expected. Evaluation of tissue perfusion and blood flow are some of the areas where DSA may find future application.[42]

Intravenous DSA will most likely become the outpatient procedure of choice for the evaluation of localized vascular problems or for the follow-up of patients after surgery or angioplasty. The image quality is acceptable for the assessment of abnormalities of most vessels that are accessible to angioplasty or bypass surgery. With increasing emphasis upon cost reduction, routine outpatient angiography using intraarterial DSA will soon become a reality.

## REFERENCES

1. Kruger RA, Riederer SJ: Basic Concepts of Digital Subtraction Angiography. Boston, GK Hall Medical Publishers, 1984.
2. Vizy KN: Electronic imaging fundamentals: Basic theory. Cardiovasc Intervent Radiol 6:174–182, 1983.
3. Kruger RA: Image data acquisition, processing, storage and display. Cardiovasc Intervent Radiol 6:183–186, 1983.
4. Mistretta CA, Ort MG, Cameron JR, et al: A multiple image subtraction technique for enhancing low contrast, periodic objects. Invest Radiol 8:43–49, 1973.
5. Ovitt TW, Capp MP, Christenson P, et al: Development of a digital video subtraction system for intravenous angiography. Proc SPIE 206:73–76, 1979.
6. Ovitt T: Personal communication.
7. Brody WR: Hybrid subtraction for improved arteriography. Radiology 141:828–831, 1981.
8. Earnest F IV, Houser OW, Forbes GS, et al: The accuracy and limitations of intravenous digital subtraction angiography in the evaluation of atherosclerotic cerebrovascular disease: angiographic and surgical correlation. Mayo Clin Proc 58:735–746, 1983.
9. Saddekni S, Sos T, Sniderman KW, et al: Optimal injection technique for intravenous digital subtraction angiography. Animal and clinical studies of right atrial injection using small volumes (25 ml) at a high rate (35 ml/sec). Radiology 150:655–659, 1984.
10. Hawkins IF: Carbon dioxide digital subtraction arteriography. AJR 139:19–24, 1982.
11. Hawkins IF: Personal communication.
12. Becker GJ, Holden RW: Sodium dehydrocholate circulation times in digital subtraction angiography. AJR 140:817–818, 1983.
13. Kaufman SL, Chang R, Kadir S, et al: Intraarterial digital subtraction angiography: a comparative view. Cardiovasc Intervent Radiol 6:271–279, 1983.
14. Kadir S: Unpublished data.
15. Kinnison M, Perler BA, White RI, et al: Tailored approach for evaluation of peripheral vascular disease: intravenous digital subtraction angiography. AJR 142:1205–1209, 1984.
16. Shehadi WH, Toniolo G: Adverse reactions to contrast media. A report from the committee on Safety of Contrast Media of the International Society of Radiology. Radiology 137:299–302, 1980.
17. Chilcote WA, Modic MT, Pavlicek WA, et al: Digital subtraction angiography of the carotid arteries: a comparative study in 100 patients. Radiology 139:287–295, 1981.
17a. Wood GW, Lukin RR, Tomsick TA, et al: Digital subtraction angiography with intravenous injection. Assessment of 1000 carotid bifurcations. AJR 140:855–859, 1983.
18. Hesselink JR, Teresi LM, Davis KR, et al: Intravenous digital subtraction angiography of arteriosclerotic vertebrobasilar disease. AJR 142:255–260, 1984.
19. Hoffman MG, Gomes AS, Pais SO: Limitations in the interpretation of intravenous carotid digital subtraction angiography. AJR 142:261–264, 1984.
20. Christenson PC, Ovitt TW, Fisher HD III, et al: Intravenous angiography using digital video subtraction: intravenous cervicocerebrovascular angiography. AJNR 1:379–386, 1980.
21. Grossman LB, Buonocore E, Modic MT, et al: Digital subtraction angiography of the thoracic aorta. Radiology 150:323–325, 1984.
22. Guthaner DF, Miller DC: Digital subtraction angiography of aortic dissection. AJR 141:157–161, 1983.
23. Buonocore E, Meaney TF, Borkowski GP, et al: Digital subtraction angiography of the abdominal aorta and renal arteries. Comparison with conventional angiography. Radiology 139:281–286, 1981.
24. Schwarten DE: Percutaneous transluminal angioplasty of the renal arteries: intravenous digital subtraction angiography for follow-up. Radiology 150:369–373, 1984.
25. Lee KR, Cox GG, Price HI, et al: A metric ruler for digital subtraction angiography. Radiology 148:296, 1983.
26. Witte G, Grabbe E, Buecheler E: Digitale Subtraktionsangiographie (DSA) bei akuter Lungenembolie. Fortsch Roentgenstr 139:616–619, 1983.
27. Ferris EJ, Holder JC, Angtuaco EJ, et al: Angiography of pulmonary emboli: Digital studies and balloon occlusion cineangiography. AJR 142:369–373, 1984.
27a. Reilley RF, Smith CW, Price RR, et al: Digital subtraction angiography: Limitations for the detection of pulmonary emboli. Radiology 149:379–382, 1983.
28. Ludwig JW, Verhoeven LAJ, Kersbergen JJ, et al: Digital subtraction angiography of the pulmonary arteries for the diagnosis of pulmonary embolism. Radiology 147:639–645, 1983.
29. Goodman LR, Golkow RS, Steiner RM, et al: The right mid-lung window. A potential source of error in computed tomography of the lung. Radiology 143:135–138, 1982.
30. Smith CW, Winfield AC, Price RR, et al: Evaluation of digital venous angiography for the diagnosis of renovascular hypertension. Radiology 144:51–54, 1982.
31. Clark RA, Alexander ES: Digital subtraction angiography of the renal arteries. Prospective comparison with conventional arteriography. Invest Radiol 18:6–10, 1983.

32. Rabe FE, Smith EJ, Yune HY, et al: Limitations of digital subtraction angiography in evaluating potential renal donors. AJR 141:91–93, 1983.

33. Flechner SM, Novick AC, Meaney TF, et al: Simultaneous structural and functional imaging of the transplant kidney using digital subtraction angiography. J Urol 129:248–252, 1983.

34. Irving JD, Khoury GA: Digital subtraction angiography in renal transplant recipients. Cardiovasc Intervent Radiol 6:224–230, 1983.

35. Passariello R, Rossi P, Simonetti G, et al: Digital subtraction angiography for examination of vessels of the leg: Use of a 40 cm image intensifier. Radiology 149:669–674, 1983.

36. Harder Th, Lackner K, Franken Th: Digitale Subtraktionsangiographie (DSA) der oberen Extremitaet. Fortschr Roentgenstr 139:609–615, 1983.

37. Schuler M, Rath M, Baumer K, et al: Kontrolle rekonstruktiver Gefaesseingriffe durch digitale Substraktionsangiographie. Fortschr Roentgenstr 139:602–608, 1983.

38. Turski PA, Stieghorst MF, Strother CM, et al: Digital subtraction angiography "road map." AJR 139: 1233–1234, 1983.

39. Rath M, Schuler M, Lissner J: Digitale subtraktionsphlebographie. Fortschr Roentgenstr 139:619–625, 1983.

40. Yeh E-L, Pohlman GP, Ruetz PP, et al: Jugular venous reflux in cerebral radionuclide angiography. Radiology 118:730–732, 1976.

41. Boxt LM: Intravenous digital subtraction angiography of the thoracic and abdominal aorta. Cardiovasc Intervent Radiol 6:205–213, 1983.

42. Buersch JH: Use of digitized functional angiography to evaluate arterial blood flow. Cardiovasc Intervent Radiol 6:303–310, 1983.

# REGIONAL ANGIOGRAPHY OF THE AORTA

## TWO

## Arteriography of the Thoracic Aorta

### ANATOMY

The ascending aorta, which is approximately 5 to 6 cm in length in the average adult, lies behind the sternum. It begins at the level of the third intercostal space on the left and continues obliquely to the first intercostal space on the right.[1] It continues as the aortic arch, coursing from right to left, anterior to the trachea at the level of the fourth thoracic vertebral body and descends along the left side of the trachea. The upper margin of the aortic arch is usually at the level of the manubrium sterni (Figs. 8–1 and 8–2).

The isthmus is the segment of aorta between the last great vessel and the point of attachment of the ductus arteriosus. The ductus diverticulum is an occasional fusiform dilatation of the proximal descending aorta (Fig. 8–3). It represents the most distal segment of the embryonic right aortic arch and does not result from traction of a left ductus.[2] The descending aorta lies in the posterior mediastinum, slightly anterior and to the left of the spine, and enters the abdominal cavity through the hiatus aorticus of the diaphragm at the level of the 12th thoracic vertebral body. As it passes into the abdominal cavity, the aorta lies posterior and to the right of the esophagus. Rarely, the descending aorta may cross over to the right side, behind the esophagus, to continue as a right descending aorta.[3] This finding is frequently associated with other developmental anomalies.[4, 5]

The coronary arteries are the first branches of the ascending aorta, arising from the upper portions of the aortic sinuses. The left coronary artery arises from the left and the right coronary from the right aortic sinus.

The brachiocephalic artery, which is the first branch of the aortic arch, arises behind the mid-portion of the manubrium sterni. It is usually 3 to 4 cm in length, lies anterior to the trachea, and is the most frequent cause of the anterior indentation of the tracheal air shadow in normal infants and small children.[6] It courses craniad along the right side of the trachea and bifurcates into the right common carotid and right subclavian arteries at the right sternoclavicular joint. Branches off the brachiocephalic artery are very infrequent. Occasionally, the arteria thyroidea ima arises from it. Less frequently, a bronchial artery may arise from it. The left common carotid artery is the second branch of the aortic arch. This vessel pursues a craniad course without giving off any branches. The left subclavian artery is the last major branch of the aortic arch.

**Arteria Thyroidea Ima.** This artery sup-

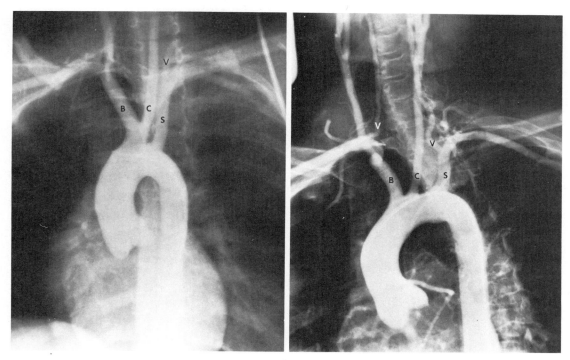

**Figure 8–1.** Normal AP (*left*) and RPO (*right*) arch aortograms from two different young individuals. B = brachiocephalic, C = left common carotid, S = left subclavian, V = vertebral arteries.

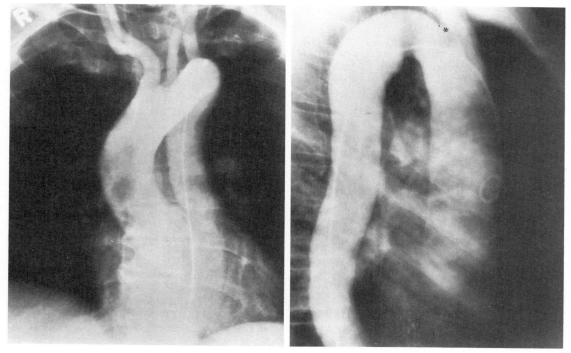

**Figure 8–2.** Normal AP (*left*) and lateral (*right*) thoracic aortogram in an elderly individual. There is some tortuosity of the aorta. The origin of the left subclavian artery (*) is displaced anteriorly.

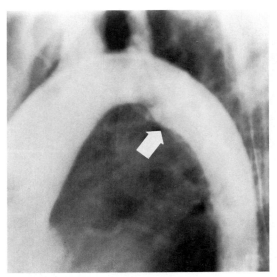

*Figure 8–3.* Arteriographic appearance of the ductus diverticulum (*arrow*).

## Anatomical Variants

1. The normal aortic arch configuration (ie, right brachiocephalic, left common carotid, and left subclavian arteries) is seen in approximately 70% of individuals.[7]

2. The most frequent variant is a common origin of the right brachiocephalic and left common carotid arteries, which occurs in up to 22% of individuals (Fig. 8–6).[7, 8]

3. The second most frequent variation of the normal left aortic arch is the left vertebral artery arising directly from the aorta, which occurs in 4 to 6% of individuals (Fig. 8–6).[7, 8]

4. Both common carotid arteries have a common origin in fewer than 1% of individuals (Fig. 8–7).

5. There are two brachiocephalic arteries in less than 1% of individuals.

6. All four great vessels have a separate origin from the aortic arch in approximately 0.1% of individuals.[7]

plies the thyroid isthmus in approximately 6% of individuals (Fig. 8–4). It arises directly from the aortic arch in 1% of individuals, from the brachiocephalic artery in 3%, and from the right common carotid artery in 1% of individuals.[7] It may also arise from the right subclavian artery and rarely from the internal mammary, suprascapularis, or inferior thyroid arteries.

**Intercostal Arteries.** In 83% of individuals, there are nine pairs of segmental dorsal intercostal arteries arising from the descending aorta along the lower nine intercostal spaces (3rd through 11th intercostal spaces) (Fig. 8–5).[7] The two (occasionally three) upper intercostal spaces are supplied by the superior intercostal artery, which is a branch of the costocervical trunk. A common origin of the left and right intercostal arteries occurs in 2% of individuals. A common origin of multiple intercostal arteries on one side is seen in 13 to 15% of individuals. This configuration occurs more frequently in the upper intercostal arteries, ie, at T3 and T4. A further discussion of the anatomic variations of the intercostal artery origins can be found in reference 7a.

**Bronchial Arteries.** The bronchial arteries vary in size, origin, and number. Most frequently there are between two and four bronchial arteries. For a detailed discussion see later in this chapter (page 162).

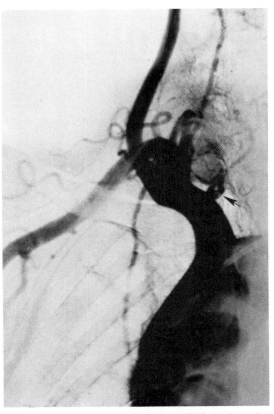

*Figure 8–4.* Arteria thyroidea ima. RPO arch aortogram shows the arteria thyroidea ima arising from the brachiocephalic artery (*arrow*). (From Janevski BK: Angiography of the Upper Extremity. Martinus Nijhoff Publishers, The Hague, 1982. Used with permission.)

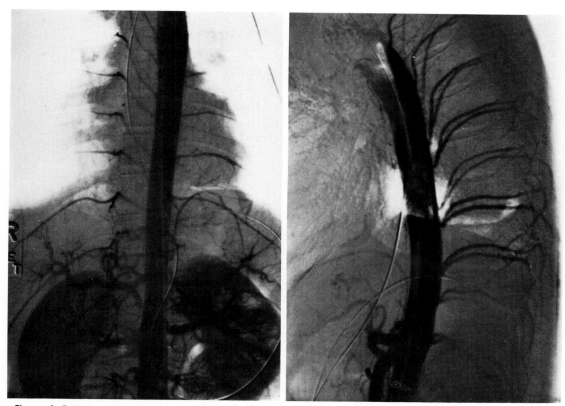

*Figure 8–5.* Normal AP (left) and lateral (right) descending thoracic aortogram. *Note:* The initial course of some of the intercostal arteries is inferiorly directed. This explains why it is often difficult to advance the catheter tip deep into these vessels.

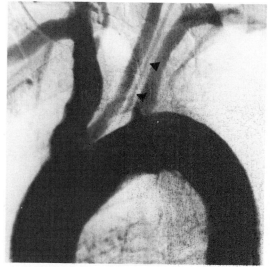

*Figure 8–6.* Common origin of the left common carotid and the brachiocephalic arteries. The left vertebral artery arises directly from the aortic arch (*arrowheads*).

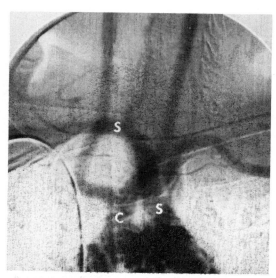

*Figure 8–7.* Intravenous DSA shows a common origin of both common carotid arteries (C). In addition, there is an aberrant right subclavian artery that arises as the last branch of the aortic arch (S).

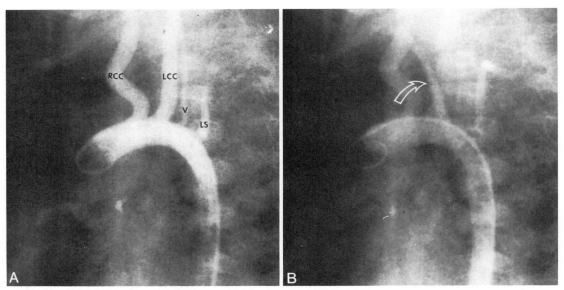

*Figure 8–8.* Left aortic arch with aberrant right subclavian artery. Early (*A*) and late (*B*) frames from a cine arch aortogram in the RPO projection show an aberrant right subclavian artery arising as the last great vessel (*arrow*). The left vertebral artery also arises separately from the aortic arch (V). RCC = right common carotid, LCC = left common carotid, LS = left subclavian artery.

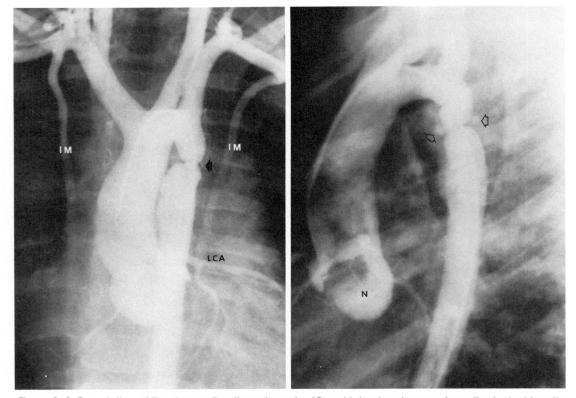

*Figure 8–9.* Coarctation of the descending thoracic aorta. AP and lateral aortogram shows the typical location of aortic coarctation (*black arrow*). There is a bicuspid aortic valve with a large noncoronary sinus (N) and mild ectasia of the ascending aorta. The left coronary (LCA) and both internal mammary (IM) arteries are hypertrophied. Small aneurysms are seen proximal to the coarctation (*open arrows*).

## Congenital Malformations

**Left Aortic Arch with Aberrant Right Subclavian Artery** (Fig. 8–8). This is the most common malformation of the aortic arch, occurring in up to 1% of individuals.[7] Unless it is tortuous or aneurysmal, the aberrant right subclavian artery rarely causes symptoms (dysphagia lusoria, dyspnea lusoria). In most cases the recurrent laryngeal nerve does not develop.

The branches of the aortic arch occur in the following sequence: right common carotid, left common carotid, and left subclavian, with the right subclavian artery as the fourth branch arising from the proximal descending aorta. The right subclavian artery courses upward, obliquely toward the right arm, crossing behind the esophagus in 80% of persons. In 15% of individuals it lies between the esophagus and the trachea, and in 5% it crosses the trachea or mainstem bronchus anteriorly.[7]

This malformation may be associated with a congenital heart disease in 10 to 15% of patients.[8] In patients with coarctation of the descending aorta, if the origin of the aberrant right subclavian artery is distal to the coarctation, blood flow may be reversed to the low-pressure descending aorta, and rib notching is unilateral on the left side (see Fig. 9–17, Chapter 9). Origin of the aberrant vessel above the coarctation gives rise to bilateral upper extremity hypertension and bilateral rib notching. Occasionally, the origin of the aberrant vessel is from an aortic diverticulum.

**Right Aortic Arch.** The ascending aorta arches posteriorly to the right side of the trachea and esophagus, thereby passing anterior to the right mainstem bronchus.[9] In the majority of individuals it continues as a right descending aorta. This malformation is observed only in 1 to 2% of humans, but is very common in birds and reptiles.[7, 10]

There are two main types:

1. Right aortic arch with mirror image branching (no retroesophageal component), ie, three main branches (left brachiocephalic, right common carotid, and right subclavian arteries), occurs in approximately 60% of persons. In the majority there is a left ductus or ligamentum arteriosum.[9, 11] Ninety-eight per cent of individuals with this type of right aortic arch have cyanotic congenital heart disease, and in about 90% of these patients the congenital defect is tetralogy of Fallot.[9]

2. Right aortic arch with aberrant left subclavian artery (retroesophageal segment) and left ductus or ligamentum arteriosum occurs in approximately 35% of patients. This type is associated with vascular rings. Only 12% of these individuals have associated congenital heart disease, most frequently tetralogy of Fallot.[9]

Expressed another way, 25% of patients with tetralogy of Fallot have a right aortic arch.[9, 10] Of these, 93% have mirror image branching, whereas the remainder have an aberrant left subclavian artery.[9]

**Cervical Aortic Arch.** This is a rare anomaly in which the aortic arch lies in the neck, above the clavicle. Clinically, a pulsatile mass is palpable and may be mistaken for an aneurysm.[12] There is no association with intracardiac malformations. A cervical aortic arch occurs more commonly on the right side.[2]

**Coarctation** (Fig. 8–9). This is a localized narrowing of the aorta that is due to infolding of the lumen as a result of an abnormality in the media. The narrowing is located at or adjacent to the insertion of the ligamentum arteriosum. In approximately half the patients, aortic coarctation is an isolated lesion. In the remainder, it is associated with congenital cardiac lesions. One of the most frequently associated lesions is a bicuspid aortic valve.[13] Other less commonly associated congenital defects include patent ductus arteriosus and ventricular septal defect. Berry aneurysms of the circle of Willis also occur in some patients with aortic coarctation.

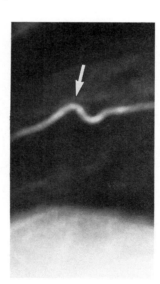

*Figure 8–10.* Intercostal arteriogram shows the relationship between the tortuous vessel and rib notching (*arrow*).

Rib notching is seen as a result of enlargement and tortuosity of the intercostal arteries, which serve as a collateral pathway (Fig. 8–10). It may be unilateral if the coarcted segment is proximal to a subclavian artery.

## ARTERIOGRAPHY OF THE THORACIC AORTA

Arch and thoracic aortography is performed via the femoral or axillary approach. A translumbar technique for arch aortography has been described but has not found widespread use.[14]

**Femoral Approach.** From the femoral approach, after percutaneous catheterization, a 100 cm long, 7 Fr pigtail catheter with 8 to 12 side holes is inserted into the abdominal aorta. The pigtail is allowed to re-form by removing the guide wire, and the catheter is flushed. It is then advanced over the aortic arch into the ascending aorta. As the pigtail approaches the arch, often a counterclockwise rotation facilitates passage into the arch. In young individuals, the catheter will occasionally not make the bend but continues into the left subclavian or common carotid artery. In this situation, it is pulled back into the mid-descending aorta and a J guide wire is advanced 4 to 6 cm beyond the catheter tip, thus straightening the pigtail. Both the guide wire and the catheter are then readvanced as a unit. The system is torqued in a counterclockwise direction to avoid entering the brachiocephalic vessels. Alternatively, the pigtail catheter is used to direct the guide wire into the aortic arch.

**Axillary Approach.** In older individuals with elongation of the thoracic aorta, the origin of the left subclavian artery is displaced to the right (see Fig. 8–2). Thus, from the left axillary approach, the guide wire usually enters the ascending aorta without difficulty. Because of the same anatomical peculiarity, catheterization of the ascending aorta from the right axillary approach is not difficult. If the guide wire does not enter the ascending aorta but goes down the descending aorta, the pigtail catheter is inserted and the pigtail is allowed to re-form in the aortic arch. After flushing the catheter, the J guide wire is reinserted so that the J protrudes beyond the catheter tip by 2 to 3 cm, partially uncoiling the pigtail. The catheter is then rotated so that the guide wire points in the direction of the ascending aorta. The wire is advanced into the ascending aorta and the catheter is inserted over it (Fig. 8–11). If the catheter does not follow the wire into the ascending aorta but flips back into the descending aorta, the following maneuver is

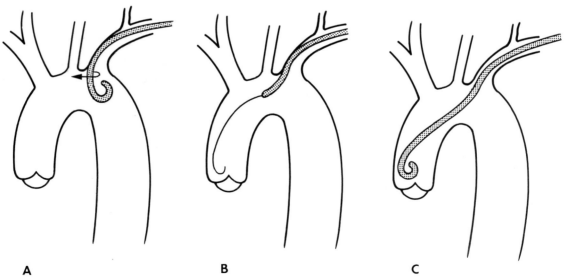

**A**                                        **B**                                        **C**

*Figure 8–11.* Technique for catheterization of the ascending aorta from the left axillary approach. *A,* The pigtail catheter is allowed to re-form in the arch. It is rotated so that it opens toward the ascending aorta. *B,* A J guide wire is inserted and is directed into the ascending aorta with the aid of the pigtail catheter. *C,* The pigtail catheter is advanced into the ascending aorta over the guide wire.

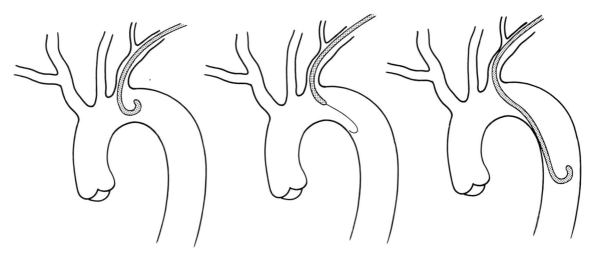

**Figure 8–12.** Technique for catheterization of the descending thoracic aorta from the left axillary approach. The pigtail catheter is used to direct a J wire into the descending aorta.

used: As the guide wire is advanced into the ascending aorta, the pigtail is straightened out by withdrawing the catheter into the subclavian artery. Once the pigtail has been straightened out, the wire is advanced up to the aortic sinuses and the pigtail catheter is inserted over it. If this maneuver is unsuccessful, a C1 cobra or hook catheter is inserted into the aortic arch and is used to torque the guide wire in the desired direction. Once the wire is in place, the cobra is exchanged for a pigtail. Other alternatives are the use of a tip deflecting wire to direct the pigtail catheter or a sidewinder-shaped pigtail catheter.[14a]

For evaluation of the ascending aorta, the catheter tip is positioned approximately 2 cm above the aortic valve. If only the brachiocephalic vessels or the aortic arch or both are to be studied, the catheter tip may be placed higher (3 to 4 cm above the aortic valve).

For evaluation of the descending aorta, the catheter is placed in the proximal descending aorta. In younger individuals, the guide wire usually enters the descending aorta without difficulty. In the older individual with an elongated aortic arch, the guide wire and catheter enter the ascending aorta preferentially. In this situation, the pigtail catheter is used to torque the guide wire into the descending aorta in the same fashion as described for catheterization of the ascending aorta (Fig. 8–12). Alternatively, either a C1 cobra or hook catheter, the sidewinder pigtail

catheter, or a catheter tip deflecting wire system is used to guide the catheter into the descending aorta. Subsequently, catheter exchange should be accomplished over a J-tipped exchange guide wire.

While attempting to catheterize the ascending or the descending aorta, the U arm, cradle table top, or the patient is positioned in a left anterior oblique position. This uncoils the arch anatomy and facilitates assessment of the direction in which the catheter or guide wire is advanced.

From the right axillary approach, the same maneuvers used for the left axillary approach are applied for catheter placement. When using these maneuvers, a standard J wire should be used. LT or LLT wires are often too flimsy and may flip back as the pigtail catheter is advanced over them.

Rapid hand injection of 5 to 10 ml of contrast medium is used to assess catheter position. When using the axillary approach, after the catheter has been positioned and secured at the skin, the arm may be brought into a more comfortable position (horizontal position or parallel to the body). Subsequently, the catheter position **must** be rechecked, since this maneuver may advance the catheter into the artery, and if necessary the catheter should be repositioned.

**Contrast Injection and Filming** (Tables 8–1 and 8–2). A total of 60 ml of contrast medium is injected at a rate of 30 ml/sec. In an unusually large, voluminous, ectatic aorta,

**TABLE 8–1. Standard Arch Aortogram**

| | |
|---|---|
| Catheter: | 7 Fr pigtail |
|    Position | Ascending aorta |
| Guide wire | 0.035 inch fixed core J |
| Contrast medium | 76% diatrizoate meglumine sodium |
| Injection rate/volume | 30 ml/sec, total 60 ml |
| Films: | 13 films per projection |
|    Filming rate | 3 per second for 9 films |
| | 1 per second for 4 films |
|    Projections | a. Biplane (AP/lateral) |
| | or |
| | b. LAO (45°) |

such as in Marfan's syndrome, or in the presence of aortic regurgitation, a larger total volume of contrast medium is necessary (70 to 80 ml) at the same flow rate. In older individuals and patients with aortic regurgitation who have slow forward flow, the filming rate may be slower: two films/sec for six films and one film/sec for seven films.

The projection in which films are obtained is dictated by several factors, such as the patient's age, availability of biplane changers, and type of information desired, and should be determined individually.

Biplane aortography is performed in the anterior-posterior (AP) and lateral projections. These are the projections of choice for evaluating aneurysms, trauma, and dissections. In the elderly and when only a single projection is available, a 45° left anterior oblique projection is used. For evaluation of atherosclerosis and occlusive diseases of the neck vessels and some cases of trauma, arch

**TABLE 8–2. Standard Descending Aortogram**

| | |
|---|---|
| Catheter: | 7 Fr pigtail |
|    Position | Proximal descending aorta |
| Guide wire | 0.035 inch fixed core J |
| Contrast medium | 76% diatrizoate meglumine sodium |
| Injection rate/volume | 25 ml/sec, total 50 ml |
| Films: | 9 films per projection |
|    Filming rate | 3 per second for 6 films |
| | 1 per second for 3 films |
|    Projections | a. Biplane (AP/lateral) |
| | or |
| | b. AP |

aortography is performed in the left and right anterior oblique projections. If an abnormality is not readily identified on the projections used, another projection should be obtained. Similarly, film subtraction should be used if no abnormality is seen on the unsubtracted arteriogram.

Digital subtraction angiography (DSA) can also be used as an alternative for the evaluation of aneurysms and atherosclerotic occlusive diseases of the aortic branches. In some patients, it can also be used for determining the extent of aortic dissection and for the assessment of vascular injury.

## ANEURYSMS

Dilatation and elongation of the aorta with increased tortuosity may occur as a result of longstanding systemic hypertension or may be due to increased volume load in patients with aortic insufficiency (Fig. 8–13). Dilatation of the ascending aorta also occurs as a result of turbulence distal to an aortic valve stenosis (see Fig. 8–9).

Aneurysms may be classified as true (all layers of the wall intact), false (all layers of the wall disrupted), or pseudo-aneurysms (one or two layers of the wall intact). They may be fusiform (circumferential involvement) or saccular (involving predominantly a portion of the wall). In general, true aneurysms are fusiform, whereas false and pseudo-aneurysms are saccular.

### Clinical Aspects

Most thoracic aortic aneurysms are asymptomatic.[15] Symptoms are usually indicative of a large aneurysm. Pain, which is substernal but occasionally occurs in the back or shoulders, is present in 26% of patients; in some patients, pain may be present only in the supine position.[15] Other symptoms may be secondary to venous obstruction (superior vena cava syndrome), esophageal compression (dysphagia), tracheobronchial compression (stridor, dyspnea), and recurrent laryngeal nerve compression (hoarseness, vocal cord fixation).

### Pathology

Thoracic aortic aneurysms may be atherosclerotic, syphilitic, posttraumatic, mycotic, congenital, or due to an arteritis.

In one study, 73% of aneurysms of the thoracic aorta were atherosclerotic, 19% sy-

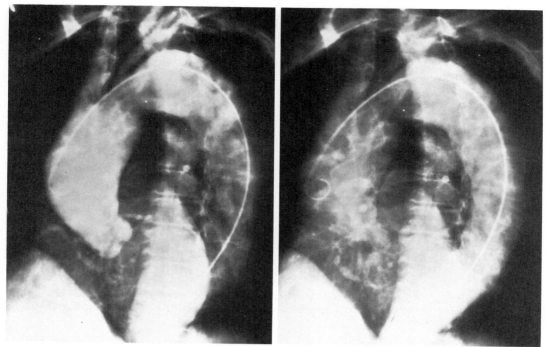

*Figure 8–13.* Aortic ectasia. Early (*left*) and late (*right*) films from a left anterior oblique arch aortogram show a fusiform aneurysm of the ascending aorta and ectasia of the arch and descending aorta. There is slow antegrade flow, which leads to poor opacification of the descending aorta as a result of mixing of contrast material with the blood. Note that the origins of the arch vessels are displaced to the right (compare with Fig. 8–1).

philitic, 5% post-traumatic, and 2% congenital.[15] Thoracic aortic aneurysms occur most frequently in patients in the sixth and seventh decades and predominantly in men, with a ratio of 3:1.[16]

## Radiology

The chest radiograph offers a clue by demonstrating a wide, tortuous aorta. Occasionally this has been mistaken for a mediastinal tumor. Demonstration of curvilinear calcification in the periphery strengthens the suspicion of an aneurysm. Differentiation from other mediastinal masses may require a computed tomography (CT) scan, magnetic resonance imaging (MRI), or dynamic nuclear medicine imaging. The calcification in syphilitic aneurysms is usually fine and pencil-like but can be coarse, as in atherosclerotic disease (Fig. 8–14). On chest fluoroscopy, aortic pulsations may be absent or inapparent because of the presence of a laminated blood clot.

## Arteriography

The indications for arteriography in patients with thoracic aneurysms are for eval-

uation of extent of the aneurysm, evaluation of aortic valvular competence in ascending aortic aneurysms, and evaluation of the presence and extent of mural thrombi and arterial blood supply to the spinal cord.

For aneurysms of the ascending aorta, either a biplane (AP/lateral) or single plane aortogram in a 45° left anterior oblique projection is obtained with the catheter in the proximal ascending aorta. In most aneurysms, the blood flow is slow and the intraluminal volume of the aorta is increased; therefore, the filming rate and volume of contrast injection are adjusted accordingly. In large aneurysms and those with significant aortic regurgitation, a larger volume of contrast medium (70 ml) is necessary because of the dilution.

For aneurysms of the aortic arch, the catheter is placed in the mid-ascending aorta for a 45° left anterior oblique aortogram. For aneurysms of the descending thoracic aorta, a biplane aortogram should be performed with the pigtail catheter placed distal to the left subclavian artery orifice. Additional projections may be required if the extent of the aneurysm and its relationship to the brachiocephalic vessels are not satisfactorily defined.

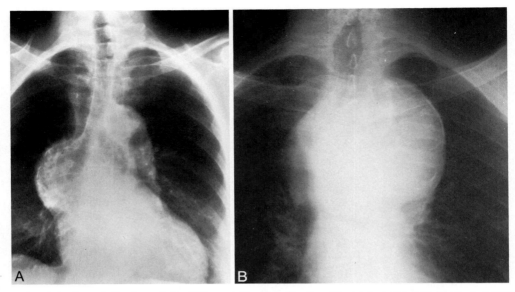

**Figure 8–14.** Aortic calcification. *A,* Syphilitic calcification. On the AP chest radiograph there is calcification outlining an ascending aortic aneurysm. *B,* Atherosclerotic calcification. There is thick calcification outlining a portion of the arch aneurysm.

Tables 8–1 and 8–2 list the details of standard arch and descending aortography.

Biplane descending thoracic aortograms may also be indicated in the evaluation of patients with embolic occlusion of lower extremity vessels.[17] In such patients, mural thrombi of the aorta are the source of thromboemboli. In some patients, the source of thromboemboli may lie in the venous system, and paradoxical arterial embolization occurs via a patent foramen ovale, which is found in 6% of normal individuals, or through arteriovenous shunts in the pulmonary circulation.[18] Although CT scanning is a valuable aid in the detection of aortic abnormalities, it may not always permit differentiation of a clot from the false lumen of a dissection.[19]

## Types of Aneurysms

**Atherosclerotic Aneurysms.** Gradual weakening of the aortic wall due to impaired nutrition (compromised vasa vasorum) and the loss of muscle fibers and turbulent blood flow lead to aneurysm formation, which is enhanced by the presence of arterial hypertension. The majority of atherosclerotic aneurysms are fusiform but can be saccular in up to 20% of patients.[15]

On arteriography, the lumen may appear

to be of normal diameter because of the presence of a thick mural thrombus. The wide soft tissue shadow and mural calcification, if present, offer a clue to the true diameter. This mural thrombus is occasionally the source for distal thromboembolism.

In the thorax, atherosclerotic aneurysms occur most frequently in the descending thoracic aorta.[16] The most common locations are the distal aortic arch and lower descending aorta (Figs. 8–15 and 8–16).[20] The latter aneurysms may extend into the abdomen (thoracoabdominal aneurysm) (Fig. 8–17).[21]

The prognosis for thoracic aortic aneurysms is poorer than that for abdominal aortic aneurysms.[22] The 1, 3, and 5 year survival rates are 57.1%, 25.9%, and 19.2%, respectively. The prognosis is poorer if the aneurysm is large, if the patient is older than 50 years, and if there is diastolic hypertension.[16] Otherwise, the location of the aneurysm in the thorax does not have a bearing upon prognosis.[16] Aneurysm rupture is the cause of death in one third of the patients and may be into the pleural cavity, retroperitoneum (in thoraco-abdominal aneurysms), tracheobronchial tree, esophagus, pericardial cavity, or vena cava (Figs. 8–18 and 8–19).[15, 16]

Aneurysms of the brachiocephalic vessels are most often traumatic and less frequently

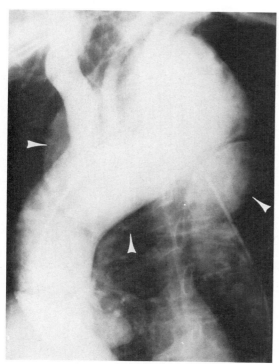

*Figure 8–15.* RPO arch aortogram shows a saccular aneurysm of the aortic arch (*arrowheads*) arising distal to the left subclavian artery.

1. Aneurysms (Fig. 8–22): 36% of syphilitic aneurysms are located in the ascending aorta, 24% in the aortic arch, 5% in the descending thoracic aorta, and less than 1% in the sinuses of Valsalva.[24] Lesions of the aortic arch may involve the brachiocephalic artery.[16] Infrarenal aortic aneurysms due to syphilis are uncommon. The sinus of Valsalva aneurysms give rise to an asymmetrical enlargement of the sinuses and have a tendency for extrapericardial rupture.[25] These can be differentiated from other forms of sinus enlargement, such as that associated with Marfan's syndrome, because in the latter, the sinus enlargement is symmetrical (which has been likened to a tulip bulb). Syphilitic aneurysms are commonly saccular but may be fusiform in 25% of patients.[23] The saccular type may attain a progressively large size, leading to pressure erosion of contiguous structures. Approximately 15% of these aneurysms have a fine, pencil-like, dystrophic calcification and may contain a mural thrombus.

2. Aortic insufficiency: This occurs either due to dilatation of the aortic annulus secondary to an aneurysm of the ascending aorta or as a result of syphilitic valvulitis.[23] The intimal thickening may further give rise to coronary ostial stenosis leading to angina.

mycotic or atherosclerotic.[16] Longstanding hypertension may give rise to extreme tortuosity (buckling) of the carotid or brachiocephalic arteries (Fig. 8–20). On physical examination, this may simulate an aneurysm. Cranio-caudad angulated imaging of the brachiocephalic artery defines the course and anatomy of this vessel (Fig. 8–21).

**Aneurysms and Other Cardiovascular Manifestations of Syphilis.** Cardiovascular manifestations of syphilis are observed in 10 to 15% of untreated patients and account for approximately one third of the deaths due to syphilis.[23-25] Arteritis is a late manifestation of syphilis. The most common sites of involvement are the ascending aorta, aortic arch, and pulmonary arteries. Less frequently, syphilitic arteritis involves the descending aorta and rarely other segments of the aorta. Syphilitic periaortitis (via lymphatics) and mesoaortitis (via the vasa vasorum) causes destruction of the arterial muscle fibers, which leads to weakening of the wall with subsequent development of aneurysms. The cardiovascular manifestations of syphilis include:

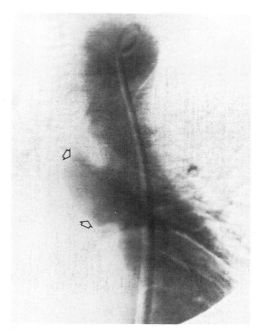

*Figure 8–16.* Intraarterial DSA using approximately 20% concentration of contrast medium shows an eccentric, partially thrombosed saccular atherosclerotic aneurysm of the descending thoracic aorta (*arrows*).

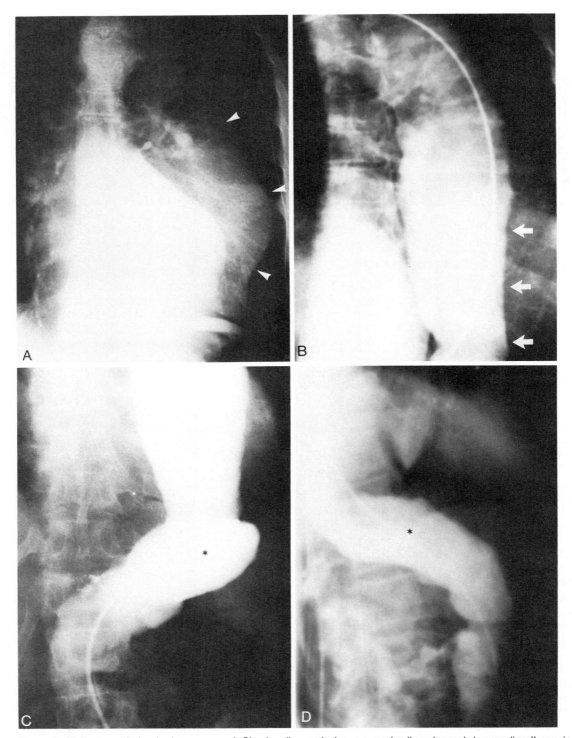

*Figure 8–17.* Thoracoabdominal aneurysm. *A,* Chest radiograph shows a markedly enlarged descending thoracic aorta extending to the lateral chest wall (*arrowheads*). *B* and *C,* AP descending aortogram shows a wide aortic lumen. The lateral portion of the aneurysm, which is filled with clot, provides a smoother margin than the remainder of the aortic wall (*arrows*). The upper abdominal aorta (*) is seen end on. *D,* Lateral abdominal aortogram shows the abdominal extension of the fusiform aneurysm. Asterisk marks the segment of the aorta that is seen on the AP aortogram.

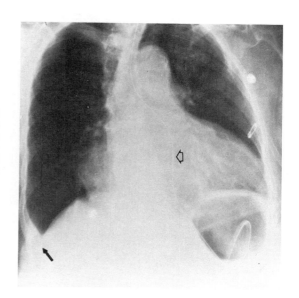

*Figure 8–18.* Ruptured thoracic aortic aneurysm. Plain radiographic findings. PA radiograph of the chest shows cardiac enlargement and lateral displacement of the nasogastric tube by a descending thoracic aortic aneurysm (*open arrow*). Fluid collection is seen in the right costophrenic angle (*solid arrow*). A ruptured aneurysm was found at operation.

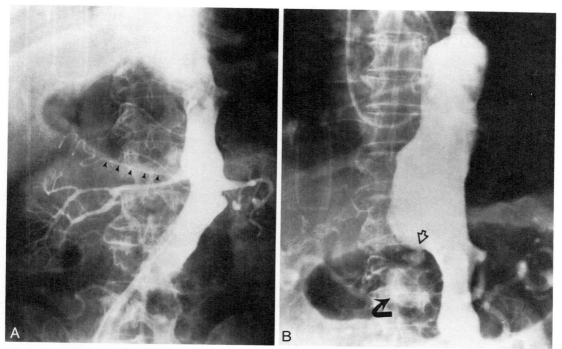

*Figure 8–19.* Ruptured atherosclerotic thoracoabdominal aortic aneurysm. Arteriographic findings. *A,* AP abdominal aortogram shows stretching of the right renal and inferior adrenal arteries (*arrowheads*) with inferior displacement of the right kidney. *B,* AP descending thoracic aortogram shows a fusiform aneurysm extending into the upper abdominal aorta. Extravasation of contrast medium (*curved arrow*) is seen from the abdominal portion of the aneurysm (*open arrow*).

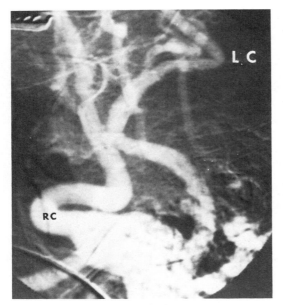

Figure 8–20. "Buckling" of the carotid arteries. Intravenous DSA in a patient with a pulsatile left neck mass. There is extreme tortuosity of carotid arteries. LC = left internal carotid, RC = right common carotid artery.

However, the majority of these patients have associated atherosclerotic coronary artery lesions.[23]

3. Aortitis: Syphilitic aortitis may occur in the absence of aortic insufficiency or aneurysm and is manifested by dilatation of the ascending aorta.[25] This must be differentiated from senile aortic ectasia and other causes of ascending aortic dilatation such as Marfan's syndrome, coarctation, and aortic valvular disease. Occasionally, atherosclerotic degeneration and syphilitic aortitis may be present concomitantly.[16]

**Mycotic Aneurysms** (Figs. 8–23 and 8–24). The term "mycotic" was coined by Osler.[26] Such aneurysms can occur anywhere and are being seen more frequently. There are four possible mechanisms for the development of mycotic aneurysms.[16]

1. Septicemia leading to abscess formation in the arterial wall by seeding via the vasa vasorum.

2. Infection within an atheromatous lesion as a result of septicemia (seeding through contamination of the blood stream).

3. Contiguous infection.[27]

4. Trauma and infection (hematoma with secondary infection, eg, postoperative).[28]

In an older report reviewing over 200 patients, the majority of whom had bacterial endocarditis, the ascending aorta was the most common location for mycotic aneurysms. The abdominal visceral, intracranial, lower and upper extremity vessels were next involved, in descending order of frequency.[29] In a more recent study, mycotic aneurysms of the aorta occurred three times as frequently as peripheral aneurysms.[30] The source remained undetermined in about 50%

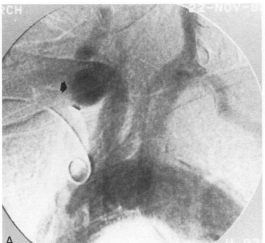
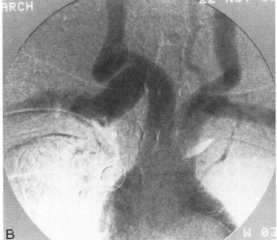

Figure 8–21. Value of angulated beam technique for the evaluation of brachiocephalic and proximal right subclavian artery abnormalities. A, Intravenous DSA of the aortic arch in the left anterior oblique projection. The distal brachiocephalic artery is seen on end (arrow) and the bifurcation is obscured. B, Repeat intravenous DSA in the AP projection with 20° craniocaudad beam angulation delineates the brachiocephalic artery bifurcation and unveils a fusiform aneurysm of the proximal subclavian artery.

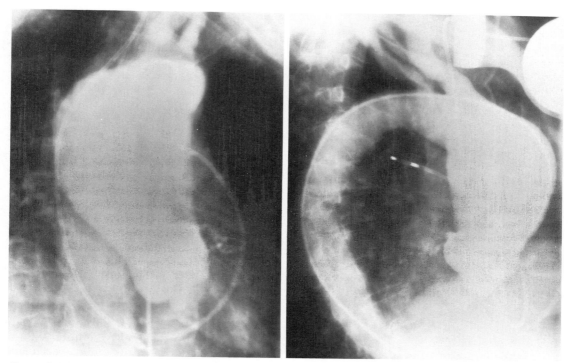

*Figure 8–22.* AP and lateral aortogram shows a syphilitic aneurysm of the ascending aorta. The aortic sinuses appear normal.

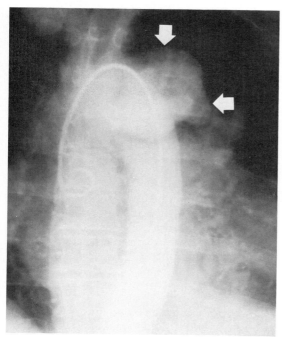

*Figure 8–23.* Mycotic aneurysm of the aortic arch (*arrows*).

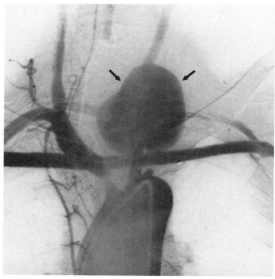

*Figure 8–24.* Mycotic aneurysm after extra-anatomic arterial bypass (*arrows*). In addition, there is a stenosis of the brachiocephalic artery and the left subclavian artery is occluded.

of the patients and only 12% had bacterial endocarditis. Rarely, false aneurysms may develop spontaneously in patients on long-term steroid therapy.[31]

**Congenital Aneurysms** (Fig. 8–25). Aneurysms that form as a result of an absent or poorly developed media are seen most commonly in the intracranial circulation. Rarely, these may also develop in the splenic, pulmonary, renal, and extremity vessels.[16] Approximately 2% of thoracic aortic aneurysms may have a congenital etiology.[15] Most frequently, these arise in the aortic sinuses and involve the right, noncoronary, and left coronary sinuses, in descending order of frequency.[32] Aneurysms of the coronary sinuses are asymptomatic until they rupture.[20]

**Arteritis.** The types of arteritis that may lead to aortic aneurysm formation are listed in Table 8–5 and include Takayasu's arteritis, giant cell arteritis, and a focal arteritis of unknown etiology (see Fig. 8–46).[33] Approximately 10% of patients with aortitis associated with relapsing polychondritis may also develop aneurysms (also see section on Aortitis).[34]

## DISSECTION

Dissection of the thoracic aorta may be seen in as many as one of every 363 cases at

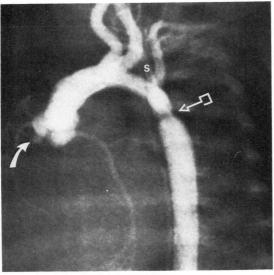

*Figure 8–25.* Congenital aneurysm of the sinus of Valsalva. Left anterior oblique aortogram shows an aneurysm of the right coronary sinus (*curved arrow*) and coarctation of the proximal descending aorta (*open arrow*). An aberrant right subclavian artery (S) is also seen.

autopsy.[35] It occurs predominantly in males in a 2 to 4.5:1 ratio and affects individuals between the ages of 30 and 85 years.[36, 37] A history of hypertension can be obtained in only 60% of patients.[36]

### Clinical Aspects

Aortic dissection may be acute, chronic, or clinically silent. Classically, acute aortic dissection presents with a sudden onset of severe chest and back pain, which progresses to hemodynamic shock in about 25% of patients.[35] Chest pain, which is the most characteristic feature, may be absent in up to 25% of patients.[38, 39] Neurological symptoms occur in 25% of patients and include hemiplegia, paraparesis, and painful ischemia of the peripheral and spinal nerves.[37, 40, 41] Murmurs and bruits are reported in 65% and asymmetrical peripheral pulses in 59% of patients.[35, 37]

The femoral pulses are absent in 25% of patients,[35] and occasionally the initial clinical presentation may simulate embolic occlusion of an extremity vessel or peripheral vascular insufficiency.[39, 41-43] The loss of peripheral pulses may be transient in some cases, with reappearance of the pulses as reentry is established.[43] Thus, according to some authors, aortic dissection should be considered in the differential diagnosis of all arterial occlusive diseases.[42]

The clinical picture can be so variable that the diagnosis on hospital admission is incorrect in a significant number of cases.[37, 44] Often the chest radiograph offers the first clue as to the correct diagnosis, but this may also be normal in approximately one fifth of patients.[36, 45]

Silent dissections are rare and are usually of limited extent without involvement of the great vessels.[41, 46] The pain associated with acute dissection is most likely due to the rapid distention of the subadventitial tissue by blood and may be absent if the dissection occurs slowly.[46] In patients with Marfan's syndrome, minor deceleration injuries (sports injuries, minor traffic accidents) may precipitate a dissection.[47]

### Pathology

Dissection occurs as blood enters the media through a tear in the weakened intima or due to a ruptured vas vasorum. In the latter case, the intimal tear may occur as a secondary event. However, in about 4% of dissections, a medial tear is not found despite a careful search.[35] The dissection occurs along the natural cleavage plane, which lies between the middle and outer third of the media. In most instances the etiology is the degenerative process occurring in a normally aging aorta, which is accelerated by hypertension.[48] Aortic dissection also occurs with a higher frequency in patients with a bicuspid aortic valve and aortic coarctation. Pregnancy and collagen vascular diseases such as Marfan's syndrome are associated with an increased incidence of aortic dissection in younger patients.[49-51] Thus, approximately half the dissections in women under 40 years of age occur in association with pregnancy.[49]

Aortic dissection also occurs with a higher frequency in patients with skeletal abnormalities such as scoliosis, pigeon breast, and funnel chest. Dissection may also occur in association with mycotic aneurysms, giant cell arteritis, and aortic laceration. Syphilis, on the other hand, does not predispose to dissection, since syphilitic aortitis leads to adhesive scarring of all layers of the aortic wall.

In the majority of patients, infarction of the mid-portion of the aortic media develops 12 to 48 hours after the dissection begins.[52] The most likely etiology is the disruption of the nutrient blood supply from the vasa vasorum. This "mid-zonal" medial infarction is localized to the intrathoracic aorta and may be responsible for the development of aneurysms occurring as a late sequela of aortic dissection.

In the vast majority of cases, two lumina are present. Rarely, a three-channel dissection may be present if a secondary dissection occurs within one of the channels, giving rise to an unusually wide aortic shadow.[53] A type I or II dissection usually begins close to the aortic root and lies anterolaterally in the ascending aorta. It may continue into the aortic arch, where it lies superiorly along the convexity. In the descending aorta, it lies posterolaterally until it reaches the diaphragm. In the abdominal aorta, it may continue anteriorly to occlude the mesenteric vessels or spiral posteriorly into the aortic bifurcation.[39, 54]

## Classification (Fig. 8–26)

According to DeBakey et al,[55] aortic dissection is classified into three types:

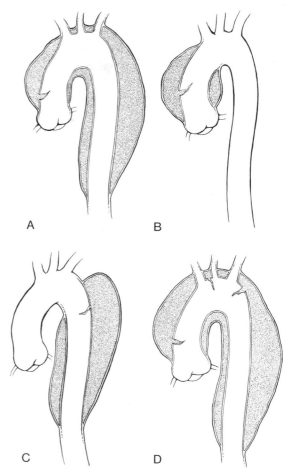

**Figure 8–26.** Classification of aortic dissection. A, DeBakey Type I. B, DeBakey Type II. C, DeBakey Type III and Stanford Type B. D, Stanford Type A. The location of the tear may be in any of the locations shown.

*Type I:* The dissection begins in the ascending aorta and extends across the aortic arch for a variable distance into the descending thoracic and abdominal aorta and occasionally into the iliac arteries. This type accounts for 29 to 34% of dissections.[36, 37]

*Type II:* The dissection is localized to the ascending aorta. This type accounts for 12 to 21% of aortic dissections.

*Type III:* The dissection begins at the isthmus, ie, distal to the left subclavian artery origin, and extends into the thoracic or abdominal aorta and distally for a variable distance. This is the most common type and accounts for approximately 50% of dissections.

According to the Stanford Classification, the dissections are divided into two groups, based upon involvement of the ascending aorta and irrespective of origin or extent of the dissection.

*Type A:* The dissection involves the ascending aorta but may extend into the arch and descending aorta. Descending aortic dissection with retrograde extension into the ascending aorta is also classified in this category.

*Type B:* The dissection involves the aortic arch and distal aorta.

## Radiology

The plain chest radiographs may demonstrate:[36, 37]

1. A widened mediastinum in up to 81% of patients. This may be due to the dissection itself or may result from displacement of the nondissected aorta by a large false channel or hematoma.

2. A double contour in up to 40% of patients. However, overlapping of ascending and descending aortic limbs may simulate this finding.[37]

3. An irregular or indistinct aortic outline with a wavy contour.

4. Displacement of the tracheal air shadow or endotracheal tube.

5. An enlarged cardiac silhouette.

6. A pleural fluid collection in up to 27% of patients.

7. Displacement of the calcified intima by more than 1 cm. This is seen in about 7% of patients. As the only finding, it is an unreliable sign of aortic dissection, since it may be seen in tortuous, atherosclerotic aortas without dissection.[36, 37, 56]

8. Enlargement of the aortic silhouette demonstrated by serial chest radiographs.

## Arteriography

Arteriography is performed to evaluate the type of dissection, its extent, its communication with the true lumen, and the status of the coronary and visceral arteries. Tables 8–1 and 8–2 list the details for aortography.

The status of the peripheral pulses should determine whether an axillary or a femoral artery approach is used. In the presence of a good femoral pulse the latter is the route of choice, not only because it is the easiest (most people have the most experience with this approach) but also because it is the safest. The left axillary approach has been advocated by some; however, it does not offer any advantages. On the other hand, the axillary approach may be disadvantageous in the presence of diastolic hypertension, because of the potential for an axillary hematoma. However, in the absence of good femoral pulses, the left axillary approach should be used. The right axillary approach may become necessary if both the left axillary and the femoral arteries are compromised by the dissection. From the axillary approach, catheterization of the descending aorta may occasionally be difficult. Extensive catheter manipulations must be avoided and another artery selected for percutaneous puncture if the catheter cannot be positioned appropriately for arteriography, owing to entry into the false channel. If arterial puncture is difficult, intravenous DSA, levo phase of pulmonary arteriography with film subtraction, CT, or MRI may be attempted in order to establish the diagnosis.

A pigtail catheter is used, and the pigtail is not allowed to re-form in the abdominal aorta. Instead, a soft-tipped J (LLT) guide wire is inserted beyond the catheter tip (5 to 10 cm) and is used to lead the catheter into the ascending aorta. If the wire does not go beyond the arch, a Type III dissection may be present. In this situation, the guide wire has entered the false channel. The guide wire and catheter are pulled back into the mid-

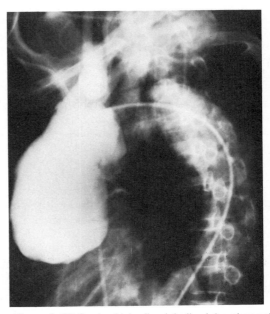

**Figure 8–27.** Contrast injection into the false channel. There is dense contrast opacification because of absent washout. The coronary arteries do not opacify. The brachiocephalic vessels opacify from the false channel.

abdominal aorta and are torqued and readvanced in an attempt to gain entry into the true lumen. If the catheter has entered the false channel in the femoral artery, this maneuver attempts to gain entry into the true lumen through one of the reentry points (if present) between the two lumina.

Catheterization of the false channel is recognized by inability to pass the guide wire tip or catheter beyond the isthmus or by resistance to guide wire and catheter advancement more proximally. A small test injection confirms catheter location in the false channel if there is slow washout of contrast medium and absent filling of branch vessels. In the ascending aorta, a test injection will opacify a blind ending pouch with slow flow, without visualization of the aortic valve, or the coronary arteries (Fig. 8–27).

If there is satisfactory flow in the false channel, an arteriogram may be performed and films are obtained over 8 to 10 seconds. Satisfactory opacification of the entire thoracic aorta is usually obtained by injecting 35 to 50 ml of contrast medium at a rate of 15 to 20 ml/sec into the ascending aorta using a pressure injector. The injection rate is determined by observation of the washout on the hand test. If washout is slow, a slower rate and smaller contrast volume are injected. The longer duration of filming serves to opacify the entry site and the true lumen. Alternatively, the catheter is pulled back to the reentry point, and a second set of films is obtained while injecting into the true lumen. As an alternative to cut film aortography, intraarterial DSA can be performed using 20% contrast medium.

If a reentry point is not demonstrated in dissections beginning in the ascending aorta, a second arteriogram should be performed with injection into the ascending aorta and filming over the abdomen. This serves to identify the extent of the dissection if a reentry point is not present in the lower thorax, in which case the descending thoracic and high abdominal aortograms would not demonstrate the second channel. Similarly, in Type III dissection a second arteriogram with the catheter tip at the isthmus and filming over the abdomen may become necessary, since this may be the only way to evaluate the extent of the dissection.

The arteriographic findings of aortic dissection are (Figs. 8–28 to 8–34):[36, 37]

1. Demonstration of an entry site and in-

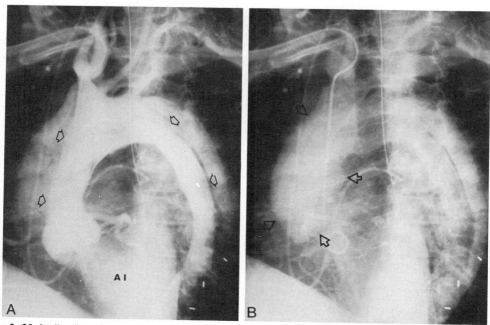

*Figure 8–28.* Aortic dissection. *A,* Left anterior oblique arch aortogram shows a DeBakey Type I or Stanford Type A dissection. The intimal flap is visualized (*arrows*). The dissection extends into the brachiocephalic artery. There is iatrogenic aortic regurgitation (AI) due to placement of the catheter in the aortic valve (see *B*). *B,* Later film from the same aortogram shows persistence of the contrast medium in the false channel in the ascending aorta (*arrows*).

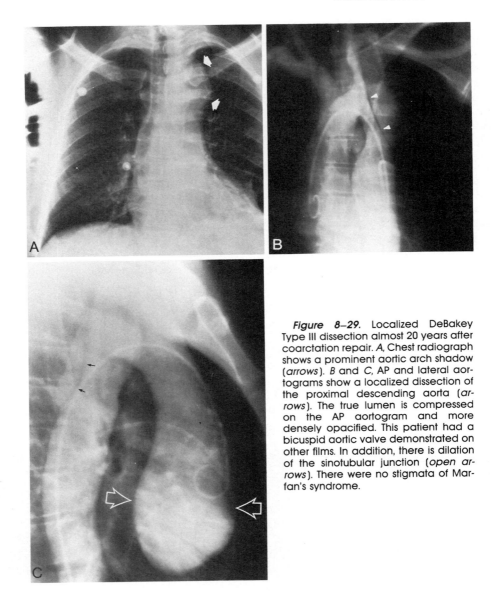

**Figure 8–29.** Localized DeBakey Type III dissection almost 20 years after coarctation repair. *A,* Chest radiograph shows a prominent aortic arch shadow (*arrows*). *B* and *C,* AP and lateral aortograms show a localized dissection of the proximal descending aorta (*arrows*). The true lumen is compressed on the AP aortogram and more densely opacified. This patient had a bicuspid aortic valve demonstrated on other films. In addition, there is dilation of the sinotubular junction (*open arrows*). There were no stigmata of Marfan's syndrome.

timal/medial flap (linear radiolucency within the opacified aorta) with opacification of a second channel, ie, "double barrel aorta" (Figs. 8–28 and 8–29): This is present in up to 87% of patients. Occasionally, only a small portion of the false channel may be opacified.[57] In approximately 13% of patients, a second channel will not be demonstrated.[37] In such cases, the false lumen may have thrombosed if a reentry did not occur or, rarely, an intimal tear may not be present[57] (Fig. 8–30). In this situation, a subtraction film may demonstrate the false channel (Fig. 8–31). Failure to opacify the second channel

may also suggest that the entry site of the dissection lies more proximal or distal to the location where the contrast medium is injected. Occasionally, a lower thoracic or abdominal aortogram may demonstrate the second channel as the contrast medium enters the other lumen via one or more communicating channels or refluxes proximally into the lower pressure false channel through the reentry site (Fig. 8–32; see also Fig. 8–38).

2. Compression of the lumen: Compression of the true lumen by the false channel is observed in 72 to 85% of patients. This may be most prominent at the hiatus aorticus

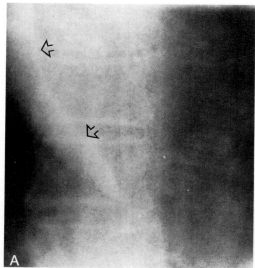

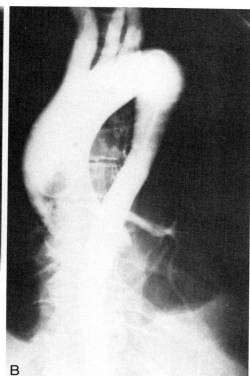

**Figure 8–30.** DeBakey Type I dissection. Spontaneous closure of the false channel in the ascending aorta. *A,* AP frame from a cine arteriogram shows crescent-shaped opacification of the false channel (*arrows*). *B,* AP aortogram obtained a few days later. There is no opacification of the false channel in the ascending aorta. Most of the branches of the descending aorta are not opacified. The false channel was opacified on a descending aortogram.

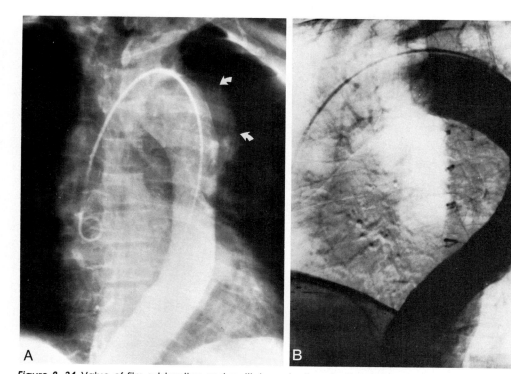

**Figure 8–31.** Value of film subtraction and multiple projections for the demonstration of the second channel. *A,* AP aortogram shows a paraaortic soft tissue density (*arrows*). A second channel is not demonstrated. *B,* Subtraction film from the RPO aortogram shows crescent-shaped opacification of the partially sealed false channel (*arrow*). This was confirmed by CT. The unsubtracted film did not demonstrate this finding.

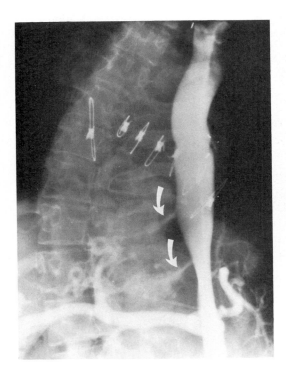

*Figure 8–32.* Aortic dissection with reentry site in the descending aorta. AP aortogram in a patient with Marfan's syndrome shows narrowing of the true lumen as it passes through the diaphragmatic hiatus. Two jets of contrast medium are seen opacifying the false channel (*arrows*).

*Figure 8–33.* Thick-walled aorta without dissection. AP descending thoracic aortogram shows a thick aortic wall (17 mm) without a dissection (*arrows*).

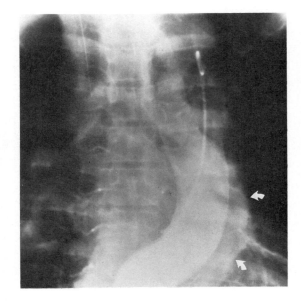

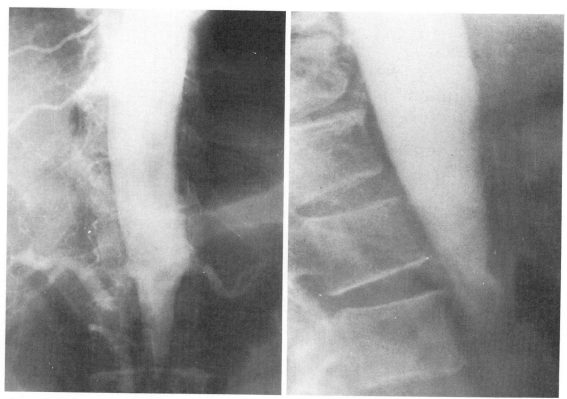

**Figure 8–34.** Aortic dissection leading to obstruction of visceral branches. AP and lateral aortogram via the left axillary approach shows occlusion of the infrarenal aorta. The anterior branches of the abdominal aorta are also occluded.

of the diaphragm (Figs. 8–29 and 8–32; see also Fig. 8–38).

3. Aortic valvular regurgitation: This is seen in up to one third of patients.

4. Abnormal catheter position, ie, outside the anticipated course of the aorta,[37] or obstruction to catheter passage: The latter usually occurs when the catheter has been placed in the false channel and does not enter the true lumen via an intimal tear. In such a situation, the catheter should be withdrawn into the abdominal aorta and repositioned with the aid of a J wire leading the catheter. Alternatively, another vessel is punctured, or intravenous DSA or MRI is performed, or a CT scan is obtained.[58]

5. Increased aortic wall thickness: The aortic wall thickness is normally about 6 mm and usually less than 10 mm. Aortic wall thickness of greater than 10 mm is occasionally seen in atherosclerotic aortas without dissection.[59, 60] This may also be due to a mural thrombus within an ectatic aorta or an aneurysm (Fig. 8–33).[61]

6. Obstruction of aortic branches (Fig. 8–34): Branches of the thoracic or abdominal aorta may be obstructed because of compression of the lumen with which they communicate or as a result of creation of an intimal flap. Any of the visceral branches may be involved. In one series, the left renal artery origin was involved in the dissection in 60% of patients.[54] In most instances, however, the involvement of the left renal artery is less frequent (about 25 to 30%). Thus, the severe hypertension observed in some of these patients may, in part, have a renovascular etiology (caused by renal ischemia). Other vessels may also be involved either by extrinsic compression (by the second channel) or by extension of the dissection (Fig. 8–35). Rarely, the magnitude of the false channel may be such that compromise of the pulmonary blood flow can occur as a result of extrinsic compression.[62]

**Criteria for Differentiating Between True Lumen and False Channel.** There are several criteria that can help to differentiate between the true lumen and the false channel:

1. Location: In most cases, the false chan-

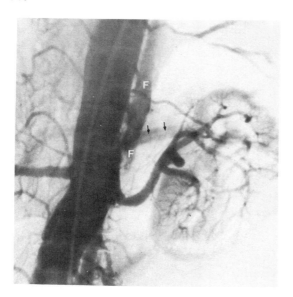

*Figure 8–35.* Extension of dissection into a branch vessel. Subtraction film from an AP aortogram shows the abdominal aortic reentry site of the DeBakey Type III dissection. The dissection extends into the splenic artery (*arrows*), which opacifies from the false channel. F = false channel.

thrombosis of the false channel or failure to establish communication with the true lumen because an intimal tear has not occurred. Often a subtraction film may aid in demonstrating the second channel (Fig. 8–31). Alternatively, intraarterial DSA and sometimes a CT scan may be of help in differentiating between thick-walled senile aortas, aneurysms, and dissection.

3. Visualization of a "pseudo" flap: A tracheo-bronchial air shadow superimposed upon the ascending or descending aorta may simulate a dissection (Fig. 8–36).

4. Visualization of a pseudodissection: Subintimal contrast injection through a side hole jet may simulate a dissection (Fig. 8–37). Unlike a true dissection, the contrast "stain" persists for several seconds after the contrast medium has cleared from the lumen.

5. Inappropriate filming techniques: Single projection aortograms may be insufficient to either establish or exclude the diagnosis (see previous discussion). In addition, 35 mm cine film cameras have the disadvantage of a small field of view and may obscure diagnosis as a result of incomplete identification.[37]

nel lies anterolaterally in the ascending aorta. In the aortic arch it lies superior and posterior and continues posterolaterally into the descending thoracic and abdominal aorta.

2. Blood flow and pressure: In most cases, the blood flow in the false channel is slower than that in the true lumen, and the blood pressure is lower than the systemic pressure.

3. Lumen size: The true aortic lumen is often compressed, whereas the false channel appears wider.

PITFALLS IN DIAGNOSIS

1. Homogeneous opacification of the aorta and nonvisualization of a false channel or intimal flap in the AP projection: This occurs when both the true lumen and the false channel are equally opacified. If the duration of filming is prolonged to approximately 8 to 10 seconds, the true lumen may be identified by more rapid clearing of the contrast medium. Thus, a rapid filming sequence (shorter than 8 seconds) and a single projection (AP) may lead to a false-negative diagnosis.[37, 59] If the biplane filming technique is used, the false channel may be identified on the lateral projection.

2. False channel not opacified: This occurs in up to 13% of patients and may be due to

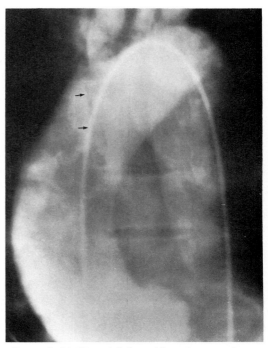

*Figure 8–36.* "Pseudo" flap. AP aortogram shows a lucent stripe projected over the ascending aorta (*arrows*), which simulates a mural flap. This lucent stripe is caused by the tracheal wall.

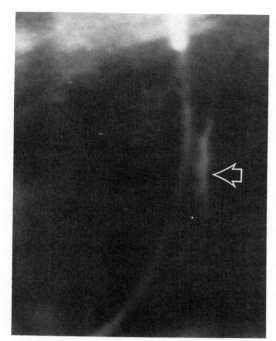

*Figure 8–37.* Subintimal contrast injection from a sidehole simulating a dissection (*arrow*).

## Prognosis and Treatment

The most common cause of death within the first 24 hours is external rupture into either the pleural cavity or the pericardium, leading to cardiac tamponade. Untreated, the mortality rate is high: 3% at onset, 30% at 24 hours, 60% at 3 weeks, and 80% at 3 months.[51] The long-term survival for patients with operatively managed dissections is similar for all types: the 5 year survival for ascending aortic dissection (Type A) is 53% and for descending aortic dissection (Type B), 55%.[63]

Opacification of the false channel on aortography has been used as a prognostic feature. Some authors believe that a failure to gain a reentry distally may lead to thrombosis of the false channel, reducing the chances of external rupture. Thus, in one report, there was a 90% survival if the false channel was not demonstrated by arteriography, whereas it was only 43% if the false channel was opacified, suggesting that spontaneous reentry may not be desirable for the survival of medically managed patients.[57] On the other hand, failure to establish a reentry may precipitate external rupture.

In general, dissections of the descending aorta (Type III or B) are managed by medical therapy. Operation is indicated for dissections involving the ascending aorta and for descending aortic dissections complicated by occlusion of visceral or lower extremity arteries.

## Chronic Dissection

Up to 10% of aortic dissections may be chronic.[35, 64, 65] Clinically, these manifest with congestive heart failure and minimal, often atypical chest pain.[35] Chronic dissections are usually Type III, and all have a reentry point distally, ie, a double barrel aorta (which has been called the "imperfect natural cure"). In one review, a reentry site was present in 90% of those patients surviving more than 5 weeks after the initial episode.[66] Such dissections are compatible with a long survival, and the increased use of arteriography often leads to their incidental, unsuspected discovery.[37]

## Aortogram After Repair of Dissection

In most cases, only the proximal portion of the aorta is replaced (ascending or proximal descending aorta). Thus, the point of reentry is not closed, and in some patients operative closure may not be desirable (if vital organs are supplied by the false channel). Thus, the false channel may persist as a low pressure second channel (Fig. 8–38).

## TRAUMA

Aortic laceration or rupture resulting from sudden horizontal deceleration injuries of the thorax, such as those associated with automobile accidents, most frequently involve the thoracic aorta. Vertical deceleration injuries occurring after a fall from great heights or airplane crashes also injure the descending thoracic aorta.[67-70]

## Clinical Aspects

Clinical findings may be vague, absent, or masked by other injuries, and often the first clue as to major vascular injury is supplied by the chest radiograph.[68, 70-73] Some of the signs of acute aortic injury include hypertension in the upper extremities (acute traumatic coarctation), alteration in peripheral pulses, murmurs, and dyspnea.[73] If no other severe injuries are present, only 20% of patients

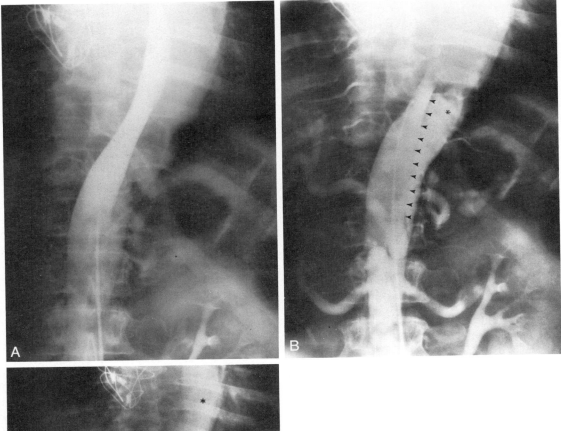

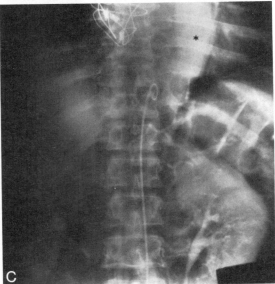

*Figure 8–38.* Patent false channel several months after repair of aortic dissection. *A,* AP aortogram shows a compressed true lumen. *B,* Later film from the same aortogram shows the mural flap (*arrowheads*) and reflux of contrast medium into the false channel (*). *C,* Late film from the same aortogram shows persistent contrast opacification of the false channel (*).

with acute aortic laceration survive the initial episode.[68] If associated cardiac injuries are present, only 14% of the victims survive.[68] Cardiac involvement in thoracic trauma may simulate complete transection of the aorta.[74] In descending order of frequency, the rupture of the cardiac chamber involves the left ventricle, right ventricle, right atrium, and left atrium.[74]

## Pathology

Deceleration injury produces torsion stress at the aorto-cardiac junction and shear stress at points of maximal fixation of the aorta. In over 80% of patients, the laceration is located at the aortic isthmus, just distal to the insertion of the ligamentum arteriosum. The second most frequent site is the proximal ascending aorta. Other areas include the descending aorta at the diaphragmatic hiatus and the transverse aortic arch. The laceration is most often transverse, and all layers of the aortic wall are involved in only 40% of patients.[75] The injury is frequently located over the anterior surface of the isthmus but can be localized to the posterior wall.[68]

## Radiology

There are several radiographic signs suggestive of severe mediastinal injury. However, none of these signs alone has any predictive value (Table 8–3).

1. Mediastinal widening: In one series, mediastinal widening of more than 8 cm was observed with almost equal frequency in patients with (75.5%) and without (73.7%) aortic laceration following blunt chest trauma.[72] In another report, mediastinal to chest width ratio, measured at the level of the aortic arch and ascending aorta, could be correlated with the presence of aortic laceration.[76] Thus, if this ratio exceeded 0.25, 95% of patients with aortic rupture could be identified, with a 25% false-positive rate. With a ratio greater than 0.28, the sensitivity was 85%, with no false-positive findings. In some patients, mediastinal widening may be due to laceration of veins and small arteries. In addition, iatrogenic causes should be excluded (eg, hydromediastinum from inappropriately placed central venous catheters or cardiovascular perforation by such catheters).[77]

2. Indistinctness of the aortic contour: This may be caused by hematoma resulting from small arterial or venous lacerations. In one series of patients with acute chest injury, this finding was present in 75.5% of those with aortic lacerations but also in 95% of patients without aortic lacerations.[72]

3. Displaced trachea: Displacement of the trachea to the right, indicative of a mediastinal hematoma, was associated with aortic laceration in approximately 61% of patients and in only 5% of patients without aortic injury in one series and approximately 32% without aortic injury in another.[72, 78] Tracheal displacement to the left may be indicative of brachiocephalic artery laceration.

4. Displaced nasogastric tube: Displacement of the nasogastric tube to the right by mediastinal hematoma or false aneurysm has been reported in 67 to 100% of patients with aortic laceration and in up to 23% of patients without laceration.[72, 78, 79] However, a combination of tracheal and esophageal displacement may be predictive of aortic laceration in 96% of patients.[78]

5. Displaced left mainstem bronchus: Inferior displacement of the left mainstem bronchus may be observed in approximately half the patients with aortic laceration.

6. Rib fractures: This finding is observed more frequently in patients without associated aortic or great vessel injury.[76, 78] Rib fractures with associated pneumothorax are more commonly associated with major airway laceration.

**TABLE 8–3.** Incidence of Chest Radiographic Signs and Aortic Laceration in Patients with Severe Blunt Thoracic Trauma*

| Radiographic Sign | Incidence of Occurrence (%) | |
|---|---|---|
| | Aortic Laceration | Normal Aortogram |
| Mediastinal widening >8 cm | 75.5 | 73.7 |
| Indistinct aortic outline (arch) (descending aorta) | 75.5 12.2 | 94.7 15.4 |
| Tracheal displacement to right | 61.2 | 31.6 |
| Esophageal displacement to right (nasogastric tube) | 66.7 | 23.1 |
| Inferior displacement of left mainstem bronchus | 53.1 | 26.3 |
| Apical pleural cap | 36.7 | 42.1 |
| Rib (1–2) fracture | 17.0 | 30.0 |

*Adapted from references 72 and 76.

Although none of these radiographic signs alone has any predictive value, nevertheless their presence reflects significant intrathoracic injury. On the other hand, the appearance of the chest radiograph cannot be relied upon to decide whether aortography should be performed, since minimal or absent abnormality on the chest radiograph can be associated with significant vascular trauma. The decision for proceeding with aortography should be based primarily on the clinical findings and assessment of severity of the injury.

## Arteriography (Table 8–4)

Arteriography is indicated to evaluate the location and extent of vascular injury. In the majority of patients, the transfemoral route can be used, as this is the safest and fastest route and facilitates a speedy examination. If femoral pulses are diminished, the axillary approach is used. A J guide wire is used to lead a pigtail catheter past the aortic isthmus and arch and into the ascending aorta. After completion of the study, the pigtail should be straightened with the aid of a guide wire before withdrawing it past the laceration. If an arterial line has to be left in the femoral artery for monitoring blood pressure, a short catheter introducer sheath should be inserted. Multiple hole catheters should not be left in the aorta, as they are not well suited to serve as indwelling arterial catheters.

The initial arteriogram is a biplane arch aortogram in the AP and lateral projections. If biplane filming is not available, a 45° left

anterior oblique arch aortogram is performed. If the ascending aorta, arch, and proximal descending aorta are normal, a biplane descending thoracic aortogram is performed in the AP and lateral projections. The descending aortogram should include the upper abdominal aorta (above the celiac artery).

If the biplane arch aortogram is unrevealing, a left anterior oblique (45°) arch aortogram should be performed. Similarly, when the left anterior oblique aortogram is the initial study (only single plane equipment) and is unrevealing, a lateral or right anterior oblique arch aortogram should be obtained.

For the arch aortograms the patient is positioned so as to include the brachiocephalic vessels. In addition, subtraction films should be obtained if the arteriograms are unrevealing.

In some patients, DSA may be used to provide a speedy examination. However, the lack of patient cooperation and the inability to detect subtle abnormalities may limit the accuracy of such an examination.

The arteriographic findings in aortic and arch vessel lacerations include (Figs. 8–39 to 8–43):

1. Traumatic aneurysm: The majority of patients develop a false aneurysm at the site

### TABLE 8–4. Aortogram for Evaluation of Aortic Laceration

| | |
|---|---|
| Catheter:<br>  Position | 7 Fr pigtail<br>Ascending aorta |
| Guide wire | J-LLT |
| Contrast medium | 76% diatrizoate meglumine<br>  sodium |
| Injection rate/volume | 30 ml/sec, total 60 ml |
| Films:<br>  Filming rate<br><br>  Projections<br><br>  Alternate | 13 films per projection<br>3 per second for 9 films<br>1 per second for 4 films<br>a. Biplane (AP/lateral)<br>b. LAO (45°)<br>a. LAO (45°)<br>b. Lateral<br>c. RAO or AP |

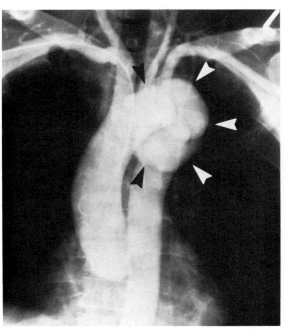

*Figure 8–39.* Traumatic aortic aneurysm following a motor vehicle accident. AP aortogram shows an aneurysm of the arch and proximal descending thoracic aorta (*arrowheads*).

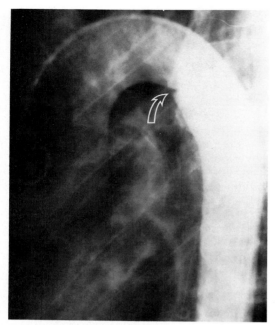

*Figure 8–40.* Aortic laceration due to deceleration injury. Lateral aortogram shows a focal intimal tear (*arrow*). This injury was confirmed at operation.

of laceration. In some patients, the aneurysm formation may be delayed by several months or years.

2. Intimal tear: In 5 to 10% of patients, only an intimal tear will be seen on aortography. In approximately 60% of patients, the laceration involves the intima and media only. On the aortogram this is seen as a linear lucency. Demonstration of contrast extravasation or complete occlusion of the aorta is rare.

3. Multiple injuries: In the majority of patients, only a single lesion is present (96.3% of 510 patients in one series).[72] In another series, 19% of patients had multiple tears.[67] Figure 8–43 shows the location of injury in 491 patients reviewed in one series.[72] Despite the relative infrequency of multiple injuries, the entire thoracic and upper abdominal aorta must be evaluated in each case. Failure to do this may leave undetected a second laceration, which may be of significance and may result in severe complications.[80] Multiple injuries are more likely if the brachiocephalic artery is involved. Thus, in one series, 74% of patients with laceration of the brachiocephalic artery had a second injury.[72]

4. Posttraumatic dissection: The injury may not be localized. In some patients, acute posttraumatic dissection, either antegrade or retrograde into the arch, may occur in addition to the laceration.[81] Significant aortic dissections may occur in up to 11% of patients with aortic lacerations (Fig. 8–42).[72, 81] Such dissections are either medial or more often

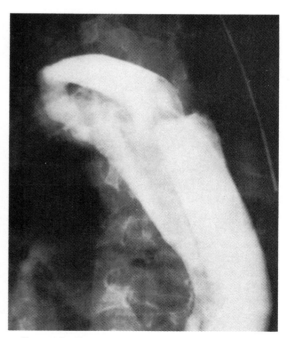

*Figure 8–42.* Traumatic aortic dissection. Contrast medium was injected into the false channel and demonstrates a transverse laceration at the aortic isthmus and dissection of the descending aorta in a 56 year old man. (From Fischer RG et al: Radiol Clin North Am 19:91, 1981. Used with permission.)

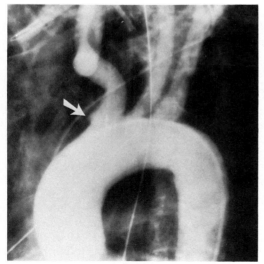

*Figure 8–41.* Traumatic aneurysm of the brachiocephalic artery (*arrow*) due to deceleration injury.

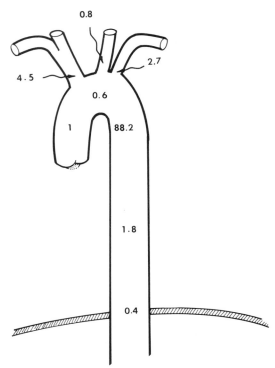

*Figure 8–43.* Distribution of nonpenetrating injuries to the aorta and major branches in a review of 491 patients with single vessel injury. (Adapted from Fischer RG et al: Radiol Clin North Am 19:91, 1981.)

subadventitial and may occur in young individuals without predisposing factors such as atherosclerosis or pregnancy.[72, 82, 83] In older individuals with atherosclerotic aortas, traumatic dissection tends to be medial.

5. Posttraumatic coarctation: The findings of (a) elevated upper extremity blood pressure and widened pulse amplitude, (b) decreased lower extremity blood pressure and narrowed pulse amplitude, and (c) widened mediastinum on the chest radiograph are considered the diagnostic triad of traumatic coarctation of the aorta.[84] Compromise of the aortic lumen with diminished distal circulation as a result of significant aortic laceration, dissection, or associated hematoma at the site of laceration is the most likely cause of this acute syndrome.[80, 85, 86] Aortic fibrosis leading to stenosis may be responsible for the delayed manifestation of this syndrome in some patients.[22, 72]

**Precautions and Complications.** Although careful passage of a soft-tipped J guide wire leading the catheter past a traumatized segment of the aorta does not increase the risk of complications, the femoral artery approach should be avoided in patients with symptoms of posttraumatic coarctation. In reports reviewing large numbers of patients and publications, no additional risks of complications from arteriography were identified.[71, 72]

PITFALLS IN DIAGNOSIS

1. Benign-appearing chest radiograph: Lesions of the descending thoracic aorta overlying the pulmonary hila and the heart may be overlooked on the chest radiograph. Thus, in presence of strong clinical suspicion, an aortogram should be performed even though the chest radiographic findings do not suggest the presence of major vessel injury.

2. Incomplete study: Single projection aortography is often not adequate for establishing the diagnosis of aortic laceration. If the first aortogram is unrevealing, another injection is made in a second projection (eg, if the left anterior oblique projection does not detect an abnormality, the aortogram is repeated in the lateral projection). If this too is unrevealing and the clinical suspicion is strong, another aortogram in a third projection (eg, an AP or a right anterior oblique) should be obtained. In all arteriograms not demonstrating a major vessel injury, subtraction films should be obtained. These will often pick up a small lesion that may have been obscured on the original aortogram.

3. Poor technical film quality: Significant abnormalities can be missed on under- or overexposed radiographs. Only good quality radiographs and patient positioning to include the proximal brachiocephalic vessels can provide an accurate diagnosis. Similarly, an abnormality may be missed if an inadequate contrast injection rate or volume is used.

## Penetrating Trauma

Approximately 20% of patients with penetrating trauma to the aorta survive the initial episode.[69] Such trauma may be due to a high or low velocity object and may lead to exsanguination, development of false aneurysms, arteriovenous fistulae, or thrombotic occlusion. Arteriography is indicated if the path of the foreign object lies in close proximity to a major vessel or if such an object actually lodges in close proximity to a major vessel.

Arterial trauma may also occur in the clinical setting, eg, during attempted subclavian vein catheterization (Fig. 8–44).

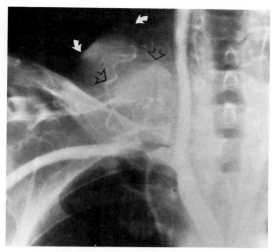

Figure 8–44. False aneurysm of the right vertebral artery. Trauma occurred during an attempt at placement of a subclavian line. AP brachiocephalic arteriogram shows a large false aneurysm. Contrast opacifies the lumen of the aneurysm (*open arrows*). Solid arrows point to the supraclavicular soft tissue mass.

## Minimal Injury

A number of patients studied for acute blunt or penetrating thoracic trauma may not have any obvious evidence of aortic injury

on the arteriogram. However, close examination of the aortogram will occasionally detect subtle signs of mural aortic injury with an intact intima.

Arteriographic signs of such injury include (Fig. 8–45):

1. Aortic displacement. This may be due to a mediastinal hematoma from venous injury and occasionally from laceration of an intercostal artery or aortic vasa vasorum.

2. Mural hematoma. A hematoma of the aortic wall may be observed after penetrating or blunt thoracic trauma. It is most likely due to direct injury to the aortic media and/or adventitia.

Since intimal injury is absent, a lumen irregularity, dissection, or false aneurysm is not observed on the arteriogram, and unless the traumatized region is seen tangentially, subtle mural injuries may go unrecognized. A careful study of the late phase of the arteriogram may detect intimal indentation due to a mural hematoma as the contrast medium begins to layer out.

Because of the apparent innocuous nature of this type of aortic injury and the absence of referable clinical signs and symptoms, such patients rarely undergo exploratory surgery or other forms of treatment for this

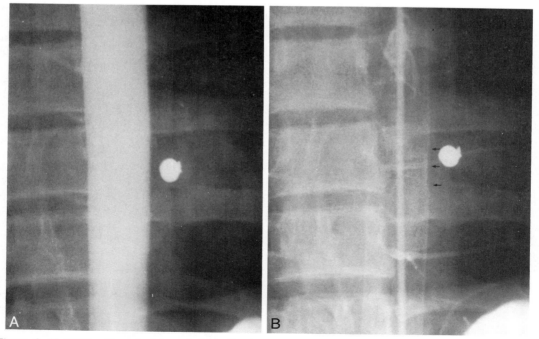

Figure 8–45. "Minimal" aortic injury. *A*, Early film from an AP descending aortogram shows a normal aortic silhouette adjacent to the bullet. *B*, Later film from the same aortogram shows minimal displacement of the intima by the mural hematoma, which is outlined by layered contrast medium (*arrows*).

injury. However, it remains undetermined whether this type of injury is responsible for the development of some late complications such as traumatic coarctation or false aneurysms.

## MISCELLANEOUS DISORDERS

### Aortitis (Figs. 8–46 to 8–48 and Table 8–5)

Aortitis may be due to an infectious agent or may occur as a manifestation of a systemic disorder. Although the incidence of syphilitic aortitis is decreasing, other infections are being seen more frequently. Suppurative and granulomatous infections of the aorta show a predilection for congenital or acquired lesions, such as coarctation, cystic medial necrosis, or atherosclerotic and syphilitic lesions, and may lead to the formation of mycotic aneurysms.[25]

In aortitis associated with rheumatic fever, aortic damage occurs rarely. In recurrent rheumatic fever, aortitis may be severe, and the abdominal aorta appears to be involved most commonly.[87] However, diffuse involvement of the aorta may also occur, and fusiform aneurysms and dissection may occasionally develop.[87, 88] Approximately 2% of

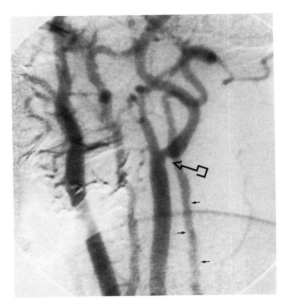

**Figure 8–47.** Giant cell arteritis. Intravenous DSA in the RPO projection in a young woman shows focal stenosis of the origin of the left internal carotid artery (*open arrow*). Alternating areas of mild stenosis of the left vertebral artery are also present (*small arrows*). Similar lesions are also seen in the right vertebral artery, which is partially obscured by a subtraction artefact.

patients with longstanding rheumatoid arthritis and ankylosing spondylitis have aortitis and valvular endocarditis, which may lead to aortic insufficiency.[89, 90] Long-term steroid therapy for rheumatoid arthritis may be responsible for spontaneous aortic rupture.[31]

Giant cell arteritis involves isolated segments of the media of large and medium-sized arteries. The aorta, coronary, carotid, vertebral, subclavian, celiac, superior mesenteric, iliac, renal, ophthalmic, and retinal arteries (leading to blindness) may be involved (Fig. 8–47).[91-96] The etiology is unknown, and giant cell arteritis is seen with equal frequency in individuals of both sexes and occurs most frequently in the fifth and sixth decades of life. Arteriography demonstrates alternating segments of smooth arterial narrowing and areas of mild dilatation. Arterial occlusions are also seen, and the involvement is characteristically bilateral.

In relapsing polychondritis, approximately 10% of patients have aortitis of the ascending aorta with dilatation of the aortic annulus.[34] Aneurysms of the descending aorta also occur.[25, 34]

Takayasu's disease, or pulseless syn-

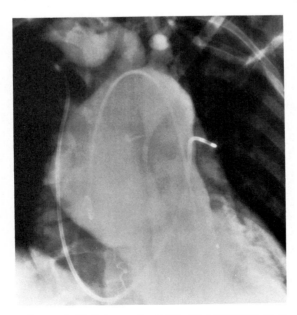

**Figure 8–46.** Takayasu's aortitis. AP aortogram in a teen-aged girl shows a massively dilated ascending and descending aorta. The arteritis also involves the arch vessels. In addition, there is cardiomegaly.

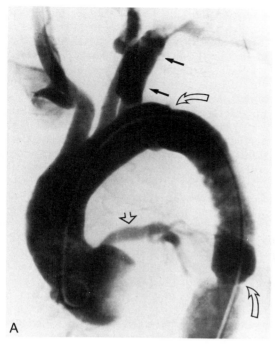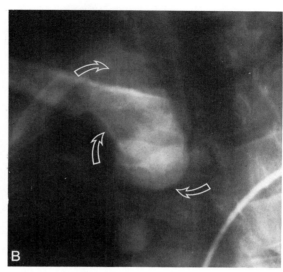

**Figure 8–48.** Diffuse arteritis leading to dissection and aneurysm formation in a 29 year old woman during the eighth month of pregnancy. *A*, Subtraction film from an aortogram after repair of a Type III dissection shows a descending aortic graft (*curved open arrows*) and a fusiform aneurysm of the left subclavian artery (*solid arrows*). There is mild ectasia of the ascending aorta and the left coronary artery (*open straight arrow*). A jet of contrast is seen entering the right subclavian artery aneurysm. *B*, Late film from an AP aortogram shows contrast medium within the right subclavian artery aneurysm (*arrows*).

drome, is an arteritis of unknown etiology with worldwide distribution, which occurs predominantly in young females. It involves the aortic arch vessels primarily but may also affect the thoracic and abdominal aorta and pulmonary arteries.[97-100] Histologically, there is intimal thickening and destruction of the muscular and elastic tissue. On arteriography, smooth segmental stenoses are seen.

### TABLE 8–5. Diseases or Agents That May Cause Aortitis

Ankylosing spondylitis
Behçet's disease
Giant cell arteritis
Hodgkin's disease
Idiopathic aortitis
Infection, suppurative
Infection, granulomatous (syphilis, tuberculosis)
Radiation
Reiter's disease
Relapsing polychondritis
Rheumatoid arthritis
Rheumatic fever
Scleroderma
Systemic lupus erythematosus
Takayasu's disease

In addition to segmental stenosis of the abdominal aorta (atypical coarctation of the abdominal aorta), there may be occlusion or aneurysm formation.[25] Aneurysms also occur in the ascending aorta, which may lead to difficulty in differentiating Takayasu's disease from other forms of aortitis (Fig. 8–46).[25] As a rule, however, other parts of the aorta are involved in Takayasu's disease, and it primarily affects younger females.

### Atherosclerotic and Occlusive Diseases

Atherosclerotic stenosis or occlusion of the brachiocephalic vessels at their origins from the aortic arch may give rise to symptoms of cerebral ischemia or arm claudication. Occasionally, a severe stenosis of the brachiocephalic artery orifice may be associated with amaurosis fugax.[101] Arteriographic evaluation of the proximal great vessels requires multiple projections, because a lesion may be missed if only the standard (AP/lateral or left anterior oblique) projections are used (Figs. 8–49 and 8–50) (also see Fig. 9–14, Chapter 9).

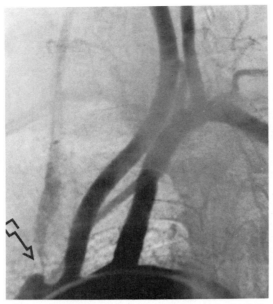

*Figure 8–49.* Severe atherosclerotic stenosis of the brachiocephalic artery *(arrow)* causing amaurosis fugax. (From Kadir S, Roberson GH: Radiology 130:171, 1979. Used with permission.)

Acute arterial occlusion may be due to either in-situ thrombus formation in areas of preexisting stenosis or an embolus (Fig. 8–51). The most common source for arterial emboli is the heart. Almost half of these patients have atrial fibrillation, and in many patients the source may be a mural thrombus after a myocardial infarction.

**Dysphagia Aortica.** "Dysphagia aortica," a term coined by Pape in 1932, may result from esophageal compression at the level of (1) the aortic arch, (2) proximal descending aorta, or (3) distal thoracic aorta.[102]

Ectasia, arch anomalies, or aneurysms of the aortic arch may be responsible for dysphagia and occasionally for hoarseness (recurrent laryngeal nerve compression).[103] Similarly, large aneurysms of the thoracic aorta may cause significant esophageal compression.[104] A more frequent cause of dysphagia aortica is an entrapment of the distal esophagus at or above the esophageal hiatus of the diaphragm by an atherosclerotic, ectatic thoracic aorta. Symptoms include substernal fullness after eating, burning chest pain, regurgitation, and inability to swallow solids. It occurs more frequently in elderly women and may be accentuated by a thoracic kyphosis.[104-106]

In most instances, the diagnosis can be made on the basis of a barium esophagogram, which has relatively characteristic appearance.[103-106] Aortography is required only if surgery is contemplated for aortic aneurysms or dissection or if aneurysm rupture is suspected.

**Dysphagia Lusoria.** Dysphagia may also be due to esophageal compression by an aneurysm or ectasia of an aberrant right subclavian artery. Rarely, a tortuous vertebral artery may be responsible for these symptoms.[107] A characteristic esophageal indentation is seen on barium swallow (see under Congenital Malformations in this chapter).[107-110]

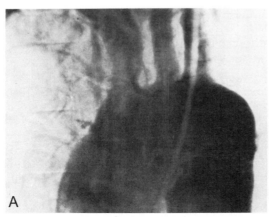
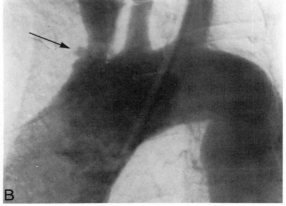

*Figure 8–50.* Ulcerated atherosclerotic plaque of the brachiocephalic artery. *A,* On the AP aortogram via the left axillary approach there is only minimal narrowing of the proximal brachiocephalic artery. *B,* Repeat aortogram in the left anterior projection reveals the ulcerated plaque *(arrow).*

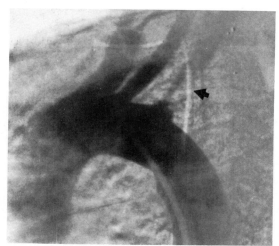

**Figure 8–51.** Left anterior oblique arch aortogram shows partial occlusion of the left subclavian artery due to in situ thrombosis (*arrow*).

## Marfan's Syndrome

Marfan's syndrome is a generalized connective tissue disorder that is manifested by

ocular, skeletal, and cardiovascular abnormalities. It is inherited as an autosomal dominant trait with variable penetrance. Approximately 15% of cases represent new mutations.[111] Cardiovascular abnormalities occur in up to 60% of patients with this disease and may be the cause of death in as many as 93% of patients.[112, 113]

Aortic disease or its complications, which account for approximately 55% of deaths,[112] may be manifested by (Figs. 8–52 and 8–53):[47, 111, 114]

1. Aortic aneurysms, predominantly of the ascending aorta.

2. Dilatation of the aortic sinuses in the region of the sinotubular junction, leading to aortic valve insufficiency. This dilatation of the aortic sinuses is the arteriographic feature that distinguishes Marfan's syndrome from atherosclerosis. However, sinotubular dilatation has also been observed in some patients with aortitis and aortic coarctation with a bicuspid aortic valve (see Fig. 8–29).

3. Aortic dissection.

4. Coarctation.

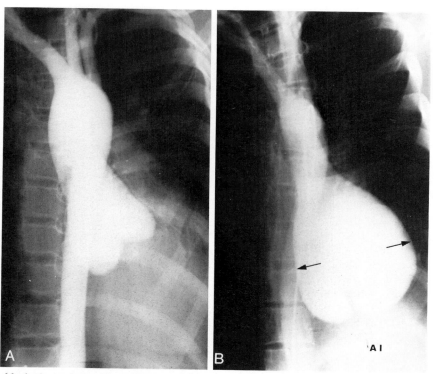

**Figure 8–52.** Marfan's syndrome. Progressive enlargement of the aortic sinuses leading to aortic insufficiency. *A*, AP aortogram in a teen-aged male patient shows dilated aortic sinuses. *B*, Aortogram obtained 5 years later shows further enlargement of the aortic sinuses and widening of the sinotubular junction (*arrows*) leading to aortic valve insufficiency (AI).

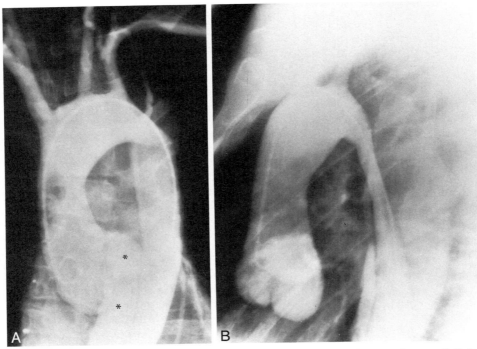

*Figure 8–53.* Aortic dissection in a patient with Marfan's syndrome. *A,* AP aortogram shows a DeBakey Type III dissection with reflux of contrast into the false channel (*) in the descending aorta. *B,* On the lateral aortogram, marked narrowing of the true lumen is present. The sinotubular junction is dilated.

Loss of vascular elastic tissue with fragmentation of the elastic fibers and accumulation of collagenous and metachromatically staining material leads to weakening of the aortic wall.[112] Progressive dilatation and aneurysm formation involve the ascending aorta most frequently but may also be seen in the abdominal aorta and iliac arteries. Eighty-one per cent of patients with an aortic root diameter exceeding 5 cm and 100% of patients with an aortic root diameter exceeding 6 cm have aortic regurgitation.[47]

In one review of 505 cases of aortic dissection, 16% of the patients, all less than 40 years of age, had Marfan's syndrome.[35] Often, old localized intimal tears have been demonstrated in the ascending aortic aneurysms of patients with Marfan's syndrome.[115] These are probably too localized and small to be detected by aortography. Not all intimal tears progress to dissection, and dissection is rare in patients without significant dilatation.

## Ehlers-Danlos Syndrome

Ehlers-Danlos syndrome is an autosomal dominant hereditary disorder of connective

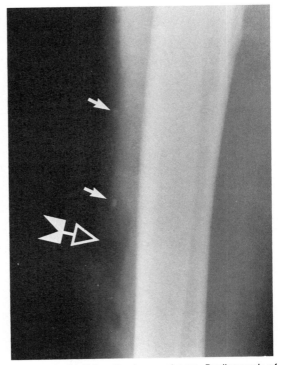

*Figure 8–54.* Ehlers-Danlos syndrome. Radiograph of the lower extremity shows a gaping soft tissue wound (*large arrow*) and spheroids (*small solid arrows*).

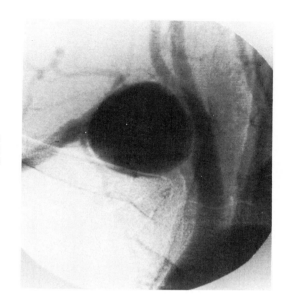

*Figure 8–55.* Intravenous DSA with contrast injection into the superior vena cava shows a large aneurysm of the right subclavian artery in a 17 year old male with Ehlers-Danlos syndrome.

tissue manifested by hyperelasticity of the skin with poor healing and gaping wounds, hyperextensibility of the joints, fragility of the blood vessels, and soft tissue calcifications (spheroids) (Fig. 8–54). There are five clinically recognizable types: gravis, mitis, benign hypermobile, ecchymotic, and X-linked. Vascular lesions include aortic dissection, aneurysms and rarely tortuosity of the arch and ectasia of the pulmonary arteries (Fig. 8–55).[116-119]

Significant complications have been reported following arteriography in some patients with Ehlers-Danlos syndrome. These include aortic rupture and hematomas of significant proportion, both of which have been linked to the tissue fragility.[120, 121] Thus, because of the potential for arterial complications, particularly in patients with the ecchymotic type, arteriography is contraindicated and carefully performed intravenous DSA, CT, or MRI may provide the necessary information.

## Pseudo-Coarctation

Pseudo-coarctation, or aortic kinking, is a rare congenital anomaly of the aortic arch.[122] It is characterized by elongation of the ascending aorta, leading to a high transverse aortic arch and redundancy of the arch and proximal descending aorta, without associated abnormalities of the arch vessels. However, associated aortic valve abnormalities such as bicuspid aortic valve, aortic insufficiency, and stenosis have been reported.[123, 124] There is no association with other congenital cardiac lesions.[125]

Clinically, an ejection type murmur, resulting from turbulence in the kink and radiating to the neck and interscapular area, may be heard.[125] The age of the individuals has ranged from 12 to 64 years.[123, 125] Often a mediastinal widening suggestive of a mass lesion is the first clue to an underlying abnormality. At surgery for erroneous diagnoses of mediastinal tumor or true coarctation and at autopsy, a redundant aorta has been found, with no evidence of a hemodynamically significant stenosis.[125]

Although the aortic valve abnormalities recorded in one series are suggestive of a similarity with obstructive coarctation,[123] pseudo-coarctation is easily differentiated from the latter by the absence of clinically referable symptoms and by the absence of hemodynamic obstruction (no collateral circulation or rib notching). Hemodynamically, a gradient may be present and is usually less than 10 mm Hg, although in some patients a gradient of 20 mm Hg has been recorded.[123-125]

The aortogram demonstrates a high aortic arch with a kink at the isthmus and proximal descending aorta resembling the numeral 3, in which the mid-portion of the 3 corresponds to the attachment of the ligamentum arteriosum (Fig. 8–56). A short ligamentum has been incriminated etiologically.[126]

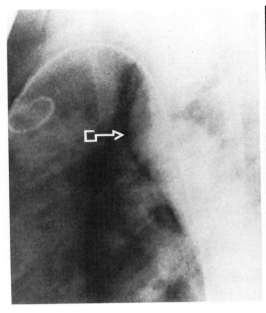 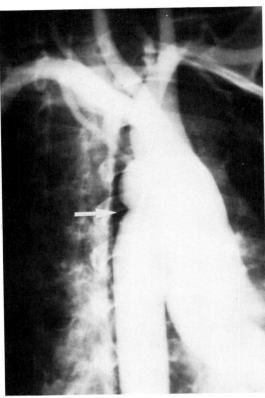

*Figure 8–56.* Pseudo-coarctation. Lateral (left) and RAO (right) aortograms from different patients show the typical "kink" at the aortic isthmus (*arrow*).

## BRONCHIAL/INTERCOSTAL ARTERIES

### Bronchial Arteries

1. Between 21 and 38% of individuals have only two bronchial arteries (one on each side).[7, 127] In up to 31%, the right bronchial artery arises from the third posterior intercostal artery and rarely from the fourth or fifth intercostal artery. The left bronchial artery arises directly from the aorta. In approximately 7% of individuals, both bronchial arteries arise from the aorta, occasionally as a common trunk.

2. Between 40 and 50% of individuals have three bronchial arteries.[7, 127] In approximately 40%, there are two left bronchial arteries arising directly from the aorta (rarely from the right third or fourth intercostal artery) and one right bronchial artery. Between 5 and 10% of individuals have two right and one left bronchial artery.

3. Approximately 24% of individuals have four bronchial arteries.[127] Twenty per cent have two left and two right bronchial arteries;

4% have three left and one right bronchial artery.

Thus, a single right bronchial artery occurs in approximately 60% of individuals, and about 70% of the time it has a common origin with an intercostal artery, thus forming an intercostobronchial trunk that arises posterolaterally from the aorta.[7, 127] Multiple bronchial arteries are more common on the left side, occurring in about 70% of individuals.[127] Only 4% of the left bronchial arteries form an intercostobronchial trunk with a right intercostal artery.[127, 128] Seventy per cent arise directly from the thoracic aorta; 15% originate from the concavity of the aortic arch; the remainder originate from the descending aorta.[127, 128]

Bronchial arteries arising directly from the aorta do so from the ventral or ventrolateral surface. The intercostobronchial trunks arise dorsolaterally or laterally on the right side.

An anomalous origin of the bronchial arteries other than the variants described is infrequent, but may be from the internal mammary, inferior thyroidal, superior intercostal, inferior phrenic, subclavian, or brachiocephalic arteries and rarely from the ascending or abdominal aorta.[7, 127, 129, 130]

Topographically, almost all bronchial arteries (except for anomalies) originate from the thoracic aorta between T4 and T7. Approximately 86% of the right and 70% of the left bronchial artery orifices are located between the undersurface of T4 and T6.[128] According to another author, approximately 90% of all bronchial arteries arise around T5–T6.[131]

Anastomoses have been demonstrated between the bronchial arteries and the pulmonary, mediastinal, and coronary arteries.[132–136] Such anastomoses serve as collateral vascular channels for the pulmonary circulation in patients with pulmonary artery atresia or stenosis and as collateral channels to the coronary arteries in patients with coronary artery stenosis.[132, 135] Bronchial and pulmonary artery anastomoses have also been demonstrated in normal lung specimens.[135, 136] In addition, spinal cord branches may arise from the central segments of the bronchial arteries. This rarely occurs on the left side. Knowledge of the presence of such collaterals is important when treating patients with hemoptysis, so that small particulate emboli, which could conceivably end up in the coronary circulation, are not used. In addition, identification of the spinal cord branch is essential for prevention of ischemic or chemical injury to the cord.

There are two groups of bronchial veins.[136] One group (true veins) drains into the pulmonary veins or left atrium; the other group anastomoses freely with the pulmonary veins but drains into the azygos-hemiazygos system.

## Intercostal Arteries

The dorsal intercostal arteries originate from the posterior aortic wall. In general, the orifices of the left and right intercostal arteries are located in close proximity to each other. Topographically, even in the presence of disease (aneurysm, dissection), the intercostal artery orifices are located adjacent to the left lateral border of the thoracic vertebral bodies.

## Arteriography of Bronchial/Intercostal Vessels

The main indication for bronchial arteriography is the evaluation of a patient with hemoptysis. In children with pulmonary atresia, bronchial arteriography serves to define the pulmonary artery anatomy prior to reconstructive surgery. Thoracic aortography may provide satisfactory information for gross evaluation of the intercostal arteries in patients with thoracic trauma or aneurysms. However, it does not provide satisfactory opacification of the bronchial arteries in patients with uncompromised pulmonary blood flow. Thus, selective arteriography is essential for accurate evaluation.

A variety of catheters have been used successfully, including the tip deflecting catheter system, 150° curved KIFA, cobra, single curve, sidewinder, and headhunter curves.[128, 137, 138] For the 15% of left bronchial arteries that arise from the concavity of the aorta, a headhunter or cobra catheter is used. For bronchial arteries originating more distally, either the sidewinder or cobra curve is used. In patients with tortuous aortas, some authors have found the Judkins right coronary catheter to be helpful.[131] Since 90% of all bronchial arteries may originate between T4 and T6, the catheter for the initial search should be either a cobra C2 or sidewinder I. In tortuous and ectatic aortas, the sidewinder II or preferably a cobra C3 curve is used.

The catheter tip is pointed posterolaterally along the right aortic wall, and the orifice of the bronchial artery is searched by moving the catheter slowly up and down the aorta between T4 and T7. For each new seeking motion, the tip of the catheter is turned slightly (by 2 to 5°) towards the lateral aortic wall. For the left bronchial artery, the catheter tip should point anterolaterally, moving anteriorly with each seeking motion. A valuable aid for localization of the area of interest is to tape small lead numbers or thin lead markers onto the skin at the level of the fourth through seventh thoracic vertebral bodies. The orifices of the upper intercostal arteries may lie in close proximity to each other, which may give rise to difficulty in separating them from each other.

When the catheter "hooks" onto a vessel, an attempt is made to aspirate blood. A hooking sensation may also be apparent as the catheter makes contact with an atheromatous plaque. If blood returns, 0.5 to 1.0 ml contrast medium (60% iothalamate meglumine or diatrizoate meglumine sodium) is injected slowly to evaluate the vessel that has been entered. If no blood can be aspirated, the catheter is either wedged into a small vessel or is hooked onto a plaque in the aorta. If the catheter is wedged in a vessel, blood will occasionally drip back when the stopcock is opened. This rarely occurs if the catheter is against the aortic wall. Alternatively, a 10 ml disposable Luer-Lok syringe filled with contrast medium is attached to the catheter before attempting selective catheterization, and air is removed from the catheter/syringe connection. In this way, if no blood returns on suction, a small volume (0.5 ml) of contrast medium can still be injected. This contrast volume is sufficient for initial identification of a bronchial or intercostal artery. Once such a test injection identifies the catheter tip in an intercostal or bronchial artery, a larger volume can be injected for confirmation.

In the presence of disease, the bronchial arteries are enlarged, and can be catheterized even with larger (6 to 7 Fr) catheters without wedging the catheter tip into the vessel, ie, permitting adequate washout of the injected contrast medium. If, however, the catheter is wedged, stasis of contrast medium is seen. The catheter should then immediately be withdrawn slightly to permit antegrade flow. Injection of contrast medium into bronchial arteries can be associated with a cough sensation. Contrast injection into the intercostal arteries is associated with back pain.

An alternative method for selective catheterization of a bronchial vessel is the use of a coaxial catheter system. A 3 Fr tapered Teflon catheter (or the open-ended guide wire) is introduced through the angiographic catheter. With this technique, a more stable catheter position can often be achieved for both diagnostic arteriography and transcatheter therapy. The coaxial catheter/guide wire can also be used to bypass spinal cord branches.

**Arteriography and Filming** (Table 8–6). Before arteriography, some authors recommend flushing with heparinized saline, histamine, or procaine or the inhalation of carbon dioxide to induce vasodilation.[138] In our own experience, this has not been necessary.

Intraarterial DSA is the preferred method for bronchial and intercostal arteriography. A hand injection of 20 to 30% contrast medium (4 to 6 ml) and 2/sec imaging for a total of 10 to 14 images provide satisfactory results. If DSA is unavailable, 100 or 105 mm spot films or 14 × 14 inch film is used for bronchial/intercostal arteriography. Four to 6 ml of 60% contrast medium is injected over

**TABLE 8–6. Bronchial/Intercostal Arteriography**

| | |
|---|---|
| Catheter | Cobra C2, sidewinder I, headhunter 1, single curve, coaxial 3 Fr teflon (with cobra) |
| Guide wire | — |
| Contrast medium | 60% iothalamate meglumine or diatrizoate meglumine sodium* |
| Injection rate/volume | 2 to 4 ml/sec, total 4 to 6 ml |
| Films: | 10 films |
|   Filming rate | 2 per second for 4 films<br>1 per second for 6 films |
|   Projections | a. AP<br>b. Ipsilateral posterior oblique |

*20 to 30% concentration with DSA.

2 seconds via hand injection or a power injector at a rate of 2 to 4 ml/sec. Films are obtained in the AP projection at two films/sec for a total of four films and then one film/sec for another six films (or a total duration of filming of 8 seconds). In most instances (also for DSA) another projection should be obtained, especially if the AP projection is uninformative. A 30 to 35° ipsilateral posterior oblique projection proves to be most useful. Magnification arteriography may be used to enhance detail.[138] In addition, subtraction films are necessary for delineating smaller branches, such as the spinal branch, which may be obscured on the unsubtracted arteriogram.

Bronchial arteries are readily distinguishable from the intercostal arteries by their meandering course toward the pulmonary hilum (Fig. 8–57). The intercostal arteries follow a slightly craniad course and then follow the undersurface of the ribs and continue on laterally. The intercostobronchial trunk also courses craniad; the bronchial artery descends toward the pulmonary hilum. Both the intercostal and the bronchial arteries give rise to multiple mediastinal, paratracheal, and paraesophageal vessels. In addition, they provide vascular branches to the mediastinal lymph nodes and vasa vasorum to the aorta, pulmonary arteries, and occasionally branches to the spinal cord.[131] These vessels can be differentiated from the bronchials by virtue of their course, which is medial (mediastinal branches) or parallel (paraesophageal branches) to the esophagus. This may not be clear on the AP view; there-

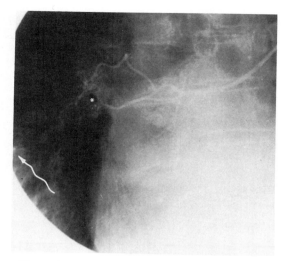

*Figure 8–57.* Bronchial arteriogram in a patient with hemoptysis. AP film from a right bronchial arteriogram shows hypertrophy of the bronchial arteries around a bronchus (\*) and extravasation of contrast medium (*arrow*).

fore, the oblique projection is used to distinguish them from the bronchial arteries. The spinal branch is identified on the AP arteriogram by its midline course (parallel to the cord, medial to the vertebral pedicle) or the characteristic hairpin bend. On the AP projection, the left bronchial artery appears shorter than the right because of foreshortening due to its AP course.

In the normal individual, the bronchial arteries are of small caliber and the peripheral branches are not visualized. The lateral extent of the opacified vessels is the medial one third to one half of the lung field. When seen end on, the bronchial wall is outlined. In patients with disease (pneumonia, bronchiectasis, granulomatous infection, pulmonary embolus, cystic fibrosis, and neoplasms), the bronchial arteries are enlarged, and branches extending to the lung periphery or to areas of abnormality are visualized,[139] and shunting into the pulmonary circulation is often demonstrated. In patients with neoplasms, the vascular supply is usually from the bronchial or parasitized intercostal arteries, and multiple feeding arteries are often present.[128, 138, 140] Similarly, in some patients with hemoptysis due to chronic lung disease, blood supply may be from the intercostal arteries (Fig. 8–58).[141, 142]

PITFALLS IN DIAGNOSIS

1. Failure to visualize the bronchial arteries: Bronchial arteries may be small and thus may not be seen well on the television monitor. Therefore, each contrast injection should be evaluated by DSA or spot films or recorded on video disc/tape. For the latter, playback helps to determine whether the appropriate vessel has been catheterized.

2. Failure to visualize both bronchial branches of a common bronchial trunk: Contrast injection may have demonstrated only one branch of a common bronchial trunk. In this case, contralateral branches may be small and not adequately demonstrated, or the catheter tip may lie beyond the orifice of one branch so that contrast medium was injected selectively into one vessel. Thus, it is desirable to have some degree of reflux of contrast medium into the aorta, which would assure that the entire vessel is opacified. If the injection is too forceful, it may dislodge the catheter.

3. Failure to visualize the abnormality: Since there is a high incidence of multiple bronchial arteries, especially on the left side, a search for additional vessels should be carried out.

4. Failure to catheterize a bronchial artery: This is observed in up to 10% of patients.[138] The most frequent reasons given are severe atherosclerosis of the aorta or pelvic vessels (access vessels) or stenosis or occlusion of the bronchial arteries.

**Precautions and Complications**

1. Catheter dislodgment: The catheter may

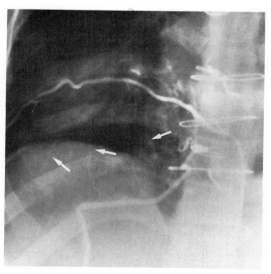

*Figure 8–58.* Intercostal-pulmonary artery communication in a patient with cyanotic congenital heart disease. On the AP intercostal arteriogram there is opacification of the peripheral pulmonary artery branches (*arrows*).

dislodge or advance inadvertently if it has not been secured at the groin. High torque catheters require relatively little motion to change their location. Thus, after a catheter is secured at the groin, injection of contrast medium should reconfirm satisfactory position.

2. Wedge position of catheter: If the catheter is wedged into the artery, stasis or very slow washout of contrast medium is observed. Wedge injection into an artery giving off a spinal cord branch may be hazardous. Therefore, if stasis is observed, the catheter is withdrawn so that antegrade flow is reestablished. Alternatively, a coaxial system is used.

3. Spinal cord complications: Persistent back pain following injection into an intercostal or bronchial artery may herald a spinal cord complication.[141] The resulting transverse myelitis is most likely a manifestation of contrast toxicity.[143-145]

4. Neurological complications: According to some authors, contrast injection into the right fifth intercostal artery may be associated with a higher risk of neurological complications.[143]

## ARTERIAL SUPPLY TO THE SPINAL CORD

The major arterial blood supply to the spinal cord is through the longitudinal anastomotic channels.[146] Segmental branches of the thoracic and abdominal aorta and vertebral, costocervical, and thyrocervical arteries in the neck contribute to this vessel. Of these segmental branches of the aorta, about four to nine vessels of significance achieve a diameter close to 1 mm (lower cervical, upper and lower thoracic, and upper lumbar). These divide into ascending and descending branches at the anterior median sulcus of the spinal cord and anastomose to form an anterior longitudinal trunk. The largest and most significant of these aortic branches is the arteria radicularis magna (artery of Adamkiewicz), which arises from either the lower thoracic or the upper lumbar aorta (from intercostal or lumbar arteries) between T8 and L4.[147-149] This is usually a single artery, originating from the left side in approximately 80% of individuals, which does not communicate with other, larger spinal cord arteries. It is responsible for blood supply to the lower two thirds of the spinal cord.[146, 147] Thus, trauma to this vessel may lead to neurological symptoms.

Since it arises from an intercostal artery in

**TABLE 8–7. Angiography of the Arteria Radicularis Magna**

| | |
|---|---|
| Catheter: | Sidewinder 1, cobra C2, single curve |
| Guide wire | — |
| Contrast medium | 60% iothalamate meglumine or diatrizoate meglumine sodium* |
| Injection rate/volume | Hand injection, 2 to 4 ml/sec, total 4 to 6 ml |
| Films: | 8 films |
|   Filming rate | 2 per second for 4 films |
| | 1 per second for 4 films |
|   Projections | a. AP |
| | b. Lateral |

*20% concentration with DSA.

the majority of individuals, the catheterization and filming technique used for the arteria radicularis magna is similar to that for bronchial and intercostal arteriography (Table 8–7). The cobra C2 or sidewinder 1 is the catheter of choice for nontortuous aortas. In ectatic and severely tortuous aortas, a cobra C3, sidewinder 2, or a single curve catheter (3 cm diameter) is used. Lead numbers are taped onto the skin to facilitate identification of the vertebral bodies.

Intraarterial DSA is the preferred method for arteriography of the arteria radicularis magna. Twenty per cent contrast medium (4 to 6 ml total) is injected by hand. Images are obtained at 2/sec for a total of 10 to 12 images. In individuals with a small arteria radicularis magna, 30% contrast medium may be required for satisfactory opacification with DSA.

On arteriography, the arteria radicularis magna is easily recognized by its characteristic appearance. The artery follows a craniad course until it reaches the mid-portion of the spinal column, where it makes a typical hairpin curve caudally (Fig. 8–59). Preoperative localization of the arteria radicularis magna is indicated in patients with thoracoabdominal aortic aneurysms, chronic aortic dissection, arteriovenous malformations, and rarely in patients with tumors of the spinal cord. In patients with thoracoabdominal aortic aneurysms, preoperative arteriographic localization of the arteria radicularis magna facilitates intraoperative identification and reimplantation to prevent spinal cord ischemia.[150]

A more detailed discussion of spinal angiography can be found in Chapter 17.

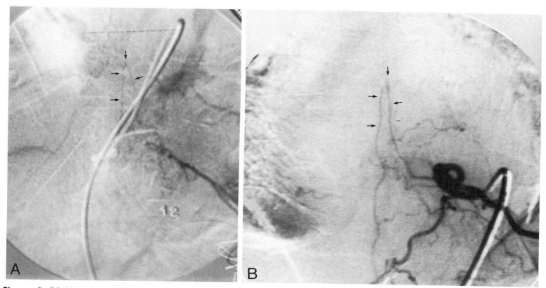

**Figure 8–59.** Normal arteriogram of the arteria radicularis magna. *A,* Subtraction film from an arteriogram of the left eleventh intercostal artery demonstrates the typical hairpin loop (*arrows*). *B,* Intraarterial DSA from another patient. Note the superior quality of the DSA image.

## Risks of Spinal Cord Trauma

In a survey of over 13,000 patients undergoing abdominal aortography, the incidence of neurological complications resulting from spinal cord injury was 0.22%.[151] A large number of reported complications occurred after translumbar aortography and may have resulted from direct needle trauma to the spinal cord arteries.[152, 153] Spinal cord ischemia during supine transfemoral aortography has also been reported and was most likely due to direct contrast toxicity.[143, 148, 152] Several of the earlier studies were done under general anesthesia, which is known to slow blood circulation and may thus have increased the contact time of the older, more toxic types of contrast media with the neural tissue.

## Management of Tetraplegia and Paraplegia Caused by Arteriography

Tetra- and paraplegias have been reported after abdominal aortography and bronchial, renal, and vertebral arteriography.[143, 154] Elevated levels of iodine were found in the cerebrospinal fluid of patients suffering neurological complications after arteriography. Thus, the treatment that has been recommended by some authors is:[154]

1. Immediate removal of spinal fluid via lumbar puncture in volumes of approximately 10 ml at a time and replacement of this fluid by an equal volume of isotonic (0.9%) saline.

2. Maintaining the head in an elevated position for several hours.

## Precautions

Avoidance of several of the factors that have been associated with spinal cord complications may prevent such complications. These include:

1. Limiting the number of contrast injections and injected contrast volume to a minimum in vessels that may give off branches to the spinal cord. A "magic number" is obviously not available, but the maximum volume per injection should be less than 4 to 6 ml.

2. Avoiding general anesthesia (prolongation of circulation time).

3. Some authors recommend using iothalamate meglumine as the contrast medium.[148] We have routinely used 60% diatrizoate meglumine sodium and have not experienced any contrast-related complications.

4. Removing the catheter from the spinal artery soon after contrast injection.

5. Using 20% contrast medium and DSA. However, prolonged contact of dilute contrast medium (wedged catheter position) may have also been responsible for neural toxicity in one of our patients.

# REFERENCES

1. Warwick R, Williams PL: Gray's Anatomy, 35th Brit. Ed. Philadelphia, WB Saunders, 1973, pp. 615–622.

2. Shuford WH, Sybers RG: The Aortic Arch and Its Malformations. Springfield, Ill, Charles C Thomas, 1974.

3. Paul RN: A new anomaly of the aorta: Left aortic arch with right descending aorta. J Pediatr 32:19–29, 1948.

4. Dominguez R, Oh KS, Dorst JP, et al: Left aortic arch with right descending aorta. AJR 130:917–920, 1978.

5. Berman W Jr, Yaber SM, Dillon T, et al: Vascular ring due to left aortic arch and right descending aorta. Circulation 63:458–460, 1981.

6. Strife J, Baumel AS, Dunbar JS: Tracheal compression by the innominate artery in infancy and childhood. Radiology 139:73–75, 1981.

7. Lippert H: Arterienvarietäten: Klinische Tabellen 2–11. Beilage Med Klin 36:1967.

7a. Khan S, Haust MD: Variations in the aortic origin of intercostal arteries in man. Ant Rec 195:545–552, 1979.

8. Stewart JR, Kincaid OW, Edwards JE: An Atlas of Vascular Rings and Related Malformations of the Aortic Arch System. Springfield, Ill, Charles C Thomas, 1964, pp. 3–129.

9. Stewart JR, Kincaid OW, Titus JR: Right aortic arch: Plain film diagnosis and significance. AJR 97:377–389, 1966.

10. Bedford DE, Parkinson J: Right sided aortic arch (situs inversus arcus aortae). Br J Radiol 9:776–798, 1936.

11. Blalock A: Surgical procedures employed and anatomic variations encountered in the treatment of congenital pulmonic stenosis. Surg Gynecol Obstet 87:385–409, 1948.

12. Lewis C, Rogers L: The cervical aortic knuckle which resembles an aneurysm. Lancet 1:825–826, 1953.

13. Tonkin ILD: The thoracic aorta and its branches. In Stanley P (ed): Pediatric Angiography. Baltimore, Williams & Wilkins, 1982, pp. 47–108.

14. Maxwell SL Jr, Kwon OJ, Millan VG: Translumbar carotid arteriography. Radiology 148:851–852, 1983.

14a. Frohlich H: Transaxillary abdominal angiography: use of the sidewinder-pigtail catheter. Radiology 150:265, 1984.

15. Joyce JW, Fairbairn JF II, Kincaid OW, et al: Aneurysms of the thoracic aorta: A clinical study with special reference to prognosis. Circulation 29:176–181, 1964.

16. Spittell JA Jr, Wallace RB: Aneurysms. In Juergens JL, Spittell JA Jr, Fairbairn JF II (eds): Peripheral Vascular Diseases. Philadelphia, WB Saunders, 1980, pp. 415–439.

17. Williams GM, Harrington D, Burdick J, et al: Mural thrombus of the aorta. An important, frequently neglected cause of large peripheral emboli. Ann Surg 194:737–744, 1981.

18. Tobin CE: The bronchial arteries and their connections with other vessels in the human lung. Surg Gynecol Obstet 95:741–750, 1952.

19. Sanders JH Jr, Malave S, Neiman HL, et al: Thoracic aortic imaging without angiography. Arch Surg 114:1326–1329, 1979.

20. Dinsmore RE, Jang GC: Roentgen diagnosis of aortic disease. Prog Cardiovasc Dis 16:151–185, 1973.

21. Crawford ES: Thoraco-abdominal and abdominal aortic aneurysms involving renal, superior mesenteric and celiac arteries. Ann Surg 179:763–772, 1974.

22. Bickerstaff LK, Pairolero PC, Hollier LH, et al: Thoracic aortic aneurysms: A population based study. Surgery 92:1103–1108, 1982.

23. Heggtveit HA: Syphilitic aortitis: A clinicopathologic autopsy study of 100 cases. Circulation 29:346–355, 1964.

24. Kampmeier RH: Saccular aneurysms of the thoracic aorta. A clinical study of 633 cases. Ann Intern Med 12:624–651, 1938.

25. Lande A, Berkmen YM: Aortitis, pathologic, clinical and arteriographic review. Radiol Clin North Am 14:219–240, 1976.

26. Osler W: The gutstonian lectures on malignant endocarditis. Lecture I. Br Med J 1:467–470, 1885.

27. Felson B, Akers PV, Hall GS, et al: Mycotic tuberculous aneurysm of the thoracic aorta. JAMA 237:1104–1108, 1977.

28. Fromm SH, Lucas CE: Obturator bypass for mycotic aneurysm in the drug addict. Arch Surg 100:82–83, 1970.

29. Stengel A, Wolforth CC: Mycotic (bacterial) aneurysms of intravascular origin. Arch Intern Med 31:527–554, 1923.

30. Mundth ED, Darling RC, Alvarado RH, et al: Surgical management of mycotic aneurysms and the complications of infection in vascular reconstructive surgery. Am J Surg 117:460–470, 1969.

31. Smith DC, Hirst AE: Spontaneous aortic rupture associated with chronic steroid therapy for rheumatoid arthritis in two cases. AJR 132:271–273, 1979.

32. Edwards JE, Burchell HB: The pathological anatomy of deficiencies between the aortic root and the heart, including aortic sinus aneurysms. Thorax 12:125–139, 1957.

33. Hines EA Jr, Kelly PJ, Barker NW: Idiopathic disseminated focal arteritis: Occurrence of false aneurysms in large and medium sized arteries. JAMA 174:848–852, 1960.

34. Cipriano PR, Alonso DR, Baltaxe HA, et al: Multiple aortic aneurysms in relapsing polychrondritis. Am J Cardiol 37:1097–1102, 1976.

35. Hirst AE Jr, Johns VJ Jr, Kime SW Jr: Dissecting aneurysm of the aorta: A review of 505 cases. Medicine (Baltimore) 37:217–279, 1958.

36. Earnest F IV, Muhm JR, Sheedy PF II: Roentgenographic findings in thoracic aortic dissection. Mayo Clin Proc 54:43–50, 1979.

37. Schmitt HE, Beck M: Die spontane Aortendissektion. Diagnostische Erfahrungen bei 32 Patienten. Fortschr Roentgenstr 126:185–192, 1977.

38. Case Records of the Massachusetts General Hospital: Case 11–1967. N Engl J Med 276:574–581, 1967.

39. Case Records of the Massachusetts General Hospital: Case 32–1974. N Engl J Med 291:350–357, 1974.

40. Heslep JH, Greening RR: Dissecting aneurysms. Rad Clin North Am 5:497–504, 1967.

41. Beresford OD: The clinical diagnosis of dissecting aneurysm of the aorta. Br Med J 2:397–400, 1951.

42. Markowitz AM: Dissecting aneurysm presenting as occlusive disease of the lower aorta. Am J Surg 103:389–393, 1962.

43. East T: Dissecting aneurysm of the aorta. Lancet 2:1017–1019, 1939.

44. Humes DM, Porter RR: Acute dissecting aortic aneurysms. Surgery 53:122–154, 1963.

45. Kaufman SL, White RI Jr: Aortic dissection with "normal" chest roentgenogram. Cardiovasc Intervent Radiol 3:103–106, 1980.

46. Hoskin J, Gardner F: Silent dissection of the aorta. Br Heart J 8:141–146, 1946.

47. Pyeritz R: Personal communication.

48. Braunstein H: Pathogenesis of dissecting aneurysm. Circulation 28:1071–1080, 1963.

49. Schnitker MA, Bayer CA: Dissecting aneurysm of the aorta in young individuals, particularly in association with pregnancy, with report of a case. Ann Intern Med 20:486–511, 1944.

50. Abbott ME: Coarctation of the aorta of the adult type. II. A statistical study and historical retrospect of 200 recorded cases, with autopsy, of stenosis or obstruction of the descending arch in subjects above the age of 2 years. Am Heart J 3:392–421, 574–618, 1928.

51. Harris PD, Malm JR, Bigger JT Jr, et al: Follow up studies of acute dissecting aortic aneurysms managed with antihypertensive agents. Circulation 35(Suppl 1):183–187, 1967.

52. Barsky SH, Rosen S: Aortic infarction following dissecting aortic aneurysm. Circulation 58:876–881, 1978.

53. McReynolds RA, Shin MS, Sims RD: Three channeled aortic dissection. AJR 130:549–552, 1978.

54. Siegelman SS, Sprayregen S, Strasberg Z, et al: Aortic dissection and the left renal artery. Radiology 95:73–78, 1970.

55. DeBakey ME, Henly WS, Cooley DA, et al: Surgical management of dissecting aneurysm involving the ascending aorta. J Cardiovasc Surg 5:200–211, 1964.

56. Itzchak Y, Rosenthal T, Adar R, et al: Dissecting aneurysm of the thoracic aorta: Reappraisal of radiologic diagnosis. AJR 125:559–569, 1975.

57. Dinsmore RE, Willerson JT, Buckley MJ: Dissecting aneurysm of the aorta. Aortographic features affecting prognosis. Radiology 105:567–572, 1972.

58. Heiberg E, Wolverson M, Sunderam M, et al: CT findings in thoracic aortic dissection. AJR 136:13–17, 1981.

59. Shuford WH, Sybers RG, Weens HS: Problems in the aortographic diagnosis of dissecting aneurysm of the aorta. N Engl J Med 280:225–231, 1969.

60. Price JE Jr, Gray RK, Grollman JH Jr: Aortic wall thickness as an unreliable sign in the diagnosis of dissecting aneurysm of the thoracic aorta. AJR 113:710–712, 1971.

61. Hayashi K, Meaney TF, Zelch JV, et al: Aortographic analysis of aortic dissection. AJR 122:769–782, 1974.

62. Charnsangavej C: Occlusion of the right pulmonary artery by acute dissecting aortic aneurysm. AJR 132:274–276, 1979.

63. Miller DC, Stinson EB, Oyer PE, et al: Operative treatment of aortic dissections. Experience with 125 patients over a 16 year period. J Thorac Cardiovasc Surg 78:365–382, 1979.

64. Ambos MA, Rothberg M, LeFleur RS, et al: Unsuspected aortic dissection: The chronic "healed" dissection. AJR 132:221–225, 1979.

65. Prior JT, Buran RT, Perl T: Chronic (healed) dissecting aneurysms. J Thorac Surg 33:213–228, 1957.

66. Jones AM, Langley FA: Chronic dissecting aneurysms. Br Heart J 8:191–199, 1946.

67. Greendyke RM: Traumatic rupture of aorta. Special reference to automobile accidents. JAMA 195:527–530, 1966.

68. Parmley LF, Mattingly TW, Manion WC, et al: Nonpenetrating traumatic injury of the aorta. Circulation 17:1086–1101, 1958.

69. Parmley LF, Mattingly TW, Manion WC: Part I. Penetrating wounds of the heart and aorta. Circulation 17:953–973, 1958.

70. Teare D: Postmortem examinations on air crash victims. Br Med J 2:707–708, 1951.

71. Fishbone G, Robbins DI, Osborn DJ, et al: Trauma to the thoracic aorta and great vessels. Radiol Clin North Am 11:543–554, 1973.

72. Fisher RG, Hadlock F, Menachem YB: Laceration of the thoracic aorta and brachiocephalic arteries by blunt trauma. Report of 54 cases and review of the literature. Radiol Clin North Am 19:91–110, 1981.

73. Schonholtz GJ, Jahnke EJ: Occult injury of the thoracic aorta associated with orthopaedic trauma. J Bone J Surg 46A:1421–1431, 1964.

74. Göbbler Th, Kaufmann H: Verbreiterung des Mediastinums in Höhe des Aortenbogens. Ein differentialdiagnostischer Beitrag. Dtsch Med Wochenschr 42:1905–1909, 1967.

75. Ayella RJ, Hankins, JR, Turney SZ, et al: Ruptured thoracic aorta due to blunt trauma. J Trauma 17:199–205, 1977.

76. Seltzer SE, D'Orsi C, Kirshner R, et al: Traumatic aortic rupture. Plain radiographic findings. AJR 137:1011–1014, 1981.

77. Fitts CT, Barnett LT, Webb CM, et al: Perforating wounds of the heart caused by central venous catheters. J Trauma 10:764–769, 1970.

78. Gerlock AJ Jr, Muhletaler CA, Coulam CM, et al: Traumatic aortic aneurysm. Validity of esophageal tube displacement sign. AJR 135:713–718, 1980.

79. Tisnado J, Tsai FY, Als A, et al: A new radiographic sign of acute traumatic rupture of the thoracic aorta. Displacement of the nasogastric tube to the right. Radiology 125:603–608, 1977.

80. Davies ER, Roylance J: Aortography in the investigation of traumatic mediastinal hematoma. Clin Radiol 21:297–305, 1970.

81. Faraci RM, Westcott JL: Dissecting hematoma of the aorta secondary to blunt chest trauma. Radiology 123:569–574, 1977.

82. O'Sullivan MJ Jr, Folkerth TL, Morgan JR, et al: Posttraumatic thoracic aortic aneurysm. Recognition and treatment. Arch Surg 105:14–18, 1972.

83. Katz S, Mullin R, Berger RL: Traumatic transection associated with retrograde dissection and rupture of the aorta. Recognition and management. Ann Thorac Surg 17:273–276, 1974.

84. Symbas PN, Tyras DH, Ware RE, et al: Rupture of the aorta—A diagnostic triad. Ann Thorac Surg 15:405, 1973.

85. Koroxenidis GT, Moschos CB, Landy ED, et al: Traumatic rupture of the thoracic aorta simulating coarctation. Am J Cardiol 16:605, 1965.

86. Gazzaniga AB, Khuri EL, Mir-Sepasi HM, et al: Rupture of the thoracic aorta following blunt trauma. Arch Surg. 110:1119–1123, 1975.

87. Klinge F: Die rheumatische Narbe (Stigmata rheumatica) das Rezidiv und die chronische (fortschwälende) Entzundung. Ergeb Allgem Path Pathol Anat 27:106–132, 1933.

88. Klotz O: Rheumatic fever and the arteries. Trans Ass Am Coll Phys 27:181–188, 1912.

89. Clark WS, Kulka JP, Bauer W: Rheumatoid aortitis with aortic regurgitation. An unusual manifestation of rheumatoid arthritis (including spondylitis). Am J Med 22:580–592, 1957.

90. Zvaifler NJ, Weintraub AM: Aortitis and aortic insufficiency in chronic rheumatic disorders. A reappraisal. Arthritis Rheumatol 6:241–245, 1963.

91. Cardell BS, Hanley T: A fatal case of giant cell or temporal arteritis. J Pathol Bacteriol 63:587–597, 1951.

92. Harrison VC: Giant cell or temporal arteritis. A review. J Clin Pathol 1:197–211, 1948.

93. Harrison JR, Harrison VC, Kopelman H: Giant cell arteritis and aneurysm. Cited in ref. 25.

94. Kimmelstiel P, Gilmour TM, Hodges HH: Degeneration of elastic fibers in granulomatous giant cell arteritis (temporal arteritis). Arch Pathol 54:157–168, 1952.

95. Ross RS, McKusick VA: Aortic arch syndromes. Diminished or absent pulses in arteries arising from arch of aorta. Arch Int Med 92:701–740, 1953.

96. Reid OVJ: Dilatation of the aorta due to granulomatous (giant cell) aortitis. Br Heart J 19:206–210, 1957.

97. Danaraj TJ, Ong WH: Primary arteritis of abdominal aorta in children causing collateral stenosis of renal arteries and hypertension. Circulation 20:856–863, 1959.

98. Inada K, Shimizu H, Kobayashi I, et al: Pulseless disease and atypical coarctation of the aorta. Arch Surg 84:306–311, 1962.

99. Lande A, Gross A: Total aortography in the diagnosis of Takayasu's arteritis. AJR 116:165–178, 1972.

100. Lande A, Bard R: Takayasu's arteritis. Unrecognized cause of pulmonary hypertension. Angiology 27:114–121, 1976.

101. Kadir S, Roberson GH: Brachiocephalic atherosclerosis. A cause of amaurosis fugax. Radiology 130:171–173, 1979.

102. Pape R: Über einen abnormen Verlauf (tiefe Rechtslage) der Mesaortitischen aorta descendens. Fortschr Roentgenstr 46:257–269, 1932.

103. Leonardi HK, Naggar CZ, Ellis FH Jr: Dysphagia due to aortic arch anomaly. Diagnostic and therapeutic considerations. Arch Surg 115:1229–1232, 1980.

104. Birnholz JC, Ferrucci JT, Wyman SM: Roentgen features of dysphagia aortica. Radiology 111:93–96, 1974.

105. Keates PG, Magidson O: Dysphagia associated with sclerosis of the aorta. Br J Radiol 28:184–190, 1955.

106. McMillan IKR, Hyde I: Compression of the esophagus by the aorta. Thorax 24:32–38, 1969.

107. Vasquez MT, Garcia MAM, Wollich FS, et al: Cervical dysphagia lusoria from vertebral artery compression. Arch Surg 118:125–126, 1983.

108. Berenzweig H, Baue AE, McCallum RW: Dysphagia lusoria. Report of a case and review of the diagnostic and surgical approach. Dig Dis Sci 25:630–636, 1980.

109. Klinkhamer AC: Aberrant right subclavian artery. Clinical and roentgenologic aspects. AJR 97:438–446, 1966.

110. Shumacker HB Jr, Isch JH, Finneran JC: Unusual case of dysphagia due to anomalous right subclavian artery. A new approach for operative treatment. J Thorac Cardiovasc Surg 61:304–308, 1971.

111. McKusick VA: The cardiovascular aspect of Mar-

fan's syndrome. A heritable disorder of connective tissue. Circulation 11:321–342, 1955.

112. Murdoch JL, Walker BA, Halpern BL, et al: Life expectancy and causes of death in the Marfan syndrome. N Engl J Med 286:804–808, 1972.

113. Steinberg I, Mangiardi JL, Nobel WJ: Aneurysmal dilatation of aortic sinuses in Marfan's syndrome, angiocardiographic and cardiac catheterization studies in identical twins. Circulation 16:368–373, 1957.

114. Boijsen E, Weiland PO: Dissecting aneurysm of the aorta in Marfan's syndrome. Acta Radiol 3:89–96, 1965.

115. Miller DC: Surgical management of aortic dissections. Indications, operative features, preoperative management and long term results. In Doroghazi R, Slater E (eds): Aortic Dissections. New York, McGraw-Hill, 1983.

116. Barabas AP: Heterogeneity of the Ehlers-Danlos syndrome: Description of three clinical types and a hypothesis to explain the defect(s). Br Med J 2:612–613, 1967.

117. Mirza FH, Smith PL, Lin WN: Multiple aneurysms in a patient with Ehlers-Danlos syndrome. Angiography without sequelae. AJR 132:993–995, 1979.

118. Bopp P, Hatam K, Bussat P, et al: Cardiovascular aspects of the Ehlers-Danlos syndrome. Circulation 32:602–607, 1965.

119. Beighton P, Thomas ML: The radiology of the Ehlers-Danlos syndrome. Clin Radiol 20:354–361, 1969.

120. Rybka FJ, O'Hara ET: Surgical significance of the Ehlers-Danlos syndrome. Am J Surg 113:431–434, 1967.

121. Schoolman A, Kepes JJ: Bilateral spontaneous carotid cavernous fistulae in Ehlers-Danlos syndrome. Case report. J Neurosurg 26:82–86, 1967.

122. Sounders CR, Pearson CM, Adams HD: An aortic deformity simulating mediastinal tumor. A subclinical form of coarctation. Dis Chest 20:35–45, 1951.

123. Soto B, Shin MS, Papapietro SE: Nonobstructive coarctation. Cardiovasc Radiol 2:231–237, 1979.

124. Steinberg I: Anomalies (pseudocoarctation) of the arch of the aorta. Report of 8 new and review of 8 previously published cases. AJR 88:73–92, 1962.

125. Nasser WK, Helmen C: Kinking of the aortic arch (pseudo-coarctation): clinical, radiographic, hemodynamic and angiographic findings in eight cases. Ann Intern Med 64:971–978, 1966.

126. Stevens GM: Buckling of the aortic arch (pseudocoarctation, kinking). A roentgenographic entity. Radiology 70:67–73, 1958.

127. Cauldwell EW, Siekert RG, Lininger RE, et al: The bronchial arteries. An anatomic study of 150 human cadavers. Surg Gynecol Obstet 86:395–412, 1948.

128. Reuter SR, Olin T, Abrams HL: Selective bronchial arteriography. Radiology 78:87–95, 1965.

129. Quain R: The Anatomy of the Arteries of the Human Body. London, Taylor & Walston, 1884. Cited in ref 128.

130. O'Rahilly R, Debson H, King TS: Subclavian origin of bronchial arteries. Anat Rec 108:227–238, 1950.

131. Hellekant Chr: Bronchialangiographie und intraarterielle Chemotherapie bei Bronchialkarzinom. Radiologe 19:521–527, 1979.

132. Björk L: Anastomoses between the coronary and bronchial arteries. Acta Radiol 4:93–96, 1966.

133. Hudson CL, Moritz AR, Wearn JT: The extracardiac

anastomoses of the coronary arteries. J Exp Med 56:919–924, 1932.

134. Robertson HF: The vascularization of the epicardial and periaortic fat pads. Am J Pathol 6:209–215, 1930.

135. Botenga ASJ: The significance of broncho-pulmonary anastomoses in pulmonary anomalies. A selective angiographic study. Radiol Clin Biol 38:309–328, 1969.

136. Marchand P, Gilroy JC, Wilson VH: An anatomic study of the bronchial vascular system and its variation in disease. Thorax 5:207–221, 1950.

137. Boijsen E, Zsigmond M: Selective arteriography of bronchial and intercostal arteries. Acta Radiol Diagn 3:513–528, 1965.

138. Viamonte M Jr, Parks RE, Smoak WM III: Guided catheterization of the bronchial arteries. Part I. Technical considerations. Radiology 85:205–230, 1965.

139. North LB, Boushy SF, Houk VN: Bronchial and intercostal arteriography in non-neoplastic pulmonary disease. AJR 107:328–342, 1969.

140. Schober R: Selective bronchialis Arteriographie. Fortschr Roentgenstr 101:337–348, 1964.

141. Vujic I, Pyle R, Parker E, et al: Control of massive hemoptysis by embolization of intercostal arteries. Radiology 137:617–620, 1980.

142. Webb WR, Jacobs RP: Transpleural abdominal systemic artery-pulmonary artery anastomoses in patients with chronic pulmonary infection. AJR 129:233–236, 1977.

143. Kardjiev V, Symeonov A, Chankov I: Etiology, pathogenesis and prevention of spinal cord lesions in selective angiography of the bronchial and intercostal arteries. Radiology 112:81–83, 1974.

144. Feigelson HH, Ravin HA: Transverse myelitis following selective bronchial arteriography. Radiology 85:663–665, 1965.

145. Broy H: Die Querschnittslähmung, eine fatale angiographische Komplikation, Kasuistik und Übersicht. Fortschr Roengenstr 114:353–366, 1971.

146. Warwick R, Williams PL: Gray's Anatomy, 35th Ed. Philadelphia, WB Saunders, 1973, pp. 839–840.

147. Doppman JZ, DiChiro G: The arteria radicularis magna: Radiographic anatomy in the adult. Br J Radiol 41:40–45, 1968.

148. DiChiro G: Unintentional spinal cord arteriography. Radiology 112:231–233, 1974.

149. Suh TH, Alexander L: Vascular system of the human spinal cord. Arch Neurol Psychiatry 41:659–677, 1939.

150. Fereshetian A, Kadir S, Kaufman S, et al: Preoperative localization of the arteria radicularis magna using DSA (in press).

151. MacAfee JG: A survey of complications of abdominal aortography. Radiology 68:825–838, 1957.

152. Efsen F: Spinal cord lesions as a complication of abdominal aortography. Report of 4 cases. Acta Radiol 4:47–61, 1966.

153. Evans AT: Renal arteriography. AJR 72:574–585, 1954.

154. Mishkin MS, Baum S, DiChiro G: Emergency treatment of angiography induced para- and tetraplegia. (Letter to the Editor.) N Engl J Med 288:1184–1185, 1973.

# Arteriography of the Upper Extremities

## ANATOMY

The right subclavian artery is a branch of the brachiocephalic artery; the left subclavian artery arises directly from the distal aortic arch. Major branches of the subclavian artery are the (Fig. 9–1):

1. Vertebral artery: This is the first branch, arising from the proximal part of the subclavian artery convexity. In 4 to 6% of individuals, the left vertebral artery arises directly from the aortic arch, proximal to the origin of the left subclavian artery. In 0.6% of individuals, the vertebral artery may have a bifid origin on the left side.[1]

2. Internal mammary artery (Fig. 9–2): This vessel originates from the ventral aspect of the subclavian artery, opposite the orifice of the vertebral artery. The proximal portion (extrathoracic segment) does not give off any branches. The intrathoracic segment lies behind the cartilages of the upper six ribs. It gives off medial branches to the thymus, bronchi, and pericardium, and laterally it gives off the anterior intercostal arteries and occasionally a lateral costal branch. The internal mammary artery divides into two terminal branches: the musculophrenic and the superior epigastric arteries.[2] The superior epigastric artery anastomoses with the inferior epigastric artery (from the external iliac artery) on the ventral surface of the anterior abdominal wall. This serves as a collateral pathway for the lower extremities in occlusive diseases of the aorta. Branches from the internal mammary artery also anastomose with branches of the lateral thoracic and subscapular arteries and provide collateral circulation to the arms in occlusive diseases of the subclavian artery.

3. Thyrocervical artery: This is a short trunk arising from the superior wall of the subclavian artery at the medial border of the anterior scalene muscle. Almost immediately it divides into three to four branches:
   a. Inferior thyroid artery: The ascending cervical artery is usually a branch of the inferior thyroid artery. It gives off one or two branches to the spinal cord.
   b. Suprascapular artery: This vessel anastomoses with the circumflex scapular, circumflex humeral, and subscapular arteries and the descending branch of the transverse cervical artery.[3]
   c. Superficial cervical artery: This vessel anastomoses with branches of the occipital artery. The transverse cervical artery is present in about one third of individuals and represents a common origin of the superficial cervical and dorsal scapular arteries from the thyrocervical trunk.[3] In approximately 8% of individuals, the transverse cervical artery arises directly from the subclavian artery.[1]

   Any or all the branches of the thyrocervical artery may arise independently from the subclavian artery. In addition, a wide variety of common origins may be encountered. In 52.5% of individuals, the thyrocervical artery exists as a single trunk; in 31%, all branches arise separately; and in 16.5%, one or more branches originate independently from the subclavian artery.[1]

4. Costocervical trunk: This is a short trunk that arises from the dorsal aspect of the distal subclavian artery and divides into the deep cervical and superior intercostal arteries.[3] The former provides branches to the spinal cord and anastomoses with branches of the vertebral and occipital arteries. The costocervical trunk is present in approximately 90% of individuals.[1] In the remainder, its branches arise independently or together with other branches of the subclavian or axillary artery.

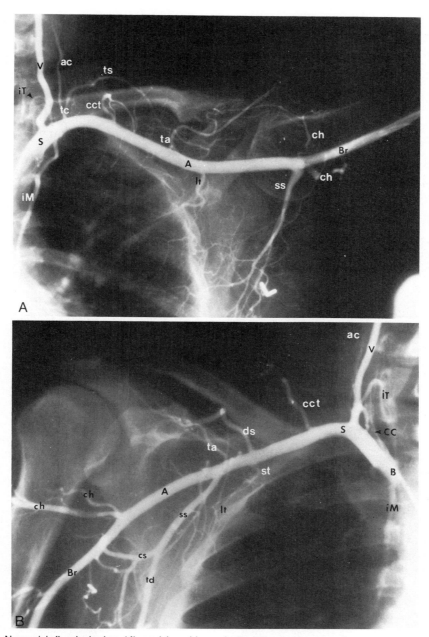

**Figure 9–1.** Normal left subclavian (*A*) and brachiocephalic (*B*) arteriograms. A = axillary; ac = ascending cervical; B = brachiocephalic; Br = brachial; CC = common carotid (faintly opacified); ch = anterior and posterior circumflex humeral; cs = circumflex scapular; cct = costocervical trunk; ds = dorsal (descending) scapular; iT = inferior thyroid; iM = internal mammary; lt = lateral thoracic; S = subclavian; ss = subscapular; st = superior thoracic; ta = thoracoacromial; tc = thyrocervical; td = thoracodorsal; ts = transverse scapular (suprascapular); V = vertebral arteries.

5. Dorsal scapular artery: This vessel arises from the third (or second) portion of the subclavian artery. Its branches anastomose with those of the subscapular, suprascapular, and posterior intercostal arteries.[3]

From the lateral aspect of the first rib, distal to the origin of the costocervical trunk, the subclavian artery continues as the axillary artery. Major branches of the axillary artery are the (Fig. 9–3):

1. Superior thoracic artery: This is a small,

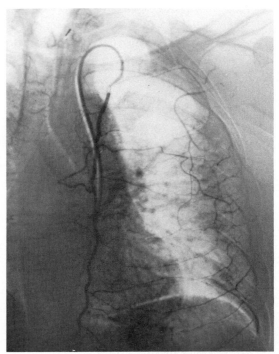

*Figure 9–2.* Internal mammary arteriogram. AP sub-traction film from a left internal mammary arteriogram shows the normal anatomy. The anterior intercostal arteries are opacified.

inconstant vessel that often arises from the thoracoacromial artery.

2. Thoracoacromial artery: This is a short vessel arising from the ventral aspect of the axillary artery, which divides into three to four branches.

3. Lateral thoracic artery: This vessel arises from the inferior aspect of the axillary artery. It courses caudally along the lateral chest wall and its branches anastomose with those of the internal mammary and intercostal arteries. The lateral thoracic artery is a single vessel in only 38% of individuals, in 28% it arises from the thoracoacromial artery and in 7% it may be a branch of the subscapular artery.[1]

4. The subscapular artery: This is the largest branch of the axillary artery. It courses inferiorly and its branches anastomose with those of the lateral thoracic, intercostal, transverse cervical, and profunda brachial arteries.

5. The anterior and posterior humeral circumflex arteries.

At the level of the anatomical neck of the

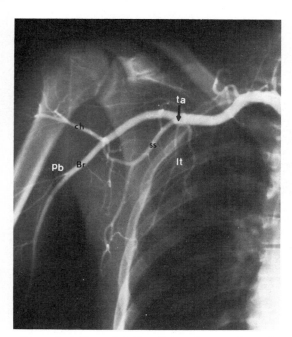

*Figure 9–3.* Normal right axillary artery anatomy. Br = brachial; ch = circumflex humeral; lt = lateral thoracic; pb = profunda brachial; ss = subscapular; ta = thoracoacromial arteries.

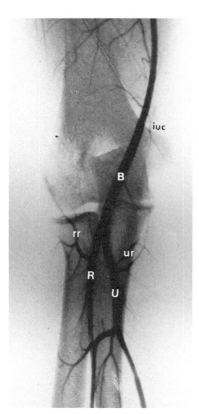

*Figure 9–4.* Normal brachial arteriogram. B = bra-chial; iuc = inferior ulnar collateral; rr = recurrent radial; R = radial; U = ulnar; ur = anterior and posterior ulnar recurrent arteries.

humerus, the axillary artery continues as the brachial artery. It lies in the medial bicipital sulcus and is accompanied by the median and ulnar nerves. Its superficial course permits easy palpation.

The major branches of the brachial artery are the profunda brachial and superior and inferior ulnar collateral arteries (Fig. 9–4). Below the elbow joint, the brachial artery bifurcates into an ulnar and a radial artery. The latter is frequently a smaller vessel and represents the direct continuation of the brachial artery. The ulnar artery gives off the

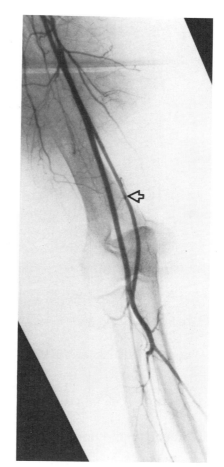

Figure 9–6. Accessory brachial artery (arrow).

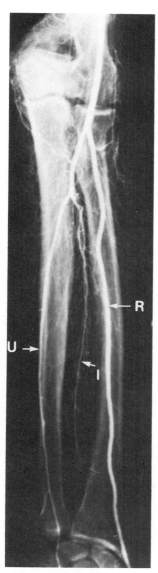

Figure 9–5. Normal arterial anatomy of the forearm. I = interosseous; R = radial; U = ulnar arteries.

anterior and posterior ulnar recurrent arteries and the common interosseous artery (Fig. 9–5).

The brachial artery may divide proximally into two trunks, which continue along the medial aspect of the arm and reunite distally (accessory brachial artery) (Fig. 9–6). In up to 19% of individuals, an early division of the brachial artery is present.[1, 4] This occurs more frequently on the right side. In such cases the first branch is usually the radial artery. The ulnar/interosseous trunk continues distally to divide below the elbow joint.

The radial artery may arise from the axillary artery in between 1 and 3% of individuals.[1, 4] Similarly, the ulnar artery may branch off at a higher level, ie, from the brachial artery, in about 1% of individuals (Fig. 9–7).[4] Knowledge of these variations is important in case a direct puncture of the brachial artery is planned. A persistent median artery (from

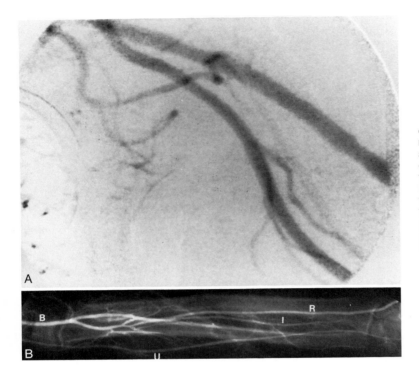

*Figure 9–7.* High origin of brachial artery branches. *A,* Intravenous DSA of the left axillary artery shows a high origin of the radial artery. *B,* Arteriogram of the left forearm in another patient. The brachial artery bifurcates into interosseous and radial arteries. The ulnar artery originates from the proximal brachial artery. B = brachial; I = interosseous; R = radial; U = ulnar arteries.

the interosseous artery) is observed in approximately 4% of individuals.[4]

## Arterial Anatomy of the Hand

The ulnar and radial arteries contribute to formation of the deep and superficial palmar arches (Fig. 9–8). A complete deep palmar arch occurs in approximately 95% of individuals.[1] It is formed primarily by the terminal portion of the radial artery, which anastomoses with the deep palmar branch of the ulnar artery and lies proximal to the superficial palmar arch.

The superficial palmar arch is complete in approximately 80% of individuals and is formed by the ulnar artery alone in about one third of individuals.[3, 5] In another one third, the arch is completed by the superficial palmar branch of the radial artery. This arch forms a distal convexity reaching down to the mid-portion of the third metacarpal bone.

The arterial supply to the fingers is through the common palmar digital arteries from the superficial palmar arch and corresponding palmar metacarpal arteries from the deep palmar arch. These continue into the fingers as the proper palmar digital arteries. The thumb and index finger receive blood supply from both arches and the ulnar and radial arteries. In addition, the dorsal carpal branches of the ulnar and radial arteries pro-

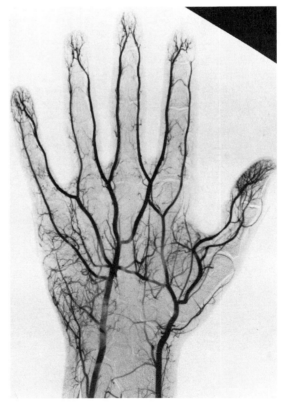

*Figure 9–8.* Subtraction film showing a normal hand arteriogram. (From Janevski BK: Angiography of the Upper Extremity. The Hague, Martinus Nijhoff, 1982. Used with permission.)

vide the dorsal metacarpal branches to the fingers.

The deep and superficial palmar arches can be divided into many subtypes. A detailed analysis of the radiographic anatomy can be reviewed in reference 1. Further review of the anatomical variations of the arteries in the forearm and hand can be found in references 5, 6, and 6a.

## Collateral Pathways

In occlusive diseases of the subclavian, axillary, or brachial arteries, the following are some of the collateral pathways to the upper extremities:

1. Stenosis or occlusion of the proximal subclavian or brachiocephalic artery:
   a. Brachiocephalic, subclavian, or thyrocervical steal. (A detailed discussion appears later in this chapter.)
   b. Anastomoses between the left and right superior and inferior thyroid arteries.
   c. Anastomoses between the vertebral arteries.
   d. Inferior epigastric → internal mammary artery.
2. Stenosis or occlusion of the distal subclavian or axillary artery:
   a. Internal mammary → intercostals → lateral thoracic → axillary or profunda brachial arteries.
   b. Thyrocervical trunk (suprascapular artery) → circumflex humeral and circumflex scapular arteries.
   c. Via branches of the dorsal scapular or subscapular arteries.
   d. Via the costocervical trunk and intercostal arteries.
   e. Via the transverse cervical artery.
3. Occlusion of the brachial artery:
   a. Superior and inferior ulnar collateral arteries → anterior and posterior ulnar recurrent arteries. In addition, the inferior ulnar collateral artery anastomoses with the medial collateral branches of the profunda brachial artery.
   b. Profunda brachial → radial collateral branch → recurrent radial artery.

## ARTERIOGRAPHY

### Arterial Catheterization

**Brachiocephalic/Right Subclavian Artery Catheterization.** From the femoral approach

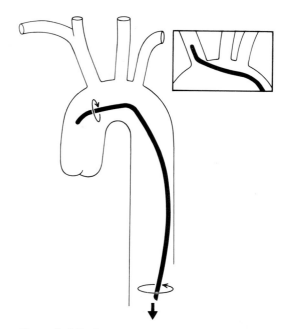

**Figure 9–9.** Technique for catheterization of the brachiocephalic artery with a headhunter catheter (see text).

a headhunter 1 catheter is used. In children and young individuals (without tortuous vessels), a hockey stick–shaped (multipurpose) catheter can also be used. The catheter is advanced into the ascending aorta over a J guide wire. The guide wire is removed and the catheter is flushed. As the catheter is pulled back slowly, it is rotated in a clockwise direction. This maneuver flips the catheter tip upward into the brachiocephalic artery orifice (Fig. 9–9).

Once the catheter tip has engaged the brachiocephalic artery, a small test injection (2 to 3 ml) of contrast medium confirms catheter position. For catheterization of the subclavian artery, a 1.5 mm LLT J guide wire is reinserted and directed into the subclavian artery by torquing the catheter. Once the guide wire is in the mid-subclavian artery, the catheter is advanced over it. Alternatively, with the J wire approximately 2 cm beyond the catheter tip, both wire and catheter are advanced as a unit. The catheter will have to be torqued into the subclavian artery, or else it tends to enter the right common carotid or vertebral artery.

In the elderly patient with elongation of the aortic arch, catheterization of the brachiocephalic artery with a headhunter 1 curve may not be possible, owing to the acute angle of origin. In such patients, a sidewinder II

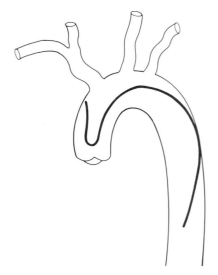

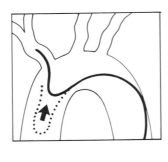

*Figure 9–10.* Technique for catheterization of the brachiocephalic artery with a sidewinder catheter. The catheter tip is pointed laterally, and as the catheter is pulled back from the ascending aorta, it engages the brachiocephalic artery.

curve is used.[7] The sidewinder catheter is advanced into the aortic arch over a J guide wire. The curve is re-formed in the aortic arch or proximal ascending aorta. As the catheter is pulled back from the ascending aorta, it engages the brachiocephalic artery (Fig. 9–10). Alternatively, a headhunter catheter can be used after formation of a loop in the left subclavian artery.[8]

**Left Subclavian Artery Catheterization.** From the femoral approach, a headhunter 1 or a multipurpose catheter (with a 45° curve) is used. In young individuals, the left subclavian artery originates from the distal portion of the aortic arch and the catheter can be advanced into it without difficulty. In individuals with advanced atherosclerosis, a 1.5 mm LLT J guide wire should be used during catheterization (unless the orifice is severely stenosed). With the J tip approximately 2 to 3 cm beyond the catheter tip, both guide wire and catheter are advanced as a unit into the left subclavian artery.

In some older individuals, the orifice of the left subclavian artery is displaced anteriorly and to the right because of elongation of the arch. In this situation, the headhunter 1 catheter is brought into the proximal arch and rotated clockwise as it is withdrawn slowly, similar to the technique for brachiocephalic artery catheterization. This maneuver will flip the catheter tip into the left subclavian orifice. If the catheter tip enters the left common carotid artery, the clockwise rotation is continued and the catheter is withdrawn further. The catheter tip enters the subclavian artery as it comes out of the common carotid orifice. If this is not successful, a sidewinder catheter is used. For arteriography, the catheter should be positioned proximal to the first rib crossing.

**Axillary and Brachial Artery Catheterization.** In most instances, the headhunter 1 catheter can be advanced into the axillary or brachial artery without the aid of a guide wire. However, in older individuals with atherosclerosis, a 1.5 mm LLT J guide wire should always be used to advance the catheter. The wire is inserted to approximately 2 to 3 cm beyond the catheter tip, and both the catheter and the guide wire are advanced together to the desired position. This will also prevent the catheter from entering branch vessels. If the catheter is to be positioned in the brachial artery, it is advanced over a straight LLT wire to avoid spasm induced by the catheter tip or J guide wire.

For arteriography of the forearm and hand, the catheter tip is positioned in the mid-brachial artery. Contrast injection should confirm position proximal to the brachial artery bifurcation. If there is a high bifurcation, the catheter must be withdrawn to lie more proximally.

**Internal Mammary Artery Catheterization.** Catheterization of this vessel may be indicated in patients being evaluated for coronary bypass surgery, for localization of parathyroid adenomas, occasionally for management of hemorrhage (postoperative, traumatic, or due to neoplastic disease) or for chemotherapy.[2]

From the femoral approach, the headhunter catheter will occasionally enter the internal mammary artery orifice. Alternatively, a right coronary, single curve or cobra C1 catheter is used. In addition, the tip deflecting wire can be used with soft, nonreinforced wall catheters.

The subclavian artery is catheterized using the techniques described above, and the catheter for internal mammary artery catheterization is inserted over an exchange wire. From the ipsilateral axillary approach, a cobra C1, single curve, or multipurpose catheter is used.

## Brachial Artery Puncture

Direct brachial artery puncture provides an alternate route for arteriography of the forearm and hand. This technique is useful if access from the femoral artery is not possible or feasible (eg, iliofemoral or subclavian artery occlusive disease). A very high origin of the ulnar or radial artery, which occurs in about 4% of individuals, is the one major drawback of this technique, since that artery cannot be studied. Thus, an intravenous DSA to define the axillary and brachial artery anatomy is advisable, prior to attempting an antegrade brachial artery puncture.

**Technique.** The arm is placed in 90° abduction. The brachial artery is entered percutaneously over the mid-portion of the humerus, in the medial bicipital sulcus (Fig. 9–11). In this region the brachial artery is accompanied by the median nerve, which

**TABLE 9–1.** Subclavian/Axillary Arteriography

| | |
|---|---|
| Catheter: | Headhunter 1 |
|   Position | Distal to vertebral artery but proximal to first rib |
| Guide wire | 0.035 inch 1.5 mm J |
| Contrast medium | 60% diatrizoate meglumine sodium* |
| Injection rate/volume | 8 ml/sec, total 24 ml |
| Films: | 10 films |
|   Filming rate | 2 per second for 4 films |
| | 1 per second for 6 films |
|   Projection | AP |

*20% concentration for DSA.

lies laterally, and the ulnar nerve, which is medial to the artery. In addition, at least two brachial veins accompany the artery. Further distally, the median nerve crosses the brachial artery anteriorly. An alternative technique is via a brachial artery cutdown. However, this technique is time consuming and more traumatic.

A Seldinger, Amplatz, or Potts needle can be used. The needle is held at a 45° angle. In most individuals, it is not necessary to insert the needle very deep, since the brachial artery is quite superficial in this region. A 0.035 inch straight LLT wire is used for placement of a 5 Fr multiple hole straight catheter.

**Patient Positioning and Arteriography** (Tables 9–1 to 9–3). Subclavian and axillary ar-

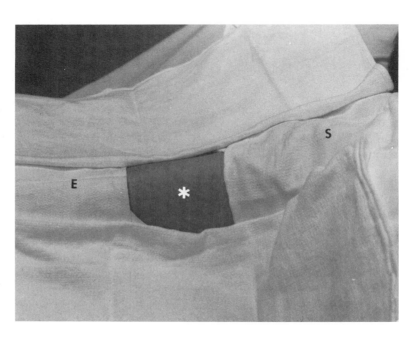

*Figure 9–11.* Arm position for brachial artery puncture (*). E = elbow; S = shoulder.

**TABLE 9–2.** Brachial Arteriography for Distal Upper Arm and Forearm

| | |
|---|---|
| Catheter: | Headhunter 1 |
| Position | Mid-brachial artery (proximal to bifurcation) |
| Guide wire | 0.035 inch 1.5 mm J and 0.035 inch straight LLT |
| Contrast medium | 60% diatrizoate meglumine sodium* |
| Injection rate/volume | 5 ml/sec, total 20 ml |
| Films: | 10 films |
| Filming rate | 1 film per second for 6 films<br>1 film every other second for 4 films |
| Projection | AP (volar side up) |
| Pharmacoangiography | 25 mg of tolazoline or 0.5 to 1.0 mg reserpine diluted in 10 to 15 ml of 5% dextrose injected intraarterially before arteriography |

*15 to 20% concentration for DSA.

teriograms are obtained in the neutral position, ie, with the arm adducted, in the AP projection. In patients with suspected thoracic outlet compression, an additional arteriogram is performed with the arm in maximal abduction.

Brachial and hand arteriograms are obtained in the AP projection with the arm in supination (volar side facing up). The tube and film changer are turned by 45° in order to facilitate utilization of the longest axis of

**TABLE 9–3.** Hand Arteriography

| | |
|---|---|
| Catheter: | Headhunter 1 |
| Position | Proximal to brachial artery bifurcation |
| Guide wire | 0.035 inch straight LLT |
| Contrast medium | 60% diatrizoate meglumine sodium* |
| Injection rate/volume | 5 ml/sec, total 20 ml |
| Films: | 10 films |
| Filming rate | 1 film per second for 6 films<br>1 film every other second for 4 films |
| Projections | AP (volar side up)/(lateral) |
| Pharmacoangiography | 25 mg of tolazoline or 0.5 to 1.0 mg of reserpine diluted in 10 to 15 ml of 5% dextrose injected intraarterially before arteriography |

*15 to 20% concentration for DSA.

the film (Fig. 9–12). For hand arteriography the fingers are spread apart and taped down. Whenever possible, hand arteriograms should be obtained using the magnification technique. The filming delay (between contrast injection and filming) should be assessed by a test injection. This should be adjusted accordingly if a vasodilator is used.

For internal mammary arteriography, 6 to 8 ml of contrast medium is injected at 3 to 4 ml/sec (or by hand). Films are obtained in the AP and ipsilateral posterior oblique (or lateral) projections at 1 film/sec for a total of 8 films.

Since contrast injection into the brachial and internal mammary arteries is very painful, analgesics should be given prior to arteriography to avoid patient motion. On the other hand, intraarterial DSA with 15 to 20% contrast medium provides a relatively pain-free study.

**Pharmacoangiography.** Placement of a catheter in the brachial artery may impede blood flow because of catheter or guide wire–induced spasm and/or partial obstruction of the arterial lumen by the catheter. In addition, some degree of vasospasm exists as a result of external stimuli (eg, cold angiographic room). Thus, an arterial injection without thermo- or pharmacovasodilatation may not visualize the distal arm and hand vessels satisfactorily. Individuals with a high flow state, ie, arteriovenous communication, are obviously an exception.

Arterial dilatation can be achieved by warming the extremity with an infrared lamp, by application of a warm compress, by oral intake of alcohol (alcoholic beverage), or by intraarterial injection of vasodilators. Vasodilators include tolazoline, 25 mg diluted in 10 to 15 ml of normal saline or 5% dextrose, injected intraarterially (over 10 to 15 seconds) immediately before the arteriogram. Alternatively, reserpine may be used for a more sustained vasodilatory response, especially in patients with vasospastic disorders. The dose of reserpine is 0.5 to 1.0 mg injected as a slow bolus or diluted in 10 to 15 ml of normal saline or 5% dextrose and injected intraarterially over 20 to 30 seconds.

**Complications and Precautions.** Inadvertent injection of a large volume of contrast medium in a branch vessel may occur as a result of catheter recoil during contrast injection. Such an injection may cause complications if the catheter tip enters the thyrocervical or the costocervical trunk, since these

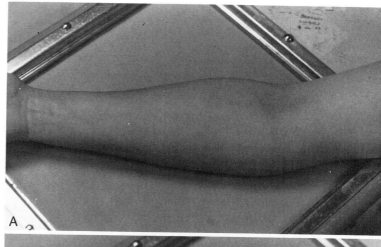

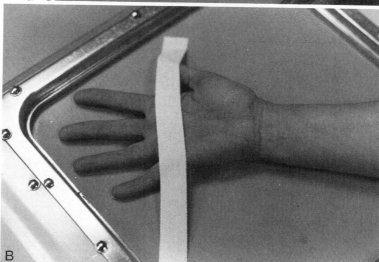

*Figure 9–12.* Position of the forearm (*A*) and hand (*B*) for arteriography.

vessels provide branches to the spinal cord. Thus, for subclavian arteriography the catheter tip should lie well beyond the vertebral artery and thyrocervical trunk but proximal to the first rib crossing, since subclavian artery stenoses often occur at this location. To check catheter position for stability, a forceful hand injection of 10 ml of saline is performed while fluoroscoping, in order to evaluate catheter recoil. Subsequently, a small contrast injection (2 to 3 ml) reconfirms catheter position.

Advancing the catheter into the brachial artery without a guide wire or over a large (3 mm) J guide wire may cause segmental arterial spasm. This may be manifested as a segmental stenosis or occlusion. If arterial spasm is observed, 25 mg of tolazoline (or 0.5 mg of reserpine) is injected intraarterially

and the catheter is withdrawn into a larger vessel. Occasionally, the spasm may be so severe that the catheter is trapped in place. If this occurs or the spasm persists, 2000 U of heparin is injected intraarterially into the extremity vessel and the catheter is attached to a power flush (heparinized 5% dextrose) for several minutes, until the spasm resolves. Once the catheter is free, it is withdrawn into the axillary artery. Catheter or guide wire manipulations are avoided until the vessel has returned to normal.

Pseudoaneurysm formation and arterial thrombosis as complications of brachial artery puncture are reported in approximately one of every 200 catheterizations[9] (Fig. 9–13). Arterial thrombosis appears to be related to multiple catheter exchanges and the use of large Fr size catheters.

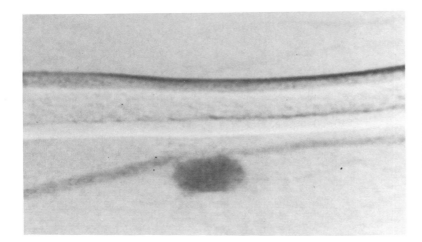

*Figure 9–13.* Aneurysm of the brachial artery demonstrated by intravenous DSA. The aneurysm developed following removal of a 5 Fr arterial catheter that had been placed for infusion of streptokinase for approximately 24 hours.

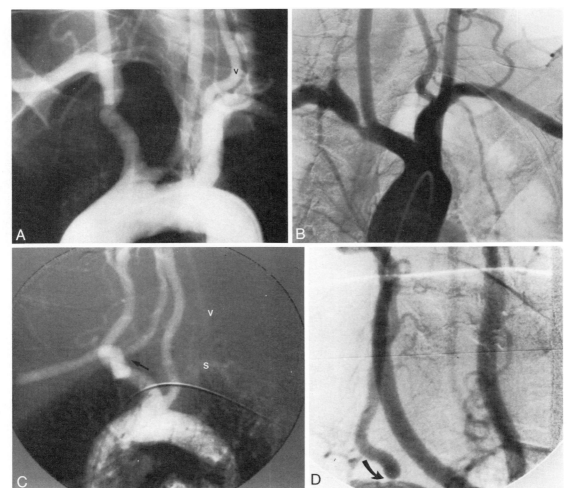

*Figure 9–14.* Occlusive disease of the brachiocephalic vessels. *A,* Left anterior oblique arch aortogram is normal. The left vertebral (V) artery is large. *B,* Subtraction film from the right anterior oblique arch aortogram shows a stenosis of the proximal right subclavian artery. *C,* Left anterior oblique arch aortogram from another patient. Intravenous DSA shows that the left subclavian artery is occluded and a subclavian steal (S) is present. A minimal stenosis of the right vertebral artery origin is seen (*arrow*). *D,* Right anterior oblique DSA of the neck vessels shows a severe stenosis of the right vertebral artery orifice (*arrow*). V = left vertebral artery. *Note:* Both these studies stress the importance of obtaining at least two projections (two opposite obliques) when evaluating the brachiocephalic vessels.

## ARTERIAL OCCLUSIVE DISEASES

Arterial insufficiency of the upper extremities is less common than that of the lower extremities. In descending order of frequency, the most common causes of upper extremity ischemia are acute trauma, thromboembolism, atherosclerotic occlusive disease, vasospastic disorders, and chronic trauma (eg, thoracic outlet syndrome).[10]

### Atherosclerosis

Areas frequently affected by atherosclerosis are the proximal segments of the extremity vessels (Fig. 9–14). Atherosclerosis of the forearm and hand vessels occurs less frequently but leads to progressive stenosis and occlusion. Multiple occlusions may be present before patients become symptomatic, as the slow progression allows the development of multiple, small, tortuous collateral channels. On arteriography, multiple segmental occlusions may be seen along with a large number of tortuous collaterals.

For the evaluation of patients with arterial insufficiency of the upper extremities, arch aortography is essential for assessment of the proximal arch vessels. Selective catheterization of the subclavian or brachial arteries is necessary for evaluation of the distal circulation. The latter may not always be possible because of the presence of severe proximal stenoses. In such patients, DSA is used with injection of contrast medium into the aortic arch. Multiple projections are necessary to determine the true extent of the disease (Fig. 9–14).

### Aneurysms

Aneurysms of the upper extremities occur less frequently than those of the lower extremities.[11] Elongation and tortuosity of the brachiocephalic arteries due to atherosclerosis and hypertension may simulate an aneurysm. This S-shaped elongation may involve the brachiocephalic, common, or internal carotid arteries (also called buckeled innominate or carotid artery).[12, 13]

Aneurysms of upper extremity vessels are most frequently secondary to arterial trauma (see Fig. 9–13).[10, 11] Less frequent causes are atherosclerosis, mycotic aneurysms, postoperative pseudoaneurysms, and aneurysms due to an arteritis (Fig. 9–15).

Subclavian artery aneurysms may be associated with the thoracic outlet syndrome. Aneurysms of the distal upper extremity vessels are most commonly posttraumatic (eg, occupational trauma, hypothenar hammer syndrome) and are rarely mycotic or due to periarteritis nodosa.[11, 14, 15]

### Steal Syndromes

**Subclavian Steal.** Severe stenosis or occlusion of the subclavian artery proximal to the vertebral artery origin may lead to reversal of blood flow in the ipsilateral vertebral artery, as this vessel provides collateral blood flow to the affected extremity. This occurs at the expense of the cerebral circulation. Other collaterals are via the thyrocervical trunk, superior and inferior thyroid arteries, internal mammary and contralateral vertebral arteries, and branches of the external carotid and the intercostal arteries.

*Figure 9–15.* Atherosclerotic aneurysm of the brachial artery. Right axillary arteriogram shows a partially thrombosed aneurysm (*arrowheads*). The brachial artery lumen is also stenosed in this region. Multiple thromboemboli originating from the aneurysm were responsible for severe ischemia of the hand. (Courtesy of Dr. CA Athanasoulis.)

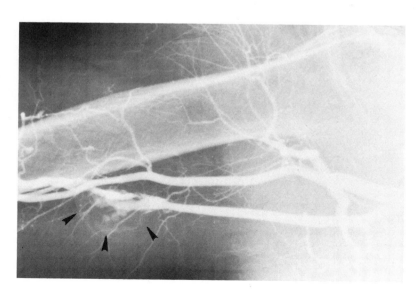

**TABLE 9–4.** Etiology of Subclavian Steal[1, 16–23]

**Acquired**
1. Atherosclerosis (most common)
2. Chest trauma
3. Extrinsic compression by tumor or fibrosis
4. Arteritis: Takayasu's, syphilitic aortitis
5. Postoperatively (Blalock-Taussig shunt or Shumacker procedure for coarctation)
6. Radiation fibrosis

**Congenital**
1. Preductal (infantile) coarctation
2. Hypoplasia of the transverse aortic arch or proximal subclavian arteries
3. Isolation of the left subclavian artery
4. Coarctation with aberrant subclavian artery arising distal to the coarctation

**Pathology.** Obstruction of blood flow from the aorta into a subclavian artery is most frequently acquired and due to atherosclerosis. Table 9–4 lists several of the acquired and congenital causes for subclavian steal.[16–23]

The syndrome occurs in the presence of severe stenosis (greater than 50% reduction of diameter) or occlusion of the subclavian artery (approximately 60% of cases) proximal to the origin of the vertebral artery.[1] In some instances, lowering of blood pressure in the affected subclavian artery by greater than 10% below systemic pressure may lead to reversal of flow in the ipsilateral vertebral artery.[24]

Symptoms depend upon the anatomical variations in the circle of Willis and upon the patency of the carotid system. Thus, if the circle of Willis is complete, cerebral ischemia may not develop. Blood flows up the unaffected vertebral artery, across the basilar artery, and retrograde down the affected vertebral artery into the subclavian artery (vertebrobasilar steal) with contributions from both internal carotid arteries.

**Clinical Aspects.** Whereas acquired lesions are frequently symptomatic (giving rise to the subclavian steal syndrome), congenital lesions are more often asymptomatic (subclavian steal).

Patients with subclavian steal syndrome are usually males, in a ratio of 3:1, in the fourth to sixth decades.[25] In 75% of patients, the left side is involved and symptoms are precipitated by exercise. On physical examination the ipsilateral radial pulse may be absent or diminished and a subclavian bruit may be present. A blood pressure difference

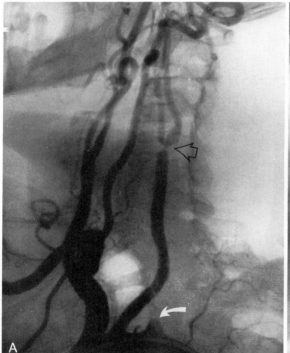
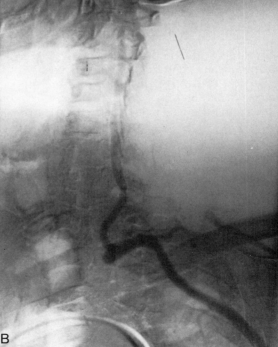

*Figure 9–16.* Subclavian steal. *A,* Subtraction film from a left anterior oblique arch aortogram shows occlusion of the left subclavian artery (*arrow*). In addition, there is a critical stenosis of the left common carotid artery (*open arrow*). *B,* Later film from the same arteriogram shows dense opacification of the left vertebral and subclavian arteries.

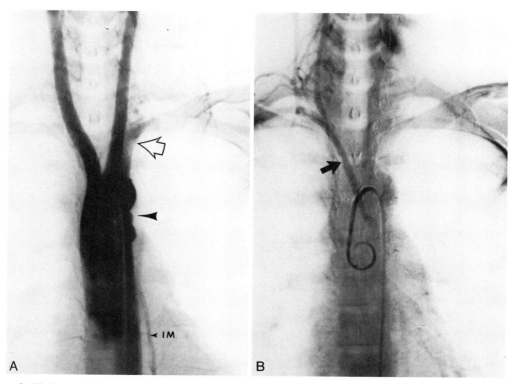

**Figure 9–17.** Congenital subclavian steal. *A,* Subtraction film from an AP arch aortogram shows a coarctation of the proximal descending aorta (*arrowhead*). Both common carotids, the left subclavian (*open arrow*), and an enlarged left internal mammary (IM) artery are opacified. *B,* Subtraction of a later film shows retrograde filling of the aberrant right subclavian artery (*arrow*) that originates below the coarcted segment of the aorta.

of greater than 40 mm Hg is usually found between the upper extremities in subclavian artery occlusion.[26]

Symptoms of vertebrobasilar ischemia are seen in approximately 40% of patients.[1] These are related to ischemia of the occipital lobe, brain stem, and upper spinal cord and may be manifested as vertigo, headache, syncope, paresis, paralysis, paresthesias, diplopia, dysarthria, and homonymous hemianopia.[1, 19, 20]

Upper extremity symptoms alone are seen in 3% of patients and may be manifested as intermittent claudication, rest pain, paresthesias, weakness, and decreased skin temperature.[1, 16] A combination of neurological and vascular symptoms is seen in approximately half the patients.[1]

**Arteriography** (Figs. 9–16 and 9–17). Arteriography is indicated to: (1) define the extent and nature of the disease, and (2) assess the pattern of blood flow.

Arch aortography or intravenous DSA (for outpatients) is performed in the AP or ipsilateral anterior oblique projection. Filming

should be carried out over at least 10 seconds in order to visualize retrograde filling of the ipsilateral vertebral and subclavian arteries. Alternatively, selective vertebral arteriography can be performed,[1] but this is usually not necessary, as the arch aortogram readily demonstrates this abnormality.

**Bilateral Subclavian Steal Syndrome.** Severe stenosis or occlusion of both subclavian arteries can give rise to the rare bilateral subclavian steal syndrome, of which only a few cases have been reported.[27, 28] The most common etiology is atherosclerosis, but the syndrome may be due to arteritis or a congenital abnormality.[20, 29] Patients with bilateral subclavian steal syndrome are usually symptomatic.

**Brachiocephalic Steal Syndrome.** This occurs rarely and is due to severe stenosis or occlusion of the proximal brachiocephalic artery. Two different flow patterns are recognized:[19, 30-33]

1. Blood flow is reversed in the right vertebral artery, which fills both the right subclavian and the right common carotid arter-

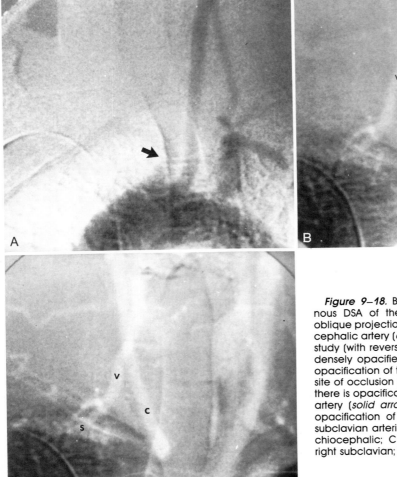

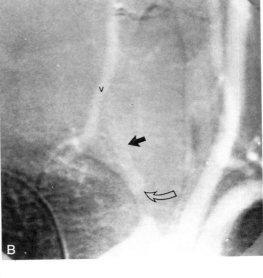

*Figure 9–18.* Brachiocephalic steal. *A,* Intravenous DSA of the aortic arch in a left anterior oblique projection shows occlusion of the brachiocephalic artery (*arrow*). *B,* Later film from the same study (with reversal of the image density) shows a densely opacified right vertebral artery with faint opacification of the brachiocephalic artery to the site of occlusion (*open curved arrow*). In addition, there is opacification of the right common carotid artery (*solid arrow*). *C,* A later film shows dense opacification of the right common carotid and subclavian arteries with antegrade flow. B = brachiocephalic; C = right common carotid; S = right subclavian; V = right vertebral arteries.

ies. The latter has antegrade flow into the head (Fig. 9–18).

2. Blood flow is reversed in both the right vertebral and the right common carotid arteries.

**Thyrocervical Steal Syndrome.** Reversal of blood flow in the thyrocervical artery is very rare and occurs if the subclavian artery is occluded or severely stenotic beyond the origin of the vertebral artery but proximal to the origin of the thyrocervical trunk. Collateral flow is mainly from the muscular and spinal branches of the vertebral arteries, which anastomose freely with the ascending cervical branch of the thyrocervical trunk. Thus, the steal may occur via the intracere-

bral circulation[1] or directly from the ipsilateral vertebral artery branches.[34, 35] Additional collateral blood supply is via the lateral branches of the thyrocervical trunk, from the occipital artery branches, and via the inferior thyroid artery (which communicates with the contralateral inferior thyroid artery). Thyrocervical steal is best demonstrated by arch aortography (Fig. 9–19).

### Thromboembolism

Thromboembolism is the most frequent cause of acute vascular insufficiency of the upper extremities in the elderly patient. The frequency of thromboembolism to the upper

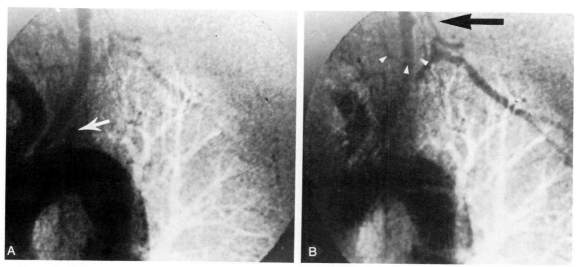

**Figure 9–19.** Thyrocervical steal. *A,* Intravenous DSA of the aortic arch in the left anterior oblique projection. The left subclavian (*arrow*) and left vertebral arteries are occluded. The distal left subclavian and thyrocervical arteries are opacified via cervical collaterals. *B,* Later film from the same study shows increasing density of opacification of the left ascending cervical (*black arrow*) and the inferior thyroid (*white arrowheads*) arteries with antegrade flow in the left subclavian artery.

extremities is between 10 and 17%.[36, 37] In over 90% of patients, the emboli originate from the heart (Fig. 9–20).[38] Approximately 50% of these patients have atrial fibrillation,[10] and approximately one third have a history of a recent myocardial infarction.[37, 38] In some

patients, the emboli may originate from a proximal vessel, ie, ulcerated plaques, aneurysms, thoracic outlet compression syndrome, and following brachial or axillary artery catheterization (Fig. 9–21).

The clinical manifestation is an acute onset

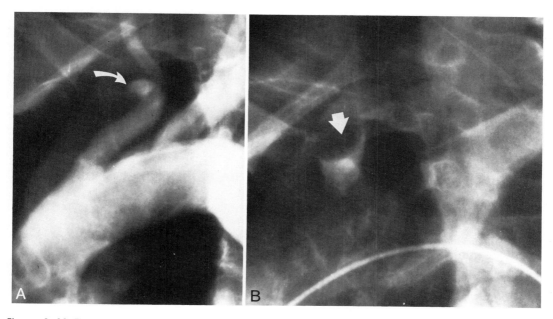

**Figure 9–20.** Thromboembolic occlusion. *A,* Early film from an arch aortogram in the left anterior oblique projection shows occlusion of the right subclavian artery (*arrow*). *B,* Close-up of a later film from the same study shows a meniscus due to the thromboembolus with stasis of contrast medium proximally (*arrow*).

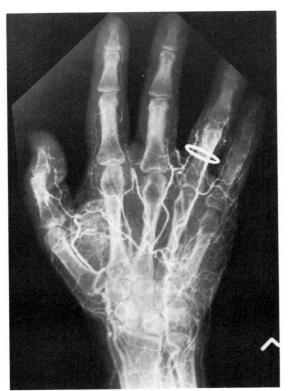

*Figure 9–21.* Thromboembolic occlusion of the hand arteries in a patient with an ipsilateral brachial artery aneurysm. Hand arteriogram following intraarterial injection of tolazoline (Priscoline) shows abrupt occlusion of common and proper digital arteries.

**TABLE 9–5.** Diseases That May Demonstrate Raynaud's Phenomenon

1. Collagen vascular diseases
2. Drug intoxication: ergotamine, methysergide
3. Endocrine: myxedema, pheochromocytoma
4. Hematological disorders
   a. Cold agglutinins
   b. Cryoglobulinemia
   c. Dysproteinemia
   d. Paroxysmal hemoglobinuria
5. Neurological disorders
   a. Carpal tunnel syndrome
6. Occlusive arterial diseases
   a. Arteriosclerosis
   b. Thromboangiitis obliterans
   c. Thromboembolism
7. Occult malignancy
8. Poisoning
   a. Lead
   b. Arsenic
9. Primary pulmonary hypertension
10. Thermal injury (cold)
11. Trauma
    a. Industrial, occupational
    b. Thoracic outlet syndrome (neurovascular trauma)

of ischemia with rest pain, absent pulses, paresthesias, decreased skin temperature, and pallor. Occasionally, a similar clinical picture can occur in in-situ thrombosis superimposed upon a severe arteriosclerotic stenosis, if the thrombotic occlusion involves a significant collateral channel, or in aortic dissection.

In one series reporting 260 cases, 55% of the emboli lodged in the brachial artery, 25% in the axillary artery, and 18% in the subclavian artery. Less than 2% of the embolizations involved the forearm vessels.[38]

The diagnosis is easily established by noninvasive methods, but arteriography is indicated for determining the location of embolic occlusion, for the evaluation of underlying diseases (eg, aneurysms, dissection), and in conjunction with intraarterial thrombolytic therapy. The arteriogram demonstrates an abrupt cutoff with a convex meniscus in the involved vessel. Atherosclerotic occlusion, on the other hand, usually demonstrates a tapered narrowing.

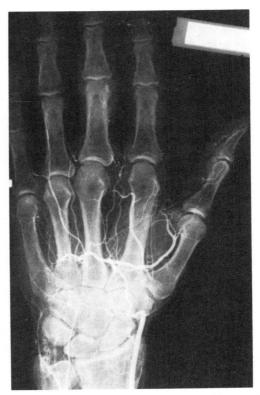

*Figure 9–22.* Raynaud's phenomenon. A 61 year old man with cyanosis and ischemic changes of the second and third fingertips. Hand arteriogram shows atherosclerotic occlusions of the ulnar, radial, and several common and proper digital arteries.

## Vasospastic Disorders

Peripheral vasospasm may be transient and may occur as a single episode such as is seen after vascular trauma or thermal stimulus (exposure to cold), or it may be due to a repetitive stimulus such as chronic drug intake (eg, ergotamine, methysergide), chronic trauma (eg, occupational), poisoning (eg, lead), collagen vascular disease, and thoracic outlet syndromes or in association with thromboangitis obliterans, thromboembolism, certain neurological disorders, and occult malignancy.[39-41]

**Raynaud's Disease and Raynaud's Phenomenon.** The disorder described by Raynaud in 1862 is characterized by an episodic constriction of small vessels of the extremities, which can be induced by cold (approximately 80% of patients) or by cold and emotional stimuli (about 20% of patients).[42] Emotional stimuli alone initiate the symptoms in less than 1% of patients. Fourteen per cent of these patients suffer from migraine and 9% have hypertension.[42] The term "Raynaud's phenomenon" is used when an underlying systemic or local disease is present.

The etiology of Raynaud's disease is unknown. A neurohumoral mechanism may be responsible by means of both local and systemic factors.[43, 44] Characteristically, the disease is bilateral; it affects young women (in a ratio of 3:1 to 5:1); underlying disease is absent; and ischemic changes are either absent or minimal.[39, 42, 45] The course of this disease is usually benign. Raynaud's phenomenon, on the other hand, may be seen in association with a number of clinical conditions (Table 9–5). Some reports suggest that patients with this disorder may

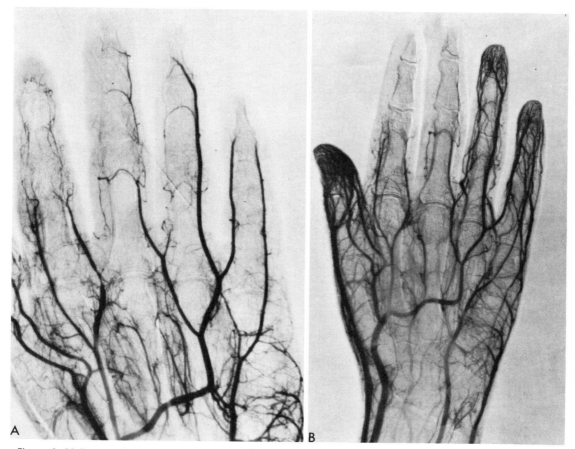

**Figure 9–23.** Raynaud's disease. A 19 year old woman with painful, cyanotic fingertips. A, Subtraction film from a hand arteriogram shows poor arterial opacification of the fingertips due to arterial spasm. The proper digital arteries of the second and third fingers are occluded. B, Repeat arteriogram after intraarterial injection of 1.0 mg of reserpine shows improved arterial filling of the thumb and fourth and fifth fingers, confirming the presence of anatomical changes in the second and third fingers. There is early venous opacification as a result of the reserpine injection. (From Kadir S et al: Peripheral vasospastic disorders. In Athanasoulis CA et al.: Interventional Radiology. Philadelphia, WB Saunders, 1982. Used with permission.)

have an underlying immunological abnormality.[46, 47]

The clinical picture consists of an initial intense vasoconstriction (digital pallor) followed by atony of the capillaries and venules (cyanosis) and reactive hyperemia (rubor). Repeated bouts of vasospasm lead to occlusion of small vessels with the development of ischemic ulcers at the fingertips.

Arteriography is indicated to:

1. Assess the extent of anatomical arterial occlusions.

2. Determine the vasodilatory response to intraarterial injections of drugs.

3. Exclude correctable anatomical lesions such as ulcerated atherosclerotic plaques, aneurysm, or a thoracic outlet compression.

After the subclavian arteriogram, the arterial catheter is placed proximal to the brachial artery bifurcation. In patients with a high origin of the radial or ulnar arteries, the catheter must be placed more proximally. A brachial arteriogram is performed first in order to evaluate the inflow vessels to the hand. For evaluation of smaller vessels of the hand, magnification arteriography ($\times 2$) and film subtraction provide the most informa-

tion. DSA can be used to evaluate the inflow vessels and occlusions of the metacarpal or digital arteries. However, cut film arteriography is necessary for assessment of subtle details.

The arteriographic findings are (Figs. 9–22 to 9–24):[46-49]

1. Patent proximal arteries.

2. Arterial occlusions at the wrist and in the palm and digits. These changes are most pronounced in the digits.

3. Multiple areas of vasospasm, which are reversible after intraarterial injection of reserpine (0.5 to 1.0 mg). This involves primarily the palmar and digital arteries.

4. Focal stenoses of veins, which are not relieved by intraarterial reserpine.

## Collagen Vascular Diseases

Periarteritis nodosa, rheumatoid arthritis, scleroderma, and systemic lupus erythematosus can give rise to abnormalities of the small and medium-sized arteries and occasionally the larger vessels.[50, 51]

**Scleroderma.** Inflammatory changes associated with scleroderma involve mainly the

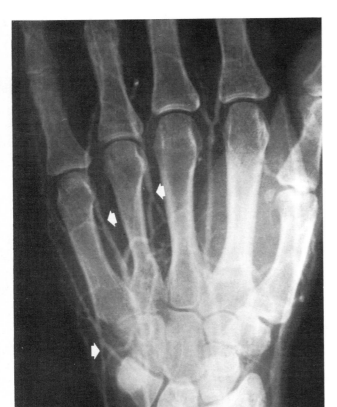

*Figure 9–24.* Focal venous stenoses in Raynaud's disease. Venous phase of a hand arteriogram shows segmental venous stenosis (*arrows*). (From Kadir S et al.: Peripheral vasospastic disorders. *In* Athanasoulis CA et al.: Interventional Radiology. Philadelphia, WB Saunders, 1982. Used with permission.)

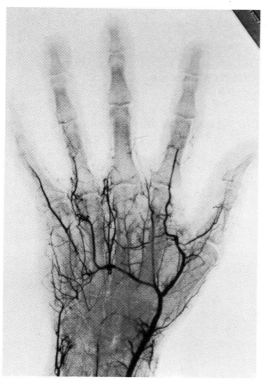

**Figure 9–25.** Scleroderma. Hand arteriogram shows occlusion of the ulnar artery, the superficial palmar arch, and multiple digital arteries. Collateral formation is absent and no arterial filling is observed distal to the occlusions in the digital arteries. (From Janevski BK: Angiography of the Upper Extremity. The Hague, Martinus Nijhoff, 1982. Used with permission.)

the presence of the disease at the arteriolar/capillary level.

3. Preservation of the radial artery. In one report evaluating 12 patients, the radial artery and deep palmar arch were never involved.[1]

**Systemic Lupus Erythematosus (SLE).** The vasculitis of SLE involves the small arteries and arterioles. There is fibrinoid degeneration with intimal proliferation, which leads to stenosis and occlusion. In addition, periarterial fibrosis may occur. Spontaneous recurrent thrombosis of large arteries and veins (about 12% of patients) may be the only clinical manifestation of the disease (Fig. 9–26).[58, 59] Approximately 20% of patients experience Raynaud's phenomenon.

The arteriographic picture is not specific, and stenosis or occlusion of the palmar and digital arteries may be seen. Unlike periarteritis nodosa, aneurysm formation is not typical in patients with SLE.[60]

## Thromboangiitis Obliterans

Thromboangiitis obliterans is an obliterative transmural arteritis that may involve the small and medium-sized arteries of the upper extremities in up to 74% of patients.[61] The vast majority of patients are males who have a history of cigarette smoking, and the most frequently involved vessels are the palmar, digital, ulnar, and radial arteries.

small vessels and the capillary bed. Large vessel involvement is rare.[52, 53] There is intimal proliferation and medial hypertrophy with concentric narrowing progressing to occlusion. A prominent feature is the loss of the capillary bed.[52] Acute thrombosis of large vessels has also been reported.[54]

Vascular abnormalities are widespread. In the extremities, multiple stenoses and occlusions may be present, leading to ischemic changes of the fingertips. The majority of patients experience Raynaud's phenomenon. Renal involvement is the most frequent cause of death.[53] Disease of the vasa vasorum of the aorta may lead to aortitis.[55]

The arteriographic findings are (Fig. 9–25):[56, 57]

1. Multiple focal stenoses and occlusions involving the ulnar, palmar, and proper digital arteries. The radial and common digital arteries are involved infrequently.

2. Sparse collateral channels. This reflects

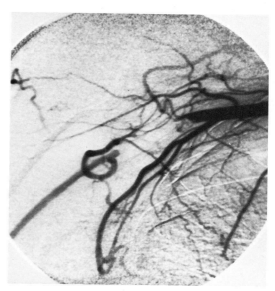

**Figure 9–26.** Spontaneous thrombosis of the axillary artery in a patient with systemic lupus erythematosus demonstrated by intraarterial DSA.

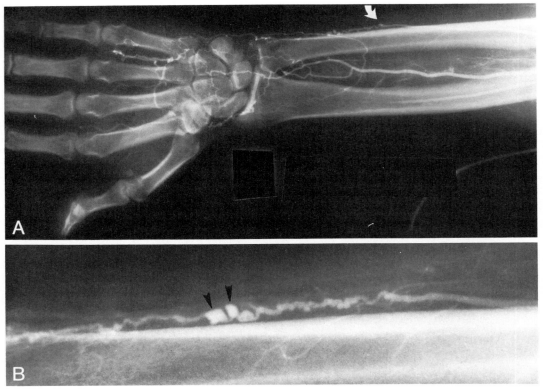

*Figure 9–27.* Thromboangiitis obliterans. *A,* Arteriogram of the distal forearm and the hand shows occlusion of the ulnar artery (*arrow*) with opacification of extremely tortuous (also described as "corrugated" appearing) collateral vessels. The flow in the radial artery is slow. Several other wrist and hand vessels are poorly opacified owing to spasm and arterial occlusions. *B,* Closeup view of the tortuous collaterals in the forearm shows the fibrotic distortion and formation of small aneurysms (*arrowheads*).

Symptoms include intermittent claudication, rest pain, ischemic and trophic changes, gangrene, decrease in skin temperature, excessive sensitivity to cold, and Raynaud's phenomenon. The last may be seen in over half the patients. Migratory thrombophlebitis is also seen in over half the patients.

Arteriography demonstrates (Fig. 9–27):

1. Fibrotic distortion of the forearm, palmar and digital arteries, or larger collaterals, resulting in a "corrugated" appearance. Severe fibrosis can lead to the formation of small saccular aneurysms.

2. Multiple areas of stenosis and occlusion that involve the forearm and hand arteries.

3. Demonstration of an extensive collateral network.

4. Areas of vascular spasm.

Pitfalls in the diagnosis of occlusive and spastic arterial diseases of the upper extremity include:

1. Undetected lesions: If the catheter tip is placed in the distal subclavian artery, a proximal lesion may be overlooked, especially if not enough contrast medium refluxes proximally.

2. Physiological compression: In muscular individuals, intense muscular contraction may cause vascular compression and simulate an anatomical stenosis or arterial spasm. This usually occurs in the brachial artery but may involve a branch vessel.

## ARTERIOVENOUS MALFORMATIONS

### Congenital Arteriovenous Communications

Congenital vascular lesions result from an abnormal development of the primitive vascular system. They have been described in association with various clinical syndromes or may occur as solitary lesions, eg, Klippel-Trenaunay-Weber syndrome, Parkes-Weber syndrome, simple capillary hemangioma, cavernous hemangioma, cirsoid aneurysm, etc.

Such anomalies can be classified according to the stage of development in which either the anomalous development occurred or the maturation process stagnated.[62] Thus, congenital arteriovenous communications are classified as: (1) cavernous and simple hemangiomas, (2) microfistulous communications, (3) macrofistulous communications (see under Arteriovenous Fistula), and (4) anomalous development in the maturation stage.

Arteriography is indicated for evaluating the type and extent of the lesion and for helping to plan therapy ("road map" for surgery or preoperative embolization). Microfistulous communications cannot be demonstrated by arteriography. In macrofistulous communications arteriography demonstrates a characteristic appearance of multiple dilated and tortuous arterial and venous channels (see Fig. 9–28). The majority of such lesions demonstrate arteriovenous shunting.[62]

## Arteriovenous Fistula

Arteriovenous fistula is an abnormal communication between an artery and a vein without an interposed capillary system. Arteriovenous fistulae can be congenital but are more often acquired.[63] Congenital arteriovenous fistulae result from a failure of differentiation between artery and vein with persistence of the communications existing in the primary anlage.[64] They may remain asymptomatic and clinically inapparent until rapid enlargement of the fistula occurs after trauma, which may be minor (see Fig. 9–28).[64, 65]

Congenital arteriovenous fistulae may be localized or diffuse, involving the entire extremity. In either type, multiple abnormal arteriovenous communications are present. Diffuse fistulae are often associated with enlargement of the involved limb.[63] References 66 to 68 provide a review of this topic.

Acquired arteriovenous fistulae are most frequently due to penetrating trauma. Blunt trauma is an infrequent cause of arteriovenous fistula formation. Approximately 3.5% of all vascular injuries result in an arteriovenous fistula.[69] Other causes that may lead to the development of an arteriovenous fistula are listed in Table 9–6.

**Pathology.** In the veins, there is intimal thickening with development of circular elastic fibers and thickening of the media with

**TABLE 9–6. Etiology of Arteriovenous Fistulae**

1. Congenital
2. Vascular trauma: external penetrating, blunt
3. Infection: mycotic aneurysm rupture
4. Access fistula for hemodialysis
5. Bone fracture (internal penetrating injury)

development of elastic and muscle fibers. These changes are similar to those seen after arterialization of veins. Thus, in a small fistula, it may be difficult to distinguish a small vein from an artery. In larger fistulae, venous aneurysms are seen. In the arteries, atrophic changes are noted, with thinning of the arterial wall due to loss of the elastic tissue and muscle fibers. This occurs as a result of the decreased resistance in the outflow, ie, through the fistula.

**Clinical Aspects.** The posttraumatic fistula may not be apparent immediately after the trauma because of temporary occlusion due to a surrounding hematoma or clot. Clinical manifestations include thrill and bruit, increased skin temperature, venous stasis, and venous insufficiency with development of stasis ulcers, similar to the postphlebitic stasis complex. If a fistula develops before epiphyseal closure, increase in limb length and girth may occur.

Large fistulae with considerable arteriovenous shunting existing over a long period of time may lead to cardiac hypertrophy and congestive heart failure. Complications include distal limb ischemia and bacterial seeding.

**Arteriography.** Arteriography is indicated:

1. To determine the site of the fistula.
2. To evaluate the arterial system for associated injuries.
3. In congenital fistulae, to evaluate the extent of disease.
4. For identification of the feeding vessels (eg, surgical road map).
5. For therapeutic embolization.

For the demonstration of arteriovenous shunting, rapid filming is required. Initially, a "survey" arteriogram is obtained to evaluate the extent of the abnormality and source of vascular supply. Subsequently, another arteriogram, with rapid filming, is obtained over the region of interest (3 films/sec for 12 films and subsequently 1 film/sec for an additional 4 to 6 films). The contrast injection rate should be adjusted after assessment of the flow by test injection (7 to 10 ml/sec for

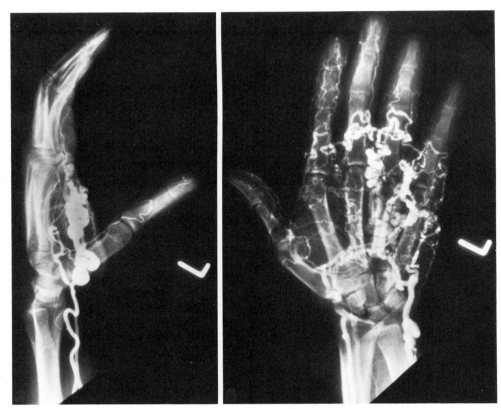

**Figure 9–28.** Arteriovenous malformation. Progressive swelling and pain following minor trauma prompted this arteriogram. Lateral and AP arteriograms of the hand show a large vascular malformation in the palm and fingers. The ulnar artery was the principal source of blood supply. On the AP film (mid-arterial phase) enlarged and tortuous early draining veins are seen.

a total of 25 to 30 ml). Intraarterial DSA provides an ideal method for the evaluation of such lesions.

The arteriographic findings are (Fig. 9–28; see also Fig. 9–34):

1. In the acquired fistula, there usually is one enlarged feeding artery. In congenital fistulae, multiple feeding arteries (or branches) are present. These are enlarged and tortuous and opacify a network of abnormal vessels (the arteriovenous malformation).

2. Arteriovenous shunting with rapid opacification of one or more veins.

3. Venous enlargement.

4. Demonstration of an arterial aneurysm (traumatic) or a venous aneurysm (secondary to high flow or trauma). Multiple venous aneurysms are seen in congenital lesions.

### Hemangioma

Cavernous hemangiomas are the most common vascular tumor of the upper extremity[1] and are usually located in the hand and occasionally in the forearm. Hemangiomas result from arrest of the normal vascular development at the capillary stage.[70] On arteriography, in contrast to other arteriovenous malformations, there is no enlargement of the feeding arteries. Cavernous vascular spaces are visualized, which remain opacified late into the venous phase (Fig. 9–29). Arteriovenous fistulous connections are infrequent. Occasionally, radiographs of the hand may demonstrate phleboliths.[65]

### THE THORACIC OUTLET SYNDROMES

**Anatomy.** The path of the subclavian vessels and the brachial plexus to and from the arm takes them through three potential compression sites:

1. Interscalene triangle: This is formed by the anterior and medial scalene muscles and inferiorly by the first rib. The subclavian artery and brachial plexus pass through the

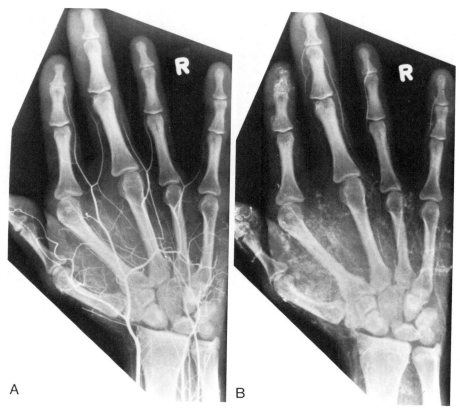

**Figure 9–29.** Hemangioma of the hand. *A*, Early arterial phase shows no arterial abnormality or arteriovenous shunting. There is increased soft tissue density over the palm (especially over the thenar prominence). *B*, Parenchymal phase shows diffuse hemangioma of the thumb, palm, and wrist with retention of contrast medium in small vascular lakes. No prominent draining veins are present.

triangle, and the subclavian vein passes anterior to the anterior scalene muscle.

2. Costoclavicular space: This is formed superiorly by the clavicle and subclavius muscle and inferiorly by the first rib. All three structures pass through this space.

3. Pectoralis minor tunnel: This is formed by the pectoralis minor tendon anteriorly and the coracoid process of the scapula. All three components of the neurovascular bundle pass through this tunnel.

**Pathology.** In the vast majority of patients, congenital or acquired abnormalities described below are present in one or more of the potential compression sites:

CERVICAL RIBS. These are seen in up to 0.5% of normal individuals.[71] Only completely developed cervical ribs are likely to be symptomatic, and less than half the individuals with complete cervical ribs have symptoms of neurovascular compression.[72] On the other hand, in about 70% of symptomatic patients, a cervical rib is responsible

for the thoracic outlet compression syndromes.[73] A cervical rib elevates the floor of the scalene triangle, thereby decreasing this and also the costoclavicular space.

SCALENUS MINIMUS MUSCLE. This is a small muscle or a fibrous band extending from the transverse process of the seventh cervical vertebra to the first rib. It inserts between the brachial plexus and the subclavian artery. This muscle is seen in one third of normal individuals, and alone it is rarely symptomatic.[73]

ANTERIOR SCALENE MUSCLE. A wide or abnormal insertion or hypertrophy of this muscle has been associated with the scalenus anticus syndrome.[73]

ANOMALOUS FIRST RIB. The unusually straight course of the anomalous first thoracic rib narrows the costoclavicular space.

ACQUIRED LESIONS. Muscular body habitus may cause neurovascular compression in the pectoralis minor tunnel; however, such patients are rarely symptomatic. Individuals with a slender body habitus, a thin long neck, and sagging shoulders are more prone to develop this syndrome.[74, 75] Other acquired lesions include clavicle or first thoracic rib fractures with nonanatomical alignment or exuberant callus and supraclavicular tumors or lymphadenopathy.[76, 77] In one series 34% of the acquired thoracic outlet syndromes were posttraumatic.[78]

**Clinical Aspects.** Thoracic outlet compression syndromes occur most frequently in women.[75] The most common type is the scalenus anticus syndrome. The chief complaint is pain in the hand, which is often increased upon elevation of the extremity. Other symptoms include numbness of the hand and fingers, paresthesias, intermittent claudication, decreased skin temperature, and ischemic changes in the digits. Approximately 40% of patients exhibit Raynaud's phenomenon.[79] Intermittent obstruction of the subclavian vein, with or without thrombosis, leads to cyanosis and edema.[80] On physical examination, an aneurysm or poststenotic dilatation of the subclavian artery can occasionally be palpated.

The diagnosis must be established using strict criteria because, in a large number of normal individuals, the radial pulse can be either obliterated or diminished by performing the diagnostic maneuvers.[73, 75, 79] Thus, in one study of normal individuals, the hyperabduction maneuver obliterated the radial pulse in 34% and diminished it significantly in another 23%.[75]

DIAGNOSTIC TESTS. In the costoclavicular maneuver, the patient's shoulders are braced posteriorly and inferiorly. In the Adson or scalenus maneuver, the patient is asked to take a deep inspiration, hyperextend the neck, and turn the face toward the extremity being evaluated. In the hyperabduction maneuver, the involved extremity is passively abducted (elevated). These tests are considered positive if a reduction or obliteration of the radial pulse occurs. In addition, a systolic bruit may be heard as the artery is compressed and disappears upon occlusion.

The compression syndromes are named after the area in which the neurovascular bundle is compressed, ie, scalenus anticus syndrome, costoclavicular compression syndrome, and pectoralis minor compression (hyperabduction) syndrome. In the last the neurovascular bundle is subjected to stretching, pinching, and torsion beneath the pectoralis minor tendon and the coracoid process of the scapula.[74, 79, 81]

**Angiography.** Angiography is performed to evaluate an anatomical vascular abnormality, the degree of vascular compression, and the status of the peripheral circulation. Arteriography is performed via the transfemoral approach. In some patients, intravenous DSA can be used for establishing this diagnosis. Two sets of films are obtained: (1) in the neutral position (arms adducted) to evaluate anatomical changes involving the subclavian, axillary, and arm vessels, and (2) in hyperabduction to evaluate the degree of vascular compression. Bilateral symptoms are evaluated by arch aortography (or intraarterial DSA) in the AP projection. In patients with unilateral symptoms, the headhunter 1 catheter is placed distal to the vertebral artery orifice. For the second set of films, the catheter position in the subclavian artery must be rechecked after the arm is maximally abducted because this maneuver may dislodge the catheter tip. Upon completion of the arteriogram, the catheter is pulled down into the distal (infrarenal) aorta, and an arm venogram is performed with the arm in a neutral (adducted) position and after maximal abduction. In patients with symptoms of distal upper extremity ischemia, arteriograms of the forearm and hand should be obtained to assess the peripheral circulation for the presence of embolic occlusion.

TECHNIQUE FOR ARM VENOGRAPHY. The cubital vein of the affected extremity is catheterized using a short Teflon sheath (eg, No. 18 angiocath). The sheath is secured in place with adhesive tape and connected via a connecting tubing (K-50) to a syringe containing 50 ml of contrast medium (60% diatrizoate meglumine sodium). For DSA, a 15% concentration is used.

With the operator (person injecting the contrast medium) standing behind a leaded screen, an arm venogram is performed using the following sequence:

1. Inject 25 ml of contrast medium rapidly.
2. Begin filming at one film/sec for a total of ten films.
3. Continue injecting contrast medium for a total of 35 to 40 ml (the injection should be completed before the last film is taken).
4. Thereafter, infuse 50 to 100 ml of heparinized flushing solution over 5 to 10 minutes.

Subsequently, the arm is placed in maximum abduction and a second venogram is performed using the same sequence. However, the total volume of contrast medium is decreased by approximately 10 ml. The arm

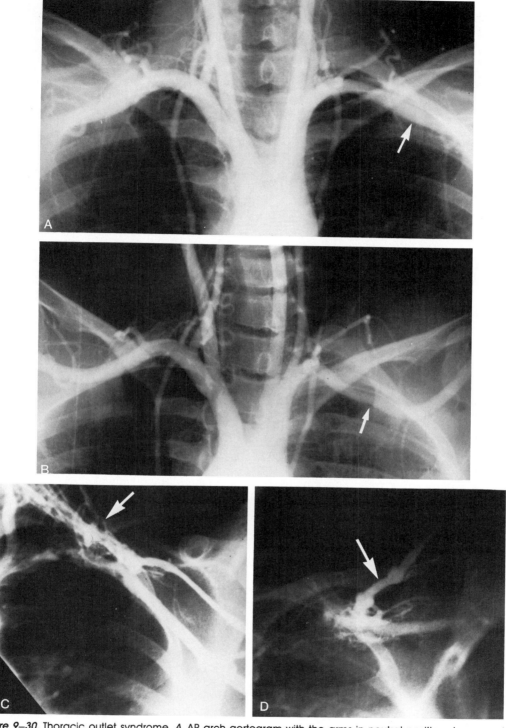

**Figure 9–30.** Thoracic outlet syndrome. *A,* AP arch aortogram with the arms in neutral position shows a minimal dilatation of the left subclavian artery (*arrow*). *B,* Repeat aortogram with the arms abducted shows an inferior indentation of the left subclavian artery (*arrow*). *C,* Left subclavian venogram in the neutral position shows partial occlusion of the subclavian vein and opacification of collaterals (*arrow*). *D,* Repeat study with the arm hyperabducted shows complete occlusion of the subclavian vein. Arrow points to distended cephalic vein.

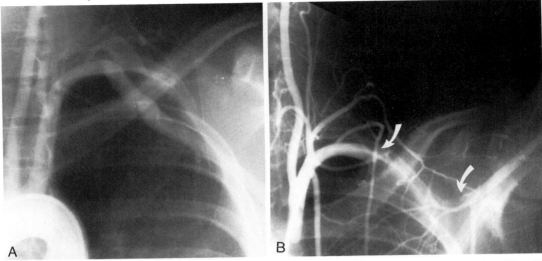

**Figure 9–31.** Thoracic outlet syndrome. *A*, AP arch aortogram with the arm in neutral position. The distal subclavian/proximal axillary artery is mildly dilated and displaced inferiorly. *B*, Left subclavian arteriogram with the arm in hyperabduction shows complete obstruction of the distal subclavian and the proximal axillary arteries (*arrows*).

is brought into a neutral position immediately after completion of the filming, in order to avoid prolonged contact of contrast medium with the vein intima. If the venogram in the neutral position demonstrates venous occlusion, the second venogram is omitted.

ANGIOGRAPHIC FINDINGS. The angiographic findings in thoracic outlet syndromes are (Figs. 9–30 and 9–31):[82, 83]

*Neutral Position:*

1. Occasionally, no arterial abnormality is present in the neutral position.

2. Mild dilatation of the distal subclavian/proximal axillary artery (poststenotic dilatation): This is the most common finding.

3. Abnormal course of the distal subclavian/proximal axillary artery (eg, displacement).

4. Focal stenosis.

5. Aneurysm.

6. Mural thrombus in an aneurysm or dilated segment.

7. Distal embolization (occlusion of forearm, palmar, and digital arteries) due to a large embolus or multiple small, recurrent emboli.

8. Arterial occlusion: This occurs very infrequently and may result in limb loss or may lead to cerebral embolization as a result of retrograde propagation of the clot.

9. Venous obstruction or thrombosis: This may be manifested clinically as edema and cyanosis (venous stasis). Proximal (eg, axil-

lary vein) occlusion may be asymptomatic because of the presence of collaterals, unless a phlebitis is superimposed.

*Maximal Abduction:*

1. Bandlike or concentric compression of the artery of varying degrees: Occasionally, an eccentric compression of the inferior wall is present.

2. Occlusion of the subclavian or axillary artery: In the costoclavicular compression syndrome, the distal subclavian and proximal segment of the axillary artery are involved.

3. Compression or occlusion of the subclavian vein: This usually occurs in the costoclavicular space.

### TRAUMA

Trauma to the upper extremity vessels may occur as a result of acute blunt or penetrating injury or chronic trauma. The vast majority of injuries are acute (blunt or penetrating), and only few injuries of the major vessels are due to chronic trauma.[84] The upper extremity vessels are injured in over 50% of cases of acute arterial injury to the extremities.[85] The most vulnerable vessel appears to be the brachial artery.

**Pathology.** Vascular trauma may be manifested as an acute event (expanding hematoma, occlusion) or may be noted later, following development of an arteriovenous

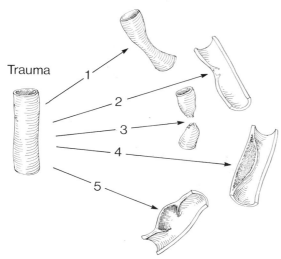

**Figure 9–32.** Diagram illustrating some of the types of arterial injuries. 1 = spasm; 2 = intimal laceration; 3 = transection; 4 = mural hematoma; 5 = pseudoaneurysm.

fistula or false aneurysm.[86] Findings include (Fig. 9–32):

1. Spasm: Blunt injury that leads to arterial spasm is usually associated with some degree of anatomical injury to the artery (eg, minor intimal laceration, mural hematoma).

2. Extrinsic compression due to a hematoma.

3. Laceration: This may involve partial or complete transection with formation of an expanding hematoma or false aneurysm, or

4. Occlusion: This may be due to an intimal disruption or contusion with mural hematoma and intravascular thrombosis. Although arterial thrombosis is usually associated with some type of intimal injury, occasionally, intravascular thrombosis may occur in severe extrinsic compression without intimal damage. In addition, circulatory stasis, due to either arterial compression or systemic shock, must be present for arterial thrombosis to develop.

5. Arteriovenous fistula.

6. Distal embolization.

**Blunt Injury.** This may cause direct vascular contusion leading to spasm or occlusion or extrinsic compression due to surrounding hematoma and/or edema. In addition, injury may occur as a result of displaced bone fragments. Blunt trauma may also lead to a stretch injury such as is seen in association with joint dislocations with and without fracture.[86–88] Such stretch injuries may be manifested by intimal/medial disruption or complete arterial transection. The latter may appear as an expanding hematoma if a large vessel (eg, subclavian) is involved or may lead to retraction and occlusion (by thrombus) of small vessels. Partial laceration of an artery may lead to development of a pseudoaneurysm.

Blunt trauma with displaced bone fractures can also cause internal penetrating injury to the blood vessels by bone fragments. This can lead to the formation of false aneurysms, expanding hematomas, or arteriovenous fistulae. Complete transection of an artery by a bone fragment can also occur.

**Penetrating Injury.** Penetrating wounds, often with minimal external signs of injury, may lead to development of an arteriovenous fistula or a pseudoaneurysm. The latter may develop over several months or years.[87]

**Iatrogenic Arterial Injury.** Iatrogenic vascular injury may be self-induced or may occur during the course of patient management. Self-induced injuries are most often related to intravascular drug abuse and result from inadvertent intra- or periarterial injections. Such injections lead to vascular spasm, gangrene, and mycotic aneurysms. Rarely, self-administered intramuscular medication may lead to false aneurysm formation.[89] Many vascular complications occurring during the course of the patient's management are unavoidable (Table 9–7).

**Clinical Aspects.** The presence or absence of peripheral pulses is an unreliable sign of

**TABLE 9–7.** Iatrogenic Vascular Trauma: Etiology and Complications of Vascular Trauma Occurring During Patient Management

1. Inadvertent intraarterial drug injection or infusion (vasospasm, chemical arteritis, arterial thrombosis)

2. Periarterial hematoma (compression, arterial spasm, thrombosis)

3. Arterial catheterization, ie, diagnostic arteriography, or interventional procedures, blood gas and blood pressure monitoring (radial artery) (vasospasm, dissection, thrombosis, peripheral embolization, arteriovenous fistula, and false aneurysm)

4. Tight plaster cast causing venous stasis and edema (arterial compression and thrombosis) or direct trauma from edge of cast to brachial artery (vasospasm, thrombosis)

5. Inadvertent arterial puncture (hematoma, false aneurysm, thrombosis)

6. Venous catheterization (thrombophlebitis, thromboembolism)

vascular injury, since up to 43% of patients with arterial injury may have normal peripheral pulses and only 39% of patients with arterial injury have absent distal pulses.[90]

Physical signs of arterial injury are absent or diminished peripheral pulses, pain, neurological deficit (sensory, motor), bruit, pulsatile mass, or bleeding.

**Arteriography.** The major indications for arteriography in acute arterial trauma are:

1. The localization of the site of arterial injury.

2. The evaluation of the extent of injuries.

3. The evaluation of patients with proximity injuries.

4. The evaluation of pulse deficits.

The last may be due to arterial spasm and cannot be differentiated from occlusion due to thrombosis or intimal injury by clinical means. In the event of an intimal tear due to a stretch injury, even visual inspection of the artery during operative exploration may not detect any evidence of injury, as the outer arterial wall may appear normal and arterial pulses may be present.

Elective arteriography is indicated for proximity injuries. However, the diagnostic yield of this procedure is very low. In one series, about 1% of 85 patients had an arterial injury and another 5% had arterial spasm and a normal physical examination.[91] On the other hand, during operation on the basis of clinical suspicion alone, approximately 20% of patients did not show evidence of arterial injury.[92] In the same series, if location of injury alone was used as an indication for operative intervention, an arterial injury would have been present in only 12% of patients.

Thus, arteriography prior to operation for suspected vascular injury can decrease the number of "negative" explorations. However, in patients with major arterial injury and hemodynamic instability, immediate operation may be indicated, without prior arteriography.

The arteriographic findings are (Figs. 9–33 to 9–40):

1. Arterial narrowing due to posttraumatic spasm or extrinsic compression by hematoma.

2. Arterial occlusion: Occasionally, intimal disruption can be visualized as a dome-shaped occlusion due to "rolling up" of the torn intima.[84] Transient arterial occlusion can also occur as a result of intense arterial spasm. In the latter, typically there is a cone-shaped narrowing proximal to the occlusion. Occasionally, the occlusion may appear as an abrupt termination of the contrast-filled artery.

3. False aneurysms.

4. Arteriovenous fistula.

5. Localized intimal defects (tears).

6. Extravasation.

Intraarterial injection of tolazoline (25 mg diluted with 10 to 15 ml of 5% dextrose and injected over 15 to 20 seconds) can be used to assist in differentiating between arterial spasm and anatomical occlusion. Alternatively, intraarterial injection of 0.5 to 1.0 mg of reserpine or 25 mg of papaverine may be used as both a diagnostic and a therapeutic measure.

Pitfalls in arteriographic interpretation include:

1. Pseudothrombosis: The "rolled up," dome-shaped intima due to laceration may simulate a thrombus or an embolus.

2. Pseudo-occlusion: Posttraumatic arterial

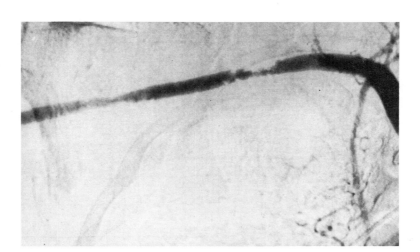

*Figure 9–33.* Stretch injury to the subclavian and axillary arteries resulting from a motorcycle accident. Subtraction film from an AP right subclavian arteriogram shows a frayed appearance of the vessel. At operation the intima and media were torn. (Courtesy of Dr. CA Athanasoulis.)

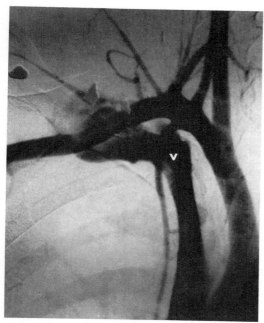

Figure 9–34. Arteriovenous fistula of the right subclavian vessels from a bullet injury. V = brachiocephalic vein.

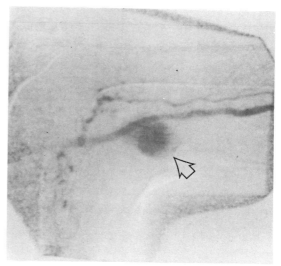

Figure 9–36. Intravenous DSA shows a false aneurysm of the left axillary artery (arrow) resulting from multiple arterial punctures.

spasm may appear as an arterial occlusion. Often, intraarterial injection of a vasodilator can relieve the spasm.

3. Failure to recognize injuries: In penetrating injuries, the intimal defect may be inapparent as a result of a dense contrast column or overlying bone. Thus, a second projection is necessary for a complete study. This pitfall is less likely to occur with the use of intraarterial DSA.

The recognition of arterial injuries is important in order to permit early therapeutic intervention so that complications can be avoided.

**Subclavian and Axillary Artery Injury** (Figs. 9–33 to 9–36). High-speed accidents

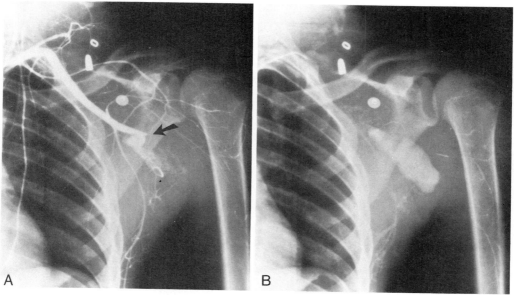

Figure 9–35. Traumatic arterial occlusion with formation of a false aneurysm. A, AP left axillary arteriogram shows abrupt occlusion of the axillary artery (arrow) with extravasation of contrast medium. B, Later film from the same study shows a false aneurysm.

may result in stretch injury to the subclavian artery. Often this is associated with a clavicular fracture, but the arterial injury can occur in the absence of such a fracture.[93] Clavicular fractures can cause laceration or transection of the subclavian artery by the sharp edge of the fracture.[94] However, the most common mechanism of arterial injury in such patients is compression and angulation of the vessels between fracture fragments.[86]

Fractures and dislocations of the humeral head may result in acute injury to the axillary and proximal brachial arteries.[95] Chronic trauma to these vessels occurs occasionally from the use of crutches or from an upper extremity cast.[84] Acute arterial occlusions or false aneurysm formation can also occur after arterial catheterization[96] or penetrating injury. The latter may also result in the development of an arteriovenous fistula.

**Brachial Artery Injury** (Figs. 9–37 and 9–38). Elbow dislocations are associated with an arterial injury in almost 7% of patients.[87] This may be manifested as arterial compression with reappearance of distal pulses after reduction of the dislocation, or an arterial laceration, avulsion or intimal stretch in-

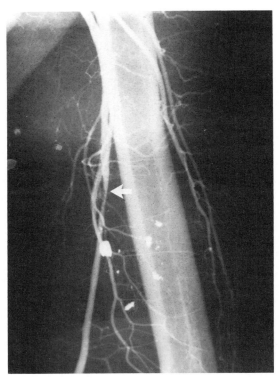

*Figure 9–38.* Intimal laceration (*arrow*) and associated spasm of the brachial artery following a bullet injury.

jury.[86, 88] Signs of peripheral ischemia may not develop after distal brachial artery interruption because of the presence of an extensive collateral system around the elbow. For this same reason, a more conservative therapeutic approach is indicated.[86]

Elbow dislocation with associated fractures can cause arterial laceration by the bone fragment. Similarly, arterial laceration or occlusion also occurs after externally penetrating trauma.

**Injury to Arteries of the Forearm and Hand** (Figs. 9–39 and 9–40). Trauma to the forearm vessels accounts for up to one third of the injuries to the upper extremity vessels, and forearm vessels are the second most common site of injury after the brachial artery.[85]

Blunt or penetrating trauma may lead to arterial occlusion or the formation of an arteriovenous fistula or a false aneurysm.[84, 97, 98] The formation of false aneurysms may also occur following iatrogenic injury (Fig. 9–39).

**Hypothenar Hammer Syndrome.** Injury to the palmar and digital arteries occurs as a result of repetitive blunt trauma or mechan-

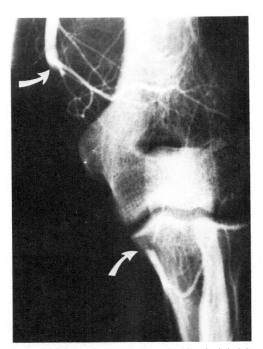

*Figure 9–37.* Arterial occlusion due to stretch injury. The distal pulses were absent following acute dislocation of the left elbow. Brachial arteriogram after reduction shows a segmental occlusion of the brachial artery (*arrows*).

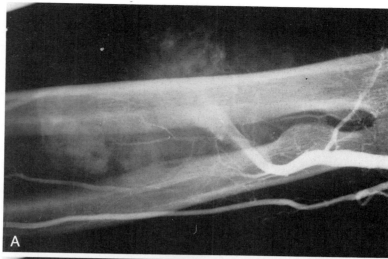

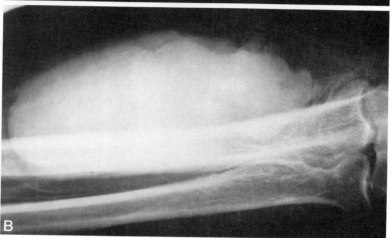

*Figure 9–39.* False aneurysm of the ulnar artery. A pulsatile mass was noted in the forearm several weeks after balloon embolectomy. *A,* Early film from a brachial arteriogram shows a markedly enlarged ulnar artery and a jet of contrast medium entering a large false aneurysm. The artery distal to the neck of the aneurysm is of normal caliber. *B,* Later film from the same arteriogram shows a large contrast-filled aneurysm.

ical pressure such as occupational trauma (eg, in vibratory/air driven tool operators, mechanics, farmers, and those individuals who use their palms for pushing, pounding, or twisting), hand trauma in persons practicing martial arts (eg, karate), or any other form of blunt trauma to the wrist and hand.[99, 100] Repetitive minor trauma (eg, in pianists, typists) may also cause digital ischemia. Such trauma leads to arterial spasm, thrombosis (usually associated with an intimal injury plus spasm), and, in the larger vessels, the formation of pseudoaneurysms (following intimal and medial injury). The ulnar artery is most vulnerable in the segment where it crosses the hamate bone. In this region, it can be compressed against the hook of the hamate.

Clinically, there is evidence of digital is-

chemia, Raynaud's phenomenon, and occasionally a pulsatile mass (occluded aneurysms may be manifested as nonpulsatile masses)[101] usually involving the dominant extremity. Symptoms are often aggravated by cold. Symptoms of digital ischemia depend upon the completeness of the palmar arch. Since the majority of individuals have a complete palmar arch, symptoms may be mild. Thus, individuals with an incomplete arch or underlying occlusive arterial disease are more likely to be symptomatic.

In the hypothenar hammer syndrome arteriography may demonstrate (Fig. 9–41):

1. Arterial occlusion: Most commonly, the ulnar and digital arteries are affected. Occasionally, the radial artery may be involved.

2. Arterial spasm.

3. Pseudoaneurysms.

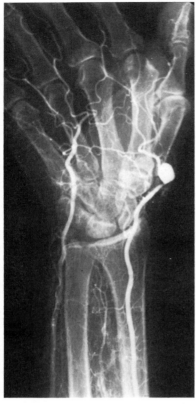

**Figure 9–40.** Brachial arteriogram shows a small, saccular aneurysm of the distal radial artery.

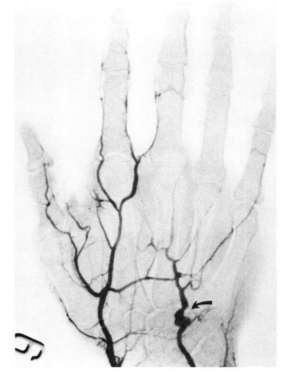

**Figure 9–41.** Hypothenar hammer syndrome. Subtraction film from a hand arteriogram shows a small aneurysm of the ulnar artery (*arrow*). The proper digital arteries of the third to fifth digits are occluded. (From Latshaw RF, Weidner WA: AJR 131:1093, 1978. Used with permission.)

## REFERENCES

1. Janevski BK: Angiography of the Upper Extremity. The Hague, Martinus Nijhoff, 1982.
2. Jonsson K, Karlsson S: Angiography of the internal mammary artery. Acta Radiol Diagn 26:113–120, 1985.
3. Warwick R, Williams PL: Gray's Anatomy, 35th Brit. Ed. Philadelphia, WB Saunders, 1973, pp. 639–656.
4. Karlsson S, Niechajev IA: Arterial anatomy of the upper extremity. Acta Radiol Diag 23:115–121, 1982.
5. Coleman SS, Anson BJ: Arterial patterns in the hand based upon a study of 650 specimens. Surg Gynecol Obstet 113:409–424, 1961.
6. McCormack LJ, Cauldwell EW, Anson BJ: Brachial and antebrachial arterial patterns. A study of 750 extremities. Surg Gynecol Obstet 96:43–54, 1953.
6a. Libersa Cl, Francke JP, Mauppin JM, et al: The arterial supply to the palm of the hand (arteriae palmae manus). Anat Clin 4:33–45, 1982.
7. Simmons CR, Tsao EC, Thompson JR: Angiographic approach to the difficult aortic arch: A new technique for transfemoral cerebral angiography in the aged. AJR 119:605–612, 1973.
8. Carlson DH, McDonald DG: Simplified catheterization of a left common carotid artery arising from the innominate trunk. Radiology 144:419, 1982.

9. McBurney RP, Lee L, Field JR: Thrombosis and aneurysms of the brachial artery secondary to brachial arteriography. Am Surg 39:115–117, 1973.
10. Schmidt FE, Hewett RL: Severe upper limb ischemia. Arch Surg 115:1188–1191, 1980.
11. Spittell JA Jr, Wallace RB: Aneurysms. *In* Juergens JL, Spittell JA Jr, Fairbairn JF II (eds): Peripheral Vascular Diseases. Philadelphia, WB Saunders, 1980, pp 415–439.
12. Brown GE, Rowntree LG: Right sided carotid pulsations in cases of severe hypertension. JAMA 84:1016–1019, 1925.
13. Honig EI, Dubilier W Jr, Steinberg I: Significance of the buckeled innominate artery. Ann Intern Med 39:74–80, 1953.
14. Spittell JA Jr: Aneurysms of the hand and wrist. Med Clin North Am 3:1007–1010, 1958.
15. Millender LH, Nalebuff EA, Kasdon E: Aneurysms and thrombosis of the ulnar artery in the hand. Arch Surg 105:686–690, 1972.
16. Newton TH, Wylie EJ: Collateral circulation associated with occlusion of the proximal subclavian and innominate arteries. AJR 91:394–405, 1964.
17. Shuford WH, Sybers RG, Schlant RC: Subclavian steal syndrome in right aortic arch with isolation of the left subclavian artery. Am Heart J 82:98–104, 1971.
18. Shumacker HB Jr: Surgical treatment of coarctation

of the aorta. Further experiences with use of subclavian arteries. Am J Surg 89:1235–1240, 1955.

19. Nemir P Jr, Bahabozorgui S, Wagner DE: Brachial-basilar insufficiency and the subclavian steal syndrome. J Thorac Cardiovasc Surg 50:534–544, 1965.

20. North RR, Fields WS, DeBakey ME, et al: Brachial-basilar insufficiency syndrome. Neurology 12:810–820, 1962.

21. Blesovsky A, Colanceski V, Ferguson J, et al: Acute subclavian steal syndrome following blunt thoracic trauma. Thorax 27:492–495, 1972.

22. Borushok MJ, White R, Oh KS, et al: Congenital subclavian steal. AJR 121:559–564, 1974.

23. Folger GM, Shah KD: Subclavian steal in patients with Blalock-Taussig anastomosis. Circulation 31:241–248, 1965.

24. Reivich M, Holling HE, Roberts B, et al: Reversal of blood flow through the vertebral artery and its effect on cerebral circulation. N Engl J Med 265:878–885, 1961.

25. Ashby RN, Karras BG, Cannon AH: Clinical and roentgenographic aspects of the subclavian steal syndrome. AJR 90:535–545, 1963.

26. Rosenburg JC, Spencer FC: Subclavian steal syndrome. Surgical treatment of three patients. Am Surg 31:307–312, 1965.

27. Coder DM, Frye RL, Bernatz PE, et al: Symptomatic bilateral "subclavian steal." Mayo Clin Proc 40:473–476, 1965.

28. Arevalo F, Katzen BT: Bilateral subclavian steal syndrome. AJR 127:668–669, 1976.

29. Skalpe IO, Semb GS: Congenital bilateral subclavian steal. Blood flow pattern. Scand J Thorac Cardiovasc Surg 4:153–158, 1970.

30. Bosniak MA: A collateral pathway through the vertebral arteries associated with obstruction of the innominate and proximal subclavian arteries. Radiology 81:89–95, 1963.

31. Blakemore WS, Hardesty WH, Bevilacqua JE, et al: Reversal of blood flow in the right vertebral artery accompanying occlusion of the innominate artery. Ann Surg 161:353–356, 1963.

32. Pratesi F, Capellini M, Macchini A, et al: The innominate steal. Vasc Dis 5:214–225, 1968.

33. Javid H, Julian OC, Dye WS, et al: Management of cerebral arterial insufficiency caused by reversal of flow. Arch Surg 90:634–643, 1965.

34. Mueller RL, Hinck VC: Thyrocervical steal. AJR 101:128–129, 1967.

35. Trevino RJ: Thyrocervical steal syndrome. Arch Otolaryngol 92:177–180, 1970.

36. Haimovici H: Peripheral arterial embolism: study of 330 unselected cases of embolism of extremities. Angiology 1:20–36, 1950.

37. Daley R, Hattingley TW, Holt CL, et al: Systemic arterial embolism in rheumatic heart disease. Am Heart J 42:566–581, 1951.

38. Savelyev VS, Zatevakhin II, Stepanov NV: Artery embolism of the upper limbs. Surgery 81:367–375, 1977.

39. Metzler M, Silver D: Vasospastic disorders. Postgrad Med 65:79–88, 1979.

40. Bergan JJ, Conn J Jr, Trippel OH: Severe ischemia of the hand. Ann Surg 173:301–307, 1971.

41. Juergens JL: Thromboangiitis obliterans (Buerger's disease, TAO). In Juergens JL, Spittell JA Jr, Fairbairn JF II (eds): Peripheral Vascular Diseases. Philadelphia, WB Saunders, 1980, pp. 469–491.

42. Gifford RW Jr, Hines EA Jr: Raynaud's disease among women and girls. Circulation 16:1012–1021, 1957.

43. Winters WL Jr, Joseph RR, Learner N: Primary pulmonary hypertension and Raynaud's phenomenon. Arch Intern Med 114:821–830, 1964.

44. Coffman JD: Diseases of the peripheral vessels. In Beeson PB, McDermott W, Wyngaarden JB (eds): Cecil Textbook of Medicine, 15th Ed. Philadelphia, WB Saunders, pp. 1299–1315, 1979.

45. Allen EV, Brown GE: Raynaud's disease: A critical review of minimal requisites for diagnosis. Am J Med Sci 183:187–200, 1932.

46. Porter JM, Snider RL, Bardana EJ, et al: The diagnosis and treatment of Raynaud's phenomenon. Surgery 77:11–23, 1975.

47. Rösch J, Porter JM: Hand angiography and Raynaud's syndrome. Fortschr Röntgenstr 127:30–37, 1977.

48. Higgins CB, Hayden WG: Palmar arteriography in acronecrosis. Radiology 119:85–90, 1976.

49. Kadir S, Athanasoulis CA: Peripheral vasospastic disorders: management with intraarterial infusions of vasodilatory drugs. In Athanasoulis CA, Pfister RC, Greene R, et al (eds): Interventional Radiology. Philadelphia, WB Saunders, 1982, pp 343–354.

50. Laws JW, Lillie JG, Scott JT: Arteriographic appearances in rheumatoid arthritis and other disorders. Br J Radiol 36:477–493, 1963.

51. Marshall TR: Radiographic changes in rheumatoid arthritis in the digits. Radiology 90:121–123, 1968.

52. Norton WL, Nardo JM: Vascular diseases in progressive systemic sclerosis (scleroderma). Ann Intern Med 73:317–324, 1970.

53. Oliver JA, Cannon PJ: Editorial. The kidney in scleroderma. Nephron 18:141–150, 1977.

54. Furey NL, Schmid FR, Kwaan HC, et al: Arterial thrombosis in scleroderma. Br J Dermatol 93:683–693, 1975.

55. Clinical Pathological Conference: Scleroderma (progressive systemic sclerosis). Am J Med 36:301–314, 1964.

56. Dabich L, Bookstein JJ, Zweifler A, et al: Digital arteries in patients with scleroderma. Arch Intern Med 130:708–714, 1972.

57. Schober R, Klüken N: Angiographische Befunde bei Sclerodermia progressiva. Fortschr Röntgenstr 105:239–244, 1966.

58. Ferrante FM, Myerson GE, Goldman JA: Subclavian artery thrombosis mimicking the aortic arch syndrome in systemic lupus erythematosus. Arthritis Rheumat 25:1501–1504, 1982.

59. Peck B, Hoffman GS, Franck WA: Thrombophlebitis in systemic lupus erythematosus. JAMA 240:1728–1730, 1978.

60. Crawford T: Blood and lymphatic vessels. In Anderson WAD, Kissane JM (eds): Pathology, 7th Ed. St. Louis, CV Mosby, 1977, pp. 879–927.

61. Goodman RM, Elian B, Mozes M, et al: Buerger's disease in Israel. Am J Med 39:601–615, 1965.

62. Szilagyi DE, Smith RF, Elliott JP, et al: Congenital arteriovenous anomalies of the limbs. Arch Surg 111:423–429, 1976.

63. Horton BT: Hemihypertrophy of the extremities associated with congenital arteriovenous fistula. JAMA 98:373–379, 1932.

64. Curtis RM: Congenital arteriovenous fistulae of the hand. J Bone Joint Surg 35A:917–928, 1953.

65. Neviaser RJ, Adams JP: Vascular lesions in the hand. Current management. Clin Orthop Res 100:111–119, 1974.

66. Seeger SJ: Congenital arteriovenous anastomoses. Surgery 3:264–305, 1938.

67. Malan E: History and different clinical aspects of arteriovenous communications. J Cardiovasc Surg 35:491–494, 1972.

68. Rienhoff WF Jr: Congenital arteriovenous fistula: an embryological study with report of a case. Bull Johns Hopkins Hosp 35:271–284, 1924.

69. Rich NM, Hobson RW II, Collins GJ Jr: Traumatic arteriovenous fistulas and false aneurysms: a review of 558 lesions. Surgery 78:817–828, 1975.

70. Szilagyi DE, Elliott JP, DeRusso FJ, et al: Peripheral congenital arteriovenous fistulas. Surgery 57:61–81, 1965.

71. Rainer WG, Vigor W, Newby JP: Surgical treatment of thoracic outlet compression. Am J Surg 116:704–707, 1968.

72. Adson AW, Coffey JR: Cervical rib: a method of anterior approach for relief of symptoms by division of the scalenus anticus. Ann Surg 85:839–857, 1927.

73. Teleford ED, Mottershead S: Pressure at the cervicobrachial junction. An operative study. J Bone Joint Surg 30B:249–265, 1948.

74. Lord JW Jr, Rosati LM: Neurovascular compression syndromes of the upper extremity. Ciba Clin Symp 10:35–62, 1958.

75. Gardner B, Hood RH Jr: Vascular compression at the shoulder girdle: analysis of normal subjects by means of radial pulse tracings. Ann Surg 153:23–33, 1961.

76. DeLaurentis DA, Wolferth CC Jr, Friedmann P: Thoracic outlet syndrome. Angiology 25:548–553, 1974.

77. van Echo DA, Sickles EA, Wiernik PH: Thoracic outlet syndrome, supraclavicular adenopathy, Hodgkin's disease. Ann Intern Med 78:608–609, 1973.

78. Roos DB, Owens JC: Thoracic outlet syndrome. Arch Surg 93:71–74, 1966.

79. Beyer JA, Wright IS: The hyperabduction syndrome: with special reference to its relationship to Raynaud's syndrome. Circulation 4:161–172, 1951.

80. Adams JT, DeWeese JA, Mahoney EB, et al: Intermittent subclavian vein obstruction without thrombosis. Surgery 63:147–165, 1968.

81. Lord JW, Stone PW: Pectoralis minor tenotomy and anterior scalenotomy with special reference to the hyperabduction syndrome and "effort thrombosis" of the subclavian vein. Circulation 13:537–542, 1956.

82. Mathes SJ, Salam AA: Subclavian artery aneurysm: sequela of thoracic outlet syndrome. Surgery 76:506–510, 1974.

83. Judy KL, Heymann RL: Vascular complications of thoracic outlet syndrome. Am J Surg 123:521–531, 1972.

84. Enge I, Aakhus T, Evensen A: Angiography in vascular injuries of the extremities. Acta Radiol Diag 16:193–199, 1975.

85. Morris GC Jr, Beall AC Jr, Roof WR, et al: Surgical experience with 220 acute arterial injuries in civilian practice. Am J Surg 99:775–781, 1960.

86. Bassett FH, III, Silver D: Arterial injury associated with fractures. Arch Surg 92:13–19, 1966.

87. Linscheid RL, Wheeler DK: Elbow dislocations. JAMA 194:1171–1176, 1965.

88. Spear HC, Janes JM: Rupture of the brachial artery accompanying dislocation of the elbow or supracondylar fracture. J Bone Joint Surg 33A:889–894, 1951.

89. Powers TA, Harolds JA, Kadir S, et al: Pseudoaneurysm of the profunda femoris artery diagnosed on angiographic phase of bone scan. Clin Nucl Med 10:422–424, 1979.

90. Saletta JD, Freearck RJ: Occult vascular injuries of the extremities. J Occup Med 12:304–307, 1970.

91. McDonald EJ Jr, Goodman PC, Winestock DP: The clinical indications for arteriography in trauma to the extremity. A review of 114 cases. Radiology 116:45–47, 1975.

92. Spencer AD: The reliability of signs of peripheral vascular injury. Surg Gynecol Obstet 114:490–494, 1962.

93. Matloff DB, Morton JH: Acute trauma to the subclavian arteries. Am J Surg 115:675–680, 1968.

94. Gryska PF: Major vascular injuries. Principles of management in selected cases of arterial and venous injury. N Engl J Med 266:381–385, 1962.

95. Shuck JM, Omer GE, Lewis CE Jr: Arterial obstruction due to intimal disruption in extremity fractures. J Trauma 12:481–489, 1972.

96. Chiavacci WE, Bucciarelli RL, Victorica BE: Aneurysm of the subclavian artery: a complication of retrograde brachial catheterization. Cath Cardiovasc Diag 2:93–96, 1976.

97. Louis DS, Simon MA: Traumatic false aneurysms of the upper extremity. A diagnostic problem. J Bone Joint Surg 56A:176–179, 1974.

98. Narsete EM: Traumatic aneurysm of the radial artery. A report of three cases. Am J Surg 108:424–427, 1964.

99. Conn J Jr, Bergan JJ, Bell JL: Hypothenar hammer syndrome: Posttraumatic digital ischemia. Surgery 68:1122–1128, 1970.

100. Latshaw RF, Weidner WA: Ulnar artery aneurysms: angiographic considerations in 2 cases. AJR 131:1093–1095, 1978.

101. Benedict KT Jr, Chang W, McCready FJ: The hypothenar hammer syndrome. Radiology 111:57–60, 1974.

# Arteriography of the Abdominal Aorta and Pelvis

## ANATOMY

The abdominal aorta extends from the diaphragmatic hiatus (T12–L1 intervertebral disc space) to the aortic bifurcation (around L4). In the young adult, the abdominal aorta follows a relatively straight course (Fig. 10–1). In older individuals, there is often some tortuosity and axial rotation that may displace the orifices of the aortic branches (Fig. 10–2).

The abdominal aorta lies anterior to the upper four lumbar vertebral bodies and slightly to the left of the midline. The pancreas and the splenic vein lie anterior to the aorta at the level of the superior mesenteric artery origin. Below this, the left renal vein crosses the aorta anteriorly. Further distally, the third portion of the duodenum lies anterior to the aorta. Posteriorly, the second to fourth lumbar veins cross the aorta. On the right side, the inferior vena cava lies adjacent to the aorta between L2 and L4.

### Branches of the Aorta

Aortic branches can be divided into four groups:[1]

1. Dorsal or body wall: lumbar and median sacral arteries.

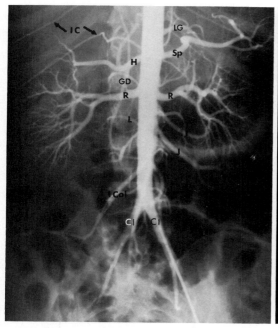
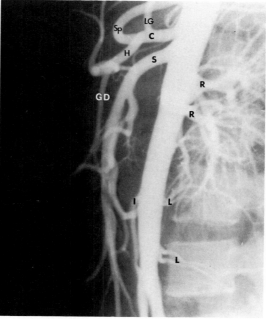

**Figure 10–1.** Normal AP (*left*) and LAT (*right*) abdominal aortogram in a young person. C = celiac; CI = common iliac; GD = gastroduodenal; H = hepatic; I = inferior mesenteric; IC = intercostal; I Col = ileocolic; J = jejunal; L = lumbar; LG = left gastric; R = renal; S = superior mesenteric; Sp = splenic arteries.

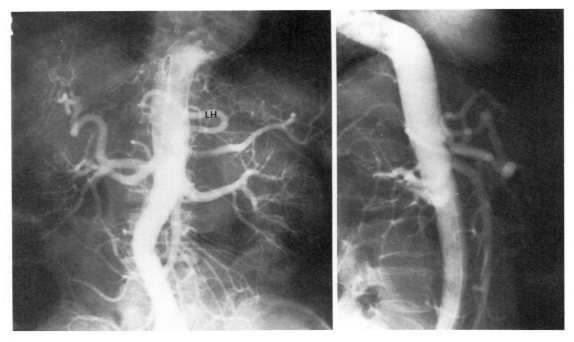

*Figure 10–2.* Normal AP (*left*) and LAT (*right*), abdominal aortogram in an older person showing tortuosity of the aorta. A large left hepatic artery (LH) is seen originating from the left gastric–left hepatic trunk off the celiac artery. The right hepatic artery is a branch of the SMA.

2. Ventral or mesenteric: celiac, superior, and inferior mesenteric arteries.

3. Lateral: phrenic, adrenal, renal, and gonadal arteries.

4. Terminal: common iliac arteries.

### Dorsal Branches

LUMBAR ARTERIES. There are usually four pairs of lumbar arteries. The lowest lumbar segment receives its vascular supply from paired lumbar branches arising off the median sacral artery or more frequently from branches of the iliolumbar arteries. Dorsal branches from the lumbar arteries provide the arterial supply to the spinal canal. The first lumbar artery gives off branches to the conus of the spinal cord. The lumbar arteries serve as important collaterals in occlusive diseases of the distal aorta and iliac arteries by means of their anastomoses with the intercostal, subcostal, iliolumbar, inferior epigastric, and deep iliac circumflex arteries.

MEDIAN SACRAL ARTERY. This is a small, inconstant branch of the terminal aorta. It arises from the dorsal surface of the aorta just proximal to the bifurcation and courses inferiorly along the ventral surface of the lumbosacral spine, terminating at the coccyx. It gives off small branches to the rectum and serves as a collateral in occlusive diseases of the aorta and iliac arteries.

**Ventral Branches.** The ventral branches are the celiac, superior, and inferior mesenteric arteries. Detailed discussion of the arterial anatomy and the anatomical variations follows in Chapter 14.

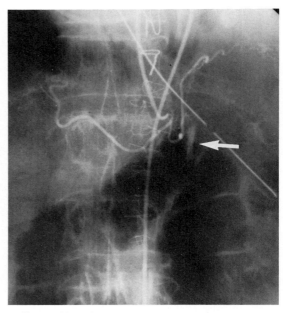

*Figure 10–3.* Common inferior phrenic trunk arising from the aorta. A normal left adrenal blush is seen (*arrow*).

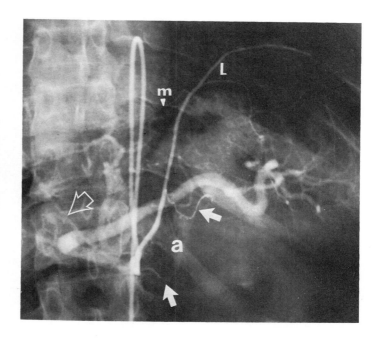

*Figure 10–4.* Left inferior phrenic artery arising from the proximal celiac artery. There are several superior adrenal branches (*arrows*). a = adrenal gland; L = lateral branch; m = medial branch of the inferior phrenic artery. Open arrow points to the right inferior phrenic artery, which arises separately from the celiac artery.

## Lateral Branches

INFERIOR PHRENIC ARTERIES. The paired inferior phrenic arteries may arise separately, but more frequently they originate as a common trunk from the ventral surface of the abdominal aorta above the celiac artery origin (Fig. 10–3). Occasionally, this trunk is a branch of the proximal celiac artery. Rarely, the inferior phrenic arteries arise separately from the aorta or the celiac or renal arteries (Fig. 10–4).

Branches of the phrenic arteries are the:

1. Diaphragmatic branches, which anastomose with the intercostal, musculophrenic, and pericardiophrenic arteries and may thus serve as collaterals in occlusive diseases of the aorta and celiac artery.

2. The left inferior phrenic artery provides branches to the distal esophagus.

3. Superior adrenal arteries.

4. Hepatic branches, which serve as collaterals in occlusion of the hepatic artery.[1]

MIDDLE ADRENAL ARTERIES. These are usually small, paired arteries arising from the lateral aortic wall at the level of the superior mesenteric artery. These vessels are infrequently visualized on abdominal aortography unless enlarged, as a result of adrenal or renal disease, or when serving as a collateral in occlusive diseases of the renal arteries.

RENAL ARTERIES. These are the largest lateral branches of the abdominal aorta. They arise from the lateral wall of the aorta, just below the origin of the superior mesenteric

artery, usually at the level of the second lumbar vertebra. Details of renal artery anatomy and its variations are discussed in Chapter 16.

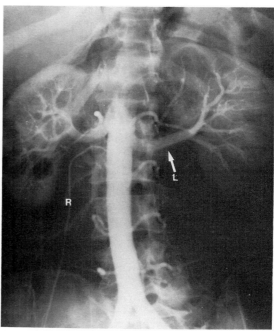

*Figure 10–5.* Normal infrarenal abdominal aortogram in a male patient showing the gonadal arteries. L = left testicular artery, which arises from the left renal artery; R = right testicular artery, which arises from the aorta. Note laterally oriented course of the right testicular artery toward the internal inguinal ring.

GONADAL ARTERIES. The paired testicular and ovarian arteries arise from the anterolateral surface of the infrarenal aorta at L2–L3 and rarely from the proximal renal artery (Fig. 10–5). The testicular artery courses inferolaterally and enters the inguinal canal. In the pelvis, the ovarian arteries follow the suspensory ligament of the ovary. Testicular arteriography is occasionally used to evaluate maldescended testes.[2]

**Terminal Branches.** At the level of the fourth lumbar vertebra, the aorta bifurcates into the left and right common iliac arteries. The left common iliac artery is usually shorter than the right. In young individuals, the iliac arteries are relatively straight; in older individuals, they are often tortuous (Fig. 10–6). The common iliac arteries do not give off any branches, except for a rare individual in whom an accessory renal artery may arise from a common iliac artery. The common iliac arteries divide into the external and internal iliac arteries at the level of the first sacral vertebra.

EXTERNAL ILIAC ARTERY. The external iliac artery is larger than the internal iliac artery except in the fetus, in whom the internal iliac

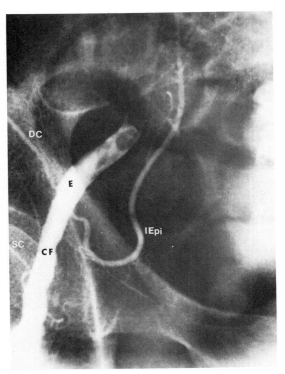

*Figure 10–7.* External iliac arteriogram. CF = common femoral; DC = deep iliac circumflex; IEpi = inferior epigastric; SC = superficial iliac circumflex arteries.

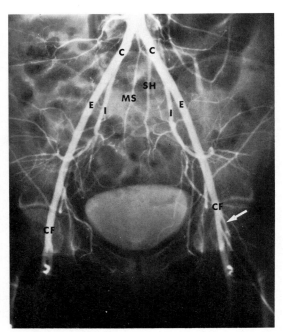

*Figure 10–6.* Normal AP pelvic arteriogram in a young person. C = common iliac; CF = common femoral; E = external iliac; I = internal iliac; MS = middle sacral; SH = superior hemorrhoidal branch of the inferior mesenteric arteries. There is an early bifurcation of the left common femoral artery. The arrow points to the profunda femoris artery.

arteries give rise to the umbilical arteries. Its branches form an important collateral route in distal aorto-iliac occlusive diseases.

*Inferior epigastric artery*: This vessel originates from the medial aspect of the external iliac artery just above the inguinal ligament and ascends into the anterior abdominal wall (Fig. 10–7). Its branches anastomose with those of the superior epigastric, lower intercostal, and obturator arteries.

*Deep iliac circumflex artery*: This artery arises from the lateral aspect of the distal external iliac artery, at the same level as the inferior epigastric artery. It courses laterally towards the anterior/superior iliac spine. Its branches anastomose with the lumbar, ascending branch of the lateral femoral circumflex, iliolumbar, and superior gluteal arteries.

INTERNAL ILIAC ARTERY. The internal iliac artery arises at an acute angle posteromedially from the common iliac artery. It is usually between 2 and 5 cm in length. From its origin, it courses inferomedially, lying anterior to the sacrum (Fig. 10–8). The branches can be divided into anterior and posterior groups (trunks). Infrequently, the internal

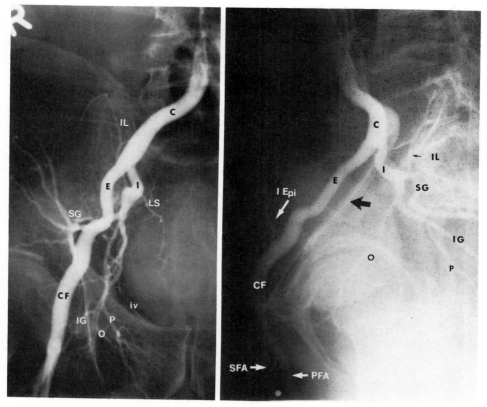

*Figure 10–8.* Normal AP and LAT common iliac arteriogram showing the pelvic branches. C = common iliac; CF = common femoral; E = external iliac; I = internal iliac; I Epi = inferior epigastric; IG = inferior gluteal; iv = inferior vesical; IL = iliolumbar; O = obturator; P = pudenal; PFA = profunda femoris; SFA = superficial femoral; SG = superior gluteal arteries. Arrow points to the arterial catheter in the contralateral iliac artery.

iliac artery divides into several branches, without forming a trunk, resulting in a large number of variations:

*Anterior branches:*

1. Superior and inferior vesical arteries: The former represents the proximal portion of the umbilical artery. Occasionally, a segment of the umbilical artery may remain patent.[3] The course of the vesical arteries varies with the fullness of the urinary bladder.

2. Middle hemorrhoidal artery: This vessel often arises together with the inferior vesical artery. It anastomoses with the superior hemorrhoidal artery from the inferior mesenteric artery and the inferior hemorrhoidal artery.

3. Obturator artery: This vessel is present as an independent branch in 70 to 80% of individuals.[1] In the remainder of individuals, it arises from the inferior epigastric artery. Its branches anastomose with those of the inferior epigastric and medial femoral circumflex arteries.

4. Internal pudendal artery: This vessel supplies the external genitalia (dorsal and deep arteries of the penis) and gives off the inferior hemorrhoidal artery. Its branches anastomose with those of the ipsi- and contralateral internal iliac arteries.

5. Inferior gluteal artery: This artery forms a lateral concave arc as it exits from the pelvis via the greater sciatic foramen. Often it arises as a common trunk with the internal pudendal artery or may arise from the superior gluteal artery in less than 30% of individuals.[3] Its branches anastomose with the medial and lateral femoral circumflex arteries. The inferior gluteal artery provides branches to the sciatic nerve.

6. Uterine and prostatic arteries and branches to the ductus deferens and seminal vesicles.

7. Persistent sciatic artery (see Fig. 11–5, Chapter 11): This is an enlarged inferior gluteal artery that represents a persistence of the embryonic vascular supply to the lower extremities. It is observed in 0.14% of indi-

viduals undergoing arteriography of the lower extremities and may occur as a unilateral or bilateral abnormality with equal frequency.[4, 5] It may be associated with absence of the profunda or superficial femoral arteries and can also be affected by disease.[6, 7] A lateral pelvic arteriogram is required to demonstrate the posterior location of this vessel, which corresponds to the position of the inferior gluteal artery.

*Posterior branches*:

1. Iliolumbar artery: This vessel lies anterior to the sacroiliac joint.

2. Lateral sacral arteries: The number of these arteries may vary between two and four. Similarly, there is significant variation in the origin of these vessels. Most frequently, two vessels are present, the superior and inferior lateral sacral arteries, arising either independently or as a common trunk. Their branches anastomose with the median sacral, contralateral lateral sacral, and superior gluteal arteries (see Fig. 10–10).

3. Superior gluteal artery: This is the largest branch of the internal iliac artery. It follows a craniad and posterior concave course

through the greater sciatic foramen into the gluteal region.

A detailed description of the arteriographic anatomy of the pelvis is provided in reference 3.

## Collateral Circulation to the Lower Extremities in Aorto-iliac Stenosis and Occlusion

**Occlusion of the Distal Aorta and Proximal Iliac Arteries** (Fig. 10–9; see also Fig. 10–19)

1. Internal mammary arteries → superior epigastric arteries → inferior epigastric arteries → external iliac arteries.

2. Superior mesenteric artery → inferior mesenteric artery → superior hemorrhoidal artery → middle and inferior hemorrhoidal arteries → internal iliac arteries → external iliac arteries.

3. Intercostal, subcostal, and lumbar arteries → superior gluteal and iliolumbar arteries → internal iliac arteries → external iliac arteries.

4. Intercostal, subcostal, and lumbar arter-

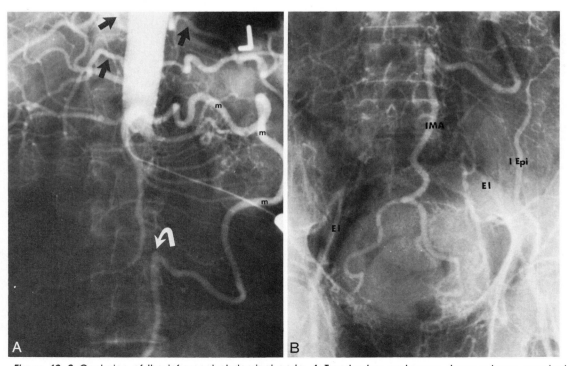

*Figure 10–9.* Occlusion of the infrarenal abdominal aorta. *A,* Translumbar aortogram shows a large marginal artery (m), which reconstitutes the inferior mesenteric artery (*curved arrow*). Enlarged inter- and subcostal arteries, which serve as collaterals, are also seen (*straight arrows*). *B,* Later frame from the same arteriogram shows reconstitution of the external iliac arteries bilaterally (EI) via numerous retroperitoneal collaterals, the inferior mesenteric artery (IMA), and the left inferior epigastric artery (I Epi).

ies → deep iliac circumflex arteries → external iliac arteries.

### Unilateral Common Iliac Artery Occlusion
(Fig. 10–10; see also Fig. 10–31)

1. Internal iliac artery → lateral sacral arteries → contralateral internal iliac artery → external iliac artery.

2. Intercostal, subcostal, and lumbar arteries → iliolumbar artery → internal iliac artery → external iliac artery.

3. External pudendal artery → contralateral external pudendal artery.

4. Internal iliac artery → obturator, superior, and inferior gluteal arteries → femoral circumflex arteries → profunda femoris artery.

5. Intercostal, subcostal, and lumbar arteries → superficial iliac circumflex and lateral femoral circumflex arteries → common and profunda femoris arteries.

6. Abdominal aorta → testicular artery → internal iliac branches, external iliac, and femoral arteries.[8]

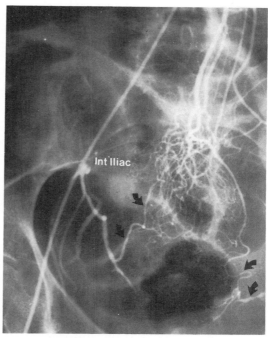

**Figure 10–11.** Superior to middle hemorrhoidal artery communications are demonstrated on an inferior mesenteric arteriogram (*arrows*).

### Unilateral Internal Iliac Artery Occlusion
(Fig. 10–11)

1. Inferior epigastric artery → obturator artery → internal iliac artery branches.

2. Inferior mesenteric artery → superior hemorrhoidal artery → middle hemorrhoidal artery → internal iliac artery branches.

3. Intercostal and lumbar arteries → iliolumbar artery.

4. Abdominal aorta → ovarian arteries → internal iliac artery branches.[9]

5. Profunda femoris artery → femoral circumflex arteries → obturator, superior, and inferior gluteal arteries → internal iliac artery branches.

6. External pudendal artery → internal pudendal artery.

7. Aorta → median sacral artery → lateral sacral arteries.

## ARTERIOGRAPHY

### Abdominal Aorta (Tables 10–1 and 10–2)

Abdominal aortography can be performed via the femoral, translumbar, or axillary approach. From the femoral approach a 60 cm thin-walled 5 or 6 Fr multiple hole pigtail catheter is inserted. From the axillary ap-

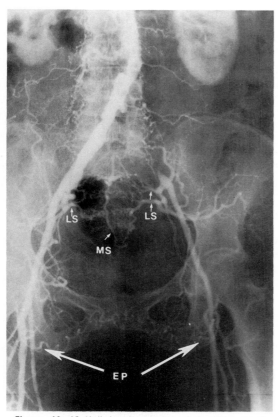

**Figure 10–10.** Unilateral common iliac artery occlusion. There is reconstruction of the external iliac artery distal to the occlusion via retroperitoneal, transsacral, and pudendal collaterals. EP = external pudendal; LS = lateral sacral; MS = middle sacral arteries.

**TABLE 10–1.** Abdominal Aortogram, Femoral or Axillary Approach

| | |
|---|---|
| Catheter:<br>    Position | 5 or 6 Fr pigtail<br>T12–L1 |
| Guide wire | 0.035 inch J |
| Contrast medium | 76% diatrizoate meglumine<br>    sodium* |
| Injection rate/volume | 20 ml/sec, total 40 ml |
| Films:<br>    Filming rate<br><br>    Projections | AP—11; lateral—9<br>2 films per second for 6 films<br>1 film per second for the rest<br>Biplane (AP and lateral, alternating exposures) |

*20% concentration for DSA.

proach an 80 or 100 cm 5 or 6 Fr pigtail catheter is used. The catheter is placed at T12–L1. From the translumbar approach the catheter is directed craniad from either a low (L2) or a high (T12) aortic puncture.

Complete evaluation of the abdominal aorta necessitates a biplane aortogram. The importance of the lateral aortogram should not be disregarded, since it provides information not available from the frontal projection alone. For example, significant atheromatous plaques or stenoses may not be appreciated unless viewed in profile. The lateral aortogram serves to:

1. Evaluate the posterior aortic wall for atheromatous disease or a mural thrombus. The latter may be a source for peripheral emboli.

2. Evaluate the orifices of the celiac, superior, and inferior mesenteric arteries for stenoses.

**TABLE 10–2.** Abdominal Aortogram, Translumbar Approach

| | |
|---|---|
| Catheter:<br>    Position | TLA needle/sheath<br>Sheath tip pointing upstream |
| Guide wire | 0.035 inch 3 mm J torque<br>    wire |
| Contrast medium | 76% diatrizoate meglumine<br>    sodium* |
| Injection rate/volume | 15 ml/sec, total 45 ml |
| Films:<br>    Filming rate<br><br>    Projections | PA—11; lateral—9<br>2 films per second for 6 films<br>1 film per second for the rest<br>Biplane (AP and lateral, alternating exposure) |

*20% concentration for DSA.

3. Search for the anterior "nipple" in patients with an aorto-enteric fistula.[10]

4. Detect anterior displacement of the aorta by retroperitoneal masses or hematoma.

## Selective Arteriography

**Inferior Phrenic Arteriogram** (Table 10–3; see also Figs. 10–3 and 10–4). The initial search for the inferior phrenic arteries should begin in the aorta with either a cobra C2 or a sidewinder catheter. The choice of sidewinder catheter, ie, Type I or II, should be determined on an individual basis. In patients with narrow vessels, the sidewinder I is used.

Inferior phrenic arteries arising from the aorta can be catheterized with a cobra C2, a cobra in loop configuration, or a sidewinder catheter. The last two catheter configurations provide a more stable catheter position. For inferior phrenic arteries arising from the celiac artery, the cobra in loop configuration or sidewinder catheter is used. If the loop technique is used, the loop should be formed in either the splenic or the hepatic artery (see Chapter 3). Once the loop is formed, the catheter tip is brought into the celiac artery in order to search for the inferior phrenic artery orifice. If the sidewinder catheter is used, after catheterization of the celiac artery, the catheter is slowly withdrawn at the groin while injecting small amounts of contrast medium. As the catheter is withdrawn, the tip is deflected upward and will seek out the inferior phrenic artery.

On test injection, the inferior phrenic artery can be differentiated from the left gastric artery by the former's course towards the diaphragm. In addition, injection of contrast medium into the phrenic arteries is associated with pain.

**TABLE 10–3.** Inferior Phrenic Arteriogram

| | |
|---|---|
| Catheter: | 5 or 6 Fr: cobra C2, sidewinder |
| Guide wire | 0.035 inch J |
| Contrast medium | 60% diatrizoate meglumine sodium* |
| Injection rate/volume | Hand injection (2–3 ml/sec, total 4–6 ml) |
| Films:<br>    Filming rate<br>    Projection | 8<br>1 film per second<br>AP |

*20% concentration for DSA.

### TABLE 10–4. Lumbar Arteriogram

| | |
|---|---|
| Catheter: | 5 or 6 Fr: cobra C2, sidewinder |
| Guide wire | 0.035 inch J |
| Contrast medium | 60% diatrizoate meglumine sodium* |
| Injection rate/volume | Hand injection (2 ml/sec, total 4–6 ml) |
| Films: | 8 |
| Filming rate | 1 film per second |
| Projection | AP |

*20% concentration for DSA.

### TABLE 10–5. Pelvic Arteriogram

| | |
|---|---|
| Catheter: | 5 or 6 Fr pigtail (transfemoral): translumbar |
| Position | 2–3 cm above aortic bifurcation |
| Guide wire | 0.035 inch J |
| Contrast medium* | 76% diatrizoate meglumine sodium† |
| Injection rate/volume | 8–10 ml/sec, total 30 ml |
| Films: | Biplane: AP—10; lateral 10; single plane: 10 films |
| Filming rate | 2 film per second for 6 films |
| | 1 film per second for 4 films |
| Projections | 1. AP |
| | 2. Biplane oblique (hip elevated 45°) |
| | *or* |
| | 3. LAO, RAO |

*Add 2 mg of lidocaine per ml of contrast medium.
†20% concentration for DSA.
*Note:* In patients with distal aortic and proximal iliac artery occlusion and individuals with slow blood flow, films are obtained at 1 film per second.

**Lumbar Arteriogram** (Table 10–4). For catheterization of the lumbar arteries, a cobra C2 or a sidewinder catheter is used. On arteriography, the lumbar arteries can be recognized by their characteristic appearance as they course posteriorly over the lumbar vertebral bodies (see Figs. 10–1 and 10–5).

**Pelvic Arteriogram** (Table 10–5). Arteriography of the pelvis utilizing a single plane (AP) technique provides sufficient information for the evaluation of patients with abdominal aortic and iliac artery aneurysms or pelvic trauma. However, in atherosclerotic occlusive disease, the single plane (AP) pelvic arteriogram offers incomplete and often misleading information (Fig. 10–12). Since significant atherosclerotic plaques may be lo-

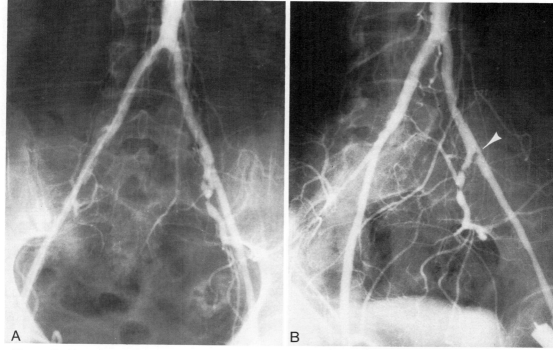

A          B

*Figure 10–12.* Importance of oblique pelvic arteriography for the evaluation of atherosclerotic occlusive disease of the pelvic arteries. *A,* AP pelvic arteriogram in a patient with left leg claudication. The proximal left internal and external iliac arteries are superimposed. *B,* LPO pelvic arteriogram shows a severe stenosis of the proximal left external iliac artery (*arrowhead*). A significant pressure gradient was measured across this lesion.

cated posteriorly, oblique arteriography of the pelvic vessels is essential.

Biplane pelvic arteriography (AP and horizontal beam) offers the most information while utilizing a single contrast injection. Alternatively, left and right anterior oblique projections (45°) may be used. For biplane pelvic arteriography, the hip on the more symptomatic side is elevated by approximately 45°. The pigtail catheter is placed approximately 2 to 3 cm above the aortic bifurcation so that the side holes lie in the distal aorta.

Filming and the volume and rate of contrast medium injected are determined by evaluating the blood flow with a hand test injection of 5 to 10 ml of diluted contrast medium. In young patients, in whom blood flow is fast, a rapid filming technique is necessary. In older individuals, in whom blood flow is slower and occlusive disease is present, films are obtained at one film/sec.

Evaluation of the internal iliac arteries can be of importance in occlusive diseases of the external iliac and common femoral arteries, pelvic trauma, and neoplasms. The proximal

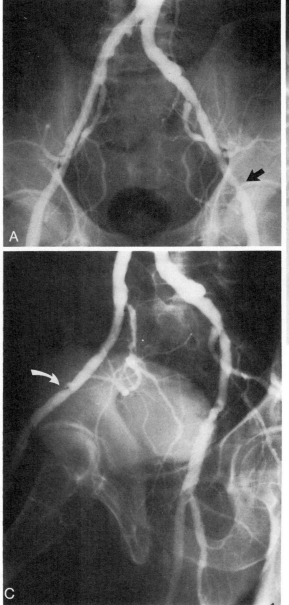

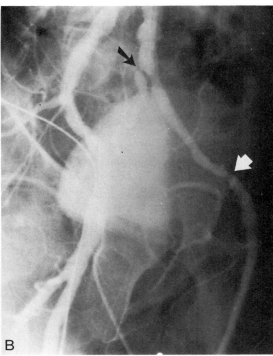

*Figure 10–13.* Importance of oblique pelvic arteriography for the evaluation of atherosclerotic occlusive disease of the pelvic arteries. *A,* The severity of the external iliac artery stenosis (*arrow*) is not apparent on the AP pelvic arteriogram. *B,* The steep LPO pelvic arteriogram shows a tight left internal iliac artery stenosis (*black arrow*) and a significant external iliac artery stenosis with a prominent posterior plaque (*white arrow*). *C,* The RPO projection shows an ulcerated right external iliac artery plaque (*arrow*).

**TABLE 10–6.** Common Iliac Arteriogram
(Contralateral Femoral Approach)

| Catheter: | 5 or 6 Fr: single curve, cobra C1, sidewinder I |
|---|---|
| Position | Proximal common iliac artery |
| Guide wire | 0.035 inch J |
| Contrast medium* | 76% diatrizoate meglumine sodium† |
| Injection rate/volume | 8 ml/sec, total 20 ml |
| Films: | 8 |
| Filming rate | 2 films per second for 6 films<br>1 film per second for 2 films |
| Projections | 1. AP<br>2. LAO, RAO |

*Add 2 mg of lidocaine per ml of contrast medium.
†20% concentration for DSA.

internal iliac artery is best demonstrated on an oblique pelvic arteriogram with the contralateral hip elevated by 45° (Fig. 10–13).

**Common and External Iliac Arteriogram** (Tables 10–6 and 10–7)

ANTEGRADE APPROACH. From the contralateral femoral artery, a 5 or 6 Fr catheter (single curve, cobra, cobra in loop configuration, or sidewinder) is placed in the proximal common iliac artery. When using the cobra in the loop configuration or the sidewinder catheter, an LLT J guide wire is used to lead the catheter into the iliac artery, to prevent it from hooking onto plaques.

RETROGRADE APPROACH. Although several techniques can be used for retrograde iliac

**TABLE 10–7.** External Iliac Arteriogram

| Catheter:* | Contralateral femoral: 5 or 6 Fr cobra C1 or cobra in loop configuration<br>Ipsilateral femoral: 5 Fr straight or Amplatz sheath |
|---|---|
| Position | Proximal external iliac artery |
| Guide wire | 0.035 inch J |
| Contrast medium† | 76% diatrizoate meglumine sodium‡ |
| Injection rate/volume | 6 ml/sec, total 15 ml |
| Films: | 8 |
| Filming rate | 2 films per second for 6 films<br>1 film per second for 2 films |
| Projections | 1. AP<br>2. LAO, RAO |

*Catheter with side ports should be used to prevent intimal trauma from the end hole jet.
†Add 2 mg of lidocaine per ml of contrast medium.
‡20% concentration for DSA.

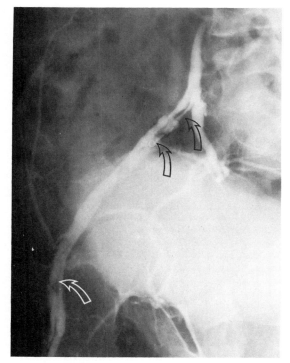

*Figure 10–14.* Arterial dissection (*arrows*) resulting from retrograde contrast injection through a short Teflon sheath placed in the external iliac artery. *Note:* Contrast material should not be injected at a high flow rate through short, single hole (end hole only) catheters placed in tortuous or atherosclerotic arteries.

arteriography from the ipsilateral femoral approach, the antegrade arteriogram provides the best results.

1. A multiple hole straight catheter (5 or 6 Fr) is placed in the mid-common iliac artery from the ipsilateral groin.

2. A short Teflon sheath is placed in the external iliac artery. The patient is asked to perform a Valsalva maneuver for 10 to 15 seconds. As this maneuver is terminated, contrast medium is injected at a rate of 15 ml/sec for a total of 30 ml. Whereas this technique provides satisfactory arteriograms, it may not be entirely safe in patients with severe atherosclerosis (Fig. 10–14).

The availability of special guide wires and alternative methods for evaluating the iliac arteries (eg, translumbar, axillary, or intravenous DSA) makes this approach unnecessary.

**Internal Iliac Arteriogram** (Table 10–8). Since the internal iliac artery arises posteromedially, placing the patient in a posterior oblique projection (eg, right posterior oblique for the right internal iliac artery) facilitates catheterization.

**TABLE 10–8.** Internal Iliac Arteriogram

| Catheter: | 5 or 6 Fr: cobra, cobra in loop configuration, sidewinder (ipsilateral femoral) |
|---|---|
| Guide wire | 0.035 inch J or straight LLT |
| Contrast medium* | 76% diatrizoate meglumine sodium† |
| Injection rate/volume | 4–6 ml/sec, total 15 ml |
| Films: | 8 |
|    Filming rate | 1 film per second for 8 films |
|    Projections | AP |
| | (Obliques) |

*Add 2 mg of lidocaine per ml of contrast medium.
†20% concentration for DSA.

IPSILATERAL APPROACH. A 5 or 6 Fr cobra C1 or C2 catheter can occasionally be advanced into the ipsilateral internal iliac artery. Alternatively, the loop technique or a sidewinder catheter is used. After formation of the loop with a cobra catheter or reforming the sidewinder curve, an LLT J guide wire is advanced past the catheter tip for a distance of 2 to 3 cm. The catheter tip is turned towards the ipsilateral iliac artery, and with the J tip leading, the catheter and wire are withdrawn at the groin as a unit. As the J enters the ipsilateral common iliac artery, the catheter is torqued to point the tip posteromedially. With this maneuver, the catheter tip can be brought into or close to the internal iliac artery orifice. The guide wire is removed, and with the aid of small contrast injections, the catheter tip is torqued into the desired position.

CONTRALATERAL APPROACH. A 5 or 6 Fr single curve or cobra catheter is placed across the aortic bifurcation. A J guide wire is advanced into the distal iliac artery. Often the wire enters the internal iliac artery and the catheter can be threaded over it. If the wire enters the external iliac artery, the catheter is advanced to the iliac artery bifurcation. The wire is removed, and a contrast injection is used to locate the internal iliac artery orifice. At this point the catheter can usually be advanced into this vessel. Alternatively, a straight LLT wire is inserted into an internal iliac artery branch, and the catheter is threaded over it.

INTERNAL ILIAC ARTERY BRANCHES (Table 10–9). Once the catheter tip is in the internal iliac artery, a straight or 15 mm LLT J guide wire is directed into the desired branch by torquing the catheter. For selective catheterization of branch vessels, either a cobra catheter is used or this can be exchanged for a headhunter (H1H) catheter. With either the cobra or the headhunter catheter, the loop technique can be used to direct the catheter tip (Fig. 10–15).

## ATHEROSCLEROSIS AND OCCLUSIVE DISEASES

### Pathology

The earliest lesion of atherosclerosis is smooth muscle proliferation, which occurs in the intima at areas of hemodynamic stress such as vascular bifurcations.[11] Subsequently, there is extracellular deposition of collagen and lipids and intimal fibrosis leading to the "fibrous plaque." Degeneration of the elastic elements leads to weakening of the arterial wall, resulting in ectasia. The development of a "complicated plaque" results from ulceration, calcification, or superimposed thrombosis.

Cigarette smoking accelerates the manifestations of atherosclerosis.[12] Hypertension, which is seen in 25% of the patients with aorto-iliac atherosclerosis, may influence the course of the disease.[13] Renovascular hypertension may also develop as a consequence of atherosclerotic renal artery stenosis.

The most common manifestations of atherosclerosis are plaque formation and arterial stenosis. Less frequently, the degenerative process may lead to arterial ectasia involving the aorta and iliac arteries and lower extremity vessels. Abdominal aortic atherosclero-

**TABLE 10–9.** Arteriogram of Internal Iliac Artery Branches

| Catheter: | 5 or 6 Fr cobra, cobra in loop configuration (headhunter H1H) |
|---|---|
| Guide wire | 0.035 inch J or straight LLT |
| Contrast medium* | 76% diatrizoate meglumine sodium† |
| Injection rate/volume | 3–5 ml/sec, total 6–10 ml |
| Films: | 8 |
|    Filming rate | 1 film per second |
|    Projections | AP |
| | (Obliques) |

*Add 2 mg of lidocaine per ml of contrast medium.
†20% concentration for DSA.

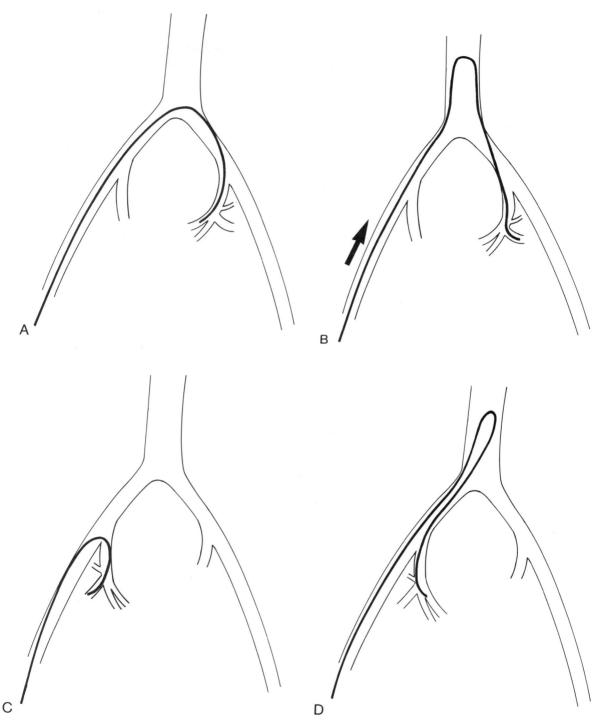

*Figure 10–15.* Technique for catheterization of internal iliac artery branches. *A,* A single or multiple curve catheter placed from the opposite groin tends to seek out the medially directed branches of the internal iliac artery. *B,* For catheterization of the lateral branches from the contralateral approach, a catheter loop is formed. *C,* From the ipsilateral approach, a single or multiple curve catheter seeks out the lateral branches of the internal iliac artery. *D,* For catheterization of the medial branches from the ipsilateral approach, a catheter loop is formed.

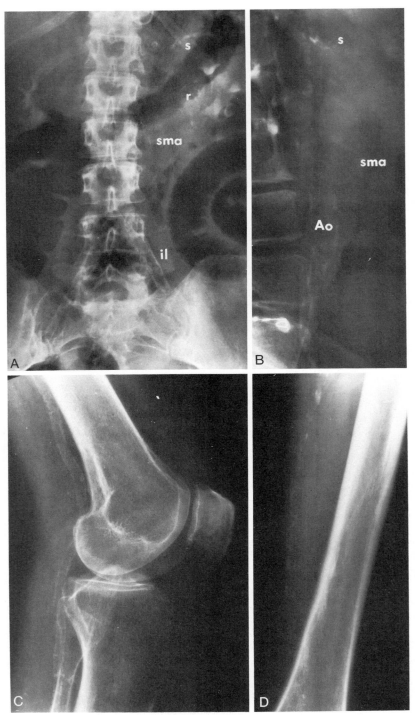

*Figure 10–16.* Vascular calcification. *A* and *B*, Diffuse, coarse vascular calcification associated with occlusive vascular disease. Ao = aorta; il = iliac; r = renal; s = splenic; sma = superior mesenteric arteries. *C*, Medial calcification, Möncheberg type. *D*, Patchy intimal calcification.

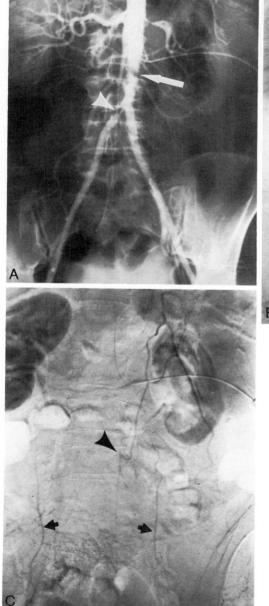

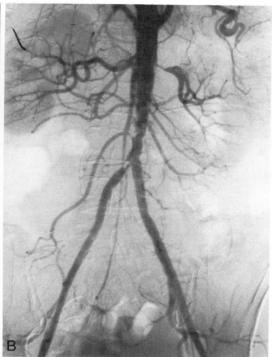

**Figure 10–17.** Moderate atherosclerosis of the aorta and branches. Value of film subtraction. *A,* An AP translumbar aortogram shows focal atherosclerosis of the infrarenal aorta (*arrow*) and severe left renal artery stenosis. A stenosis of the proximal right common iliac artery is also present (*arrowhead*). *B,* Subtraction film from the same aortogram shows the severity of the common iliac artery stenosis. In addition, there is mild stenosis of the right renal artery. The inferior mesenteric artery is occluded. *C,* Subtraction of a later film shows reconstitution of the inferior mesenteric artery (*arrowhead*). Both inferior epigastric arteries are also opacified (*arrows*).

sis may involve the orifices of the aortic branches. In such cases the disease is located in the aortic wall with extension into the proximal segments of the involved vessels. Such stenoses can be eccentric or concentric and circumferential.

## Clinical Aspects

Atherosclerosis is seen predominantly in males over 50 years of age and in postmenopausal women. In one series, the male to female ratio was 11:1.[13] Patients with metabolic disorders such as diabetes mellitus demonstrate a higher incidence and severity of atherosclerosis with premature appearance of the disease. In a large autopsy study, the incidence of gangrene of the extremities was 0.66% in nondiabetic individuals and 24.9% in diabetics.[14]

Symptoms are due to tissue ischemia. Such patients may have relatively few symptoms even in the presence of extensive occlusive disease. Symptoms of aorto-iliac occlusive disease are intermittent thigh and buttock claudication, impotence, paresthesias, is-

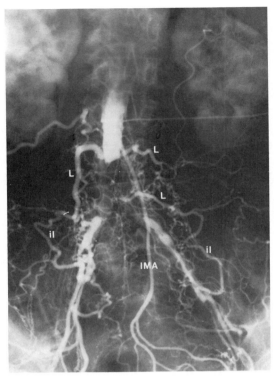

*Figure 10–19.* Translumbar aortogram shows atherosclerotic occlusion of the distal aorta with reconstitution of the common iliac arteries through well-developed lumbar and retroperitoneal collaterals and the inferior mesenteric artery (IMA). il = iliolumbar; L = lumbar arteries.

chemic neural pain (in patients with acute occlusions), and limb weakness. Acute arterial occlusion may be the first manifestation of the disease.[15]

## Radiology

Radiographically recognizable calcification of the abdominal aorta is seen in approximately 20% of individuals, occurs most frequently in white women 45 years or older, and may be related to osteoporosis of the skeleton.[16] Two types of calcifications are seen in association with occlusive disease—a coarse, patchy type and a medial calcification (Fig. 10–16). Another type, a fine, pencil-like senile calcification, is observed in patients without occlusive atherosclerosis.

## Occlusive Atherosclerosis

The most frequently affected segments are the infrarenal aorta and iliac arteries. The

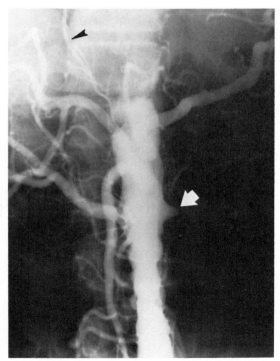

*Figure 10–18.* Severe atherosclerosis of the entire abdominal aorta with occlusion of the left renal artery (*arrow*). Arrowhead points to catheter in the inferior vena cava (introduced via the cubital vein).

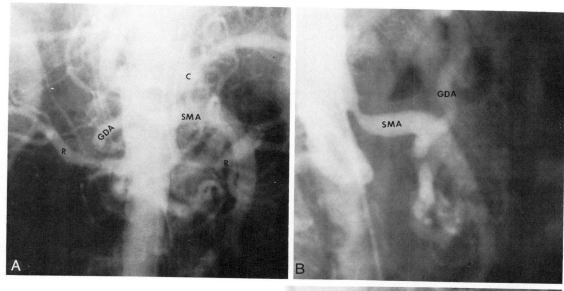

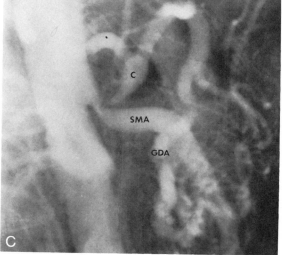

*Figure 10–20.* Value of lateral aortogram for the evaluation of celiac and superior mesenteric artery orifices. *A,* AP aortogram. The orifices of the celiac (C) and superior mesenteric (SMA) arteries are seen en face. A large gastroduodenal artery (GDA) is seen. The renal arteries (R) are seen in profile. A severe stenosis of the left renal artery is present. *B,* Early film from the lateral aortogram shows occlusion of the celiac artery and a stenotic superior mesenteric artery orifice. *C,* Later film shows reconstitution of the entire celiac artery up to the beaklike occlusion. *Note:* Although the large GDA suggests the presence of a proximal stenosis/occlusion, the diagnosis of a celiac artery occlusion or SMA stenosis could not have been established without the lateral aortogram.

spectrum of occlusive atherosclerosis extends from a shallow mural plaque with minimal lumen irregularity to complete occlusion (Figs. 10–17 to 10–19). Because of their location, the mural plaques are often appreciated only on the lateral aortogram.[17] In addition, the orifices of the mesenteric arteries are also best evaluated on a lateral aortogram (Fig. 10–20). Progression of occlusive atherosclerosis is slow, permitting the development of extensive collaterals.[18, 19]

Narrow atherosclerotic aortas are seen most frequently in women (see Fig. 10–17). Frequently, there is a focal area of severe distal aortic stenosis. This has also been referred to "atherosclerotic coarctation" of the abdominal aorta.[20] The lesion is characterized by a relatively discrete, eccentric, often diaphragm-like atherosclerotic plaque in the distal abdominal aorta (Fig. 10–21). In such patients, the distal vessels are usually small and without significant stenoses (Fig. 10–22).

If untreated, a severe stenosis progresses to arterial occlusion by superimposition of a thrombus (Fig. 10–23). In the aorta, distal occlusion may be associated with retrograde thrombosis extending proximally to the level of the renal arteries. Occasionally, the thrombus may extend to occlude both renal arteries and rarely the mesenteric arteries (Fig. 10–24).[15, 21–24] Atherosclerotic occlusion of the abdominal aorta usually begins close to the

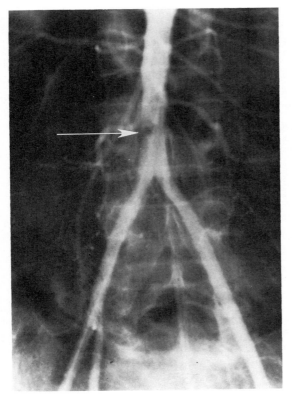

*Figure 10–21.* Atherosclerotic coarctation of the abdominal aorta in a 46 year old woman. AP aortogram shows a severe, eccentric, diaphragm-like stenosis (*arrow*). A 40 mm Hg resting pressure gradient was present.

bifurcation. Iliac artery occlusion is most frequently located in the proximal common iliac artery and is seen in 35% of patients with peripheral arterial disease.[25]

## Ectatic Atherosclerosis (Arteriomegaly, Arteria Magna)

Atherosclerosis may result in diffuse ectasia and tortuosity of the aortoiliac vessels with formation of multiple aneurysms (Fig. 10–25).[26] This type of atherosclerosis is rarely seen in women. It is associated with axial rotation of the aorta that leads to displacement of the visceral artery orifices, making visceral artery catheterization difficult. Frequently, the ectasia extends into the orifices of the major aortic branches. The iliac arteries are severely tortuous, often assuming an "M" configuration.[27] Patients with ectatic atherosclerosis show a propensity for thromboembolic complications.[28] Ectasia of the iliac and femoral arteries may also be seen in association with abdominal aortic aneurysms.

Arteriographic evaluation is difficult, as blood flow is extremely slow and often the contrast bolus can be seen moving with each systole. Arteriography demonstrates irregularity of the arterial lumen with multiple areas of focal stenoses. In some patients, the ectatic arteries may be smooth, possibly owing to the presence of laminated thrombi.

According to some authors, the histopathology is distinctively different from occlusive atherosclerosis and thus permits categorization of ectatic atherosclerosis as a distinct entity.[27] The main histological abnormality appears to be a loss of the medial elastic tissue.[26, 27]

## Occlusion

Acute occlusion of the abdominal aorta or iliac arteries may be due to trauma, thromboembolism, occlusion of an aneurysm, acute in-situ thrombosis superimposed upon atherosclerotic stenosis (Leriche's syndrome), or iatrogenic causes (following guide wire and

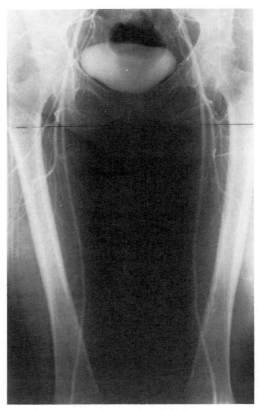

*Figure 10–22.* Same patient as in Figure 10–21. The iliofemoral arteriogram shows normal vessels distal to the abdominal aortic stenosis.

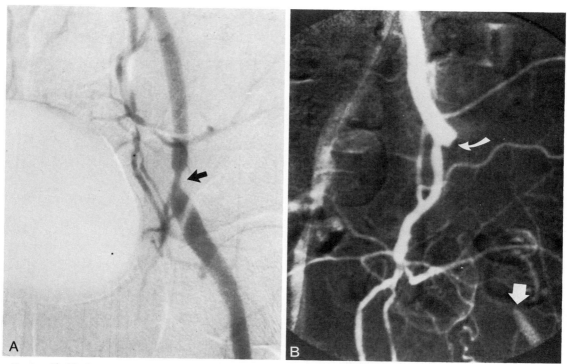

**Figure 10–23.** Progression of a severe stenosis to occlusion. *A,* Subtraction film from a left common iliac arteriogram shows a severe external iliac artery stenosis (*arrow*). *B,* Repeat arteriogram (intraarterial DSA) approximately 6 weeks later shows occlusion of the entire external iliac artery (*curved arrow*). There is reconstitution of the common femoral artery (*straight arrow*).

catheter manipulations).[29–31] Other rare causes include embolization of a prosthetic valve poppet or spontaneous thrombosis in the absence of significant intimal disease such as seen in low cardiac output states, metastatic malignancy, systemic lupus erythematosus, and coagulation disorders (Fig. 10–26).[32, 33] Acute occlusion manifests with

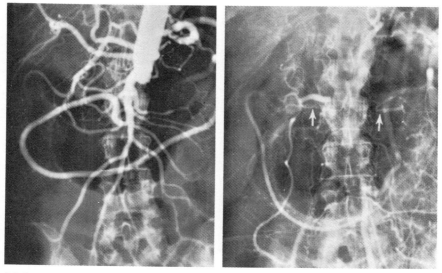

**Figure 10–24.** Suprarenal aortic occlusion. *A,* AP aortogram shows occlusion of the aorta below the superior mesenteric artery origin. *B,* Later film from the same aortogram shows reconstitution of both renal arteries (*arrows*) via collaterals. (From Sequeira JC et al: AJR 132:773, 1979. Used with permission.)

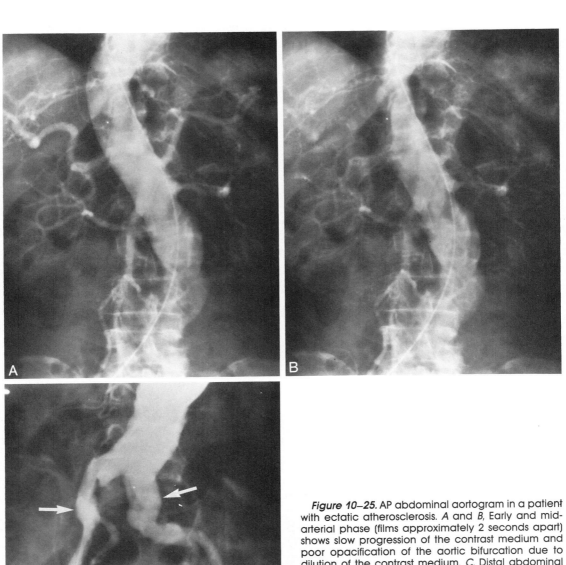

*Figure 10–25.* AP abdominal aortogram in a patient with ectatic atherosclerosis. *A* and *B,* Early and mid-arterial phase (films approximately 2 seconds apart) shows slow progression of the contrast medium and poor opacification of the aortic bifurcation due to dilution of the contrast medium. *C,* Distal abdominal aortogram opacifies the ectatic distal aorta and the pelvic vessels. Aneurysms of several vessels are seen (*arrows*).

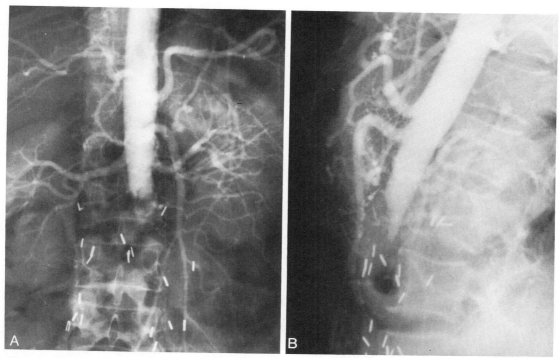

*Figure 10–26.* A and B, Spontaneous occlusion of the infrarenal abdominal aorta in 38 year old woman with a coagulopathy. The patient was a heavy smoker and had previously undergone sympathectomy and aortic endarterectomy.

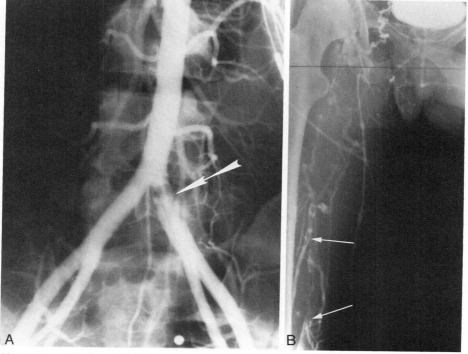

*Figure 10–27.* Paradoxical embolization to the left common iliac artery in a patient with a single ventricle. A, AP aortogram shows a nonoccluding embolus (*arrow*). B, Venogram of the right lower extremity shows extensive venous occlusion. Fresh-appearing thrombi are seen in several veins (*arrows*).

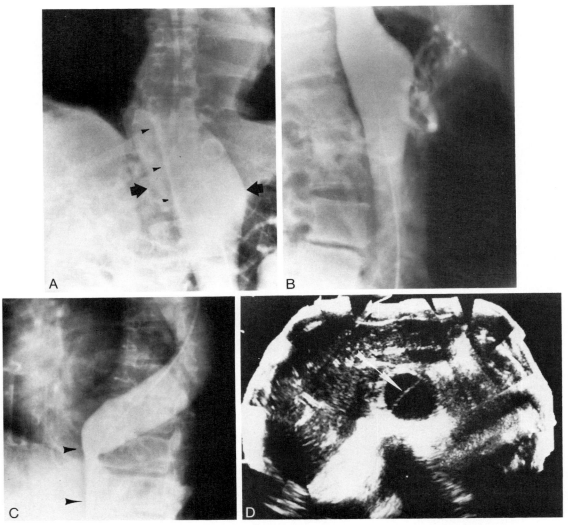

*Figure 10–28.* Localized dissection of the abdominal aorta with formation of a "dissecting aneurysm." *A,* AP aortogram shows an intimal flap (*arrowheads*) and a wide aortic lumen (*arrows*). *B,* Lateral aortogram shows the aneurysm. The initial flap is not seen. *C,* Left anterior oblique aortogram with the catheter positioned in the descending thoracic aorta shows the dissection (*arrowheads*). There is narrowing of the aortic lumen at the diaphragmatic hiatus. *D,* Transverse sonogram through the dissection shows the flap (*arrow*). At surgery, the dissection did not extend into the thoracic aorta.

pulselessness, pallor, pain, paresthesias, and paralysis (the five "P's").[31]

In thromboembolic occlusion of the lower extremities, the aorta was the site of acute occlusion in 18% and the iliac arteries in 21% of patients in one series.[31] In the majority of patients, the heart is the source of the thromboemboli. Occasionally, paradoxical embolization may occur through a patent foramen ovale or a septal defect (Fig. 10–27).[34] A patent foramen ovale (up to 0.7 cm in diameter) is found in 6% of unselected autopsies.[35]

## Dissection

Aortic dissection beginning in the thorax may extend to involve the abdominal aorta and iliac and femoral arteries. Rarely, aortic dissection may begin in the abdomen.[36–38] More frequently, a Type III dissection with an entry site in the abdominal aorta may suggest a primary abdominal aortic dissection. Spontaneous localized dissection of the abdominal aorta or iliac arteries is rare and represents a manifestation of atherosclerotic vascular disease (Figs. 10–28 and 10–29). Ab-

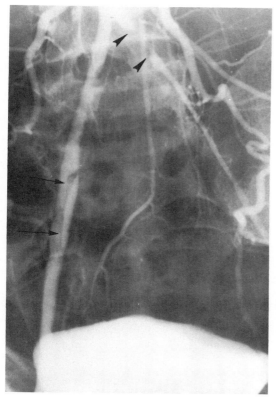

Figure 10–29

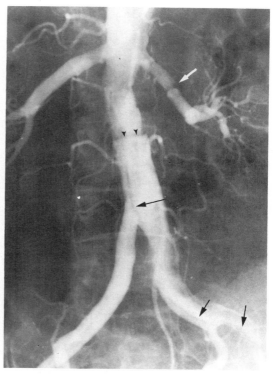

Figure 10–30

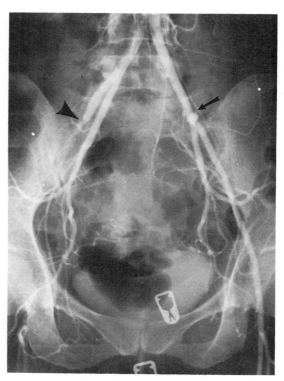

**Figure 10–29.** Translumbar aortogram showing spontaneous focal atherosclerotic dissection of the right external iliac artery (*arrows*) There is a segmental occlusion of the left common iliac artery (*arrowheads*).

**Figure 10–30.** Iatrogenic dissection of the abdominal aorta and iliac artery following aortorenal endarterectomy. AP aortogram shows dissection extending into the left external iliac artery (*black arrows*). Arrowheads point to the distal extent of the endarterectomy. There is stenosis of the left renal artery at the termination point of the endarterectomy (*white arrow*).

**Figure 10–31.** Fibromuscular disease of the iliac arteries. AP pelvic arteriogram shows the typical beaded appearance of medial fibroplasia involving the left common and external iliac arteries (*arrow*). On the right side, the disease has progressed to complete occlusion (*arrowhead*). There is reconstitution of the right common femoral artery via the obturator artery.

Figure 10–31

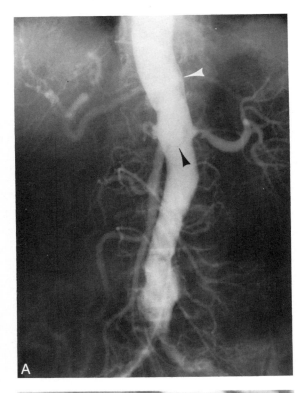

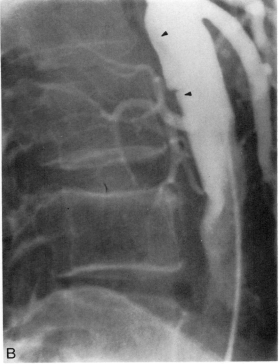

*Figure 10–32.* Atherosclerotic plaque simulating thrombus or dissection. *A,* On the AP aortogram, there is a curvilinear lucency (*arrowheads*). The right renal artery is occluded. *B,* Lateral aortogram shows a jagged-appearing posterior plaque (*arrowheads*).

dominal aortic and iliac artery dissection may be iatrogenic, occurring after arterial catheterization or aorto-iliac endarterectomy (Fig. 10–30).

## Fibromuscular Disease

Fibromuscular disease may involve the abdominal aorta and iliac arteries. Such patients usually have fibromuscular disease of other systemic arteries. Aortic involvement is rare and may be associated with the development of abdominal aortic coarctation or aneurysms.[39, 40]

The iliac arteries are affected in 1 to 5% of individuals with renal or carotid artery fibromuscular disease.[41, 42] Iliac disease may be an incidental finding in an asymptomatic patient; it may lead to the development of an aneurysm, hemodynamically significant stenosis, or iliac artery occlusion (Fig. 10–31). Microemboli originating from the diseased arterial segment have been responsible for peripheral arterial occlusions.[43]

## Arteriography
(see Tables 10–1, 10–2, and 10–5, and Figs. 10–17 to 10–31)

For the abdominal aorta, biplane aortography (AP and lateral) is performed via the femoral, translumbar, or axillary route. In addition, oblique aortography may become necessary for the evaluation of the proximal renal arteries.

In atherosclerotic disease, oblique pelvic arteriography provides the most information. Either the biplane technique or the left and right anterior oblique (45°) projections can be used. The information obtained from an AP pelvic arteriogram alone is often inadequate and occasionally misleading, except in patients with abdominal aortic aneurysms and trauma (see Fig. 10–12).

In chronic occlusive disease of the distal abdominal aorta and iliac arteries, a properly performed abdominal aortogram (with reactive hyperemia) provides satisfactory opacification of the proximal lower extremity vessels. In patients with inadequate opacification of the reconstituted lower extremity vessels, intraarterial DSA can be used. In others, intravenous DSA may be used to obtain distal opacification via the internal mammary collaterals.[44]

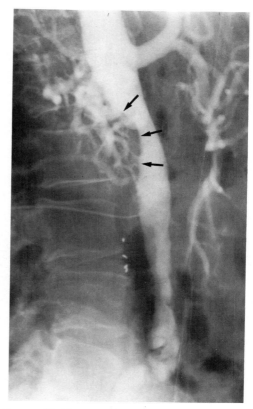

*Figure 10–33.* Posterior scalloping due to mural thrombus. Lateral abdominal aortogram shows the typical appearance of a posterior aortic wall thrombus (*arrows*).

PITFALLS IN DIAGNOSIS

1. Inhomogeneous opacification of the aorta in the AP projection: This could be due to mural thrombus, bowel gas shadow, flow artefact, or plaque (Fig. 10–32). The lateral aortogram clarifies the situation. In the presence of atherosclerotic plaques, the posterior aortic wall has a jagged appearance. The laminated posterior wall thrombus causes typical scalloping (Fig. 10–33).

2. Focal arterial stenosis: The hemodynamic significance of a lesion cannot always be determined by measuring the arterial diameter (Fig. 10–34).

3. Stenosis not demonstrated on the AP arteriogram: Renal, iliac, and femoral artery stenoses often remain obscured on the AP arteriogram (Fig. 10–35; see also Fig. 10–12). Thus, in patients suspected of having stenoses of these vessels oblique arteriography is necessary.

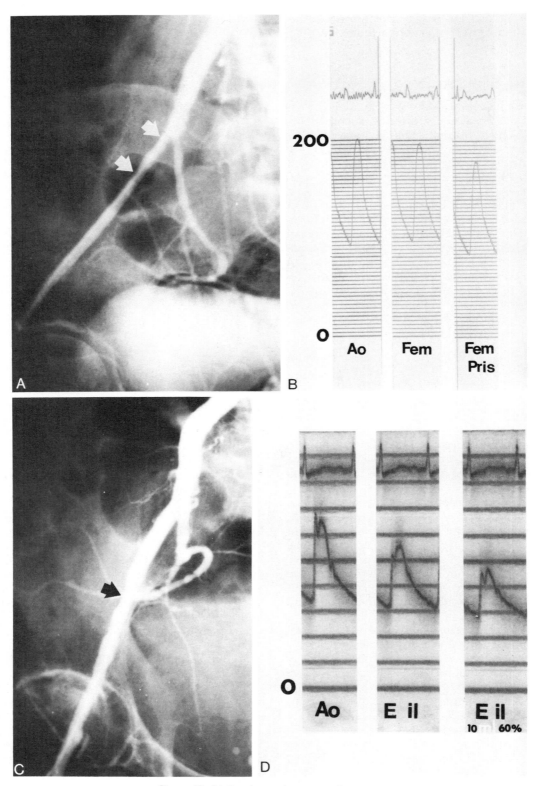

*Figure 10–34. See legend on opposite page.*

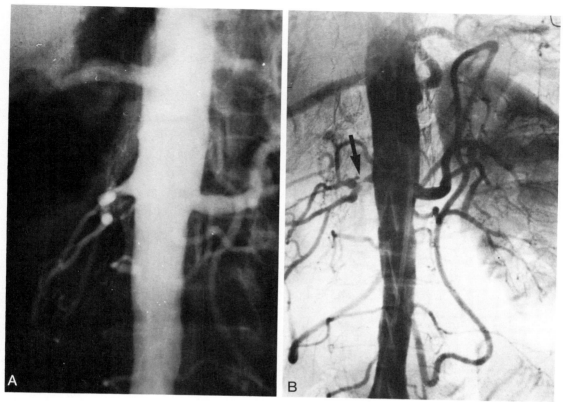

**Figure 10–35.** Critical renal artery stenosis not demonstrated on the AP aortogram. *A,* AP abdominal aortogram shows a slight stenosis of the right renal artery. *B,* Approximately 10° right posterior oblique projection reveals the critical renal artery stenosis (*arrow*).

## ANEURYSMS

### Definitions

An aneurysm is a localized segmental or diffuse dilatation of an artery. Aneurysms may develop as a result of an abnormality in one or more layers of the arterial wall:

1. Fusiform aneurysm: This type occurs as a result of dilatation of all layers of the arterial wall. It usually involves multiple segments of an artery.

2. Saccular aneurysm: This type results from thinning and stretching of the arterial media. In small saccular aneurysms, all layers of the arterial wall remain intact. In large saccular aneurysms, there may be progressive thinning and virtual disappearance of all layers of the arterial wall. The process is localized, ie, it involves a segment of the artery.

3. False aneurysm: This is a saclike structure that communicates with the arterial lumen and results from disruption of all layers of the arterial wall. It is surrounded by periarterial tissue and blood clot.

The diameter of the normal abdominal

---

**Figure 10–34.** Inability of the arteriogram to predict hemodynamic significance of an arterial stenosis. *A,* Oblique pelvic arteriogram shows two areas of stenosis (*arrows*) in the right external iliac artery. *B,* Tracing of the intraarterial pressures across the lesions shows no significant resting gradient. Following injection of 25 mg of tolazoline in the right common femoral artery, the intraarterial pressure distal to the stenosis fell by 16 mm Hg. *Note:* This response is at the upper limits of normal, considering that the intraaortic pressure also falls after intraarterial injection of a vasodilator. *C,* Oblique pelvic arteriogram in another patient with a stenosis of the right external iliac artery (*arrow*) similar to the one shown in *A. D,* Tracing of the intraarterial pressures across the stenosis reveals a significant resting pressure gradient of 25 mm Hg. Following injection of 10 ml of contrast medium into the distal external iliac artery, the distal pressure fell another 20 mm Hg.

aorta is between 2 and 3 cm. A focal widening of greater than 3 cm is called an aneurysm. However, a "gray zone" exists in some older patients with diffuse atherosclerosis in whom the diameter of the ectatic aorta exceeds 3 cm without focal aneurysm formation.

## Pathology

Atherosclerosis is responsible for more than 90% of abdominal aortic aneurysms.[45] Other causes include mycotic, syphilitic, traumatic, and anastomotic aneurysms and aneurysms developing as a result of arteritis. Ninety-one per cent of abdominal aortic aneurysms are infrarenal, and in 69% of patients the aneurysm extends into the iliac or femoral arteries.[46]

Isolated iliac and femoral artery aneurysms are found 16% and visceral and renal artery aneurysms in 2% of patients with abdominal aortic aneurysms.[46] Isolated iliac artery aneurysms are rare in patients without abdominal aortic aneurysms. In one review, they were found in only 0.6% of patients undergoing aorto-iliac angiography (Fig. 10–36).[47] Eighty-nine per cent are located in the common iliac arteries, 10% in the internal iliac artery, and only 1% in the external iliac artery.[48] Isolated internal iliac artery aneurysms occur in 0.4% of patients with abdominal aortic aneurysms.[49] Rarely, iliac artery aneurysms may assume gigantic proportions.[50] Anastomotic aneurysms after aorto-iliac or aorto-femoral

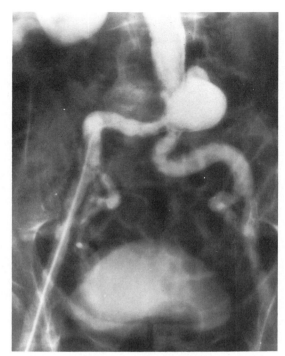

*Figure 10–37.* Anastomotic aneurysm. AP pelvic arteriogram shows an aneurysm at the distal anastomosis of an aortic tube graft.

bypass surgery are reported in 0.2% of aortic and 1.2% of iliac anastomoses.[51] The most frequent cause is a structural defect in the parent vessel (Fig. 10–37). The "growth rate" of atherosclerotic abdominal aortic aneurysms between 3 and 6 cm in diameter has been calculated as 0.39 cm/year.[52]

Because of the nature of the atherosclerotic disease, associated stenoses and occlusions of the pelvic and lower extremity vessels are seen in the majority of patients.

## Clinical Aspects

Abdominal aortic aneurysms are seen most frequently in males (ratio of 5:1) 60 years or older.[53] In children and young adults, abdominal aortic aneurysms are rare and may occur as a result of infection, trauma, or an arteritis.[54]

Seventy per cent of patients with abdominal aortic aneurysms are symptomatic.[45] The most common symptoms are abdominal pain (37%), which may be intermittent or constant, and an abdominal mass (26%). In patients with ruptured aneurysms, the pain is due to the hematoma. It may be abdominal or may radiate to the flank (mostly left), the groin, or in the lower back.

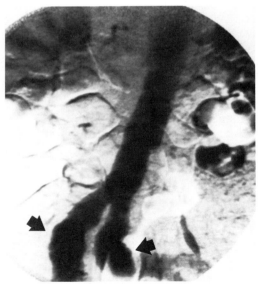

*Figure 10–36.* Isolated common iliac artery aneurysms in a patient with relapsing polychondritis (*arrows*).

In 10% of abdominal aortic aneurysms, there is perianeurysmal fibrosis, which is an inflammatory process of unknown etiology that may lead to entrapment, deviation, and obstruction of the ureters, simulating retroperitoneal fibrosis.[55] Seeding of infectious organisms in an atherosclerotic aneurysm may simulate an inflammatory aneurysm.[56]

On physical examination there is a pulsatile abdominal mass with expansile pulsations. However, in 12% of patients, this finding may be simulated by a tortuous, ectatic, senile atherosclerotic aorta, horseshoe kidney, or paraaortic masses.[57, 58] Seven per cent of patients have a normal physical examination.[45]

## Radiology

In the past, abdominal radiographs were used to assess aneurysm size and growth. The presence of mural calcification permits plain radiographic detection of an aneurysm in up to 86% of patients.[45, 59] Diagnostic ultrasonography provides an accurate and simple means of diagnosis and follow-up of patients with asymptomatic abdominal aneurysms.[60] The problems associated with this technique are the inability to distinguish the aortic wall from adherent sonolucent masses (giving rise to false measurements) and the inability to detect complete thrombosis.[61, 62] Computed tomography and magnetic resonance imaging provide other accurate methods for the detection of aortic aneurysms and postoperative complications.[63]

In ruptured abdominal aortic aneurysms, the plain radiograph may demonstrate the following (see Fig. 10–43):[64, 65]

1. Soft tissue mass with obliteration of the psoas margin.

2. Ill-defined borders of the aneurysm.

3. Disruption of the curvilinear calcification (in calcified aneurysms) with the presence of a soft tissue density beyond the calcified wall.

4. "Pseudo-gas" in the retroperitoneum, due to dissection of blood through retroperitoneal fat.

## Arteriography

Unfortunately, the misconception that arteriography is "dangerous," a carryover from the past years of the initial period of arteriography, still persists in some circles. Arteriography is an essential part of the preoperative evaluation of patients with abdominal aortic aneurysms. It is not required for the establishment of the diagnosis or for the follow-up of such patients. It is indicated in patients who are hemodynamically stable, to:

1. Evaluate the extent of the aneurysm, especially with respect to the renal arteries.

2. Evaluate the status of renal, mesenteric, and iliofemoral arteries.

3. Detect aberrant vessels.

In one series, preoperative arteriography significantly influenced therapeutic decisions in 75% of patients evaluated.[46] In this series, celiac and superior mesenteric artery stenosis or occlusion was observed in 22% of patients. Thirty-seven per cent of patients had accessory renal arteries and 7% of these arose from the aneurysm itself. Renal artery stenosis was observed in 22% of patients in one series and in 30% of patients in another series.[46, 66] In 38% of patients, the aneurysm originated close to or involved the renal arteries.[46]

Left colonic ischemia is observed in 1.6% of patients undergoing aorto-iliac surgery.[67] In this setting, the mortality associated with colonic ischemia is 48%. Seen from another perspective, 10% of operative deaths after aneurysmectomy are due to visceral ischemia.[68] Similarly, postoperative renal failure may occur in up to 14% of patients after elective aneurysmectomy.[59] Preoperative knowledge of any existing mesenteric or renal artery disease could avoid these complications.

Angiographic evaluation of an abdominal aortic aneurysm requires a biplane aortogram and an AP pelvic arteriogram. Biplane aortography is performed via the femoral or axillary approach. A pigtail catheter is placed in the upper abdominal aorta at T12–L1 (see Table 10–1). For pelvic arteriography, the catheter is positioned above the aortic bifurcation. Contrast medium can safely be injected into the aneurysm provided it is not leaking or acutely expanding. A safe contrast injection rate is between 8 and 10 ml/sec.

Angiographic findings are (Figs. 10–38 to 10–44):

1. Focally widened aortic lumen (greater than 3 cm) (Figs. 10–38 to 10–40). The majority of atherosclerotic aneurysms are single and infrarenal in location. Syphilitic aneurysms of the abdominal aorta, which are very rare, involve the suprarenal aorta more frequently and are multiple in 64% of patients.[69] Atherosclerotic aneurysms of the abdominal aorta are either saccular or fusiform with

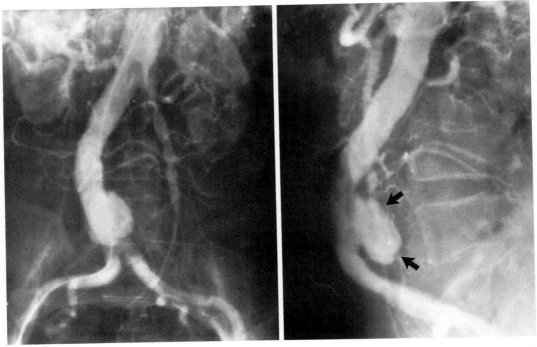

*Figure 10–38.* AP (*left*) and lateral (*right*) abdominal aortogram shows a saccular mycotic aneurysm of the infrarenal aorta (*arrows*).

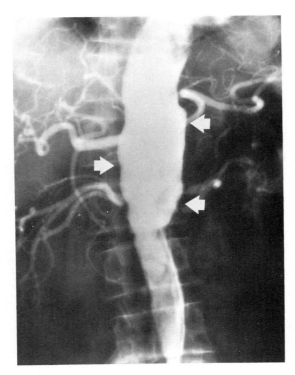

*Figure 10–39.* Fusiform atherosclerotic suprarenal abdominal aortic aneurysm (*arrows*) The patient had previously undergone resection of an infrarenal aneurysm.

equal frequency. Syphilitic aneurysms are more often saccular than fusiform (ratio of 5:1).[69]

2. Thickened aortic wall (between the opacified lumen and a mural calcification) due to a mural clot, which is present in 80% of patients (Fig. 10–40).[53] This may cause scalloping of the opacified lumen.

3. Occlusion of the lumbar arteries. This is seen in the majority of patients. In one series, only 22% of patients had patent lumbar arteries arising from an abdominal aortic aneurysm (Fig. 10–41).[46]

4. Occlusion of the inferior mesenteric artery. This is seen in close to 80% of patients.[46]

5. Extension of the abdominal aortic aneurysm into the iliac arteries. This is seen in 66% of patients.[46]

6. Slow antegrade flow of contrast medium.

7. Leaking aneurysm: Extravasation of contrast medium from a leaking aneurysm is rarely demonstrated. Such patients are usually symptomatic and seldom require preoperative arteriography.

8. Contained aneurysm rupture: Contrast opacification of an extraluminal cavity may be demonstrated. A large surrounding hematoma is usually present (Fig. 10–42).

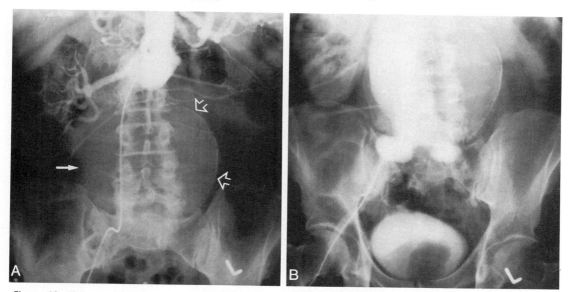

*Figure 10–40.* Large saccular atherosclerotic infrarenal aortic aneurysm. *A,* Egg-shell calcification of the aneurysm is present (*open arrows*). The right border is not calcified but can be determined by the soft tissue density (*arrow*). *B,* Contrast injection in the aneurysm opacifies the pelvic vessels. Aneurysms of both common iliac arteries are present. The opacified lumen of the distal aorta is narrowed, owing to the presence of a large left-sided mural thrombus. The left kidney was removed following blunt trauma 25 years ago.

PITFALLS IN DIAGNOSIS
1. "Normal" abdominal aorta: In some aortic aneurysms, the mural thrombus may narrow the aortic lumen to give the impression of a normal aorta (11% of patients)

(Fig. 10–45).[59] In such patients, the following signs offer a clue to the presence of an abdominal aortic aneurysm:

a. Occlusion of several or all lumbar arteries (in 78% of patients[46]).

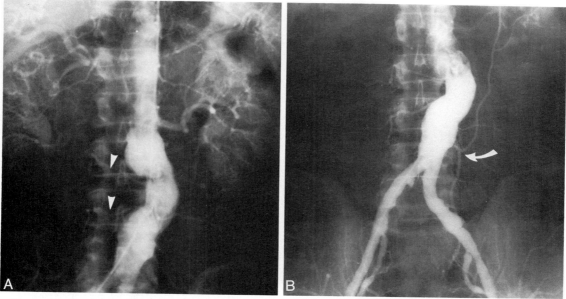

*Figure 10–41.* Abdominal aortic aneurysm with patent lumbar arteries. The inferior mesenteric artery is not demonstrated on a high aortic injection. *A,* AP aortogram with the catheter sideholes at T11 opacifies the posteriorly located lumbar arteries (*arrows*). The inferior mesenteric artery does not fill. *B,* On repeat arteriography with the catheter at the aortic bifurcation, the inferior mesenteric artery is visualized (*curved arrow*).

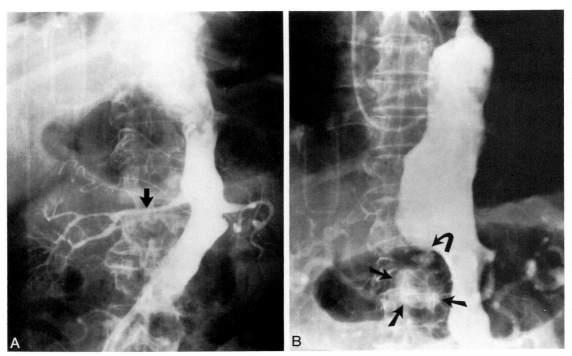

*Figure 10–42.* Contained rupture of an atherosclerotic thoracoabdominal aneurysm. *A,* AP abdominal aortogram shows stretching of the right renal artery (*arrow*). An aneurysm is not demonstrated. *B,* Repeat arteriogram with the catheter placed in the mid-descending thoracic aorta shows a fusiform aneurysm with extravasation of contrast medium (*straight arrows*). The curved arrow points to the site of rupture.

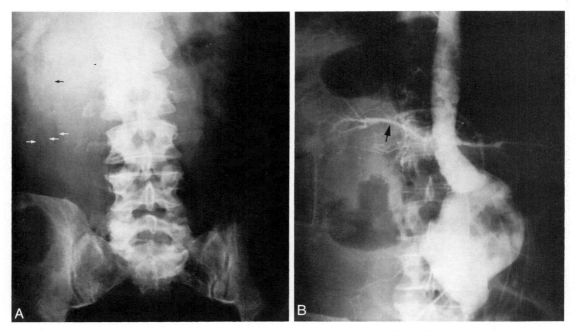

*Figure 10–43.* Ruptured atherosclerotic abdominal aortic aneurysm. *A,* Plain film of the abdomen shows obliteration of the right psoas margin and the presence of "pseudo gas" (*arrows*). *B,* AP aortogram shows a large saccular infrarenal aortic aneurysm. The right renal artery is displaced craniad (*arrow*). The renal and mesenteric vessels are constricted in response to systemic hypotension.

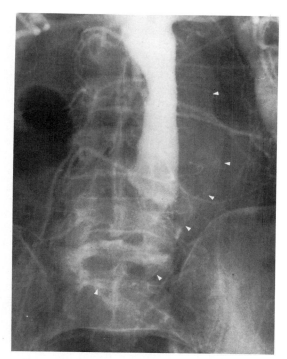

*Figure 10–44.* Spontaneous occlusion of an abdominal aortic aneurysm. Fine mural calcification is seen (*arrowheads*). Note the narrow diameter of the opacified aortic lumen.

b. Displacement and bowing of the mesenteric artery branches.
c. Zone of absent parenchymal (capillary) stain around the opacified abdominal lumen (avascular halo).
d. Displacement of the left kidney or ureter, or both.

2. Inferior mesenteric artery occlusion: A high abdominal aortogram in patients with abdominal aortic aneurysms may not opacify the inferior mesenteric artery, which arises anteriorly from the aneurysm. This is due to the posterior layering of the contrast medium in the distal aorta. A contrast injection into the lower abdominal aorta or aneurysm will opacify the inferior mesenteric artery if this vessel is patent (Fig. 10–41).

3. Short or absent "neck": This pitfall is encountered when a single (AP) aortogram is performed. The proximal-anterior portion of the abdominal aortic aneurysm is superimposed upon the renal artery and may give the impression that a "neck" of the aneurysm is either short or not present. On the lateral projection, this relationship is demonstrated clearly.

4. Contrast injection into a soft clot may

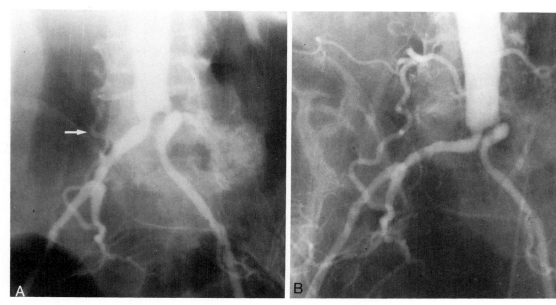

*Figure 10–45.* "Normal"-appearing distal aorta in a patient with an infrarenal abdominal aortic aneurysm and reconstitution of the lumbar arteries via the iliolumbar artery. *A,* AP distal aortogram shows absent filling of the lumbar arteries. No aneurysm is demonstrated because of the presence of a mural thrombus. A prominent right iliolumbar artery is opacified (*arrow*). *B,* On a later film from the same aortogram, the lumbar arteries are demonstrated. There is severe stenosis of the left common iliac artery. *Note:* If only the later films were evaluated, the aorta would appear normal. At operation an aneurysm of the distal aorta was found.

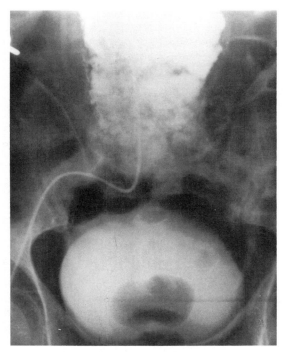

*Figure 10–46.* Contrast injection into mural thrombus in a patient with an abdominal aortic aneurysm.

result in persistent "stain" simulating extravasation (Fig. 10–46).

**Complications of Arteriography.** With proper catheterization technique, complications during or after aortography for abdominal aortic aneurysms are infrequent. The overall complication rate has been reported at 1 to 2%.[46, 66] In our own experience, no serious complications have been observed. The vast majority of complications are minor and represent groin hematomas. Properly performed contrast injection into an aneurysm (that is not expanding, leaking, or ruptured) is safe and does not precipitate aneurysm rupture. Similarly, clot dislodgment and occlusion are extremely rare.

## Complications of Abdominal Aortic Aneurysms

1. Rupture (see Fig. 10–43): This occurs most frequently into the retroperitoneum on the left side. Rarely, there is spontaneous aneurysm rupture into the gastrointestinal tract or the inferior vena cava.[53, 70, 71] Whereas the former is associated with massive gastrointestinal hemorrhage, the latter causes rapid cardiac decompensation. Mortality from untreated ruptured aneurysms is close to 100%. Aneurysm rupture usually occurs

in the body of the aneurysm and rarely at the junction of the aneurysm with the nondilated aorta.[53] Aneurysm rupture may be contained by the perivascular tissue, resulting in a perianeurysmal hematoma. In such patients, arteriography is indicated only if the diagnosis is uncertain and the patient is hemodynamically stable.

2. Spontaneous occlusion (see Fig. 10–44):[72, 73] Blunt abdominal trauma may also be responsible for occlusion of an abdominal aortic aneurysm.[74]

3. Peripheral embolization: In one report, in 10% of patients undergoing embolectomy, the embolus originated in an abdominal aortic aneurysm.[75] Peripheral thromboembolism may also occur as a complication of aneurysmectomy.

4. Infection:[76] Ulceration and thrombus deposition in an atherosclerotic aneurysm make the aneurysm susceptible to secondary infection.

The incidence of aneurysm rupture and leakage has been correlated with aneurysm size, ie, the larger the aneurysm, the greater the possibility of rupture.[77] In an autopsy study of 473 unoperated abdominal aortic aneurysms, the overall incidence of rupture was 24.9%.[78] The incidence of rupture of aneurysms relative to size was as follows: less than 4 cm, 9.5%; 4.1 to 5.0 cm, 23.4%; 5.1 to 7.0 cm, 25.3%; 7.1 to 10.0 cm, 45.6%; and greater than 10.0 cm, 60.5%.

With successful operative management, the 5 year survival of patients with abdominal aortic aneurysms was 49% versus 17.2% for unoperated patients, and the life expectancy of patients undergoing surgical repair was doubled.[77] In another series, the 5 year survival after operative repair was 61%.[79] Surgical mortality for elective repair of abdominal aortic aneurysms is less than 2%, whereas mortality for emergency operation of a ruptured abdominal aortic aneurysm is approximately 60%.[78, 80]

## TRAUMA

### Aortic Injury

**Blunt Aortic Injury.** In 63% of cases, blunt abdominal trauma occurs as the result of a motor vehicle accident.[81] In 16% of patients with significant intraabdominal injury, signs and symptoms of such injury may be absent.[82] If there is an associated head injury, such signs and symptoms may be masked by the head injury in almost half of the patients.

Blunt abdominal trauma most frequently involves the solid organs or their vascular pedicles and the intestines.[81] Injury to the abdominal aorta leading to rupture occurs in about 4% of patients with blunt aortic injury.[83, 84] Blunt aortic injury may be manifested as an aortic laceration, thrombosis, posttraumatic dissection, or false aneurysm formation.

**Penetrating Aortic Injury.** Penetrating injury to the abdominal aorta may cause aortic occlusion, arteriovenous fistula, retroperitoneal hematoma, or the formation of a traumatic or mycotic aneurysm (inoculation of bacterial agents by the injuring object). In addition, distal embolization can cccur from the site of injury.

**Arteriography.** Arteriography is indicated to localize and evaluate the extent of injury. Biplane aortography is performed from the femoral or axillary approach (see Table 10–1). The femoral approach is used if groin pulses are present. An LLT J guide wire is used to lead the pigtail catheter beyond the anticipated site of injury. The catheter is placed at T12–L1. At the time of catheter removal, the pigtail is straightened out and removed over a J guide wire. In patients with blunt trauma, the lower thoracic aorta should also be evaluated.

Arteriographic findings are (Fig. 10–47):
1. False aneurysm.
2. Arteriovenous fistula.
3. Aortic occlusion: In blunt trauma, the

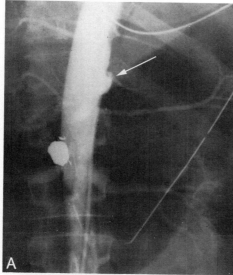

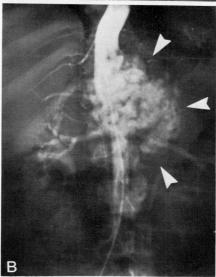

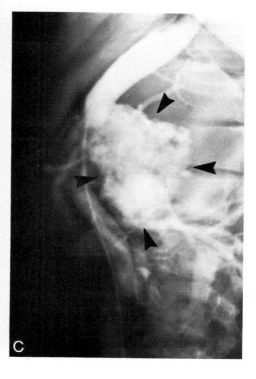

*Figure 10–47.* Traumatic abdominal aortic aneurysm. *A,* AP aortogram shows a small false aneurysm (*arrow*) following penetrating injury. *B* and *C,* AP and lateral abdominal aortograms in a patient with blunt abdominal trauma show a large aneurysm (*arrowheads*).

most frequent location of aortic occlusion is the infrarenal aorta at the level of the inferior mesenteric artery.[85]

4. Retroperitoneal hematoma with anterior and lateral displacement of the aorta.

PITFALLS IN DIAGNOSIS

The retroperitoneal hematoma may be from small vessel bleeding without associated aortic injury. Such displacement may also be due to a preexisting condition, such as a retroperitoneal mass.[86]

## Pelvic Vessel Injury

**Blunt Pelvic Trauma.** Blunt pelvic trauma is most frequently due to a motor vehicle accident and is associated with a 12% mortality.[87] The major causes of death are hemorrhage and sepsis. The mortality associated with open pelvic fractures is 50% and is 75%

if major vessel injury has occurred.[87, 88] In contrast, closed pelvic fractures are associated with only a 10% mortality. The types of fractures predisposing to a high mortality are, in descending order of frequency: open pelvic fractures, fractures of the superior and inferior pubic rami, sacroiliac joint separation, iliac wing fractures, and separation of the pubic symphysis.

The site of bleeding is most frequently in the distribution of the internal iliac artery and varies with the location of the fracture (eg, anterior branches—fractured pubic rami, separation of pubic symphysis; posterior branches—sacroiliac joint separation, iliac wing fracture).

Although a pelvic arteriogram (with a pigtail catheter in the distal aorta) may be performed as the first study to assess the extent of injury, an internal iliac arteriogram is often

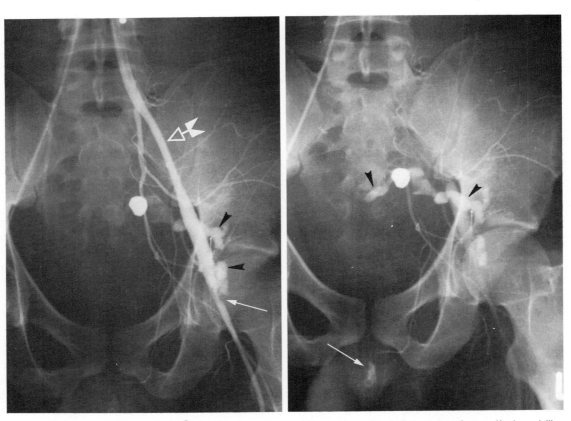

*Figure 10–48.* Penetrating trauma (bullet injury) with hemorrhage from the left common femoral/external iliac artery. Early film from an AP left common iliac arteriogram (*left*) shows a focal narrowing of the common femoral artery due to mural injury (*white arrow*). Extravasation of contrast medium is seen (*arrowheads*). There is segmental dilatation of the external iliac artery, possibly due to focal paresis as a result of injury to autonomic nerve fibers. The large white arrow points to the normal caliber of the external iliac artery. Later film from the same arteriogram (*right*) shows the extravasated contrast medium (*arrowheads*). In addition, there is a corpus cavernosum blush (*arrow*). This has occasionally been mistaken for contrast extravasation in blunt pelvic trauma.

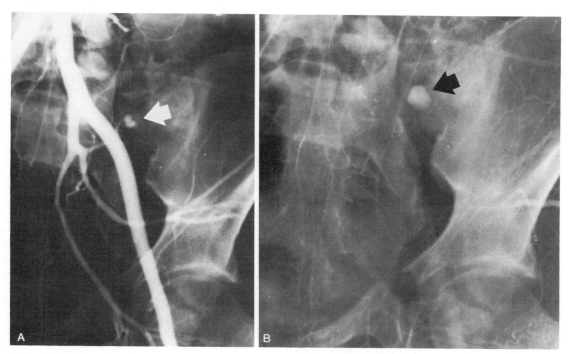

**Figure 10–49.** Blunt pelvic injury resulting in traumatic aneurysm. *A*, AP pelvic arteriogram shows a traumatic aneurysm of the left iliolumbar artery (*arrow*). There is separation of the left sacroiliac joint and a fracture through the left ischium. Branches of the left internal iliac artery are bowed around a pelvic hematoma. *B*, Later film from the same arteriogram shows persistent opacification of the false aneurysm (*arrow*).

necessary for demonstration of a bleeding site. In one report, bleeding was demonstrated by arteriography in 20 of 28 patients.[89] Seven of the 20 patients (35%) in whom bleeding was demonstrated by arteriography had multiple bleeding sites.

The most effective method for control of arterial bleeding is transcatheter embolization. This not only provides occlusion of the arteries close to the site of bleeding but also blocks potential sources of collateral blood supply to the site of the arterial injury. Operative exploration not only deprives the patient of the possibility to tamponade a hemorrhage but may also be associated with a high rate of failure to control the bleeding and an increased risk of infection. Thus, in one series, internal iliac artery ligation proved ineffective for controlling traumatic pelvic hemorrhage, leading to a 91% mortality in patients thus treated.[87] Bilateral proximal internal iliac artery ligation decreases arterial pressure by only 50%[90] which stresses the inadequacy of this form of therapy. Other authors with a large experience with the management of pelvic trauma also conclude

that "internal iliac (hypogastric) artery ligation is not indicated as a means of controlling retroperitoneal hemorrhage in patients with fractures of the pelvis."[91]

**Penetrating Pelvic Trauma.** Penetrating trauma to the pelvis occurs less frequently than blunt trauma. It may damage major vessels, leading to occlusion, false aneurysm formation, arteriovenous fistula, or extensive pelvic hemorrhage. The latter may dissect craniad into the retroperitoneum.

**Arteriography.** Arteriography is indicated for assessment of vascular injury and for transcatheter management. From the femoral approach, a pelvic arteriogram is performed using a pigtail catheter (see Table 10–5). Subsequently, selective arteriography of the involved artery is performed (see Tables 10–6 to 10–9).

Arteriographic findings are (Figs. 10–48 to 10–50):

1. Contrast extravasation.
2. False aneurysm.
3. Occlusion.
4. Hematoma: This is the most common finding in blunt trauma and may be associated

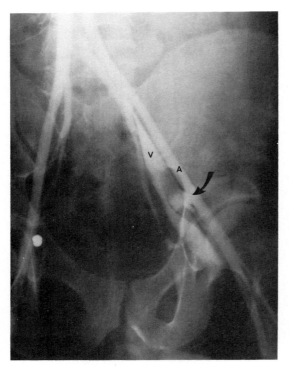

*Figure 10–50.* Penetrating injury resulting in a false aneurysm of the left external iliac artery and an arterio-venous fistula (*curved arrow*). A = artery; V = vein.

with any of the previously listed findings. Pelvic hematoma is manifested by the following signs:

    a. Displacement of major arteries (common or external iliac artery).

    b. Compression of large or small arteries.

    c. Stretching of internal iliac artery branches.

5. Arteriovenous fistula.

PITFALLS IN DIAGNOSIS

1. Pelvic arteriogram shows no bleeding: An insufficient volume of contrast medium entering a branch vessel in the distribution of the internal iliac artery may not demonstrate a bleeding site. In our experience, this is a relatively common finding since many of the internal iliac artery branches are constricted (owing to hypovolemia, shock) or compressed (by hematoma). Therefore, an internal iliac arteriogram should be performed in patients with blunt pelvic trauma if the pelvic arteriogram does not show a bleeding site. If there is a midline injury (eg, pubic fracture or postoperative bleeding after prostatectomy), both internal iliac arteries may have to be injected (consecutively) if bleeding is not demonstrated on the first arteriogram. Similarly, for the treatment of

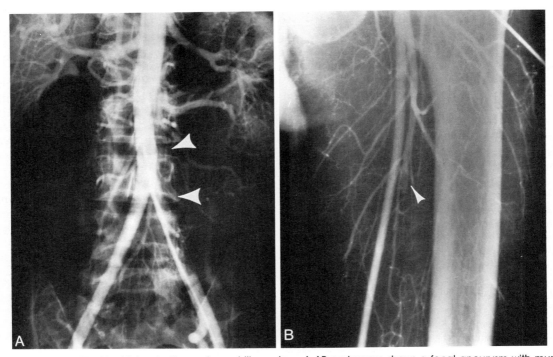

*Figure 10–51.* Electrical injury to the aorta and iliac artery. *A,* AP aortogram shows a focal aneurysm with mural thrombus involving the aorta and left common iliac artery (*arrowheads*). *B,* Left common femoral arteriogram shows embolization of a fragment of the mural thrombus into the left profunda femoris artery (*arrowhead*).

midline pelvic bleeding, both internal iliac artery branches (supplying the bleeding site) must be embolized.

2. Midline injury in which a single internal iliac arteriogram is negative: The ipsilateral vessels may have been compressed by hematoma or occluded by the injury. Therefore, a contralateral internal iliac arteriogram should be performed.

3. Male patient with a midline blush below the pubic symphysis: Contrast extravasation must be differentiated from a corpus cavernosum blush. Contrast extravasation is usually dense and persists after the venous phase, whereas the corpus cavernosum blush fades with the venous phase (Fig. 10–48; also see Fig. 14–43, Chapter 14).

### Electrical Injury

The passage of an electric current through the body generates heat that causes tissue necrosis.[92] Acutely, such injuries may cause vascular thrombosis. Late complications are arterial stenosis and formation of pseudoaneurysms (Fig. 10–51). The only clinical manifestation of such aneurysms may be peripheral thromboembolism.

### Radiation Injury

Therapeutic doses of radiation can cause endothelial injury leading to subintimal fibrosis and results in arterial stenosis or occlusion.[93] Occasionally, transmural necrosis may occur.[94] The extent of the vascular lesion corresponds to the radiation portal and is characterized by a change in arterial caliber to normal at the edge of the radiation field.

### Iatrogenic Injuries

Iatrogenic injury to the aorta and iliac arteries may be unavoidable and may occur during vascular surgery, eg, focal intimal tear from cross clamping or intimal dissection after endarterectomy (Fig. 10–52; see also Fig. 10–30). Injury may also occur as a complication of lumbar disc or hip surgery. The latter complications can result in arteriovenous fistula, occlusion, or false aneurysm formation.[95, 96] Aortic and pelvic arterial injury may also occur as a complication of diagnostic or interventional angiography. This may be manifested as a mural hematoma, dissection, arteriovenous fistula, or thrombosis.

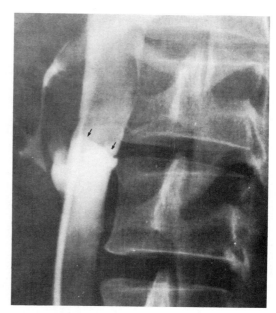

*Figure 10–52.* Iatrogenic injury to the abdominal aorta following placement of a vascular clamp (cross clamping for an aorto-renal bypass graft). An intimal tear is present (*arrows*).

## MISCELLANEOUS DISORDERS

### Abdominal Aortic Coarctation

Two per cent of aortic coarctations involve the abdominal aorta.[97] Abdominal aortic coarctation may occur as an isolated congenital anomaly or as part of a disease complex. The congenital form is due to failure or incomplete fusion of the primitive dorsal aortae, with subsequent obliteration of one of them.[98] Microscopic study of such specimens shows an absence of inflammatory elements.[99] The acquired form is seen most frequently in Orientals and Africans.[100–102] Acquired coarctation is often due to a panaortitis, which leads to stenosis or occlusion of the aorta.[103] The acquired type may be seen in association with the aortic arch syndrome.[100] Table 10–10 lists some of the dis-

**TABLE 10–10.** Diseases Associated With Abdominal Aortic Coarctation[39, 100, 105–110]

Thoracic aortic coarctation
Idiopathic hypercalcemia syndrome
Rubella syndrome
Takayasu's arteritis
Neurofibromatosis
Effects of radiation therapy
Fibromuscular disease

eases that may be associated with abdominal aortic coarctation.

The disorder affects children and young adults. Although some reports indicate a female preponderance (with a ratio close to 1.8:1),[39, 99] other reports suggest that abdominal aortic coarctation occurs more commonly in males.[104] Symptoms include intermittent claudication, renovascular hypertension, and abdominal angina.

The coarctation is most frequently of the segmental type, involving the renal arteries in 35%, infrarenal aorta in 15%, and suprarenal aorta in 13% of patients.[99] Diffuse hypoplasia of the abdominal aorta is seen in 21% of patients. In the remainder, the hypoplasia involves only the infra- or suprarenal aorta. The aorta proximal to the coarctation often shows premature atherosclerosis and, rarely, aneurysms.[98, 105]

Arteriography demonstrates smooth segmental or diffuse narrowing of the abdominal aorta (Fig. 10–53). If the inferior mesenteric artery is not affected by the stenosis, it serves as a major collateral to the lower extremities.

## Neoplasms

Computed tomography (CT) and ultrasonography provide more sensitive methods than arteriography for the detection and staging of retroperitoneal and pelvic neoplasms.

**Retroperitoneal Neoplasms.** The main indications for arteriography of retroperitoneal tumors (exclusive of pancreatic, renal, and adrenal tumors) are:

1. Preoperative evaluation of tumor vascularity and source of tumor blood supply.

2. Evaluation of major vessel involvement (eg, inferior vena cava).

3. Preoperative embolization.

4. Catheter placement for chemotherapy.

An AP abdominal aortogram usually provides sufficient information regarding tumor vascularity and vascular supply (Fig. 10–54). If a transcatheter interventional procedure is anticipated, further definition of the vascular supply to the tumor may become necessary.

**Pelvic Neoplasms.** Tumors of the pelvis may be parietal (mesenchymal, musculoskeletal), neurogenic, or visceral. CT and ultra-

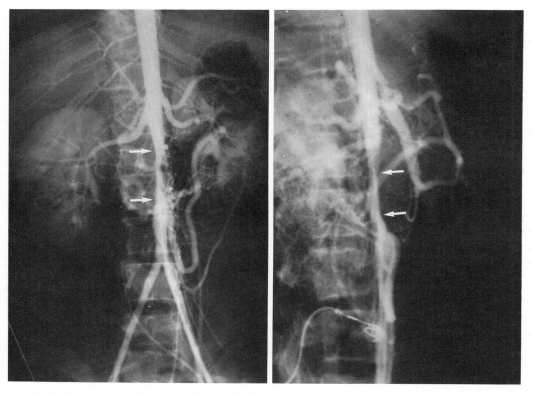

*Figure 10–53.* Abdominal aortic coarctation. AP (*left*) and lateral (*right*) aortogram in a teen-aged Oriental girl shows a smooth stenosis of the infrarenal aorta (*arrows*). The inferior mesenteric artery is enlarged as a result of collateral flow. In addition, numerous retroperitoneal collaterals are present.

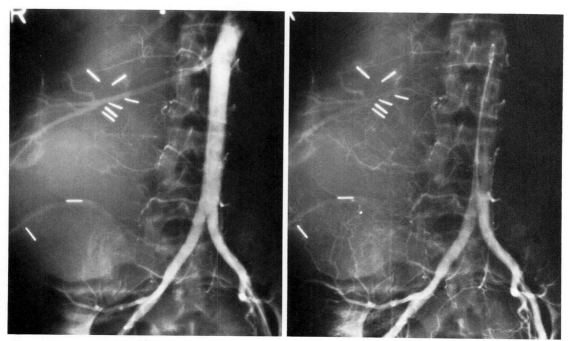

**Figure 10–54.** Retroperitoneal sarcoma. Early arterial (*left*) and parenchymal phase (*right*) from an AP aortogram shows a moderately vascular tumor that derives its blood supply from the lumbar, superior gluteal, and iliolumbar arteries. The right kidney has been displaced by the tumor.

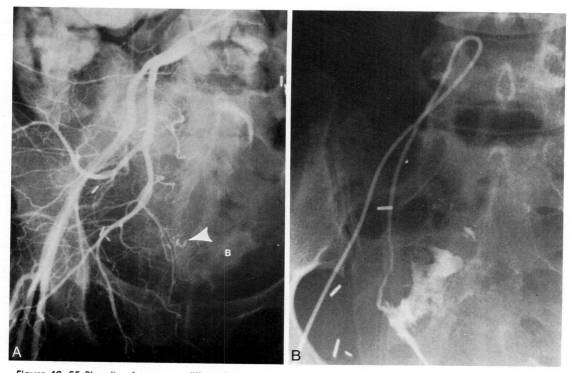

**Figure 10–55.** Bleeding from an undifferentiated mesenchymal pelvic tumor following radiation and chemotherapy. *A,* Right common iliac arteriogram shows a vascular tumor and contrast extravasation (*arrowhead*). The urinary bladder (B) has been displaced to the left. *B,* Selective catheterization of the bleeding vessel using the loop technique. Extensive contrast extravasation is seen. Bleeding was controlled by transcatheter embolization.

sonography are sensitive methods for the detection and staging of pelvic neoplasms. However, ultrasonography, unlike CT, is less useful for the evaluation of bladder tumors. Some authors have used the demonstration of neovascularity on arteriography for accurate staging of invasive pelvic neoplasms.[111, 112] In one report, the accuracy of arteriographic staging for T3B bladder cancer (extension of tumor into perivesical fat) was 87%; the sensitivity was 87% with a 95% specificity.[111] Despite this, arteriography is used infrequently for the purpose of staging.

The indications for arteriography of pelvic neoplasms are (Fig. 10–55):

1. Preoperative evaluation of tumor vascularity and source of tumor blood supply.

2. Evaluation of the inferior gluteal, inferior epigastric, and circumflex iliac arteries for a vascularized skin flap for closure after extensive resection.

3. Preoperative embolization.

4. Localization and treatment of postoperative or postbiopsy hemorrhage.[10, 113]

5. Placement of chemotherapy infusion catheters.

6. Management of intractable hemorrhage due to advanced malignancy or bleeding following chemotherapy or radiation therapy in patients with genitourinary tract neoplasms.

## Malignant Gestational Trophoblastic Disease

In approximately half the patients, malignant gestational trophoblastic disease develops after a molar pregnancy.[114] The diagnosis is made by determination of urinary or serum gonadotropin levels and is aided by ultrasonography.[115]

Arteriography may be indicated for:

1. Differentiation of gestational trophoblastic neoplasms from other gonadotropin-producing conditions in the presence of equivocal sonographic examination (eg, gonadotropin-producing anaplastic large cell carcinoma of the lung).[115–117]

2. Determination of extent of disease.

3. Transcatheter therapy.

Arteriography cannot be used for differentiating between invasive mole and choriocarcinoma.[118] Furthermore, it is not a reliable

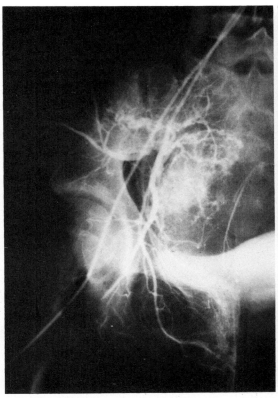
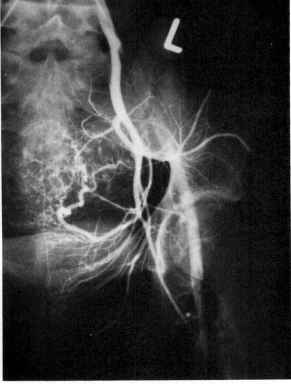

*Figure 10–56.* Left and right internal iliac arteriograms in a teen-aged girl with malignant gestational trophoblastic disease (see text for description of arteriographic findings).

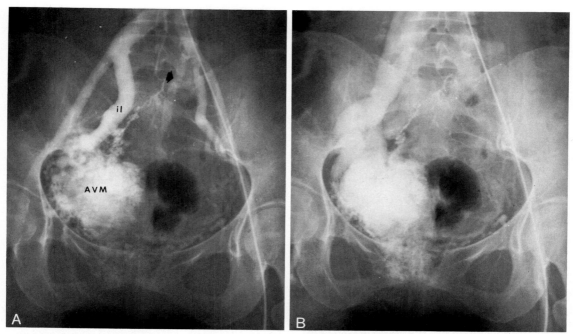

*Figure 10–57.* Arteriovenous malformation (AVM) of the pelvis. *A,* AP pelvic arteriogram shows a large AVM in the right hemipelvis. The right internal iliac (il) artery and inferior mesenteric artery (*arrow*) feed the AVM. Both vessels are enlarged markedly. *B,* Later film shows markedly enlarged draining iliac veins.

guide for assessment of success of chemotherapy, as the arteriographic abnormality may persist despite cure.[118, 119]

The arteriographic findings are (Fig. 10–56):

1. Enlargement of uterine, ovarian, and smaller myometrial arteries: This enlargement is often asymmetrical and represents a nonspecific finding.[118, 119]

2. Irregular vascular lakes.

3. Arteriovenous fistulae: These may persist even after successful chemotherapy.[119]

4. Inhomogeneous, irregular "tumor stain" with areas of relative avascularity.

According to some authors, this "stain" most likely represents increased vascularity in the actively growing segments of the tumor with the central avascular areas representing hemorrhage and fibrinoid material.[118] Not all trophoblastic tumors are hypervascular.

Arteriography may not be helpful for differentiating malignant trophoblastic disease from molar or normal pregnancy and from other vascular tumors.

## Vascular Malformations

Arteriography is the definitive diagnostic test for abdominal and pelvic vascular mal-

formations, which may be congenital or acquired. The latter can occur after blunt or penetrating trauma or following percutaneous biopsy or operation.[120]

Vascular malformations have a typical arteriographic appearance, demonstrating large tortuous arteries and veins (Fig. 10–57). Some lesions may demonstrate arteriovenous shunting. Occasionally, a neoplasm may also cause arteriovenous shunting and may thus simulate a vascular malformation (Fig. 10–58).

## Vasculogenic Impotence

In approximately 25% of affected individuals, impotence may have a vascular etiology.[121] Penile arterial pressure, which accurately reflects penile blood flow, can be assessed by measuring the Doppler-derived penile-arm index. In normal individuals, the systolic pressure in the dorsal artery of the penis is approximately 20 mm Hg lower than the pressure in the brachial artery.

Arteriography is indicated to exclude a vascular etiology for impotence by evaluating both large and small vessels. The large vessels are studied by AP and oblique pelvic arteriography (the oblique projection is used to evaluate the proximal internal iliac arteries)

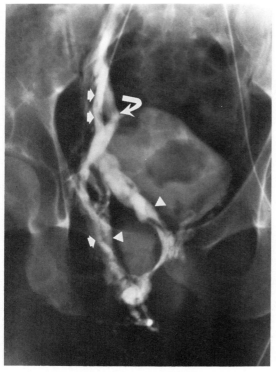

*Figure 10–58.* Arteriovenous shunting in a patient with Ewing's sarcoma of the pubic bone. Internal iliac arteriogram (*arrows*) shows early venous opacification (*arrowheads*). Curved arrow points to internal iliac vein.

(see Table 10–5). Internal pudendal arteriography is performed in the ipsilateral anterior oblique position, with the penis extended towards the contralateral thigh (see Table 10–9).

The vascular causes of impotence demonstrated by arteriography are:

1. Atherosclerotic large and small vessel disease (most common cause), eg, distal aortic occlusion, common iliac, internal iliac, or pudendal artery stenosis or occlusion (Fig. 10–59).

2. External iliac artery occlusion: pudendal steal.

3. Renal transplant: utilization of the remaining internal iliac artery for a second renal transplant.[122]

4. Internal pudendal artery trauma: pelvic fractures.

5. Operative ligation or transcatheter embolization of internal pudendal artery branches: This may be indicated for the management of trauma or priapism.[123]

## REFERENCES

1. Warwick R, Williams PL: The arteries of the trunk. *In* Warwick R, Williams PL (eds): Gray's Anatomy, 35th Ed. Philadelphia, WB Saunders, 1973, pp. 656–673.

2. Khademi M, Seebode JT, Falla A: Selective spermatic arteriography for localization of an impalpable undescended testis. Radiology 136:627–634, 1980.

3. Merland J-J, Chiras J: Arteriography of the Pelvis. Diagnostic and Therapeutic Procedures. New York, Springer Verlag, 1981.

4. Pirker E, Schmidberger H: Die Arteria Ischiadica. Eine seltene Gefässvariante. Fortschr Röntgenstr 116:434–437, 1972.

5. Senior HD: An interpretation of the recorded arterial anomalies of the human pelvis and thigh. Am J Anat 36:1–46, 1925.

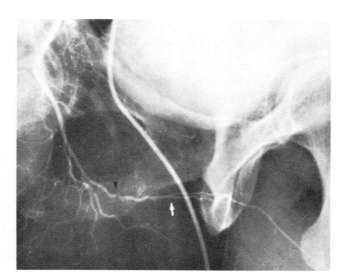

*Figure 10–59.* Vasculogenic impotence. Atherosclerotic occlusion of the deep artery and stenosis of the dorsal artery of the penis (*arrowhead*). Arrow points to bifurcation of the dorsal artery, which continues into the glans. (From Miller K et al: RadioGraphics 2:131, 1982. Used with permission.)

6. Nicholson RL, Pastershank SP, Bharadwaj BB: Persistent primitive sciatic artery. Radiology 122: 687–689, 1977.

7. Thomas ML, Blakeny CG, Browse NL: Arteriomegaly of persistent sciatic artery. Radiology 128: 55–56, 1978.

8. Conroy RM, Van der Molen RL: Scrotal "arteriocele" from iliac artery occlusion. AJR 127:670–672, 1976.

9. Siegel P, Mengert WF: Internal iliac artery ligation in obstetrics and gynecology. JAMA 178:1059–1062, 1961.

10. Kadir S, Athanasoulis CA: Angiographic diagnosis and control of postoperative bleeding. CRC Crit Rev Diag Imag 35–78, 1979.

11. Daoud A, Jarmolych J, Zumbo A, et al: Preatheroma phase of coronary atherosclerosis in man. Exp Mol Pathol 3:475–484, 1964.

12. Strong JP, Richards ML: Cigarette smoking and atherosclerosis in autopsied men. Atherosclerosis 23:451–476, 1976.

13. Juergens JL, Barker NW, Hines EA Jr: Arteriosclerosis obliterans: review of 520 cases with special reference to pathogenic and prognostic factors. Circulation 21:188–195, 1960.

14. Bell ET: Incidence of gangrene of the extremities in nondiabetic and in diabetic persons. Arch Pathol 49:469–473, 1950.

15. Bell JW: Acute thrombosis of the subrenal abdominal aorta. Arch Surg 95:681–684, 1967.

16. Boukhris R, Becker KL: Calcification of the aorta and osteoporosis. JAMA 219:1307–1311, 1972.

17. Simon H, Fairbank JT: Biplane translumbar aortography for evaluation of peripheral vascular disease. Am J Surg 133:447–452, 1977.

18. Edwards EA, LeMay M: Occlusion patterns and collaterals in arteriosclerosis of the lower aorta and iliac arteries. Surgery 38:950–963, 1955.

19. Muller RF, Figley MM: The arteries of the abdomen, pelvis and thigh. I. Normal roentgenographic anatomy. II. Collateral circulation in obstructive arterial disease. AJR 77:296–311, 1957.

20. Raaf JH, Shannon J: Atherosclerotic coarctation of the abdominal aorta in women. Surg Gynecol Obstet 150:715–720, 1980.

21. Sequeira JC, Beckmann CF, Levin DC: Suprarenal aortic occlusion. AJR 132:773–776, 1979.

22. Lipchick E, Rob CG, Schwartzberg S: Obstruction of abdominal aorta above the level of renal arteries. Radiology 82:443–445, 1964.

23. Starrett RW, Stoney RJ: Juxta-renal aortic occlusion. Surgery 76:890–897, 1974.

24. Johnson JK: Ascending thrombosis of abdominal aorta as fatal complication of Leriche's syndrome. Arch Surg 69:663–668, 1954.

25. Loose KE: Die Aortographie in der Diagnostik peripherer Gefässleiden. Quoted by Felson B: Translumbar arteriography in intrinsic disease of the abdominal aorta and its branches. AJR 72:597–608, 1954.

26. Staple TW, Friedenberg MJ, Anderson MS, et al: Arteria magna et dolicho of Leriche. Acta Radiol Diag 4:297–305, 1966.

27. Randall PA, Omar MM, Rohner R, et al: Arteria magna revisited. Radiology 132:295–300, 1979.

28. Carlson DH, Gryska P, Seletz J, et al: Arteriomegaly. AJR 125:553–558, 1975.

29. Leriche R, Morel A: The syndrome of thrombosis of the aortic bifurcation. Ann Surg 127:193–206, 1948.

30. Johnson JM, Gaspar MR, Movius HJ, et al: Sudden complete thrombosis of aortic and iliac aneurysms. Arch Surg 108:792–794, 1974.

31. Fairbairn JF II, Joyce JW, Pairolero PC: Acute arterial occlusion of the extremities. In Juergens JL, Spittell JA, Fairbairn JF II (eds): Peripheral Vascular Diseases. Philadelphia, WB Saunders, 1982, pp. 381–401.

32. Kemeny MM, Martin EC, Lane FC, et al: Abdominal distention and aortic obstruction associated with phenothiazines. JAMA 243:683–684, 1980.

33. Shapiro ME, Rodvien R, Bauer KA, et al: Acute aortic thrombosis in antithrombin III deficiency. JAMA 245:1759–1761, 1981.

34. Meister SG, Grossman W, Dexter L, et al: Paradoxical embolism: diagnosis during life. Am J Med 53:292–298, 1972.

35. Thompson T, Evans W: Paradoxical embolism. Q J Med 23:135–150, 1930.

36. Sniderman KW, Sos TA, Gay WA Jr, et al: Aortic dissection beginning in the abdomen. AJR 130:1115–1118, 1978.

37. Burch GE, DePasquale N: Quoted in reference 36.

38. Weston TS, Ardagh JW: Infrarenal dissection of the aorta. NZ Med J 82:302–304, 1975.

39. Riemenschneider TA, Emmanouilides GC, Hirose F, et al: Coarctation of the abdominal aorta in children: Report of three cases and review of the literature. Pediatrics 44:716–726, 1969.

40. Walter JF, Stanley JC, Mehigan JT, et al: External iliac artery fibroplasia. AJR 131:125–128, 1978.

41. Wylie EJ, Brinkley FM, Palubinskas AJ: Extrarenal fibromuscular hyperplasia. Am J. Surg 112:149–155, 1966.

42. Stanley JC, Gewertz BL, Bove EL, et al: Arterial fibroplasia: Histopathologic character and current etiologic concepts. Arch Surg 110:561–566, 1975.

43. Mehigan JT, Stoney RJ: Arterial microemboli and fibromuscular dysplasia of the external iliac arteries. Surgery 81:484–486, 1977.

44. Chait A: The internal mammary artery: an overlooked collateral pathway to the leg. Radiology 121:621–624, 1976.

45. Estes JR Jr: Abdominal aortic aneurysm: a study of one hundred and two cases. Circulation 2:258–264, 1950.

46. Rösch J, Keller FS, Porter JM, et al: Value of angiography in the management of abdominal aortic aneurysm. Cardiovasc Radiol 1:83–94, 1978.

47. Steinberg I: Isolated arteriosclerotic aneurysm of a common iliac artery. Report of three cases. AJR 90:166–168, 1963.

48. McCready RA, Pairolero PC, Gilmore JC, et al: Isolated iliac artery aneurysms. Surgery 93:688–693, 1983.

49. Kasulke RJ, Clifford A, Nichols WK, et al: Isolated atherosclerotic aneurysms of the internal iliac arteries. Report of two cases and review of the literature. Arch Surg 117:73–77, 1982.

50. Clees A, Awender R: Kindskopfgrosses Aneurysma der Arteria iliaca communis sinistra. Fortschr Röntgenstr 128:92–93, 1978.

51. Szilagyi DE, Smith RF, Elliott JP, et al: Anastomotic aneurysms after vascular reconstruction: problems of, incidence, etiology and treatment. Surgery 78:800–816, 1975.

52. Bernstein EF, Dilley RB, Goldberger LE, et al: Growth rates of small abdominal aortic aneurysms. Surgery 80:765–773, 1976.

53. Crane C: Arteriosclerotic aneurysm of the abdom-

inal aorta: some pathological and clinical correlations. N Engl J Med 253:954–958, 1955.

54. Rose JS, Hotson WC, Levin DC: Abdominal aortic aneurysm in childhood. A noninvasive approach to the diagnosis. AJR 123:708–711, 1975.

55. Walker DI, Bloor K, Williams G, et al: Inflammatory aneurysms of the abdominal aorta. Br J Surg 59:609–614, 1972.

56. Marty AT, Webb TA, Subbs KG, et al: Inflammatory abdominal aortic aneurysm infected by *Campylobacter fetus*. JAMA 249:1190–1192, 1983.

57. Kadir S, Athanasoulis CA, Brewster DC, et al: Tender pulsatile abdominal mass. Abdominal aortic aneurysm or not? Arch Surg 115:631–633, 1980.

58. Robicsek F, Daugherty HK, Mullen DC, et al: The value of angiography in the diagnosis of unruptured aneurysms of the abdominal aorta. Ann Thorac Surg 11:538–550, 1971.

59. May AG, DeWeese JA, Frank I, et al: Surgical treatment of abdominal aortic aneurysms. Surgery 63:711–721, 1968.

60. Hertzer NR, Beven EG: Ultrasound aortic measurement and elective aneurysmectomy. JAMA 240:1966–1968, 1978.

61. Anderson JC, Baltaxe HA, Wolf GL: Inability to show clot: One limitation of ultrasonography of the abdominal aorta. Radiology 132:693–696, 1979.

62. Leopold GR, Goldberger LE, Bernstein EF: Ultrasonic detection and evaluation of abdominal aortic aneurysms. Surgery 72:939–945, 1972.

63. Brown OW, Stanson W, Pairolero PC, et al: Computerized tomography following abdominal aortic surgery. Surgery 97:716–722, 1982.

64. Nichols GB, Schilling PJ: Pseudo-retroperitoneal gas in rupture of aneurysm of abdominal aorta. AJR 125:134–137, 1975.

65. Janower ML: Ruptured arteriosclerotic aneurysms of the abdominal aorta. Roentgenographic findings on plain films. N Engl J Med 265:12–15, 1961.

66. Brewster DC, Retana A, Waltman AC, et al: Angiography in the management of aneurysms of the abdominal aorta. Its value and safety. N Engl J Med 292:822–825, 1975.

67. Ottinger LW, Darling RC, Nathan MJ, et al: Left colon ischemia complicating aorto-iliac reconstruction. Causes, diagnosis, management and prevention. Arch Surg 105:841–846, 1972.

68. Johnson WC, Nabseth DC: Visceral infarction following aortic surgery. Ann Surg 180:312–318, 1974.

69. Gliedman ML, Ayers WB, Vestal BL: Aneurysms of the abdominal aorta and its branches: a study of untreated patients. Ann Surg 146:207–214, 1957.

70. Beall AC, Cooley DA, Morris GC, et al: Perforation of arteriosclerotic aneurysms into inferior vena cava. Arch Surg 86:809–818, 1963.

71. Ala-Ketola L, Kärkölä P, Koivisto E: Aorto-caval fistula as complication of abdominal aortic aneurysm. A case report. Fortschr Röntgenstr 128:93–94, 1978.

72. Johnson JM, Gaspar MR, Movius HJ, et al: Sudden complete thrombosis of aortic and iliac aneurysms. Arch Surg 108:792–794, 1974.

73. Costandi YT, Gates WH, Khan JA, et al: Abdominal aortic aneurysm presenting as retroperitoneal fibrosis. Urology 11:74–76, 1978.

74. Roehm EF, Twiest MW, Williams RC Jr: Abdominal aortic thrombosis in association with an attempted Heimlich maneuver. JAMA 249:1186–1187, 1983.

75. Lord JW, Rossi G, Daliana M, et al: Unsuspected abdominal aortic aneurysms as the cause of peripheral arterial occlusive disease. Ann Surg 177:767–771, 1973.

76. Gore I, Hirst AE Jr: Arteriosclerotic aneurysms of the abdominal aorta. A review. Prog Cardiovasc Dis 16:113–150, 1973.

77. Szilagyi DE, Smith RF, DeRusso FJ, et al: Contribution of abdominal aortic aneurysmectomy to prolongation of life. Ann Surg 164:678–698, 1966.

78. Darling RC, Messina CR, Brewster DC, et al: Autopsy study of unoperated abdominal aortic aneurysms. Circulation 56(Suppl 2):161–164, 1977.

79. Baker AG, Roberts B: Longterm survival following abdominal aortic aneurysmectomy. JAMA 212:445–450, 1970.

80. Ottinger LW: Ruptured arteriosclerotic aneurysms of the abdominal aorta. Reducing mortality. JAMA 233:147–150, 1975.

81. Williams RD, Yurko AA Jr: Controversial aspects of diagnosis and management of blunt abdominal trauma. Am J Surg 111:477–482, 1966.

82. Wilson CB, Vidrine A Jr, Rives JD: Unrecognized abdominal trauma in patients with head injuries. Ann Surg 161:608–613, 1965.

83. Parmley LF, Mattingly TW, Manion WC: Nonpenetrating traumatic injury of the aorta. Circulation 17:1086–1101, 1958.

84. Strassman G: Traumatic rupture of the aorta. Am Heart J 33:508–515, 1947.

85. Mozingo JR, Denton IC: The neurological deficit associated with sudden occlusion of the abdominal aorta due to blunt trauma. Surgery 77:118–125, 1975.

86. Spirt BA, Skolnick L, Carsky EW, et al: Anterior displacement of the abdominal aorta. A radiographic and sonographic study. Radiology 111:399–403, 1974.

87. Rothenberger DA, Fischer RP, Strate RG: The mortality associated with pelvic fractures. Surgery 84:356–361, 1978.

88. Rothenberger D, Velasco R, Strate R, et al: Open pelvic fracture: a lethal injury. J Trauma 18:184–187, 1978.

89. Matalon T, Athanasoulis CA, Margolies MN, et al: Pelvic fractures with hemorrhage: Efficacy of transcatheter embolization. AJR 133:859–864, 1979.

90. Burchell RC: Arterial physiology of the human pelvis. Obstet Gynecol 31:855–860, 1968.

91. Patterson FP, Morton KS: The cause of death in fractures of the pelvis: with a note on treatment by ligation of the hypogastric (internal iliac) artery. J Trauma 13:849–856, 1973.

92. Pearl FL: Electric shock. Presentation of cases and review of the literature. Arch Surg 27:227–249, 1933.

93. Warren S: Effects of radiation on normal tissues. IV: Effects of radiation on the cardiovascular system. Arch Pathol 43:1070–1079, 1942.

94. Thomas E, Forbus WD: Irradiation injury to the aorta and the lung. Arch Pathol 67:256–263, 1959.

95. Aust JC, Bredenberg CE, Murray DG: Mechanisms of arterial injury associated with total hip replacement. Arch Surg 116:345–349, 1981.

96. Brewster DC, May ARL, Darling RC, et al: Variable manifestations of vascular injury during lumbar disc surgery. Arch Surg 114:1026–1030, 1979.

97. Wood P: Diseases of the heart and circulation.

Quoted by DeBakey ME, Garrett HE, Howell JF, et al: Coarctation of the abdominal aorta with renal artery stenosis: surgical considerations. Ann Surg 165:830–843, 1967.

98. Maycock WA: Congenital stenosis of the abdominal aorta. Am Heart J 13:633–646, 1937.

99. Ben-Shoshan M, Rossi NP, Korns ME: Coarctation of the abdominal aorta. Arch Pathol 95:221–225, 1973.

100. Ueda H, Morooka S, Ito I, et al: Clinical observations of 52 cases of aortitis syndrome. Jap Heart J 10:277–288, 1969.

101. Sen PK, Kinare SG, Engineer SD, et al: The middle aortic syndrome. Br Heart J 25:610–618, 1963.

102. Isaacson C: An idiopathic aortitis in young Africans. J Pathol Bacteriol 81:69–79, 1961.

103. Roberts WC, MacGregor RR, DeBlanc HJ Jr, et al: The prepulseless disease, or pulseless disease with pulses. Am J Med 46:313–324, 1969.

104. Scott HW Jr, Dean RH, Boerth R, et al: Coarctation of the abdominal aorta: pathophysiologic and therapeutic considerations. Ann Surg 189:746–757, 1979.

105. Baird RJ, Evans JR, Labrosse CL: Coarctation of the abdominal aorta. Arch Surg 89:466–474, 1964.

106. Fortuin NJ, Morrow AG, Roberts WC: Late vascular manifestations of the rubella syndrome. A roentgenolographic-pathologic study. Am J Med 51: 134–140, 1971.

107. Colquhoun J: Hypoplasia of the abdominal aorta following therapeutic irradiation in infancy. Radiology 86:454–456, 1966.

108. Doberneck RC, Varco RL: Congenital coarctation of the abdominal aorta. J Lancet 88:143–150, 1968.

109. Blitznak J, Bargainer JD: Coarctation of the abdominal aorta with aneurysms of the middle cerebral artery. AJR 122:29–31, 1974.

110. Siassi B, Klyman G, Emmanouilides GC: Hypoplasia of the abdominal aorta associated with rubella syndrome. Am J Dis Child 120:476–479, 1970.

111. Lang EK: Angiography in the diagnosis and staging of pelvic neoplasms. Radiology 134:353–358, 1980.

112. Braedel HU, Krautzun K: Die Gefässdarstellung bösartiger Harnblasen Geschwülste unter besonderer Berücksichtigung ihrer örtlicher Ausbreitung. Fortschr Röntgenstr 100:209–214, 1964.

113. Lang EK: Transcatheter embolization of pelvic vessels for control of intractable hemorrhage. Radiology 140:331–339, 1981.

114. Jacobs EM, Johnson FD: Gestational choriocarcinoma. Oncology 26:231–237, 1972.

115. Levin DC, Staiano S, Schneider M, et al: Complementary role of sonography and arteriography in the management of uterine choriocarcinoma. AJR 125:462–468, 1975.

116. Fusco FD, Rosen SW: Gonadotropin-producing anaplastic large cell carcinomas of the lung. N Engl J Med 275:507–515, 1966.

117. Shimkin PM, vanThiel DH, Ross GT: Selective hypogastric arteriography in uterine choriocarcinoma. AJR 111:535–540, 1971.

118. Brewis RAL, Bagshawe KD: Pelvic arteriography in invasive trophoblastic neoplasia. Br J Radiol 41: 481–495, 1968.

119. Cockshott WP, de V Hendrickse JP: Persistent arteriovenous fistulae following chemotherapy of malignant trophoblastic disease. Radiology 88: 329–333, 1967.

120. Gaylis H, Levine E, vanDorgen LGR, et al: Arteriovenous fistulae after gynecologic operations. Surg Gynecol Obstet 137:655–658, 1973.

121. Miller K, Kaplan L, Weitzman AF, et al: The radiology of male impotence. Radiographics 2: 131–152, 1982.

122. Gittes RF, Waters WB: Sexual impotence: the overlooked complication of a second renal transplant. J Urol 121:719–720, 1979.

123. Wheeler GW, Simmons CR: Angiography in post-traumatic priapism. A case report. AJR 119:619–620, 1973.

# Arteriography of the Lower Extremity Vessels

## ANATOMY

**Common Femoral Artery** (Fig. 11–1). Distal to the inguinal ligament, the external iliac artery continues as the common femoral artery. It is best palpated immediately below the inguinal ligament because of its superficial location in this region, lying anterior to the psoas major tendon.[1] This region, also called the femoral triangle, provides the most appropriate location for percutaneous puncture and compression. The common femoral artery is flanked laterally by the femoral nerve and medially by the femoral vein. Further distally, the vein lies posterior to the artery.[1] Thus, a low needle puncture is more likely to traverse both artery and vein. A small nerve, the femoral branch of the genitofemoral nerve, accompanies the common femoral artery.

Major branches of the common femoral artery are:

1. The superficial iliac circumflex artery: Occasionally, this vessel has a common origin with the superficial epigastric artery. It anastomoses with the deep iliac circumflex, superior gluteal, and lateral femoral circumflex arteries. This artery is frequently used for microvascular free tissue transfer in the management of bone tumors.[2]

2. One or two external pudendal arteries.

**Profunda Femoris Artery** (Fig. 11–2). This vessel arises posterolaterally from the common femoral artery approximately 4 cm be-

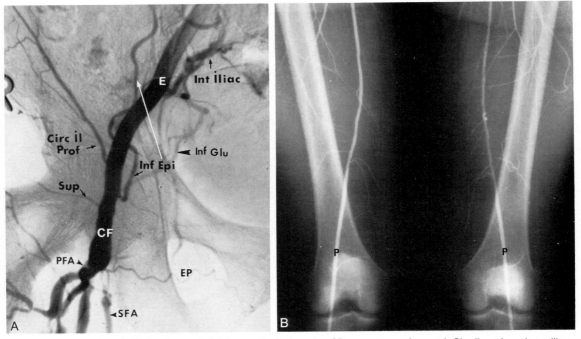

**Figure 11–1.** *A,* Iliac; *B,* Bilateral superficial femoral arteriogram. CF = common femoral; Circ il prof = deep iliac circumflex; E = external iliac; Ep = external pudendal; Inf epi = inferior epigastric; Inf Glu = inferior gluteal; Int Iliac = internal iliac; P = popliteal; PFA = profunda femoral; SFA = superficial femoral; Sup = superficial iliac circumflex arteries.

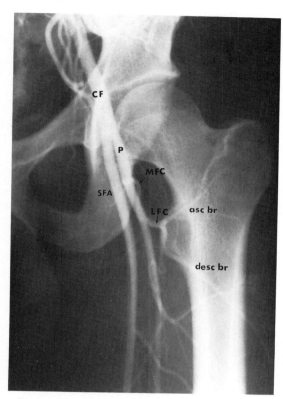

**Figure 11–2.** Common femoral arteriogram demonstrating the branches of the profunda femoris artery (P). CF = common femoral; LFC = lateral femoral circumflex; asc br = ascending branch of LFC; desc br = descending branch of LFC; MFC = medial femoral circumflex; SFA = superficial femoral arteries.

low the inguinal ligament.[3] It often lies posterior to the superficial femoral artery.

Major branches of the profunda femoris artery are:

1. The medial femoral circumflex artery. Branches from this artery anastomose with those of the gluteal and obturator arteries.

2. The lateral femoral circumflex artery. This divides into three branches: large ascending and descending branches and a small transverse branch. The descending branch serves as an important collateral to the lower extremity in occlusion of the superficial femoral artery. Occasionally, one or both femoral circumflex arteries may arise directly from the superficial femoral artery.

3. Muscular branches.

**Superficial Femoral Artery (SFA)** (see Fig. 11–1). After giving off the profunda femoris, the common femoral artery continues along the anterior medial aspect of the thigh as the superficial femoral artery. It gives off several unnamed muscular branches and the de-

scending genicular artery before entering the adductor canal. Rarely, the proximal SFA may divide into two trunks, which reunite at the adductor canal.[1] If a sciatic artery is present, the SFA is absent.

**Popliteal Artery** (Fig. 11–3). The popliteal artery begins distal to the adductor canal and continues into the calf through the popliteal fossa between the lateral and medial heads of the gastrocnemius muscle. It lies ventromedial to the popliteal vein. At its terminal portion, the popliteal artery bifurcates into the anterior and posterior tibial arteries. Rarely, a trifurcation is present. Occasionally, the bifurcation occurs proximally, at the level of the knee joint space or even higher.

Major branches of the popliteal artery are the:

1. Superior genicular arteries (lateral and medial).

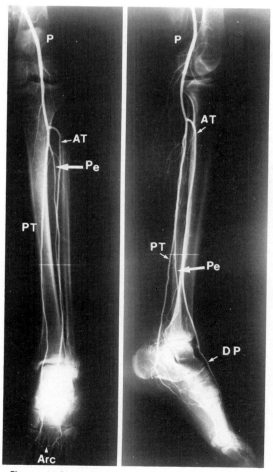

**Figure 11–3.** AP (*left*) and lateral (*right*) distal lower extremity arteriograms. Arc = arcuate; AT = anterior tibial; DP = dorsalis pedis; P = popliteal; Pe = peroneal; PT = posterior tibial arteries.

2. Medial genicular artery.

3. Inferior genicular arteries (lateral and medial).

4. Anterior tibial artery: This artery passes through the interosseous membrane, lying medial to the fibular neck, and descends anterior to the interosseous membrane, along the medial border of the fibula. In the distal leg, it moves towards the midline and continues into the foot as the dorsalis pedis artery.

5. Posterior tibial artery: Approximately 2 to 3 cm from its origin at the popliteal bifurcation, the posterior tibial artery gives off the peroneal artery. The posterior tibial artery continues into the foot, passing behind the medial malleolus, and divides into the lateral and medial plantar arteries.

Occasionally, the peroneal artery may arise from the popliteal artery, and rarely it may be larger than the posterior tibial artery. At the ankle, the peroneal artery terminates, giving off a communicating branch, which anastomoses with the posterior tibial artery, and a perforating branch, which anastomoses with the anterior lateral malleolar artery from the anterior tibial artery.

The genicular, peroneal, and tibial arteries and the descending branch of the lateral femoral circumflex artery contribute to the formation of an intricate anastomotic arterial network around the knee. This provides collateral circulation for the distal lower extremity in occlusive diseases of the superficial femoral and popliteal arteries.

**Arteries Around the Ankle and Foot** (Fig. 11–4). The dorsalis pedis artery gives off the arcuate artery, which anastomoses with the lateral tarsal artery to form a type of dorsal arch. A true superficial plantar arch does not exist.[3] The dorsal metatarsal arteries arise from the arcuate and the dorsalis pedis arteries.

The plantar arch is formed by the lateral plantar artery and the deep plantar branch of the dorsalis pedis artery. It is convex distally and lies beneath the metatarsal bones, extending from the base of the fifth to the proximal third of the first metatarsal bone. The arch gives off four plantar metatarsal arteries and several perforating vessels. The latter anastomose with the dorsal metatarsal arteries. Each metatarsal artery gives rise to two plantar digital arteries. A rich collateral network, similar to the one around the knee, also exists around both malleoli and the calcaneus.[3]

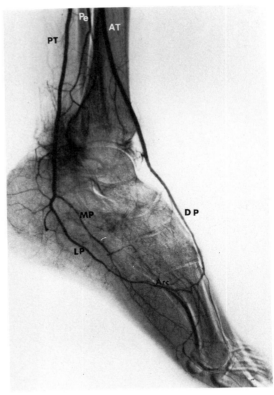

*Figure 11–4.* Arterial anatomy of the ankle and foot. Arc = arcuate; AT = anterior tibial; DP = dorsalis pedis; LP = lateral plantar; MP = medial plantar; Pe = peroneal; PT = posterior tibial arteries.

## Anatomical Variants

**Femoral Artery** (Fig. 11–5)

1. The common femoral and superficial femoral arteries may be absent in 0.14% of normal individuals. In such persons there is a persistence of the sciatic artery.[4]

2. Rarely, the SFA may be duplicated.

**Popliteal Artery** (Fig. 11–6)

1. A high bifurcation of the popliteal artery occurs in approximately 4% of individuals.[5]

2. A high bifurcation of the popliteal artery with the peroneal artery arising from the anterior tibial artery is observed in close to 2% of individuals.[5]

3. The popliteal artery may bifurcate into a peroneal and an anterior tibial artery.[1]

4. The posterior tibial artery is absent in 1 to 5% of individuals.[5, 6]

5. A trifurcation of the popliteal artery occurs in 0.4% of individuals.[5]

**Arteries of the Ankle and Foot.** Although the posterior tibial artery pulse is always present in the absence of clinically mani-

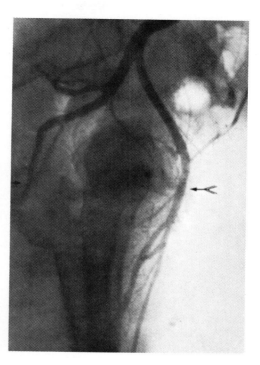

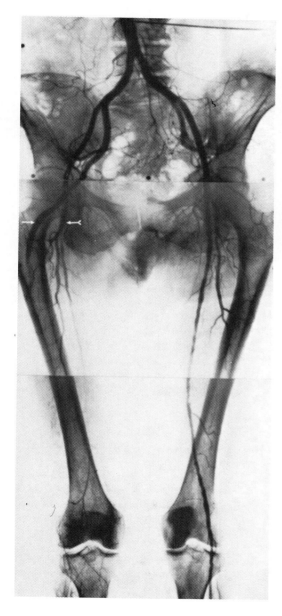

*Figure 11–5.* Persistent sciatic artery. AP pelvis and lateral right iliac arteriograms show a persistent sciatic artery on the right side (*arrow*). *Triple arrow* points to the femoral artery. There is atherosclerotic occlusion of the distal sciatic artery. (From Pirker E, Schmidberger H: Fortschr Roentgenstr 116:434–437, 1972. Stuttgart, Georg Thieme Verlag. Used with permission.)

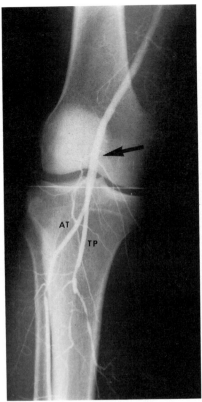

*Figure 11–6.* High bifurcation of the popliteal artery (*arrow*). There is atherosclerotic occlusive disease involving the anterior tibial artery (AT) and the tibioperoneal trunk (TP).

fested occlusive vascular disease,[7] the proximal posterior tibial artery may be absent, with the peroneal artery reconstituting the distal posterior tibial artery at the ankle.[5] The dorsalis pedis pulse may be absent because of hypoplasia or aplasia of the anterior tibial artery, which is observed in 4 to 12% of individuals.[6, 7] In another 8% of individuals, the dorsalis pedis artery has an anomalous location.[6]

## Development of Collateral Circulation

The development of arterial collaterals in response to an obstruction occurs in two phases:

1. In one phase, preexisting underutilized communications enlarge spontaneously in response to an acute occlusion.[8, 9] Laboratory experiments and clinical observation have shown that such a collateral circulation goes into effect within minutes of occlusion.[10]

2. The other phase involves a slower and more complex process, which develops over weeks or months and is responsible for the improvement of the collateral circulation.

**Stimulus for Development.** The stimulus for the development of arterial collaterals may come from several factors, which probably act in combination, ie, the pressure gradient above and below the obstruction, the degree of vasodilatation of the distal vessels, and the possible effects of metabolites accumulating in the ischemic tissue.

1. Pressure gradient: The presence of a pressure gradient across an obstruction in a main artery is probably the single most important factor responsible for the opening of collateral channels immediately after an occlusion has occurred.[8, 11] However, since the resting pressure gradient decreases shortly after collateral circulation has been established, it does not contribute to the growth of these collaterals over the ensuing months.[8] Intermittent muscular activity causes a decrease in the arterial pressure distal to an obstruction, thereby increasing the pressure gradient and thus providing a stimulus for the growth of collaterals. Exercise-induced fall in peripheral arterial pressure is also observed in normal individuals.

After acute occlusion of the femoral artery, the blood flow falls to zero initially, but within 30 minutes it reaches 30% of the preocclusion flow, and within 90 minutes it increases to approximately 80% of the preocclusion flow.[8] A similar response occurs with the blood pressure.

2. Vasodilatation: Vasodilatation in the vessels distal to the obstruction augments blood flow through the collaterals.[12] The mechanism involved may have a neurovascular basis.[10, 13]

3. Accumulation of metabolites: The accumulation of metabolites in the ischemic tissue is also considered responsible for vasodilatation.[12]

**Growth of Existing Collaterals.** Passive enlargement of collateral channels occurs in the immediate post-obstruction period. Later, the collateral vessels enlarge by means of active growth, which may extend over several months.[14, 15]

**Efficiency of the Collateral Circulation.** The volume of blood flow reaching the circulation distal to an obstruction is determined by the capacity of the collaterals. Regardless of their number and size, collaterals are, for the most part, inefficient substitutes for the normal vascular channels. They may provide sufficient blood flow at rest, but the increased demand during exercise gives rise to symptoms, indicating the limits of their capacity.

Evaluation of the efficiency or adequacy of the collateral circulation on the basis of an arteriogram may not be possible. However, in general, fewer large vessels provide a more efficient collateral system than numerous small vessels.

In addition to size and number, other factors that influence the efficiency of the collateral circulation are the length and location of the arterial occlusion and the time required for the collaterals to develop fully.[15] In general, the more distal the occlusion on the extremity, the less efficient the collateral system.

Relief of the obstruction (eg, after transluminal angioplasty) leads to the disappearance and subsequent regression of the collateral vessels, which occurs almost as quickly as their appearance following obstruction.

## ARTERIOGRAPHIC TECHNIQUES

Evaluation of peripheral vascular disease due to occlusive atherosclerosis is the most common indication for arteriography of the lower extremities. Since atherosclerosis is a generalized disease, the inflow vessels, ie, the distal abdominal aorta and iliac arteries, must also be evaluated in all patients.

### Types of Studies

The lower extremities can be studied by the retrograde femoral, translumbar, or axillary artery approach or by intravenous digital subtraction angiography (DSA). Intraarterial DSA can also be used in conjunction with standard arteriography and provides an excellent means for evaluating the distal circulation (lower calf and foot). Both lower extremities should be studied, since most diseases are bilateral. Single leg arteriograms are indicated for disorders limited to the one side, such as arterial trauma, embolic occlusion, or amputation of the contralateral extremity.

**Femoral Approach.** Retrograde femoral artery puncture is performed, and a 65 cm 5 or 6 Fr pigtail catheter is placed in the distal abdominal aorta for an AP arteriogram of the lower extremities.

For the sake of convenience, most vascular radiologists use the right femoral artery (for arterial puncture) if the pulse is not significantly diminished. As a rule, the femoral artery with the better pulse should be used, unless both femoral artery pulses are equal. A bruit in the presence of a good femoral pulse should not be a deterrent to puncturing the vessel. However, in this situation additional precautions must be taken to avoid subintimal passage of the guide wire.

For selective arteriography, eg, antegrade arteriography, the contralateral femoral artery puncture is preferable. From the ipsilateral side, either the loop technique is used if there is no significant ipsilateral iliac artery disease or an antegrade femoral artery puncture is performed. With the antegrade puncture, the study is limited to one extremity.

**Translumbar Approach.** From a low (L2) or high (T12) lumbar aortic puncture, the catheter is directed caudad. The tip is positioned at least 3 cm above the aortic bifurcation. This distance is necessary to prevent subintimal injection and dissection from the catheter end hole jet or selective contrast injection into one common iliac artery.

**Axillary Approach.** From the left or right axillary approach, a 100 cm 5 or 6 Fr pigtail catheter is placed at the aortic bifurcation.

**DSA.** Intraarterial DSA provides a method for outpatient evaluation to survey the peripheral vascular tree. On the other hand, intravenous DSA provides a less invasive method for the focused evaluation of peripheral vascular disease in outpatients. With the latter, in some cases conventional arteriography or intraarterial DSA may be required for confirmation of the arterial abnormality prior to operation or an interventional procedure.

### Contrast Injection

Blood flow in the aorta varies with the age of the patient, tortuosity and diameter of the aorta, cardiac output, and presence and severity of atheromatous disease. Thus, the rate of contrast injection must be individualized on the basis of the test injection. It is a misconception that high injection rates (>12 ml/sec) provide better lower extremity arteriograms in all patients. Although such a contrast injection rate will no doubt provide excellent opacification of the peripheral vascular tree in younger individuals with high blood flow velocity, in older individuals, such as patients with arteriomegaly or severe atherosclerotic occlusive disease, a high rate will result in proximal reflux and loss of contrast medium in other circulations, such as the kidneys. In addition, increased mixing of the contrast medium with blood will result in poorer opacification of distal vessels.

In younger individuals with fast blood flow, the contrast injection rate should be between 8 and 12 ml/sec. In older individuals, the appropriate contrast injection rate is between 6 and 8 ml/sec. In an average-sized patient, the minimal volume of contrast medium necessary for a good bilateral lower extremity arteriogram is 60 ml. Our experience suggests that a total contrast volume of 60 to 70 ml provides the best arteriograms. A smaller volume of contrast medium provides incomplete opacification of the distal vessels, which may either result in the erroneous diagnosis of a stenosis[16] or obscure a stenosis as a result of incomplete opacification.[17] For a single leg arteriogram (contrast injection into the common or external iliac artery), 35 to 40 ml of contrast medium is injected at 6 to 8 ml/sec.

Either 60 or 76% contrast medium can be used. However, the 76% contrast medium provides better arterial opacification and patient discomfort is not significantly increased. Moreover, if 2 mg of lidocaine is added per ml of contrast medium, the discomfort associated with arteriography is reduced very significantly.

**Phasic Contrast Injection.** Contrast medium may be injected as either a single or a biphasic injection. During single phase injection, a predetermined volume of contrast medium is injected at one predetermined flow rate, eg, 10 ml/sec for a total volume of 70 ml.

Biphasic contrast injection can be performed manually[18] or with the aid of a specially designed injector (Medrad Mark IV with Universal Flow Module, FMO 965), which is programmed to inject as follows:

First phase: 8 ml/sec for 48 ml total.
Second phase: 12 ml/sec for 36 ml total.

Intraarterial injection of contrast medium provides a dose-dependent vasodilatation of the skin and musculature.[19, 20] Thus, the use of larger volumes of contrast medium may contribute to the enhanced visualization of distal vessels. The biphasic technique utilizes vasodilatation induced by the first phase of the contrast injection. A higher contrast injection rate is required during the second phase in order to adjust to the increased blood flow. In our own experience, the bi-

phasic injection technique offers no advantages over a conventional high volume arteriogram.

### Filming

**Stepping Table.** With this system, between four and five filming positions are programmed (Table 11–1). Scout films should be obtained prior to contrast injection to confirm appropriate patient positioning and filming techniques.

When calculating the filming delay for this technique, it must be kept in mind that each table shift requires 1 second. If reactive hyperemia is used, the filming delay is decreased to 1 second.

If a section of the vascular tree is inadequately visualized, a stationary or an abbreviated run (eg, two steps) can be performed for demonstration of the area of interest, after calculation of the appropriate filming delay. The filming can also be prolonged over the distal lower extremity by filming at one film every other second.

**Long Film Changers.** Long film changers for extra-large field angiography utilize three films end to end in a long cassette (14 by 51 inch). These permit evaluation of the entire lower extremity on each set of films. The films can be exposed only at one film/sec.

Filming is timed to coincide with the appearance of the contrast medium in the popliteal artery, but at least 2 seconds before

**TABLE 11–1. Program for Lower Extremity Arteriography With a Stepping Table Top**

| | |
|---|---|
| Total number of films | 19 |
| Filming rate | 1 film per second |
| Filming delay* | 2–3 seconds |
| Contrast medium | 76% diatrizoate meglumine sodium† |
| Injection rate/volume | 6–10 ml/sec, 60–70 ml total |
| Number of filming positions | 5 (4 in short individuals) |
| First position | Pelvis (3 films) |
| Second position | Thighs (2–3 films) |
| Third position | Knees (5 films) |
| Fourth position | Calves (4 films) |
| Fifth position | Feet (4 films) |

*Filming delay is 4 to 5 seconds if only 4 filming positions are used.
†Add 2 mg of lidocaine per ml of contrast medium.

**TABLE 11–2.** Program for Lower Extremity Arteriography With a Long Film Changer

| | |
|---|---|
| Contrast medium* | 76% diatrizoate meglumine sodium |
| Injection rate/volume | 6–10 ml/sec, 60–70 ml total |
| First film | Filming delay calculated on the basis of the test injection (~5–7 sec) |
| Second film | 4 seconds later |
| Third film | 5 seconds later |
| Fourth film | 5 seconds later |
| Fifth film | 5 seconds later |

*Add 2 mg of lidocaine per ml of contrast medium.

completion of the contrast injection. In this way, the entire arterial system from the aortic bifurcation to the popliteal arteries is opacified on the first set of films. After calculation of the appropriate filming delay, four to five films are obtained (Table 11–2).

**Calculation of the Filming Delay and Duration of Filming.** With the exception of young patients with fast blood flow, the duration of filming for evaluation of the lower extremities for peripheral vascular occlusive disease should be extended for at least 25 seconds after the contrast injection is begun. In some patients with severe occlusive atherosclerosis, filming must be carried out to at least 30 seconds to permit opacification of the distal vessels. In young individuals, the duration of filming is usually less than 20 seconds. However, in some patients, a longer duration is necessary because of the presence of peripheral arterial constriction.

With the catheter at the aortic bifurcation, 10 ml of contrast medium is injected rapidly. The image intensifier is positioned over the proximal tibia of the more symptomatic leg. Using a clock or a watch, the time interval is determined in which the contrast medium appears in the popliteal artery (ie, time interval between injection of contrast medium and its appearance in the popliteal artery). Approximately another 15 seconds are required for the contrast medium to appear in the plantar arches.

The time delay between the beginning of the contrast injection and the filming varies with the type of filming equipment used. For the stepping table, a 2 to 3 second delay is used, and for the long film changers, a 5 to 7 second delay is required. Since the contrast medium is injected over several seconds (between 8 and 10 seconds), filming with long film changers can be delayed for several seconds, in order to permit filming at the time of maximal arterial opacification. As a rule, filming should begin at least 2 seconds before the completion of the contrast injection, in order to demonstrate the iliac arteries. If hyperemia or vasodilators are used, the delay must be decreased by 2 or 3 seconds.

## Techniques for Enhancement of Distal Vessel Opacification

There are several ways to obtain optimal visualization of the distal vessels (below the popliteal artery). With the exception of intraarterial DSA and dry field and antegrade arteriography, these methods lead to better opacification of the distal circulation by inducing vasodilatation and augmenting distal blood flow. Thus, with each one of these vasodilatory methods, the rate and volume of contrast injection must be adjusted. A rule of thumb that we have found helpful is: increasing the rate of contrast injection by 25 to 50% and increasing the total contrast volume by approximately 25%. Failure to adjust these parameters will lead to poorer opacification with a washed out appearance of the blood vessels.

The techniques for enhancement of the distal arterial opacification are:

1. Injection of contrast medium at an appropriate rate and volume. Contrast medium itself is a vasodilator, and immediately after injection there is a fall in the peripheral resistance and a steep rise in blood flow lasting for several minutes.[21]

2. Intraarterial injection of vasodilators:
*Tolazoline*: 25 mg of tolazoline diluted in 10 to 15 ml of a 5% glucose solution is injected over 10 to 15 seconds. Arteriography is then performed within 1 to 2 minutes. According to some authors, tolazoline must be injected over 5 minutes in order to be effective.[22] Other studies indicate that the arteriogram should be completed within 5 minutes of the tolazoline injection in order to utilize the vasodilatation maximally.[19] To effect improved visualization of the distal lower extremity vessels, tolazoline requires patency of the SFA and popliteal arteries. Intraarterial injection is associated with a sensation of warmth in the extremities. Side reactions that

have been observed with the use of tolazoline include chilliness, nausea, and epigastric pain.[23, 24] In our own experience, these side reactions have not been noted.

*Papaverine*: 30 mg of papaverine is injected over 60 seconds. Arteriography is performed immediately thereafter. Papaverine is a myovascular relaxant that has a direct paralyzing action on the arterial smooth muscle. This property makes it useful for the treatment of vascular spasm. Papaverine is not a satisfactory vasodilator for peripheral arteriography.[22]

*Lidocaine*: 50 mg of lidocaine diluted in 5 to 10 ml of a 5% glucose solution is injected as a slow intraarterial bolus immediately before arteriography.

*Reserpine*: 0.5 to 1.0 mg of reserpine is used primarily in peripheral vasospastic disorders.

The vasodilatation induced by intraarterial injection of pharmacological agents is most pronounced in the proximal vessels, leading to early venous opacification in the thigh (Fig. 11–7), and often the distal calf and foot vessel opacification is either unchanged or poorer if a higher volume of contrast medium has not been used. This observation has also been made by others.[22, 25]

3. Reactive hyperemia: The legs are elevated for approximately 60 seconds to enhance venous drainage and prevent venous congestion. Blood pressure cuffs are applied over the lower portion of the calf and are inflated to approximately 50 mm Hg over the systolic brachial artery pressure, and the extremity is brought into a horizontal position. The pressure cuffs remain inflated for approximately 7 minutes. The cuffs are deflated and removed from the field, and the contrast medium is injected immediately thereafter for arteriography. Higher cuff inflation pressures (>50 mm Hg) and long inflation periods (longer than 10 minutes) are not necessary. On the contrary, these could be hazardous (Fig. 11–8).

Reactive hyperemia is the best and most consistent method for the improved visualization of the distal small vessels. With this method, an increase in the peripheral blood flow of up to 500% has been reported (after 10 minutes of arterial occlusion).[19] In general, the time needed for the contrast medium to reach the popliteal artery is decreased by about 50%.[24] This necessitates adjustment of the timing for the filming program. The maximal reactive hyperemia is obtained after 5 to 10 minutes of occlusion.[26] The duration of

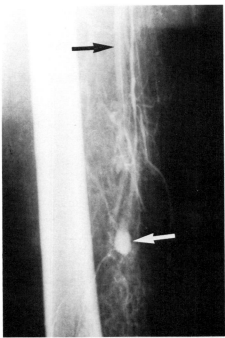
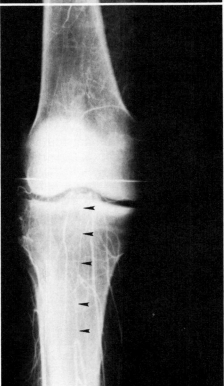

**Figure 11–7.** Pharmacological enhancement techniques for distal vessel opacification. Following intraarterial injection of 25 mg of tolazoline, there is early venous opacification (*arrows*) without significant improvement in the demonstration of distal vessels. Severe spasm of the popliteal artery (*arrowheads*) was subsequently relieved by intraarterial reserpine.

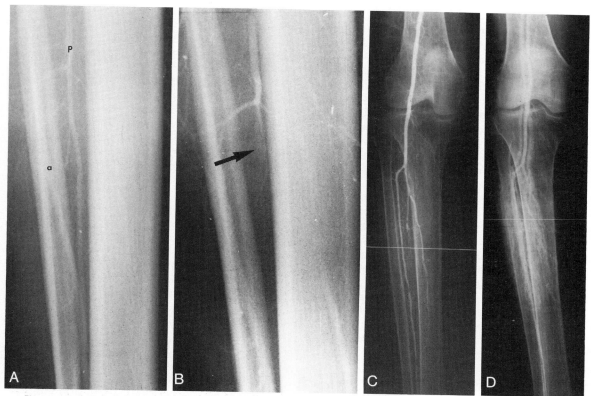

*Figure 11–8.* A and B, Arterial occlusion occurring as a result of high inflation pressure. A, Left leg arteriogram shows patent anterior tibial (a) and peroneal (p) arteries. B, Repeat arteriogram after reactive hyperemia using a blood pressure cuff shows occlusion of the peroneal artery (*arrow*). C and D, Arteriovenous shunting due to high position of pressure cuff. Arteriogram before (*C*) and after (*D*) reactive hyperemia using a pressure cuff placed over the proximal calf. There is hyperemia of the calf with arteriovenous shunting. Opacification of the distal vessels is not improved.

hyperemia is usually short, lasting only for 2 to 3 minutes.[26, 27]

Application of the blood pressure cuff over the distal calf permits selective vasodilatation in the distal portion of the leg and has provided us with the best results. Applying the blood pressure cuff above the knee or over the proximal calf has provided us with results similar to those obtained after intraarterial injection of vasodilators (Fig. 11–8). The improved visualization of the foot vessels reported by others using this technique has not been our experience.[24] In patients with severe occlusive disease and poor collateral circulation, the response to reactive hyperemia is often poor.

4. Reflux hyperemia: Temperature elevation to induce vasodilatation as an adjunctive technique for improved small vessel opacification has been used for hand arteriography.[28] The same technique can also be applied to the lower extremities. By warming the opposite extremity to 109° F for 10 to 15 minutes, a 100% increase in blood flow can be induced in the ipsilateral extremity.[19] However, because of the availability of simpler and better methods, this technique has not found much use.

5. Antegrade arteriography: Failure to adequately demonstrate the distal vessels (eg, of the foot) by the methods just described may necessitate antegrade injection into the femoral artery. This technique may be used either with or without the aid of peripheral vasodilatation and in conjunction with standard arteriography or DSA.

6. Intraarterial DSA.

7. Film subtraction.

8. Dry limb arteriography (Fig. 11–9):[29] With the aid of a double lumen balloon catheter, the artery is occluded to arrest circulation distal to the balloon. Subsequent contrast injection results in excellent opacification of the distal circulation. This technique can be used during antegrade or retrograde femoral arteriography. For the *retrograde* ap-

plication, a 6 Fr double lumen balloon catheter with multiple side holes (Berman angiographic balloon catheter, Critikon, Inc., Tampa, Florida) is inserted into the external iliac artery through a 6 Fr introducer sheath. The balloon is inflated with diluted contrast medium (30%) to occlude the artery. Overinflation of the balloon must be avoided in order to prevent traumatization of the artery. The appropriate inflation volume is determined by injecting a small amount of contrast medium as the balloon is inflated. Stasis of the injected contrast medium indicates the correct inflation volume. Heparin, 1500 mg, diluted in 20 to 30 ml of 5% dextrose, is injected through the catheter, followed by injection of 76% contrast medium (with 2 mg of lidocaine per ml of contrast medium) at 6 ml/sec for a total of 60 ml (for the entire extremity), and films are obtained over 25 seconds. For the *antegrade* application, a 6 Fr double lumen balloon wedge catheter (end hole only) is placed in the distal SFA or proximal popliteal artery. After balloon inflation, contrast medium is injected at 5 ml/sec

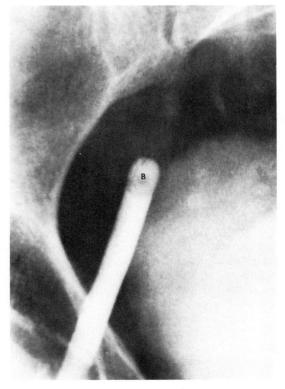

*Figure 11–9.* Retrograde dry limb arteriography using an angiographic balloon catheter. The balloon (B) is inflated with dilute contrast medium (30%). Note the dense opacification of the external iliac artery.

for a total of 40 ml. Films are obtained over 20 seconds. The antegrade application is less useful, since an antegrade contrast injection through a regular angiography catheter placed in the distal SFA provides the same result. The best results are obtained if dry limb arteriography is combined with reactive hyperemia.

9. Epidural anesthesia.[29a] In addition to providing effective analgesia, epidural anesthesia leads to a peripheral vasodilatation as a result of the sympathetic blockade.

## Analgesia

Many factors are responsible for the perception of pain during arteriography: the patient's pain threshold, anxiety, stress, and attitude; the patient-physician relationship; the severity of the occlusive disease; and the patient's understanding of the procedure.[30, 31] Almost all patients find extremity arteriograms to be quite painful. Therefore, several methods have been used in an attempt to reduce or eliminate pain caused by intraarterial injection of contrast medium.

1. General or spinal anesthesia: The risks and potential complications, cost, and length of time associated with these procedures do not justify their use for routine arteriography.

2. Premedication with strong analgesics such as morphine and meperidine: When these agents are used in combination with tranquilizers such as diazepam, there is marked reduction in the perception of pain.

3. Inhalation of nitrous oxide gas.[31a]

4. Epidural anesthesia.[29a]

5. Contrast agents that are nonionic or have a lower osmolality.[32, 33]

6. Intraarterial analgesics.

Several studies have demonstrated the usefulness of intraarterial lidocaine for the prevention of pain associated with lower extremity arteriography.[30, 32, 34, 35] The almost instantaneous analgesia provided by intraarterial lidocaine is incompletely understood. Likely sites of action are the arterial osmoreceptors and a stabilizing action on the neuronal membrane.[30]

A solution of 20% lidocaine (Lidocaine HCl, Bristol Laboratories, Syracuse, New York) is mixed with the contrast medium in the injector syringe in a ratio of 2 mg of lidocaine per ml of contrast. The maximal safe dose is 300 mg/hour. At this dose we have not observed any adverse reactions.

Injection of a mixture of 1 mg/ml of contrast

medium or a 50 to 100 mg lidocaine bolus immediately before arteriography is much less effective.

## Selective Catheterization

Selective catheterization of the femoral artery may become necessary to obtain better arterial detail in patients with occlusive atherosclerosis, trauma, tumors, or vascular malformations and for interventional procedures or the preoperative evaluation of patients for microvascular free tissue transfer.

### Common and Superficial Femoral Arteries (Tables 11–3 and 11–4)

**Contralateral Approach.** From the contralateral femoral artery a 5 or 6 Fr cobra catheter with side holes is placed over the aortic bifurcation. A J guide wire is inserted into the common femoral artery. The catheter is advanced to the external iliac or common femoral artery. For catheterization of the SFA, the cobra is exchanged for a 5 or 6 Fr headhunter catheter that is advanced to the desired position. Alternatively, a multiple hole straight catheter can be inserted over an exchange guide wire.

**Ipsilateral Approach.** There are four different techniques from the ipsilateral femoral artery:

**TABLE 11–3. Common Femoral Arteriogram**

| Approach | Ipsi- or contralateral femoral artery (axillary or translumbar) |
|---|---|
| Catheter: | Ipsilateral approach (retrograde catheterization): 5 or 6 Fr multiple hole straight catheter<br>Contralateral approach: 5 or 6 Fr cobra,* H1H, or multiple hole straight catheter |
| Position | Common femoral/external iliac artery |
| Guide wire | 0.035 inch J |
| Contrast medium† | 76% diatrizoate meglumine sodium‡ |
| Injection rate/volume | 5–6 ml/sec, total 25 ml |
| Films:<br>Filming<br>Projections | 8 films<br>1 per second<br>a. AP<br>b. Oblique (ipsilateral anterior) |

*C1 or C2 cobra with two side holes.
†20% concentration for DSA.
‡Add 2 mg of lidocaine per ml of contrast medium.

**TABLE 11–4. Superficial Femoral Arteriogram**

| Approach | Ipsilateral femoral artery (antegrade puncture)<br>Contralateral femoral artery |
|---|---|
| Catheter: | Ipsilateral approach: 5 Fr multiple hole straight catheter<br>Contralateral approach: 5 or 6 Fr cobra,* H1H, or multiple hole straight catheter |
| Position | Proximal superficial femoral artery |
| Guide wire | 0.035 inch J<br>0.035 inch J exchange wire (for contralateral approach) |
| Contrast medium† | 76% diatrizoate meglumine sodium‡ |
| Injection rate/volume | 5 to 6 ml/sec, total 20 ml |
| Films: | Long film changer, stepping table, or stationary run (6 to 8 films) |
| Projection | AP |

*C1 or C2 cobra with two side holes.
†20% concentration for DSA.
‡Add 2 mg of lidocaine per ml of contrast medium.

1. Antegrade femoral artery puncture (Fig. 11–10; for a detailed description, see Chapter 3).

2. Retrograde catheterization of the ipsilateral common femoral/external iliac artery.

3. The conversion technique using the loop catheter technique (see Chapter 3).

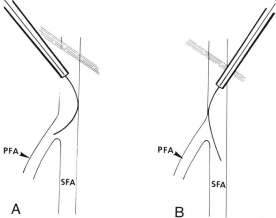

*Figure 11–10.* Technique for catheterization of the profunda femoris and superficial femoral arteries from an antegrade approach. *A,* Profunda femoris artery (PFA): During antegrade femoral artery puncture from the ipsilateral side, the needle tip is directed medially. This tends to direct the guide wire laterally, into the profunda femoris artery. *B,* Superficial femoral artery (SFA): If the needle tip is pointed laterally, the guide wire can be directed medially, into the SFA.

4. The conversion technique using a side-winder catheter (see Chapter 3).

**Axillary Artery Approach.** If the femoral approach (contra- or ipsilateral) is not possible, a 5 or 6 Fr 100 cm headhunter catheter is inserted from the axillary artery approach.

### Profunda Femoris Artery (Table 11–5)

**Contralateral Approach.** A cobra catheter is placed over the aortic bifurcation, a J guide wire is inserted into the SFA or common femoral artery, and the catheter is advanced over it. In this position the catheter tip points medially, but occasionally a guide wire can be manipulated into the profunda femoris artery. Alternatively, the loop catheter technique is used. The guide wire is pulled back proximal to the aortic bifurcation, and the catheter is torqued clockwise and advanced at the groin. With this maneuver, a loop will form in the distal aorta, and the catheter tip begins to retract and flips to point laterally. A 7.5 mm J or a straight LLT guide wire is inserted and advanced into the profunda femoris artery by torquing the catheter. Once the guide wire is in the vessel, the catheter is withdrawn at the groin. This will straighten out the loop and advance the catheter into the profunda femoris. If a loop is no longer present, the catheter is simply advanced over the guide wire.

A useful aid for catheterization of the profunda femoris artery is to place the patient (or the image intensifier) in an oblique posi-

### TABLE 11–5. Profunda Femoris Arteriogram

| | |
|---|---|
| Approach | Ipsilateral femoral artery (loop technique) Contralateral femoral artery |
| Catheter: | Ipsilateral approach: 5 or 6 Fr cobra catheter Contralateral approach: 5 or 6 Fr cobra or H1H catheter |
| Position | Profunda femoris artery |
| Guide wire | 0.035 inch J LLT 0.035 inch J exchange wire (for contralateral approach) |
| Contrast medium* | 76% diatrizoate meglumine sodium† |
| Injection rate/volume | 4–5 ml/sec, total 20 ml |
| Films: Filming Projection | 8 films (stationary run) 1 per second AP |

*20% concentration for DSA.
†Add 2 mg of lidocaine per ml of contrast medium.

tion to lay out the common femoral bifurcation (eg, RAO for the right side and LAO for the left side). As an alternative to the cobra, a headhunter catheter can also be used.

**Ipsilateral Approach Using the Loop Catheter Technique** (see Chapter 3 under catheterization of the ipsilateral superficial femoral artery or conversion of a retrograde into an antegrade puncture). The loop technique is used, and as the catheter tip approaches the profunda femoris orifice, it is torqued to point posterolaterally. Once the catheter tip is in the profunda femoris, the catheter is further withdrawn at the groin in order to advance the tip deeper into the vessel.

**Axillary Artery Approach.** From the axillary approach, either a headhunter or multipurpose catheter is used.

## ANEURYSMS

Aneurysms of the extremity vessels occur much less frequently than those of the aorta. In over 90% of cases the etiology is atherosclerosis, followed by trauma and anastomotic and mycotic aneurysms. Atherosclerotic aneurysms are frequently multiple and are often associated with aorto-iliac aneurysms. Detection of an extremity artery aneurysm is an indication for a careful search for other aneurysms, since 59% of these patients have additional aneurysms.[36] Similarly, because of the associated complications, demonstration of such an aneurysm also constitutes an indication for operation. A search for other aneurysms should include a sonogram of the aorta and iliac arteries, since the physical examination alone may fail to detect aorto-iliac aneurysms in a significant number of patients.[36] The most common locations for atherosclerotic aneurysms of the peripheral vessels are the femoral and popliteal arteries. Atherosclerotic aneurysms of the distal vessels (distal to the popliteal artery bifurcation) are extremely rare. Such aneurysms are most frequently anastomotic or traumatic.

### Femoral Artery Aneurysms

The normal diameter of the common femoral artery on arteriography is between 0.7 and 1.0 cm. Diffuse or focal widening of the common femoral artery diameter by 50% or more compared with the diameter of the distal external iliac artery is defined as an aneurysm.

**Atherosclerotic Aneurysms.** Atherosclerosis is responsible for most aneurysms of the femoral arteries. The majority of the aneurysms involve the common femoral artery; in 15% the disease may also involve the profunda femoris and SFA, and in 85% aorto-iliac aneurysms are an associated finding.[37] The aneurysms are bilateral in 47 to 72% of patients, and 44% of patients also have aneurysms of the popliteal arteries.[37, 38] Isolated aneurysms of the profunda femoris artery are observed in 2% of patients.[37]

Atherosclerotic femoral artery aneurysms are rare in women. In one report, all 100 patients were males.[37] Symptoms may be local (pain, swelling, tenderness, and venous obstruction), may be manifested as distal occlusive disease (due to distal embolization), or may be related to concomitant occlusive atherosclerosis. Symptoms referable to the aneurysm may be absent in 30 to 40% of patients.[37, 38]

Aneurysm rupture has been reported in as many as 14% and thrombotic occlusion in 16% of aneurysms.[38] Other complications are distal embolization, femoral neuropathy, venous compression, and infection.

**Traumatic Aneurysms.** Traumatic aneurysms of the femoral artery or its branches are most often due to penetrating trauma. They have been observed after bullet and knife wounds, operative trauma, arterial catheterization, fractures, and intramuscular injection of medication.[39–41] Occasionally, blunt trauma may also give rise to false aneurysms.[42]

Because of its superficial location in the femoral triangle, the femoral artery is susceptible to injury. Frequently, the wound appears superficial, and a vascular injury is not suspected.[40] Aneurysms are usually a late manifestation of vascular trauma. Although small aneurysms may be demonstrated on arteriography shortly after the trauma, most large aneurysms may take several weeks to years to develop and become symptomatic. On physical examination, the aneurysm can be palpated as a mass, which is pulsatile in only half the cases.[43]

**Mycotic Aneurysms.** A painful, tender, pulsatile mass in the groin with fever, bacteremia, and femoral neuropathy is highly suggestive of a mycotic femoral artery aneurysm.[44, 45] Mycotic aneurysms of the femoral arteries may occur after bacterial sepsis, parenteral drug abuse, and other penetrating injuries. Such aneurysms may also occur as a result of an infected hematoma after arterial catheterization or arterial reconstruction.

In patients with *Salmonella* sepsis, the femoral arteries are the second most frequent location for mycotic aneurysm formation (preceded only by mycotic aortic aneurysms).[46] *Staphylococcus* is the most frequent causative agent in patients who are parenteral drug users.

**Other Aneurysms.** Other types of aneurysms that may involve the femoral arteries are anastomotic aneurysms after arterial reconstruction (see Chapter 12) and aneurysms arising adjacent to exostoses.[47]

## Popliteal Artery Aneurysms

Diffuse or focal widening of the popliteal artery greater than 50% compared with the diameter of the distal SFA is defined as an aneurysm. The diameter of the normal popliteal artery on arteriography is between 0.5 and 0.7 cm.

**Atherosclerotic Aneurysms.** Approximately two thirds of limb vessel aneurysms occur in the popliteal arteries. The vast majority of these aneurysms are atherosclerotic and are most frequently located immediately below the adductor hiatus.[48] The distal popliteal artery and the bifurcation are almost never involved. Ninety per cent are fusiform and may extend over a distance of 10 cm or more.[48]

Only 25% of popliteal artery aneurysms are solitary; the rest are associated with aneurysmal disease elsewhere.[49] Fifty-nine per cent are bilateral,[50] and patients with bilateral aneurysms are more likely to have aneurysms elsewhere (ie, aorta and iliac and femoral arteries).[51, 52] Abdominal aortic aneurysms are seen in approximately one third of the patients with popliteal artery aneurysms.[48, 50]

As many as 45% of patients may be asymptomatic.[49, 52] Symptoms are most frequently referable to peripheral ischemia due to peripheral vascular occlusion and include intermittent claudication, rest pain, and gangrene. Other symptoms include local pain, nerve compression, and popliteal vein occlusion.[53, 54] Occasionally such aneurysms may be misdiagnosed as a Baker's cyst or thrombophlebitis.

Unlike other aneurysms, rupture of a popliteal artery aneurysm is rare and has been reported in only 4% of patients.[53] Thrombosis accounts for over half the total complications.[48, 50] In patients with thrombosed popliteal artery aneurysms, the amputation rate can be as high as 50%, stressing the need for an early diagnosis.[51] Other complications include peripheral embolization with digital ischemia, venous thrombosis, neuropathy, and infection.

**Other Aneurysms.** Less than 10% of popliteal artery aneurysms are nonatherosclerotic.[48–50] Such aneurysms may be due to acute trauma, syphilis, infection (mycotic), or chronic vascular trauma (osteochondroma, jogging) or may develop at vascular anastomoses (anastomotic aneurysms).[55, 56]

## Arteriography

The diagnosis of an extremity artery aneurysm, which is suspected on physical examination, can be confirmed or excluded by ultrasonography.[57] The main indication for arteriography is to define the arterial anatomy prior to operation and to evaluate the peripheral circulation for the feasibility of arterial reconstruction.

Arteriography can be performed from the femoral, translumbar, or axillary approach. In some patients intravenous DSA can be used for screening. In patients with atherosclerotic and mycotic aneurysms, both lower extremities must be evaluated, in addition to a biplane abdominal aortogram. In patients with traumatic and other types of aneurysms,

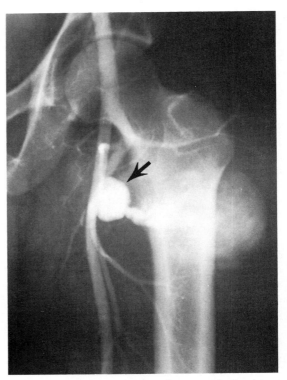

**Figure 11–12.** False aneurysm from penetrating injury to the thigh. Left common femoral arteriogram shows a traumatic aneurysm of the profunda femoris artery (*arrow*). A systolic jet of contrast material is seen entering a large false aneurysm.

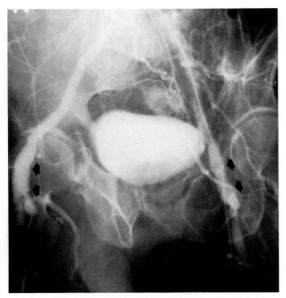

**Figure 11–11.** Bilateral atherosclerotic femoral artery aneurysms (*arrows*). The aneurysms extend into the profunda femoris artery and SFA.

an arteriogram is obtained of the region of interest and of the distal circulation if symptoms of ischemia are present. For femoral artery aneurysms, arteriography in the oblique projection may be necessary to define the extent and involvement of the profunda femoris and the superficial femoral arteries. Intraarterial DSA is extremely helpful for determining the site of injury in traumatic aneurysms. Most popliteal artery aneurysms require only an AP arteriogram.

**Arteriographic Findings** (Figs. 11–11 to 11–14)

1. True atherosclerotic aneurysms may be fusiform or saccular. The former are most frequently seen in association with aorto-iliac aneurysms and arteriomegaly. Mycotic and traumatic aneurysms are saccular.

2. In occluded aneurysms, the arteriogram shows an abrupt termination of the main artery with draping of the branches around the thrombosed aneurysm.

3. Abrupt termination of the arteries distal to the aneurysm may be seen if thromboembolization has occurred (Fig. 11–15).

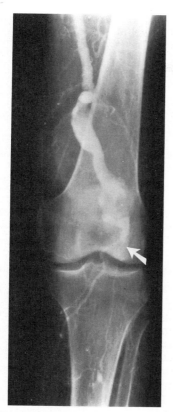

*Figure 11–13.* Atherosclerotic popliteal artery aneurysm with distal occlusion (*arrow*). Faint calcification outlines the aneurysm.

### PITFALLS IN DIAGNOSIS

In aneurysms with mural thrombi, the arteriogram may demonstrate a normal or only slightly widened arterial lumen. In such cases, there is draping of the muscular branches around the aneurysm, which corresponds to the outer dimension of the aneurysm.

## ARTERIAL OCCLUSIVE DISEASES

Ischemia of the peripheral lower extremities depends upon several factors: (1) location of the obstruction, (2) degree and extent of the obstruction, (3) status of the collateral vessels, (4) rapidity of onset of the obstruction, and (5) status of the arterioles and capillaries (ie, vasodilatation or vasoconstriction).

In the lower extremities, a relatively long occlusion of a major vessel may be compatible with relatively few symptoms, owing to the presence of numerous collaterals. Thus, the efficiency of the collateral system determines the extent of symptoms. However, the collateral circulation cannot be as efficient as the normal vascular channels in maintaining limb blood flow.

### Clinical Aspects

The incidence of occlusive peripheral vascular disease (PVD) is approximately 3% for persons between 45 and 54 years and 6% for persons between 55 and 64 years.[58] Males are affected more frequently than females. Symptoms typical of occlusive PVD may be absent in over half the patients.[58] Such symptoms are due to tissue ischemia, and the onset is usually unilateral, gradual, and episodic. Acute exacerbation of symptoms is due either to an occlusion of a severely stenotic lesion by superimposition of a thrombus or to embolic occlusion (Fig. 11–16). Rarely, aorto-iliac dissection may simulate peripheral vascular disease. Patients with occlusive PVD can be divided into several categories, which

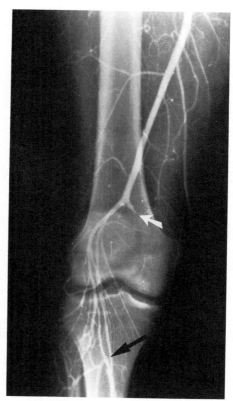

*Figure 11–14.* Occluded popliteal artery aneurysm in a male jogger (jogger's aneurysm). The popliteal artery terminates abruptly (*white arrow*) and reconstitutes at the bifurcation (*black arrow*). The genicular arteries are draped around the occluded aneurysm. (From Lundell C, Kadir S: J. Cardiovasc Intervent Radiol 4:239, 1981. Used with permission.)

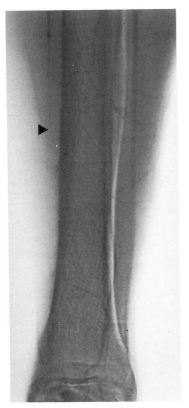

*Figure 11–15.* Peripheral embolization from a popliteal artery aneurysm causing distal leg ischemia. Subtraction film from a lower leg arteriogram shows an abrupt termination of the posterior tibial artery (*arrowhead*). There is a paucity of collateral vessels as a result of microembolization.

reflect the severity of the symptoms and the extent of the anatomic abnormality.

**Absent or Atypical Symptoms.** In some individuals, there is an absence of the typical symptoms of PVD, both at rest and after exercise. The occlusive disease is usually localized, and well-developed collaterals are present. The skin perfusion test is normal. In other individuals, the symptoms of PVD are masked by the presence of other diseases.

**Intermittent Claudication.** At rest, patients with PVD have an adequate muscular blood supply. During stress (eg, exercise or walking), the muscular blood supply is insufficient, giving rise to symptoms of fatigue, aching, numbness, pain, and cramps. The group of muscles involved (ie, the location of the pain) indicates the level of the obstruction (Table 11–6). As the activity is continued, the symptoms become progressively more severe, forcing the patient to stop. The symptoms subside within a few minutes of rest

**TABLE 11–6.** Location of Pain as an Indicator for Level of Arterial Obstruction

| | |
|---|---|
| Aorta and common iliac artery | Buttock and thigh claudication Occasionally calf claudication Painless paresis relieved by rest |
| External iliac and common femoral arteries | Thigh claudication Painless paresis relieved by rest |
| Internal iliac artery | Impotence, pudenal and obturator steal |
| SFA | Calf claudication |
| Popliteal artery and branches | Foot and plantar surface claudication, paresthesias |

and permit resumption of the activity until renewed symptoms occur. The distance that initiates the onset of symptoms may vary from several feet to several hundred yards.

Intermittent claudication is the initial symptom of PVD in approximately 75% of patients. Several other conditions that may simulate intermittent claudication due to PVD are listed in Table 11–7.

**Rest Pain.** More severe ischemia due to advanced occlusive disease leads to pain at rest. This usually begins in the foot and may extend to involve the distal leg. The pain may be in the form of a persistent dull ache or a severe pain requiring analgesics. Dependent position of the extremity usually alleviated the pain by means of gravity-induced increase in the arteriolar pressure. The pain is worse in the horizontal position.

Pain is due to a decrease in skin perfusion and is often nocturnal as a result of decreased

**TABLE 11–7.** Diseases That May Simulate Intermittent Claudication Due to Occlusive PVD[87–95]

Abdominal aortic aneurysm
Acute aortic dissection
Acute embolic occlusion
Adventitial cystic disease of the popliteal artery
Erythromelalgia
Extrinsic vascular compression
Metabolic (gout, muscle glycogen metabolism deficiency)
Musculoskeletal disorders
Neuroclaudication (meiopragmie medullaire Déjérine)
Neurological disorders (lumbar disc, amyotrophic lateral sclerosis, multiple sclerosis, polyneuritis, etc)
Popliteal artery entrapment syndrome
Vasospastic disorders
Venous diseases

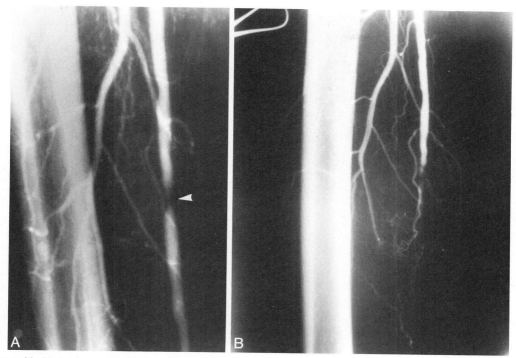

**Figure 11–16.** Acute exacerbation of symptoms due to thrombotic occlusion of a severe stenosis. *A,* Femoral arteriogram shows a severe stenosis of the superficial femoral artery (*arrowhead*). *B,* On repeat arteriography 6 weeks later, there is occlusion of the superficial femoral artery. Worsening of the intermittent claudication had occurred approximately 2 weeks prior to the second arteriogram.

hydrostatic pressure in the horizontal position. Physical examination reveals skin marmoration, pallor, decreased skin temperature, increased sensitivity to touch, and muscle atrophy.

**Ulceration and Gangrene** (Fig. 11–17). This stage represents severe and often endstage disease. In one series, approximately 10% of patients with PVD who were less than 60 years old were in this group at the time of diagnosis.[59] The incidence of gangrene and the amputation rate are four times higher in diabetics than in nondiabetics with clinically manifested PVD.[60] In an autopsy study of a larger population, the incidence of gangrene was 0.66% for nondiabetic males and 24.9% for diabetic males over 50 years of age.[61] A similar ratio was also found for females.

There is severe skin and muscle ischemia, skin ulceration, and acral gangrene, in addition to intense rest pain. With the exception of some diabetics, the peripheral pulses are usually absent. In diabetics with patent major vessels, peripheral neuropathy and small vessel disease may lead to ischemic ulceration and gangrene.

The skin ulceration and gangrene are usu-

ally not due to ischemia alone but result from infection and often avoidable minor trauma (mechanical or thermal) and impaired healing.

## Atherosclerosis

Atherosclerosis is by far the most common cause of occlusive PVD and occurs predominantly in men in a 9:1 to 11:1 ratio.[59, 60] The onset of symptoms occurs a decade earlier in men than in women.[62]

Diabetes mellitus predisposes to atherosclerosis, and approximately 15% of patients with clinically manifested atherosclerotic PVD have diabetes.[60] Atherosclerosis also occurs a decade earlier and about 11 times more frequently in diabetics than in nondiabetics.[63] The incidence and severity of complications of PVD are also higher in diabetics.[60, 61] The majority of patients with atherosclerotic PVD are smokers. The frequency of limb amputation is also higher among diabetics and smokers.[59, 60]

Clinical and arteriographic follow-up shows that the disease is progressive despite therapeutic intervention (surgery or translu-

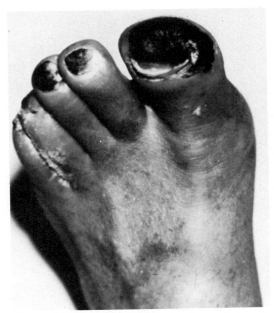

*Figure 11–17.* Severe atherosclerotic occlusive disease with gangrene.

minal angioplasty).[64–68] Anatomical progression of atherosclerotic PVD may not correlate with clinical symptoms. In one study, anatomical progression of disease occurred in 52% of patients over a 3 year observation period.[64] However, 39% of these patients were unaware of the progression of their disease.

**Arteriography.** Arteriography is indicated for definition of the anatomy, evaluation of severity of the disease, assessment of the distal circulation, and the search for unsuspected lesions, such as thromboemboli and aneurysms.

The femoral, translumbar, or axillary approach may be used. The inflow vessels (distal aorta and pelvic arteries) and vessels of both extremities must be evaluated. Although symptoms may be unilateral, atherosclerosis is a generalized disorder and involves both extremities. In addition, the absence of symptoms does not exclude the presence of occlusive disease. Every effort should be made to visualize the ankle and foot vessels. The latter are of particular importance if a distal bypass procedure is being considered.[69] Failure to demonstrate the distal vessels on the standard arteriogram requires intraarterial DSA or other adjunctive methods to enhance distal vessel opacification.

Oblique pelvic arteriography should be performed routinely in all patients. This is particularly important in patients suspected of having proximal disease. If a stenotic lesion of the iliac vessels is demonstrated, an effort should be made to obtain intraarterial pressures (resting and after injection of a vasodilator).

**Arteriographic Findings** (Figs. 11–18 to 11–21)

Three basic arteriographic patterns are recognized. However, not all arteriograms can be classified according to these types.

1. Diffuse stenotic pattern: There is diffuse disease involving the SFA and the popliteal artery and its major branches. Multiple areas of stenoses are present and occasionally, there is a short SFA or popliteal artery occlusion. Progression of disease leads to extensive occlusions.

2. Occlusive pattern: Short or long occlusions are present. The remaining vessels show evidence of atherosclerosis, but the arterial lumen is generally uncompromised. An occasional severe stenosis may be present.

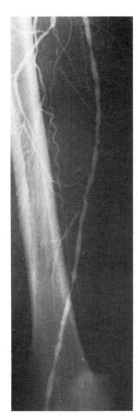

*Figure 11–18.* Diffuse stenotic type of atherosclerosis. Superficial femoral arteriogram shows diffuse stenosis without focal occlusion.

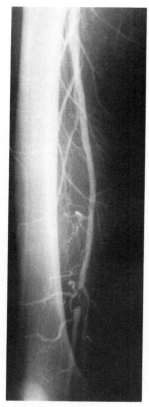

*Figure 11–19.* Occlusive type of atherosclerosis. Right femoral arteriogram shows a short segmental occlusion of the distal SFA and proximal popliteal artery. The remainder of the vessels are relatively normal appearing.

3. Diffuse ectatic pattern: The ectatic type of atherosclerosis (arteriomegaly) is seen in association with aortic and iliac artery ectasia and aorto-iliac aneurysms. In this type there is a tendency for formation of popliteal and femoral artery aneurysms.

Stenoses and occlusions are most frequently located at bifurcations and in arterial segments exposed to mechanical stress (adductor canal, popliteal artery). In the thigh, the most frequent location of arterial occlusion is the adductor canal, followed by SFA occlusion in the proximal thigh.[65] In the distal lower extremity, the posterior tibial artery is the most frequently occluded vessel; the peroneal artery is the least frequently occluded. Occlusion of the profunda femoris artery is observed in 9% of patients.[65]

PITFALLS IN DIAGNOSIS

1. Long versus short occlusion (Fig. 11–22): Repeat arteriography in patients with short SFA occlusions reveals the tendency of these lesions to progress.[65] In our own experience, incomplete filling of the SFA distal to an occlusion may simulate a long occlusion. In a review of SFA occlusions greater than 10 cm, there was retrograde opacification of a portion of the occluded segment of the SFA in 10% of the patients.[70] This suggests that not all long-appearing occlusions are indeed long. Retrograde filling can be demonstrated if appropriate filming techniques are employed, ie, if an adequate vol-

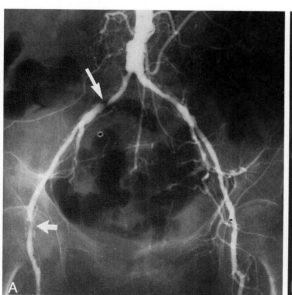
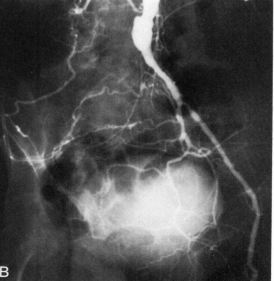

*Figure 11–20.* Progression of severe stenosis to arterial occlusion. *A,* Focal severe atherosclerotic stenosis of the right common iliac and common femoral arteries is present (*arrows*). *B,* Repeat arteriogram 3 months later shows extensive occlusion of the right iliac and femoral arteries. There is a stenosis of the proximal left external iliac artery.

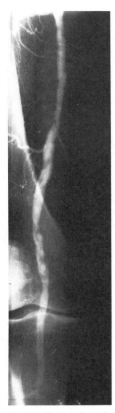

*Figure 11–21.* Ectatic atherosclerosis or arteriomegaly of the right superficial femoral and popliteal arteries. Diffuse ectasia and atherosclerotic plaques are present.

ume of contrast medium is injected and the duration of filming over the thighs is prolonged. A careful evaluation of the point at which the SFA or popliteal artery is reconstituted distal to the occlusion permits the prediction of a long or short occlusion (Fig. 11–23).

2. Pseudo-stenosis (Fig. 11–24): Incomplete opacification of a distal vessel may simulate a stenosis. This occurs because the volume of contrast medium reaching that segment of the vessel is inadequate for complete opacification of the arterial lumen and therefore layers on the dependent wall, providing the impression of a hemodynamically significant stenosis.

3. Deceptive stenoses (Figs. 11–25 and 11–26): Superimposition of vessels may obscure significant stenoses. This is particularly true for arterial bifurcations. Thus, oblique arteriography should be performed routinely to define the anatomy at the femoral bifurcations. Similar deceptive stenoses may also be encountered in the distal vessels. A dense

contrast column or a superimposed branch may obscure an eccentric arterial stenosis. Evaluation of several radiographs often provides the diagnosis. Alternatively, if a lesion is suspected, oblique or lateral arteriograms should be obtained of the region in question. A technique for biplane arteriography of the lower extremities has been desribed.[71] However, we have not found it necessary to obtain routine biplane arteriograms of the lower extremities distal to the femoral bifurcations.

4. Stenosis versus occlusion (Fig. 11–27): During diagnostic arteriography, passage of a catheter through a critical iliac or femoral artery stenosis may temporarily occlude the lumen. Thus, a segment of the vessel may not opacify, simulating passage of the catheter through an occluded vessel.

If left untreated, during the course of the examination a thrombus may form proximal to the segment that is occluded by the catheter. This thrombus is a potential source for distal embolization at the time of catheter removal or may continue to occlude the critical stenosis. Therefore, as soon as this situation is recognized, heparin (3000 Units) is administered as an intraarterial bolus, and upon completion of the arteriography, an attempt is made to suction out the thrombus through a 7 or 8 Fr tapered catheter. The lumen of the critical stenosis is enlarged by the larger catheter, and therefore the chance of thrombosis decreases; furthermore, the larger catheter provides a better suction. Alternatively, the stenosis is dilated with an appropriate-sized balloon angioplasty catheter. Catheter thromboembolectomy can also be employed in the SFA and popliteal arteries if an antegrade technique has been used (see Chapter 23 for details).

## Thromboangiitis Obliterans (Winiwarter-Buerger Disease)

This disease was first described by von Winiwarter in 1879. It is an inflammatory disease of unknown etiology involving the medium and small arteries of the extremities and leading to segmental occlusions. The underlying abnormality is a panarteritis with thrombotic occlusion.

Thromboangiitis obliterans occurs predominantly in young males less than 40 years of age. There is a definite association with cigarette smoking. Symptoms occur as a result of arterial and venous insufficiency. The re-

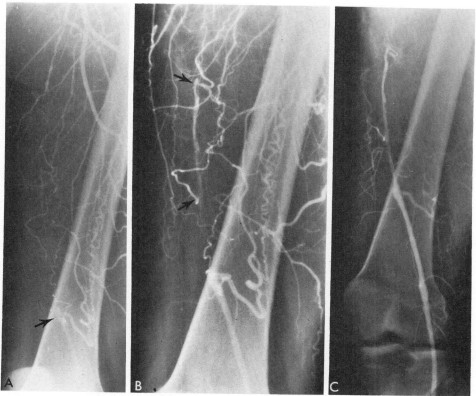

*Figure 11–22.* Deceptively long SFA occlusion. *A,* Early film from a superficial femoral arteriogram shows a long-appearing occlusion and reconstitution of the popliteal artery (*arrow*). *B,* An isolated-appearing segment of the SFA is reconstituted on a repeat arteriogram (*arrows*). *C,* Later film shows that the distal SFA and popliteal artery are continuous and that the SFA occlusion is short. (From Kadir S et al: Selected Techniques in Interventional Radiology. Philadelphia, WB Saunders, 1982.)

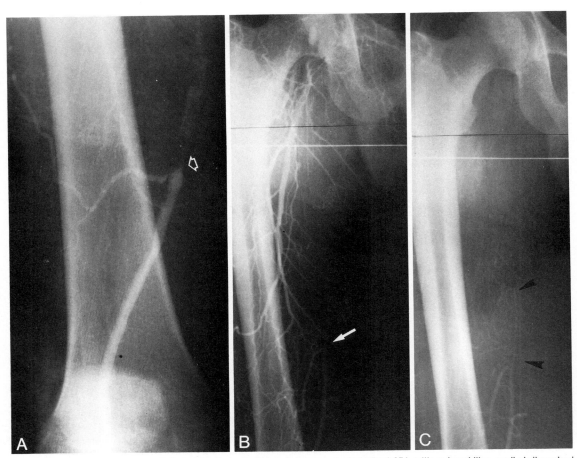

*Figure 11-23.* Recognition of deceptively long SFA occlusions. *A,* Calcified SFA with a beaklike, well-delineated occlusion (*arrow*). Such an appearance suggests that retrograde filling is unlikely. *B,* In a long SFA occlusion, the distally reconstituting vessel is poorly opacified (*arrow*). *C,* Later film from the same arteriogram (as in *B*) shows refilling of a segment of the distal SFA (*arrowheads*). The poor delineation of the reconstituted vessel is an indicator that retrograde filling may occur.

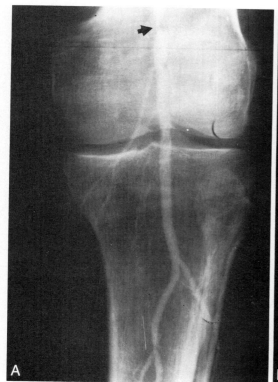

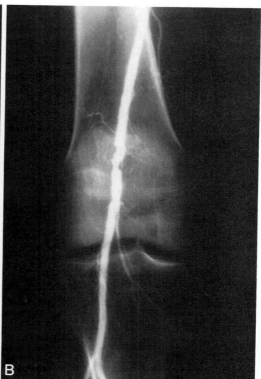

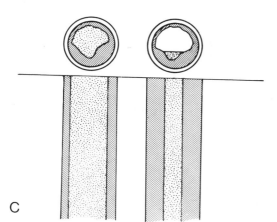

**Figure 11–24.** Pseudo-stenosis due to incomplete opacification of the arterial lumen. *A,* Arteriogram obtained at another hospital shows a severe popliteal artery stenosis (*arrow*) for which the patient was referred for angioplasty. *B,* Repeat arteriogram via antegrade catheterization of the SFA shows that the stenosis is not severe. *Note*: Antegrade contrast injection leads to superior opacification of the distal extremity vessels. (*A* and *B,* From Kadir S et al: Selected Techniques in Interventional Radiology. Philadelphia, WB Saunders, 1982.) *C,* Diagram illustrating this angiographic phenomenon. On arteriography, if the entire lumen is opacified by contrast medium, the lumen appears wider, thereby obscuring smaller plaques that are not in profile. Thus, a vessel appears "better" if completely opacified. Incomplete opacification of the arterial lumen with posterior layering of the contrast medium, which is commonly the case with retrograde femoral arteriography, will give the appearance of a severe stenosis.

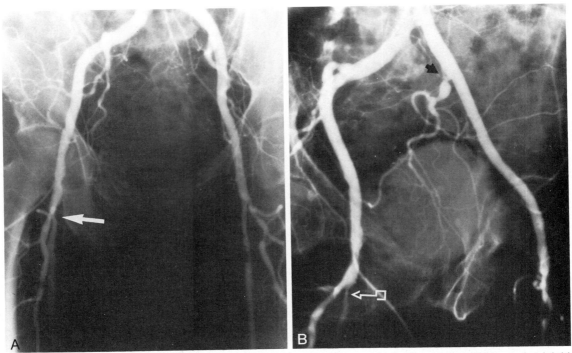

*Figure 11–25.* Deceptive arterial stenosis. *A,* AP pelvic arteriogram shows minimal narrowing of the proximal right SFA (*arrow*). The right common femoral bifurcation is not well demonstrated. *B,* Left posterior oblique pelvic arteriogram defines the right common femoral bifurcation and reveals a tight SFA stenosis (*white arrow*). In addition, this oblique view also defines the left internal iliac artery orifice, which is also stenotic (*black arrow*).

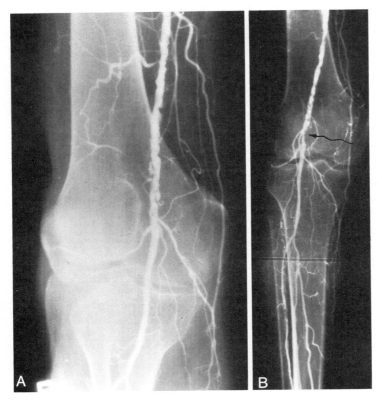

*Figure 11–26.* Deceptive arterial stenosis. *A,* Arteriogram with the leg externally rotated shows diffuse atherosclerosis of the popliteal artery without a focal stenosis. *B,* Repeat arteriogram with the leg AP. A tight mid-popliteal arterial stenosis is present (*arrow*). In *A,* this stenosis was obscured by a genicular artery.

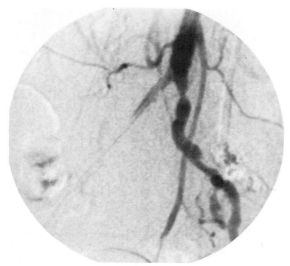

**Figure 11–27.** Stenosis vs occlusion. Passage of a catheter through a severe stenosis may simulate arterial occlusion. AP intraarterial DSA of the pelvis shows severe atherosclerosis of the left common and external iliac arteries. There is no opacification of the distal right iliac artery. An arterial pulse was present before catheterization. The pulse was not palpable during the procedure but returned following removal of the catheter.

duction of blood flow is due to a combination of an anatomical obstruction and arterial spasm.[72] The foot and calf vessels are affected most frequently; popliteal and superficial femoral artery occlusions are less frequent.

Intermittent claudication of the foot and lower calf is the most frequent initial symptom. Rest pain, ulceration, and gangrene also occur. The dorsalis pedis and posterior tibial artery pulses are often absent. A painful migratory superficial thrombophlebitis occurs in close to half the patients.

Thromboangiitis obliterans may be differentiated from arteriosclerosis by the absence of predisposing factors such as diabetes mellitus and hyperlipidemia, the young age of the patients (always under 50 years), and the high frequency of involvement of the upper extremity. In addition, the arteriogram provides a fairly typical picture.

**Arteriography.** Unlike atherosclerotic PVD, routine arteriography is not necessary in patients with thromboangiitis obliterans. However, it may be required for the definition of the anatomy and localization of the occlusions. In certain cases, arteriography may be required to establish the diagnosis. In addition, it may be indicated preoperatively to predict the level of amputation.

**Arteriographic Findings** (Fig. 11–28)

1. Multiple segmental occlusions: There is an abrupt transition from a normal caliber

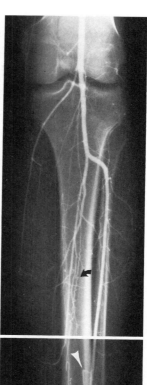
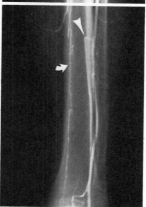
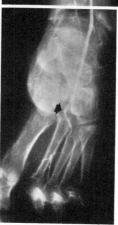

**Figure 11–28.** Thromboangiitis obliterans. Young male patient with ischemic changes of the left foot. Arteriogram shows occlusion of the peroneal and posterior tibial arteries. The peroneal artery reconstitutes distally (*arrowhead*). The dorsalis pedis artery terminates abruptly (*straight arrow*). Tortuous collaterals are seen (*curved arrows*).

vessel to an occlusion or rarely to a thready, partially recanalized vessel. The occlusion ends as abruptly as it begins, with continuation of a normal caliber vessel. Occlusions involve the foot and calf vessels primarily.

2. Multiple segmental stenoses or occlusions of the metatarsal and digital arteries.

3. Opacification of an extensive, tortuous collateral network. These collaterals may not be demonstrated in all cases without the aid of vasodilators, because of the presence of arterial spasm.

4. Areas of arterial spasm.

## Thromboembolic Occlusion

Fifty-eight per cent of peripheral embolizations occur to the lower extremity vessels distal to the inguinal ligament.[73] Thirty-eight per cent of the emboli to the lower extremity lodge at the common femoral artery bifurcations.[74] The most common source for such emboli is the heart. Other sources include mural thrombi from the thoracic or abdominal aorta, aortic or peripheral arterial aneurysms, atheromatous plaques or debris from the aorta or iliac arteries, and paradoxical embolization through a patent foramen ovale or an intracardiac septal defect.[75-78] In addition, peripheral thromboembolization may occur as a complication of aortic aneurysmectomy or of diagnostic or interventional angiography.

Peripheral embolization may be associated with spasm of the arteries distal to the obstruction and of the collateral channels.[73] Vasospasm, in association with slowed arterial circulation in the distal vessels, also predisposes to in-situ thrombus formation.

The severity of the complications associated with embolic occlusion of the extremity vessels is determined by the type of embolus and the site of lodgment. Saddle emboli at arterial bifurcations not only occlude the main artery but also block the collateral pathways.

Clinically, only 81% of peripheral embolizations have a sudden onset.[73] In the remaining patients, the symptoms develop gradually. Of importance is the observation that approximately 6% of peripheral embolizations are clinically silent.[73]

**Arteriography.** The indications for arteriography are for definition of the arterial anatomy of the affected limb, in particular, the distal circulation, and for the localization of a potential source for the emboli (aneurysm, mural thrombi). Arteriography may also be required to aid in differentiating between in-situ thrombosis of a severe atherosclerotic stenosis and thromboembolism.[79]

**Arteriographic Findings** (Figs. 11–29 and 11–30)

1. Abrupt occlusion of a uniform caliber vessel. In the presence of large emboli, collateral channels (branches) are also occluded.

2. Superior convex meniscus.

3. In larger vessels with nonoccluding or partially occluding emboli, the embolus may be outlined by the contrast medium and may appear as an unopacified defect.

4. Diffuse and often severe vasospasm of the vessels distal to the obstruction. This occurs with large, occluding emboli and can be reversed by intraarterial injection of vasodilators.

5. If contrast medium is injected into the occluded segment (eg, for confirmation that the catheter is embedded in the clot) prior to thrombolytic therapy, a focally widened arterial lumen is demonstrated.

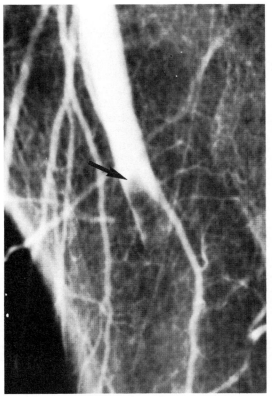

*Figure 11–29.* Thromboembolic occlusion. Occlusion of the distal popliteal artery by thrombus. A typical superior convex meniscus is present (*arrow*). All three run-off vessels are occluded. Collateral vessels are opacified as a result of intraarterial injection of a vasodilator.

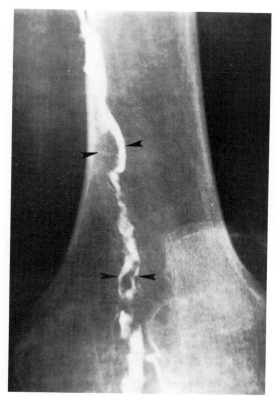

*Figure 11–30.* Focal widening of the popliteal artery due to thromboemboli (*arrowheads*). The patient developed leg ischemia following surgery for a large thoracic aortic aneurysm.

**Differentiation Between Atherosclerotic Occlusion, Thromboembolism, and Low Flow States** (Figs. 11–30 and 11–31). In most cases, embolic occlusions can be differentiated from atherosclerotic occlusion. However, difficulty may arise in patients with thromboembolism superimposed upon atherosclerotic occlusive disease. Rarely, extrinsic compression may simulate embolic occlusion.[80] In atherosclerotic occlusion, the artery usually tapers to an occlusion and there is a collateral vessel just proximal to the occlusion. In addition, numerous other collateral channels are usually present, confirming the chronic nature of the disease. Acute embolic occlusion (with large emboli) on the other hand, is characterized by a paucity of collaterals, since these are either blocked by the embolus or do not opacify because of severe spasm.

Low cardiac output and hypovolemia may lead to ischemia of the lower extremities in the absence of occlusive disease. The symptoms may be asymmetrical and the clinical picture may simulate acute arterial occlusion (thrombosis or thromboembolism).[81] A similar picture may also be observed in the presence of minimal occlusive disease. In such patients, the symptoms are out of proportion to the extent of disease.

On arteriography, the blood flow is markedly slowed and the distal arterial bed is inadequately defined by·retrograde femoral arteriography.

### Atheroma Embolization

Atheromatous microemboli to the lower extremities are found at autopsy in 4% of individuals older than 50 years of age.[82] Four types of emboli may originate from proximal arteries: mural thrombi from the aorta or aneurysms, fibrin-platelet thrombi from ulcerated atherosclerotic plaques, cholesterol emboli, and atheromatous plaques. Embolization of mural thrombi from the aorta and aneurysms has been discussed in the previous section on Thromboembolic Occlusion.

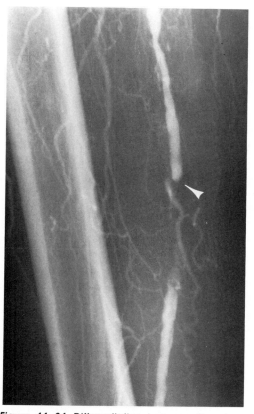

*Figure 11–31.* Differentiation between thromboembolic and atherosclerotic occlusion. Superficial femoral arteriogram shows a typical atherosclerotic occlusion. The artery tapers to an occlusion (*arrowhead*) just distal to a collateral vessel. The occlusion is concave superiorly.

**Fibrin-Platelet Thrombi.** Fibrin-platelet emboli may originate from ulcerated plaques in the aorta (aortic arch to bifurcation) and iliac and femoral arteries.[83] Occasionally, a piece of atheromatous material may embolize with the thrombus. Such emboli occlude larger vessels and may not be distinguishable clinically from other thromboemboli.

**Cholesterol Emboli.** Embolization of cholesterol crystals from ulcerated aorto-iliac plaques gives rise to a characteristic clinical picture. Microembolization develops to the small arteries of the feet (arteries between 55 and 665 μ, average 100 to 200 μ), leading to painful cyanotic skin spots (Figs. 11–32 and 11–33).[84] In some of these cases, the clinical picture is that of acute livedo reticularis, whereas in others it has been called the "blue toe syndrome."[85, 86] The larger vessels of the foot are usually patent, and the pulses at the ankle are palpable.

Most frequently, cholesterol embolization occurs spontaneously, but it has also been observed after arteriography. Histologically, necrotizing angiitis may be present, simulating polyarteritis nodosa.[84]

**Atheromatous Plaques.** Embolization of atheromatous plaques from the aorta or iliac

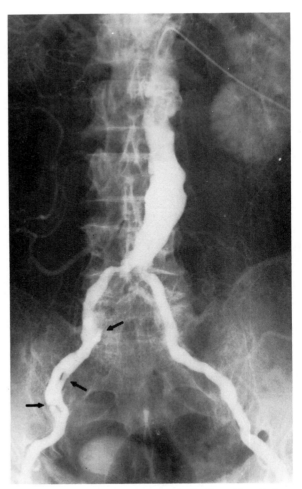

*Figure 11–33.* Cholesterol embolization. AP arteriogram from the same patient as in Figure 11–32 shows severe atherosclerosis of the aorta and iliac arteries. Several ulcerated plaques are seen in the right iliac artery (*arrows*).

arteries may occur as a complication of arteriography or percutaneous transluminal angioplasty (Fig. 11–34).

## Foreign Body Embolization

Foreign bodies introduced into the arterial system for diagnostic or therapeutic purposes (catheter or guide wire fragments, arterial dilators, steel coils, and other materials for transcatheter occlusion) or as a result of arterial trauma may embolize into the peripheral circulation (Fig. 11–35).

## Tumor Embolization

Arterial invasion, intraarterial growth, and subsequent embolization of extracardiac neo-

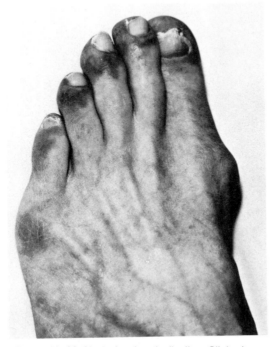

*Figure 11–32.* Cholesterol embolization. Clinical manifestations. Typical mottled, cyanotic appearance of the toes in a patient with cholesterol embolization. Compare with Figure 11–17.

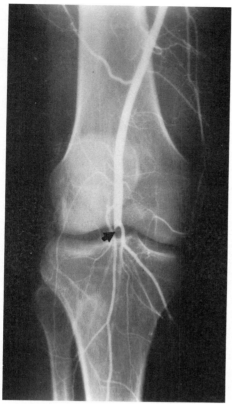

*Figure 11–34.* Atheroma embolization. Occlusion of the popliteal artery (*arrow*) due to embolization of an atheromatous plaque following iliac artery angioplasty. (From Kadir S et al: Selected Techniques in Interventional Radiology. Philadelphia, WB Saunders, 1982.)

plasms is a rare cause of embolic arterial occlusion of the peripheral vessels. We have observed two such cases during the past 5 years. In one patient, embolization of an angiosarcoma led to embolic occlusion of the abdominal aorta. In the other patient, the iliac artery was invaded by a pelvic neoplasm and tumor fragments embolized into the peripheral circulation (Fig. 11–36).

## TRAUMA

Early recognition of acute vascular trauma is the most important factor in the successful management of such injuries. Lower extremity vessels are affected in one third of the patients with acute arterial trauma.[96] The femoral arteries are the most frequent site of injury. Penetrating injury of the extremity is the most frequent indication for arteriography of trauma.

### Pathology

Externally nonpenetrating trauma is responsible for 10% of vascular injuries.[97] It occurs most frequently in association with fractures and dislocations of the extremities.[98, 99] The mechanism of arterial injury may be:

1. Stretch injury: In minor arterial trauma, focal arterial spasm may be seen. Severe trauma may result in intimal disruption, medial tears, and arterial thrombosis. Severe stretch injury may also lead to complete arterial disruption and false aneurysm formation. In the traumatized patient, arterial spasm may also be a manifestation of systemic hypotension.

2. Internal penetrating injury: This type of vascular injury is seen in association with fractures of the long bones. The sharp edges of the fractured bone may lacerate or transect an artery. Such injuries may lead to thrombosis or formation of a false aneurysm or an arteriovenous fistula.[100]

The majority of externally penetrating arterial injuries are due to gunshot wounds and less frequently to stab wounds.[101] Such injuries may result in:

1. Arterial laceration or transection. This can lead to thrombosis or the formation of a false aneurysm or an arteriovenous fistula.

2. Occlusion.

3. Arteriovenous fistula.

4. False aneurysm formation.

In addition, associated venous injuries may be present in close to half the patients with arterial injuries.[97]

### Clinical Aspects

Clinical signs and symptoms may be absent in the presence of significant vascular injury. The physical findings that may be associated with vascular injury are listed in Table 11–8.

Pulsatile bleeding and an expanding hematoma are the most reliable signs of arterial injury.[101, 102] A weak or absent pulse distal to the site of injury is a less reliable sign of arterial injury. In the presence of significant vascular injury, 43% of patients have normal pulses.[103] The location of trauma (proximity) is one of the least reliable signs of vascular injury.[102]

Although arteriovenous fistula and false aneurysm may develop acutely, they are more often a late manifestation of vascular injury. Simultaneous arterial and venous in-

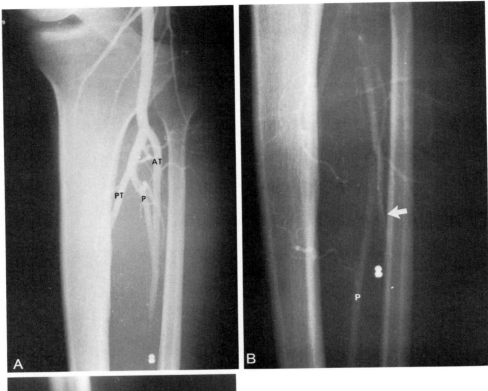

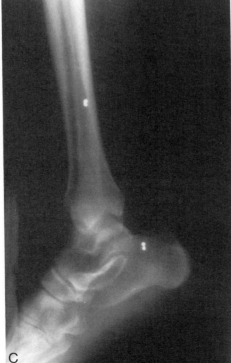

*Figure 11–35.* Foreign body embolization. Typical appearance of intravascular buckshot located in the anterior tibial (AT) and posterior tibial arteries (PT). P = peroneal artery. *A,* In the early arterial phase the anterior tibial and peroneal arteries are superimposed. Slow antegrade flow did not opacify the distal circulation sufficiently to permit localization. *B,* Repeat arteriogram localizes the buckshot to the anterior tibial artery. A superimposed thrombus is present (*arrow*). *C,* Scout film from the lateral arteriogram localizes the buckshot to the anterior tibial artery. Other emboli are seen in the distal posterior tibial artery. *Note:* Antegrade contrast injection, the aid of vasodilators, and lateral filming may be required to localize such intravascular foreign bodies.

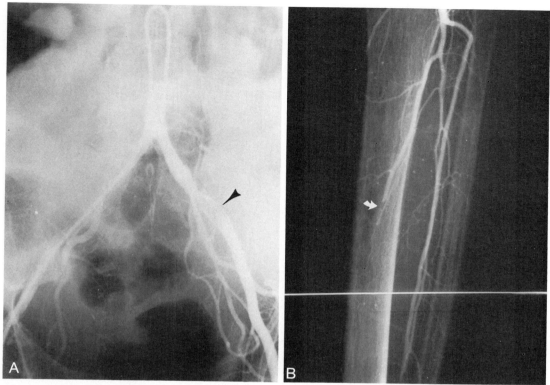

**Figure 11-36.** Tumor embolization in a woman with a pelvic malignancy. *A,* Pelvic arteriogram shows an intraluminal lesion with focal widening of the left external iliac artery (*arrowhead*). *B,* Distal left leg arteriogram shows tumor embolus in the posterior tibial artery (*arrow*).

jury may occur as a result of a penetrating trauma, but a communication does not develop immediately because of the presence of a hematoma. As the hematoma resolves, the fistula is opened (see Fig. 11-42).

## Arteriography

Emergency arteriography is indicated in patients with diminished or absent pulses, distal ischemia, a bruit, and an expanding hematoma. Elective arteriography is indicated in patients with proximity injuries and normal arterial pulses. In this situation, the

**TABLE 11-8.** Physical Findings That May Be Associated With Peripheral Arterial Injury

Normal peripheral vascular examination
Absent pulses distal to the site of injury
Diminished pulses distal to the site of injury
Ischemia distal to the site of injury (pallor, decreased skin temperature, rest pain)
Expanding hematoma
Pulsatile bleeding
Bruit
Concomitant venous injury

incidence of significant arterial injury is 1%.[101] Arteriography should be considered prior to exploratory surgery for suspected arterial injury in patients who are hemodynamically stable. In patients with late manifestations of arterial trauma, arteriography is indicated for the planning of the vascular reconstructive procedure.

An arteriogram is obtained of the traumatized limb. AP arteriography usually provides satisfactory information. If the arteriogram demonstrates arterial occlusion or intimal disruption, the distal circulation must also be evaluated to assess the extent of damage and distal embolization. In shotgun injuries, the distal circulation should also be evaluated for the detection of embolized buckshot (see Fig. 11-35). The accuracy of arteriography for the detection of traumatic arterial lesions is about 90%, with false-negative arteriograms in fewer than 1% of patients.[104] The accuracy can be further increased by accepting only good quality arteriograms (AP and oblique) and by the use of intraarterial DSA (see Fig. 11-43).

If arterial spasm is demonstrated, the arteriogram should be repeated after intraarterial injection of tolazoline, 25 mg diluted in 15 to 20 ml of 5% dextrose and injected over 30 seconds, or reserpine, 0.5 to 1.0 mg diluted in 15 to 20 ml of 5% dextrose and injected over approximately 30 seconds. Resolution of the arterial spasm permits improved distal vessel opacification and excludes extrinsic compression or mural injury.

**Arteriographic Findings** (Figs. 11–37 to 11–42)

1. Segmental arterial narrowing: This may be due to spasm or extrinsic compression by a hematoma. Diffuse narrowing may be due to reflux vasospasm (eg, shock, exposure to cold).

2. Focal intimal tear.

3. Arterial occlusion.

4. Contrast extravasation into the soft tissues.

5. False aneurysm formation: Identification of the traumatized artery is necessary for proper management. The arteriographic sign of the systolic jet and diastolic washout aids in identifying the traumatized vessel.[105]

6. Arteriovenous fistula.

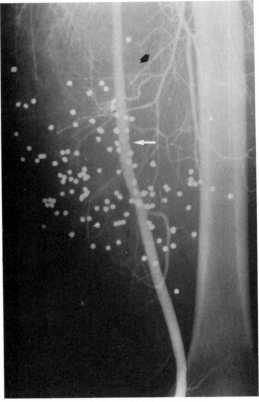

*Figure 11–38.* Focal intimal tear of the superficial femoral artery due to shotgun injury (*white arrow*). There is spasm of a profunda femoris artery branch (*black arrow*).

PITFALLS IN DIAGNOSIS (Fig. 11–43)

1. Pseudo-occlusion: Trauma-induced arterial spasm or extrinsic compression by a hematoma may occasionally simulate arterial occlusion.

2. Pseudothrombus: The "rolling up" of the torn intima may simulate a thrombus.

3. Obscured intimal injury: A subtle intimal lesion may be obscured by the dense contrast column. Later frames from the same arteriogram should be evaluated for the detection of subtle injuries. Similarly, an arterial injury may be obscured by overlying bone. Therefore, in some types of injuries, especially multiple stab wounds or shotgun injuries, an arteriogram in a second projection should be obtained.

Why is it important to detect subtle arterial injuries? Arterial injuries may appear subtle on the arteriogram, but in fact the damage may be significant. Such injuries may progress to arterial occlusion, false aneurysm formation, and distal embolization. These complications are often more difficult to manage.

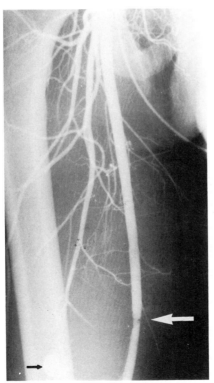

*Figure 11–37.* Arterial trauma. Segmental intimal tear of the superficial femoral artery (*white arrow*) due to a bullet injury. *Black arrow* points to the bullet.

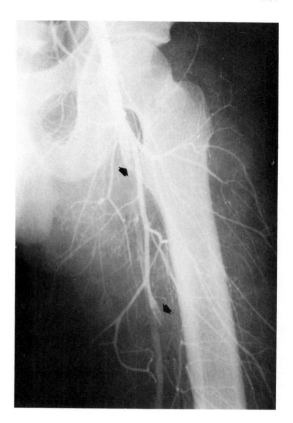

*Figure 11–39.* Traumatic arterial occlusion. There is occlusion of the superficial femoral and profunda femoris arteries due to bullet injury (*arrows*). The distal SFA is reconstituted via collaterals.

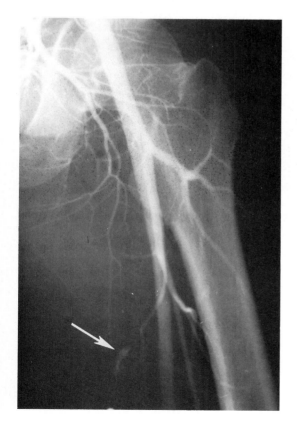

*Figure 11–40.* Extravasation of contrast medium (*arrow*) is seen from a branch of the profunda femoris artery in a patient with a stab wound to the thigh.

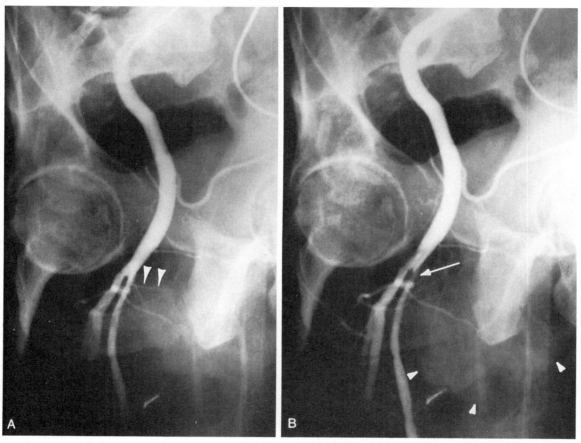

***Figure 11–41.*** Traumatic "false" aneurysm or pulsating hematoma of the superficial femoral artery following insertion of an intraaortic counterpulsation balloon. *A*, During systole a jet of contrast medium is seen at the arterial puncture site in the SFA (*arrowheads*). *B*, During diastole a negative defect is present at the arterial puncture site (*arrow*). This is due to a "wash out" of the contrast medium in the femoral artery by the unopacified (or less opacified) blood from the aneurysm (*arrowheads*).

*Figure 11–42.* Delayed manifestation of an arteriovenous fistula following stab injury. *A,* Early film from a femoral arteriogram obtained a week after the injury shows transient, early opacification of the posterior tibial and popliteal veins (*arrows*). *B,* Late arterial film shows dense opacification of the popliteal and femoral veins.

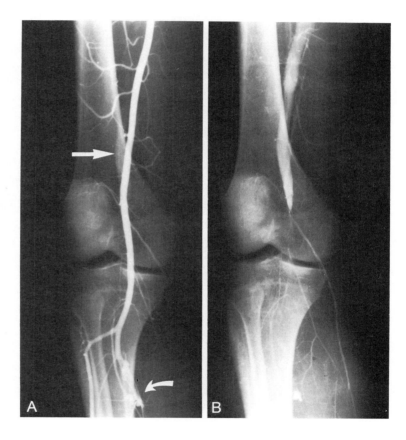

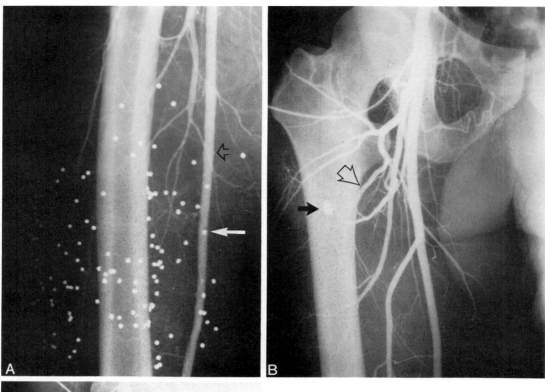

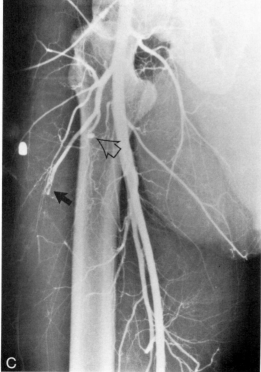

*Figure 11–43.* Pitfalls in angiographic diagnosis of peripheral arterial injury. *A,* Subtle arterial trauma. Femoral arteriogram after shotgun injury shows subtle intimal tears in the superficial femoral artery. The lesions seen in profile appear as minimal intimal irregularities (*open arrow*). En face lesions, which appear as "punched-out" defects, may be obscured by dense contrast column or overlying foreign bodies (*white arrow*). Distal embolization should be suspected if such punched-out lesions are observed. *B* and *C,* Obscured injury. *B,* AP right common femoral arteriogram in a patient with a gunshot wound to the thigh demonstrates some arterial spasm (*open arrow*). No other arterial injury is seen. Solid arrow points to the bullet. *C,* Repeat arteriogram in the oblique projection shows a traumatic aneurysm (*open arrow*) and occlusion of a profunda femoris artery branch (*solid arrow*).

## Iatrogenic Arterial Injuries

Arterial injury may occur as a result of a diagnostic or therapeutic intraarterial procedure. Complications of diagnostic arteriography are discussed in Chapter 23. Iatrogenic arterial injuries may also be self-induced, as a consequence of attempted parenteral drug abuse (Fig. 11–44).

**Peripheral Arterial Complications of Intraaortic Counterpulsation Balloons** (see Fig. 11–41). Vascular complications after percutaneous insertion of intraaortic counterpulsation balloons are observed in 13% of patients.[106] These include reversible peripheral arterial ischemia, arterial dissection, thrombosis, and distal embolization. False aneurysm formation is observed in less than 1% of patients.[106] These complications appear to be related to balloon insertion into the SFA and may be avoided by cannulation of the relatively larger common femoral artery.

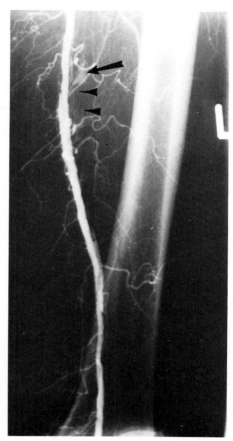

**Figure 11–45.** Iatrogenic arterial injury following angioplasty. Superficial femoral arteriogram following angioplasty shows contrast opacification of the vasa vasorum (*arrowheads*) and the superficial femoral vein (*arrow*). This injury is self-limited and does not result in any complications.

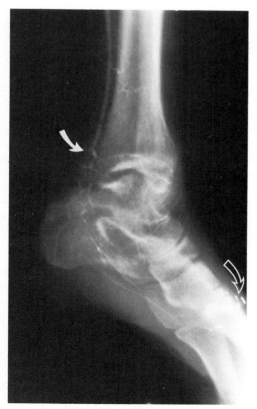

**Figure 11–44.** Self-induced arterial injury in a drug addict. The anterior and posterior tibial arteries were used as sites for parenteral drug injection. There is abrupt termination of the posterior tibial artery (*solid arrow*). Metallic densities from a previous injury are seen over the instep (*open arrow*).

**Arterial Injury Following Angioplasty and Fogarty Balloon Embolectomy** (Figs. 11–45 and 11–46). Significant pressures can be generated inside angioplasty and embolectomy balloons.[107] As this pressure is applied to the arterial wall, it leads to intimal and medial tears. Such medial tears are an accepted consequence of balloon angioplasty and are a common observation on post-angioplasty arteriograms. Rarely, the tear is transmural and is associated with extravasation of contrast medium. Opacification of vasa vasorum on post-angioplasty arteriograms is also a manifestation of the mural injury. Such injury is usually self-limited and does not lead to any complications. Balloon rupture may be associated with transmission of a significant force on the arterial wall and may lead to the formation of a false aneurysm or to arterial occlusion.

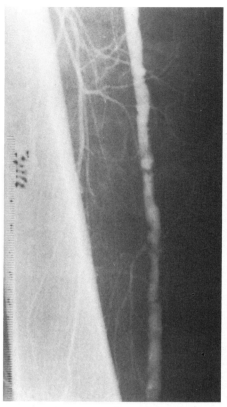

*Figure 11–46.* Iatrogenic arterial injury following Fogarty balloon embolectomy for a paradoxical embolus. Postoperative arteriogram after embolectomy
shows the severely traumatized, irregular intimal surface
of the superficial femoral artery in a young male patient.

Intimal injury also occurs during balloon
embolectomy, as the inflated embolectomy
balloon is withdrawn. On arteriograms performed after balloon embolectomy, the intimal surface appears uneven. Arterial disruption with false aneurysm formation has also
been observed (see Fig. 9–39, Chapter 9).

## VASOSPASTIC DISORDERS

The arterial tonus is maintained by continuous asynchronous contractions of the
smooth muscles in the peripheral arteries.
This muscle activity underlies the vasoconstrictive influence of the sympathetic inner-
vation and can also be altered by the action
of local regulating mechanisms.[108, 109] These
include vasoactive peptides, prostaglandins,
nicotine, physical agents (thermal stimuli),
and oxygen tension.[110]

**TABLE 11–9. Conditions That May Be Associated
With Peripheral Arterial Spasm**[101, 102, 111–117, 121–125]

Arterial catheterization
Arterial trauma
Collagen vascular diseases
Drugs (ergotamine, methysergide, propranolol, vaso-
 pressin)
Hematological disorders·
Hypothermia, frostbite
Inadvertent intraarterial injection of drugs
Neurological disorders
Occlusive arterial diseases
Occult malignancy
Poisoning
Psychological trauma
Systemic hypotension

Peripheral vasospasm may be due to a
primary vasospastic disorder or may occur as
a manifestation of a local or systemic disease.
Conditions that may have peripheral vasospasm as part of their clinical manifestations
are listed in Table 11–9. Primary vasospastic
diseases include acrocyanosis, arterial hypertonus, livedo reticularis, and Raynaud's disease.

### Drug-induced Vasospasm

**Vasopressin.** Intraarterial and intravenous
infusion of vasopressin is frequently used in
the management of gastrointestinal bleeding.
Peripheral vasoconstriction and acral gangrene have been reported in 0.5% of patients
receiving vasopressin therapy.[111] In older
persons, vasopressin-induced spasm of the
distal extremity vessels may simulate thrombotic or thromboembolic occlusion. Symptoms of peripheral ischemia are most prominent in patients with underlying occlusive
peripheral vascular disease.

**Ergot Derivatives** (Fig. 11–47). Ergotamine
tartrate and methysergide maleate are prescribed for the treatment of migraine headaches and in obstetrics. The mode of action
is an alpha-adrenergic blockage and peripheral vasoconstriction. Symptoms may be due
to chronic intake, acute overdose, or hyper-
sensitivity to therapeutic doses.[112]

Ergot-induced vasoconstriction affects primarily the lower extremities. Occasionally,
the upper extremities, mesenteric and neck
vessels, and systemic veins are also affected.[113–116] Symptoms include peripheral vasoconstriction associated with intermittent
claudication, rest pain, and occasionally acral
gangrene.[112] The peripheral arterial pulses are
severely diminished or absent. The vast ma-

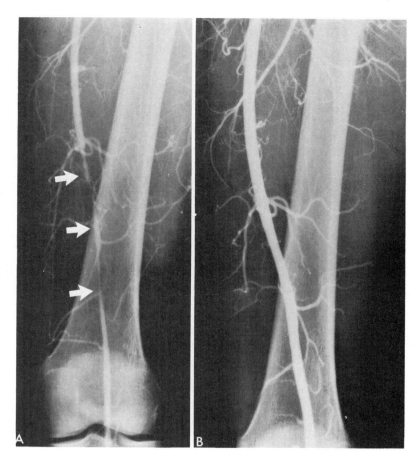

*Figure 11–47.* Severe arterial spasm due to chronic ergot intake. *A,* Femoral arteriogram shows severe spasm and occlusion of the superficial femoral artery (*arrows*). *B,* Repeat arteriogram 2 weeks after the drug was discontinued shows a normal artery. (From Kadir S et al: *In* Athanasoulis CA et al (Eds.): Interventional Radiology. Philadelphia, WB Saunders, 1982.)

jority of patients are young women. A history of ingestion of ergot preparations may not be obtainable in some patients; in such patients, the arteriogram indicates the diagnosis.[117]

Diagnostic arteriography is indicated only if the clinical diagnosis is uncertain. Intraarterial infusion of vasodilator drugs may be indicated in some patients not responding to discontinuation of ergot-containing medication.[118] The arteriographic findings are:[112, 117, 119, 120]

1. Arterial spasm: There is bilateral, symmetrical vasoconstriction that begins abruptly. The artery may appear threadlike or may be completely occluded. The arterial spasm may be diffuse or focal and involves the SFA and the popliteal and distal vessels most frequently, but more proximal vessels may also be affected. The diagnosis of ergot-induced arterial spasm may first be suspected after arteriography.

2. Arterial thrombosis: This is observed infrequently and may be related to the ergot-induced endothelial damage.

3. Demonstration of a collateral network:[112] This is most likely a nonspecific finding representing a physiological response to arterial occlusion.

## Posttraumatic Vascular Spasm
(Fig. 11–48)

A self-limited, severe arterial spasm may be observed after arterial catheterization in some young adults and children. This is most often related to the use of relatively large catheter size (ie, relative to arterial diameter) or to excessive catheter manipulation. In addition, arterial trauma may occur as a result of inadvertent intramural injection of local anesthetic or after multiple unsuccessful attempts at arterial puncture.

Arterial spasm is also observed after peripheral arterial trauma. If focal, arterial spasm is usually indicative of some arterial injury. Diffuse spasm may be due to reflux vasoconstriction, ie, a manifestation of systemic hypotension, or due to exposure of the traumatized extremity.

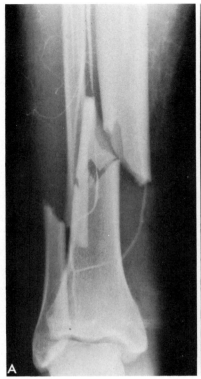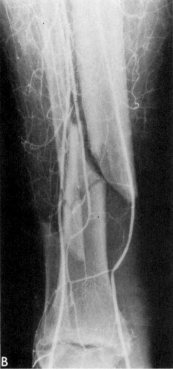

*Figure 11–48.* Vascular spasm following leg trauma. *A,* Lower extremity arteriogram shows spasm and poor opacification of the peroneal posterior and anterior tibial arteries and their branches. *B,* Arteriogram after intraarterial injection of tolazoline (12 mg) shows reversal of the spasm. (From Kadir S et al: *In* Athanasoulis CA et al (Eds.): Interventional Radiology. Philadelphia, WB Saunders, 1982.)

## Raynaud's Disease and Raynaud's Phenomenon

Raynaud's disease is a vasospastic disorder of the extremities of unknown etiology. It affects the upper extremities most frequently, and the symptoms can be induced by cold and by emotional stimuli. Raynaud's phenomenon, on the other hand, is the term used for such symptoms when they occur in association with underlying systemic or local disease.

The clinical picture consists of three phases: In the initial phase, there is an intense vasoconstriction leading to digital pallor. This is followed by atony of the capillaries and venules, which results in acrocyanosis. The final phase is that of reactive hyperemia, which is manifested as rubor. Arteriography shows focal areas of arterial spasm and occlusion involving the small and medium-sized arteries.

## Collagen Vascular Diseases
(Fig. 11–49)

Raynaud's phenomenon is seen as part of the clinical picture in collagen vascular diseases. The small- and medium-sized arteries are affected by the vasospasm. This may progress to anatomical arterial occlusion.[121]

## Peripheral Arterial Hypertonus
(Fig. 11–50)

Symmetrical spasm of the muscular-type arteries has been observed after emotional trauma.[122, 123] This may be associated with intermittent claudication and rest pain and can also lead to gangrene.[122, 124] The peripheral pulses may be intermittently absent or diminished. Arteriography is indicated to differentiate between functional (spastic) and anatomical occlusion. In the former, intraarterial vasodilatory drug infusions may provide relief of spasm and prevent tissue ischemia.[125]

### MISCELLANEOUS DISORDERS

## Arteriovenous Malformations

The lower extremities are one of the most frequent locations for congenital vascular malformations.[126] (For classification and pathology of arteriovenous malformations, see Chapter 9.)

An arteriovenous malformation (AVM) of the lower extremities may be congenital, traumatic, neoplastic, infectious, or secondary to a vascular disease.[127] With the rare

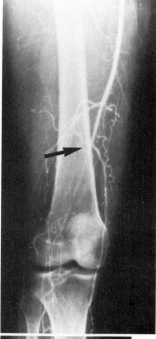

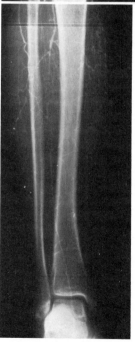

*Figure 11–49.* Vascular spasm and occlusions in a patient with collagen vascular disease. Femoral arteriogram in a 26 year old woman shows occlusion of the popliteal artery (*arrow*) and spasm and occlusion of the run-off vessels.

exception of a benign intraosseous AVM, all limb AVMs affect the soft tissues.

Arteriography is indicated for:[128, 129]

1. Localization of the vascular supply.

2. Definition of the extent of the lesion for the assessment of resectability.

3. Evaluation of the adequacy of the surgical resection.

4. Performance of transcatheter occlusion, either preoperatively or as the primary therapeutic procedure.

Initially, a survey arteriogram is obtained to assess the extent of the lesion and identify the main arterial feeders. Subsequently, selective arteriography is performed for assessment of the arteriovenous communications and for transcatheter therapy. If only selective arteriography is performed, assessment of the true extent of the lesion may not be possible. Demonstration of large arteriovenous communications is important, as this represents a contraindication to transcatheter embolization with small particulate material.

In lesions without arteriovenous shunting, the contrast injection rate is not increased. However, the contrast volume should be increased by approximately 50% compared with the volume that would normally be used for arteriography of that particular vessel (eg, for profunda femoris arteriography, use a total of 30 ml instead of 20 ml).

**Arteriographic Findings** (Fig. 11–51)

1. Enlarged, tortuous feeding arteries: Acquired arteriovenous fistulae usually have a single artery-to-vein communication. Occasionally, multiple fragment injuries may give rise to several arteriovenous communications, which may simulate a congenital lesion.

2. Opacification of multiple tortuous small vessels, dilated vascular spaces, or venous aneurysms.

3. Arteriovenous shunting.

The entire lesion is best appreciated during the late phase of the arteriogram. Arteriovenous malformations cannot always be differentiated from a hypervascular malignancy.

## Hemangioma

Hemangiomas constitute 7% of all benign tumors.[130] Most hemangiomas are of the cavernous type (75%) and only 1% originate in skeletal muscle, most frequently in the thigh.[131] The lesions are usually asymptomatic during childhood and early adult life. They may manifest as a mass, local pain, or

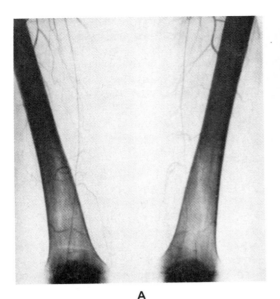
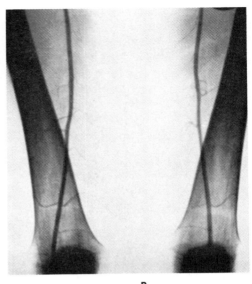

A                                                                                           B

*Figure 11–50.* Arterial hypertonus. *A*, Lower extremity arteriogram in a 34 year old woman shows extreme arterial spasm. *B*, Repeat arteriogram 4 weeks later shows normal vessels. (From Hegglin R: Differentialdiagnose innerer Krankheiten, 12th ed. Stuttgart, Georg Thieme Verlag, 1972. Used with permission.)

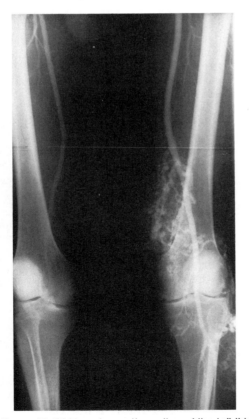

*Figure 11–51.* Vascular malformation of the left thigh and calf. The left SFA is enlarged. Multiple, enlarged, tortuous vessels and dilated vascular spaces are seen. Also note the earlier opacification of the left popliteal and distal arteries, resulting from increased blood flow in the left SFA.

swelling. Women are affected more frequently than men. Hemangiomas may occur as an isolated abnormality or in association with one of several clinical syndromes.

Arteriography is indicated to localize a lesion and define its extent, vascularity, and vascular supply. The arteriographic picture of a hemangioma may vary from only minimally increased vascularity to a markedly hypervascular lesion (Figs. 11–52 and 11–53). In the latter, dilated, tortuous feeding vessels and pooling of contrast medium are seen in dilated vascular spaces (vascular lakes). Angiographically demonstrable arteriovenous shunting is usually absent. Although some distinguishing features may be present in malignant lesions (eg, coarse, irregular feeding arteries), arteriography cannot always be used to differentiate between a benign hemangioma and a malignancy.[132]

## Klippel-Trenaunay-Weber Syndrome

The Klippel-Trenaunay syndrome consists of (1) hypertrophy of the soft tissues and bones of one extremity (infrequently, the abnormality can be bilateral), (2) portwine hemangiomas, and (3) varicose veins.[133] The classic triad is present in only 75% of patients. In the Klippel-Trenaunay-Weber syndrome, arteriovenous shunting is present in addition to this triad. The disease is not familial and is usually diagnosed in children

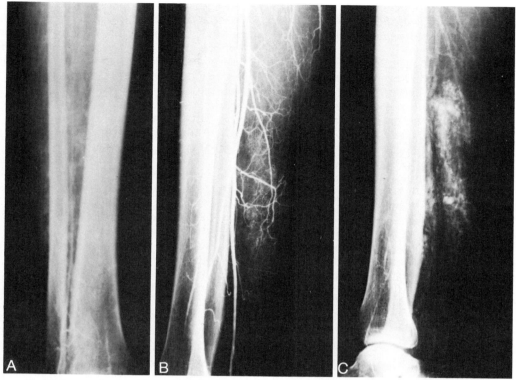

*Figure 11–52.* Hemangioma of the calf. *A,* On the AP arteriogram, the lesion is difficult to identify because of the superimposition of the tibia. *B* and *C,* Early arterial and parenchymal phase of the lateral arteriogram shows a typical hemangioma. The arterial branches supplying the lesion are slightly enlarged. Vascular lakes are present, and there is no arteriovenous shunting.

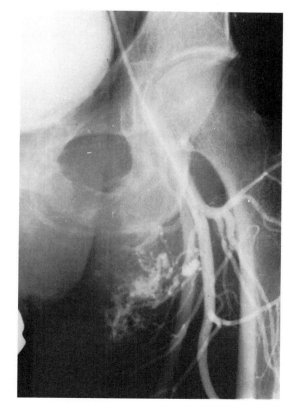

*Figure 11–53.* Intramuscular hemangioma of the left thigh. The lesion is supplied by branches from both the profunda femoris artery and the SFA.

or young adults. Clinically, the first indication may be the presence of a cutaneous hemangioma and subsequently the development of varicose veins.

Venography is necessary for establishing the diagnosis in patients suspected of having this disease. Arteriography is indicated for evaluation of arteriovenous fistulae. The technique for leg venography is described in Chapter 19. Retrograde femoral arteriography provides satisfactory results, and selective arteriography is usually not necessary. The arteriogram should include the pelvis and the proximal thighs.

**Angiographic Findings** (Figs. 11–54 and 11–55)

*Venous abnormalities:*

1. Hypoplasia or aplasia of the deep veins of the calf, thigh, or pelvis: The deep venous system may not opacify on intravenous or intraosseous venography because of preferential filling of the superficial varicosities

through the incompetent venae comitantes. In such patients, the opacification of the deep venous system may be demonstrated on the venous phase of a lower extremity arteriogram.[134] The deep venous system may not opacify on venography also because of competitive blood flow into this system through arteriovenous fistulae.

2. Superficial varicose veins.

3. Absent or abnormal vein valves.

4. Venous aneurysms.

*Arteriocapillary abnormalities* (Fig. 11–56):

1. Hemangioma:[135] Associated hemangiomas of other organ systems may also be present.[136]

2. Arteriomegaly of the involved limb with or without an angiographically demonstrable arteriovenous fistula: Occasionally, an aneurysm may be present.

3. Arteriovenous fistulae: Elevated venous oxygen saturation suggests the presence of microfistulae in the affected limb when arteriovenous fistulae are not demonstrable on arteriography.

## Adventitial Cystic Disease of the Popliteal Artery

Adventitial cystic disease has been observed in the arteries of the forearm, the iliac artery, and, most frequently, the popliteal arteries.[137–139] The exact etiology of the disease is not known. Chronic trauma and a developmental abnormality (heterotopic mucin cells) have been postulated. In one review, adventitial cystic disease of the popliteal artery was found in 1 of 1000 lower extremity arteriograms.[139]

Histologically, mucin-containing multilocular cysts are found in the outer media and adventitia of the popliteal artery.[140] There is no communication with the arterial lumen, but a communication with the knee joint capsule has been demonstrated.[141]

Clinically, there is an abrupt onset of cramplike calf pain, followed by progressively worsening intermittent claudication. Spontaneous, temporary improvement of symptoms and regression of the arteriographic abnormality have been observed.[141] This has been attributed to spontaneous emptying of the cysts. In most cases, there is no history of trauma.

On physical examination, the popliteal and distal pulses are diminished or absent. Occasionally, a pulsatile mass is palpable.[140] In

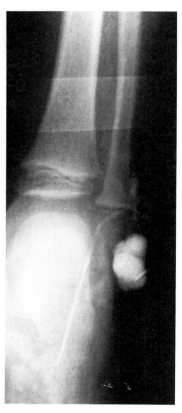

*Figure 11–54.* Venous abnormality in the Klippel-Trenaunay-Weber (KTW) syndrome. Leg venogram in a child with KTW syndrome shows a large premalleolar varix.

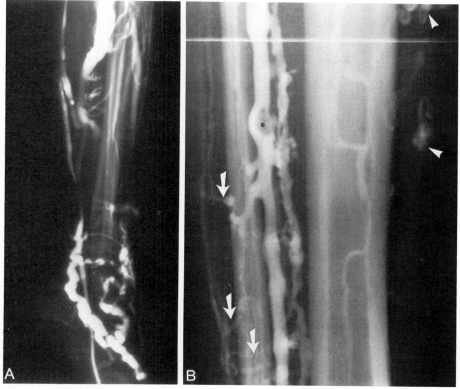

**Figure 11–55.** Venous abnormalities in the Klippel-Trenaunay-Weber syndrome. *A,* Leg venogram in the same patient as in Figure 11–54 shows absent valves, a large posterior tibial vein (venous aneurysm) and enlarged plantar veins. *B,* Right leg venogram from another patient shows an abnormal vein valve (*) and incompetent perforating veins (*straight arrows*) with opacification of superficial veins and varicosities (*arrowheads*).

patients with palpable distal pulses, sharp flexion of the knee causes the pulses to disappear.[142] Most patients are in the third and fourth decades of life (age range, 11 to 70 years), and men are affected more frequently than women (ratio of 6:1).[143] This disease must be considered in the *differential diagnosis* of intermittent claudication in young individuals. Other causes of intermittent claudication in such patients include (1) popliteal artery entrapment syndrome, (2) jogger's aneurysm, (3) thromboangiitis obliterans, (4) embolic occlusion, and (5) popliteal fossa masses.

Arteriography is necessary for the establishment of the diagnosis and for evaluation of the distal circulation.

**Arteriographic Findings** (Fig. 11–57)[140, 141, 143, 144]

1. Segmental stenosis of the popliteal artery: This is the most frequent abnormality and may be in the form of an eccentric, concentric, or spiral-shaped smooth indentation.

2. Segmental occlusion of the popliteal artery.

3. Normal caliber of the artery proximal and distal to the abnormal segment.

4. Normal course of the popliteal artery in the popliteal fossa: This helps to differentiate adventitial cystic disease from the popliteal artery entrapment syndrome.

PITFALLS IN DIAGNOSIS

Extrinsic compression of the popliteal artery may also occur from masses in the popliteal fossa.

## Popliteal Artery Entrapment Syndrome

Popliteal artery entrapment syndrome due to an abnormal course of the popliteal vessels or to an abnormal attachment of the medial head of the gastrocnemius or popliteus muscle is a rare cause of peripheral ischemia of

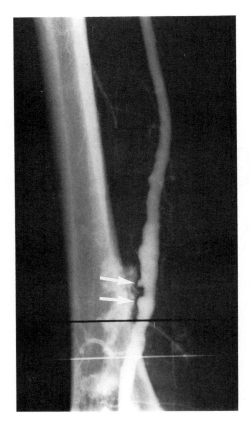

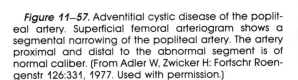

Figure 11–56. Arterial abnormalities in the Klippel-Trenaunay-Weber syndrome. Superficial femoral arteriogram shows diffuse abnormality of the distal SFA and popliteal arteries. There is arteriomegaly and focal aneurysm formation (*arrows*).

Figure 11–57. Adventitial cystic disease of the popliteal artery. Superficial femoral arteriogram shows a segmental narrowing of the popliteal artery. The artery proximal and distal to the abnormal segment is of normal caliber. (From Adler W, Zwicker H: Fortschr Roengenstr 126:331, 1977. Used with permission.)

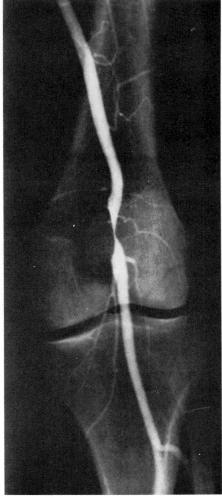

the leg.[145, 146] The etiology is a congenital developmental abnormality and is rarely acquired.[147]

The congenital form can be divided into four types (Fig. 11–58):[91, 146]

*Type I*: The popliteal artery loops medially around the medial head of the gastrocnemius muscle. The latter arises in a normal position. The popliteal vein also follows a normal course and is thus separated from the artery by the medial head of the gastrocnemius muscle.

*Type II*: Also in this type, the popliteal artery loops around the medial head of the gastrocnemius muscle. Since the muscle attachment itself is abnormal (arises more laterally than usual), the deviation of the popliteal artery is not as pronounced as in the Type I abnormality.

*Type III*: The popliteal artery is compressed beneath accessory slips of the medial head of the gastrocnemius muscle. In some instances, a portion of the plantaris muscle may arise together with the medial head of

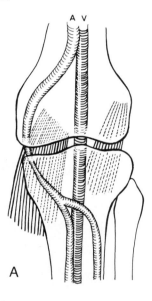

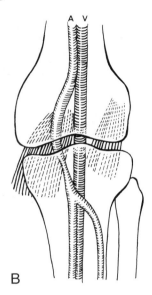

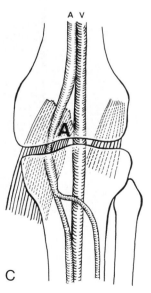

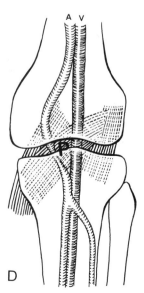

*Figure 11–58.* Popliteal artery entrapment sydnrome. *A*, Type I. *B*, Type II. *C*, Type III. Large A = accessory slip of gastrocnemius muscle. *D*, Type IV. P = popliteus muscle. A = Popliteal artery; V = popliteal vein.

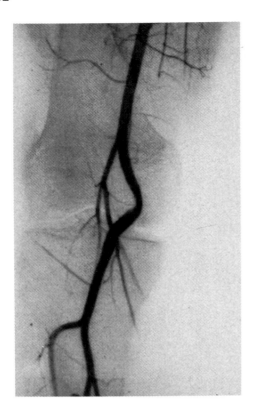

*Figure 11–59.* Popliteal artery entrapment syndrome (Type III). Compression of the popliteal artery is due to an accessory slip of the gastrocnemius muscle. (From Rich NM et al: Arch Surg 114:1377, 1979. Copyright 1979, American Medical Association. Used with permission.)

*Figure 11–60.* Popliteal artery entrapment syndrome. Popliteal artery is normal in the neutral position (*left*). Arterial compression from fibrous bands is seen during plantar flexion (*right*). (From Rich NM et al: Arch Surg 114:1377, 1979. Copyright 1979, American Medical Association. Used with permission.)

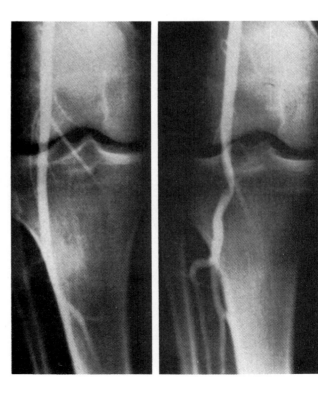

the gastrocnemius muscle, which may also lead to popliteal artery compression.

*Type IV*: The popliteal artery is compressed by the popliteus muscle or fibrous bands. The artery may follow a normal or a deviated course.

The Type I abnormality is the most common form and is found in 57% of patients. The Type II abnormality is the second most common form and is seen in 28% of patients.[148] The popliteal vein may also be involved in the entrapment.[91] A similar entrapment syndrome has also been reported involving the femoral artery at the inguinal ligament.[149]

In one third of the patients, the onset of symptoms is acute, following an episode of exertion.[148] This is followed by progressively increasing intermittent claudication. Males are affected more frequently than females (ratio of 8:1), and the disease is bilateral in 20% of patients.[145, 148] The age of the patients ranges from 12 to 64 years.[91, 145] On physical examination the popliteal and distal pulses may be normal, diminished, or absent. In patients with normal or only minimally diminished distal pulses, passive plantar flexion of the foot leads to compression of the popliteal artery with diminishment or obliteration of the pulse.

Arteriography is indicated for the establishment of the diagnosis and assessment of the complications. Retrograde femoral arteriography provides satisfactory information and permits evaluation of both lower extremities. If symptoms are unilateral, antegrade femoral arteriography may be performed with a multiple hole straight catheter placed in the mid-SFA. The anatomical complications associated with the popliteal artery entrapment syndrome are most likely due to chronic traumatization.[91]

**Arteriographic Findings** (Fig. 11–59)

1. Medial deviation of the mid-portion of the popliteal artery: Occasionally, lateral deviation may be seen.[148]

2. Thrombosis of the popliteal artery.

3. Aneurysm formation.

PITFALLS IN DIAGNOSIS (Fig. 11–60)

1. No arterial abnormality: In this situation, the arteriogram is repeated with the foot in dorsal (plantar) flexion. This maneuver will result in extrinsic compression of the popliteal artery in patients with the entrapment syndrome.[91, 148]

2. Popliteal artery occlusion with apparent

bowing of the artery or collaterals: This may be due to an occluded popliteal artery aneurysm in a patient without the entrapment syndrome. In addition, a slight obliquity of the distal lower extremity may simulate bowing of the collaterals.

## REFERENCES

1. Warwick R, Williams PL: Gray's Anatomy, 35th Brit. Ed. Philadelphia, WB Saunders, 1973, pp. 673–684.
2. Weiland AJ, Kleinert HE, Kutz JE, et al: Free vascularized bone grafts in surgery of the upper extremity. J Hand Surg 4:129–144, 1979.
3. Sobotta J, Becher H: Atlas der Anatomie des Menschen. 3 Teil: Blutkreislauf, Herz, Periphere Nerven und Blutgefaesse, Lymphgefaesse, Zentralnervensystem, Sinnesorgane, Haut. Muenchen–Berlin, Urban & Schwartzenberg 1962, pp. 173–192.
4. Pirker E, Schmidtberger H: Die Arteria Ischiadica. Eine seltene Gefaessvariante. Fortschr Roentgenstr 116:434–437, 1972.
5. Bardsley JL, Staple TW: Variations in branching of the popliteal artery. Radiology 94:581–587, 1970.
6. Reich RS: The pulses of the foot. Their value in the diagnosis of peripheral circulatory disease. Ann Surg 99:613–622, 1934.
7. Barnhorst DA, Barner HB: Prevalence of congenitally absent pedal pulses. N Engl J Med 278:264–265, 1968.
8. John HT, Warren R: The stimulus to collateral circulation. Surgery 49:14–25, 1961.
9. Longland CJ: Collateral circulation in the limb. Quoted in reference 8.
10. Latschenberger J, Deahna A: Beitraege zur Lehre von der reflectorischen Erregung der Gefaessmuskeln. Arch Gesamt Physiol 12:157–204, 1876.
11. Hess WR: Die physiologischen Grundlagen fuer die Enstehung der reaktiven Hyperaemie und des Kollateralkreislaufes. Beitr Klin Chir 122:1, 1921.
12. Folkow B: Pathophysiological aspects of blood flow distal to an obliterated main artery with special regard to the possibilities of affecting the collateral resistance and the arterioles in the distal low pressure system. Scand J Clin Lab Invest 99 (Suppl):211–218, 1967.
13. Mulvihill DA, Harvey SC: The mechanism of the development of collateral circulation. N Engl J Med 204:1032–1034, 1931.
14. Shaper W, De Brabander M, Lewi P: DNA synthesis and mitoses in coronary collateral vessels of the dog. Circ Res. 28:671–679, 1971.
15. Bollinger A: Periphere zirkulation. Pathophysiologie des arteriellen systems. *In* Siegenthaler W (ed): Klinische Pathophysiologie. Stuttgart, Georg Thieme Verlag, 1970, pp. 563–594.
16. Kadir S, Kaufman SL, Barth KH, et al: Selected Techniques in Interventional Radiology. Philadelphia, WB Saunders, 1982, pp. 142–207.
17. Thomas ML, Lintott DJ: Large volume aortography in atherosclerotic peripheral vascular disease. A comparative investigation with conventional aortography. Acta Radiol Diagn 14:56–64, 1973.
18. Glenn JH: Biphasic injection for femoral and aor-

tofemoral arteriography utilizing a standard pressure injector. Radiology 115:479–480, 1975.

19. Murphy RA Jr, McClure JN Jr, Cooper FW, et al: The effect of priscoline, papaverine and nicotinic acid on blood flow in the lower extremity of man. A comparative study. Surgery 27:655–663, 1950.

20. Lindgren P, Tornell G: Blood circulation during and after peripheral arteriography: experimental study of the effects of Triurol (sodium acetrizoate) and Hypaque (sodium diatrizoate). Acta Radiol 49:425–440, 1958.

21. Sako Y: Hemodynamic changes during arteriography. JAMA 183:253–256, 1963.

22. Kahn PC, Callow AD: Selective vasodilatation as an aid to angiography. AJR 94:213–220, 1965.

23. Abramson DI: Drugs used in peripheral vascular diseases. Am J Cardiol 12:203–215, 1963.

24. Kahn PC, Boyer DN, Moran JM, et al: Reactive hyperemia in lower extremity arteriography: an evaluation. Radiology 90:975–980, 1968.

25. Hishida Y: Peripheral arteriography using reactive hyperemia. Jap Circ J 27:349–358, 1963.

26. Hillestad LK: The peripheral blood flow in intermittent claudication: V. Plethysmographic studies. The significance of the calf blood flow at rest and in response to timed arrest of the circulation. Acta Med Scand 174:23–41, 1963.

27. Beckmann CF, Levin DC, Kubicka RA: Reactive hyperemia vs. pharmacologic hyperemia in the canine iliac circulation. A comparison. Invest Radiol 18:254–256, 1983.

28. Rosch J, Antonovic R, Porter JM: The importance of temperature in angiography of the hand. Radiology 123:323–326, 1977.

29. Chermet J: Arteriography of lower limbs with blocked circulation ("dry-limb" arteriography). Radiology 140:826–830, 1981.

29a. Spigos DG, Akkineni S, Tan W, et al: Epidural anesthesia: effective analgesia in aortoiliofemoral arteriography. AJR 134:335–337, 1980.

30. Guthaner DF, Silverman JF, Hayden WG, et al: Intraarterial analgesia in peripheral arteriography. AJR 128:737–739, 1977.

31. Editorial: Attitude to pain. Br Med J 3:261, 1975.

31a. Katzen BT, Edwards KC: Nitrous-oxide analgesia for interventional radiologic procedures. AJR 140:145–148, 1983.

32. Hagen B, Clauss W: Kontrastmittel und Schmerz bei der peripheren Arteriographie. Randomisierter, intraindividueller Doppelblindversuch: Ioglicinat, Ioglicinat-Lidocain, Ioxaglat. Radiologe 22:470–475, 1982.

33. Nyman U, Nilsson P, Westergren A: Pain and hemodynamic effects in aortofemoral angiography. Clinical comparison of iohexol, ioxaglate and metrizamide. Acta Radiol 23:389–399, 1982.

34. Gordon IJ, Westcott JL: Intraarterial lidocaine: An effective analgesic for peripheral angiography. Radiology 124:43–45, 1977.

35. Widrich WC, Singer RJ, Robbins AH: The use of intra-arterial lidocaine to control pain due to aortofemoral arteriography. Radiology 124:37–41, 1977.

36. Dent TL, Lindenauer SM, Ernst CB, et al: Multiple arteriosclerotic arterial aneurysms. Arch Surg 105:338–344, 1972.

37. Graham LM, Zelenock GB, Whitehouse WM, et al: Clinical significance of arteriosclerotic femoral artery aneurysms. Arch Surg 115:502–507, 1980.

38. Cutler BS, Darling RC: Surgical management of arteriosclerotic femoral artery aneurysms. Surgery 74:764–773, 1973.

39. Powers TA, Harolds JA, Kadir S, et al: Pseudoaneurysm of the profunda femoris artery diagnosed on angiographic phase of bone scan. Clin Nucl Med 10:422–424, 1979.

40. Engelman RM, Clements JM, Herrmann JB: Stab wounds and traumatic false aneurysms in the extremities. J Trauma 9:77–87, 1969.

41. Stock JR, Athanasoulis CA: Musculoskeletal trauma: Control of bleeding with transcatheter embolization. In Athanasoulis CA, Pfister RC, Greene R, et al (eds): Interventional Radiology. Philadelphia, WB Saunders, 1982, pp. 174–195.

42. Enge I, Aakhus T, Evensen A: Angiography in vascular injuries of the extremities. Acta Radiol 16:193–199, 1975.

43. Love L, Braun T: Arteriography of peripheral vascular trauma. AJR 102:431–440, 1968.

44. Feinsod FM, Norfleet RG, Hoehn JL: Mycotic aneurysm of the external iliac artery. A triad of clinical signs facilitating early diagnosis. JAMA 238:245–246, 1977.

45. Yellin AE: Ruptured mycotic aneurysm. A complication of parenteral drug abuse. Arch Surg 112:981–986, 1977.

46. Wilson SE, Gordon E, Van Wagenen PB: Salmonella arteritis. A precursor of aortic rupture and pseudoaneurysm formation. Arch Surg 113:1163–1166, 1978.

47. Solhaugh JH, Olerud SE: Pseudoaneurysm of the femoral artery caused by osteochondroma of the femur. J Bone Joint Surg 57A:867–868, 1975.

48. Bouhoutsos J, Martin P: Popliteal aneurysm: a review of 116 cases. Br J Surg 61:649–675, 1974.

49. Szilagyi DE, Schwartz RL, Reddy DJ: Popliteal arterial aneurysms: Their natural history and management. Arch Surg 116:724–728, 1981.

50. Wychulis AR, Spittell JA Jr, Wallace RB: Popliteal aneurysms. Surgery 68:942–952, 1970.

51. Baird RJ, Sivasankar R, Haywood R, et al: Popliteal aneurysms: a review and analysis of 61 cases. Surgery 59:911–917, 1966.

52. Whitehouse WM, Wakefield TW, Graham LM, et al: Limb-threatening potential of arteriosclerotic popliteal artery aneurysms. Surgery 93:694–699, 1983.

53. Edmunds LH Jr, Darling RC, Linton RR: Surgical management of popliteal aneurysms. Circulation 32:517–523, 1965.

54. Giustra PE, Root JA, Mason SE, et al: Popliteal vein thrombosis secondary to popliteal artery aneurysm. AJR 130:25–27, 1978.

55. Greenway G, Resnick D, Bookstein JJ: Popliteal pseudoaneurysm as a complication of an adjacent osteochondroma: angiographic diagnosis. AJR 132:294–296, 1979.

56. Lundell C, Kadir S: The jogger's aneurysm. Unusual manifestation of popliteal artery trauma. J Cardiovasc Intervent Radiol 4:239–241, 1981.

57. Davis RP, Neiman HL, Yao JST, et al: Ultrasound scan in diagnosis of peripheral aneurysms. Arch Surg 112:55–58, 1977.

58. Widmer LK: Der chronische Verschluss von Gliedermassenarterien. Haeufigkeit, Aetiologie, Bedeutung. In Widmer LK, Waibel P (eds): Arterielle Durchblutungsstoerungen in der Praxis. Bern, Verlag Hans Huber, 1972, pp. 10–14.

59. Juergens JL, Barker NW, Hines EA Jr: Arteriosclerosis obliterans: Review of 520 cases with special reference to pathogenic and prognostic factors. Circulation 21:188–195, 1960.

60. Schadt DC, Hines EA Jr, Juergens JL, et al: Chronic atherosclerotic occlusion of the femoral artery. JAMA 175:937–940, 1961.

61. Bell ET: Incidence of gangrene of the extremities in nondiabetic and diabetic persons. Arch Pathol 49:469–473, 1950.

62. Kannel WB, Skinner JJ Jr, Schwartz MJ, et al: Intermittent claudication. Incidence in the Framingham Study. Circulation 41:875–883, 1970.

63. Dry TJ, Hines EA Jr: The role of diabetes in the development of degenerative vascular disease: with special reference to the incidence of retinitis and peripheral vessels. Ann Intern Med 14:1893–1902, 1941.

64. Strandness DE Jr, Stahler C: Arteriosclerosis obliterans. Manner and rate of progression. JAMA 196:1–4, 1966.

65. Warren R, Gomez RL, Marston JAP: Femoropopliteal arteriosclerosis obliterans. Arteriographic patterns and rates of progression. Surgery 55:135–143, 1964.

66. Kuthan F, Burkhalter A, Baitsch R, et al: Development of occlusive arterial disease in the lower limbs. Arch Surg 103:545–547, 1971.

67. Morris, PE, Hessel SJ, Couch NP, et al: Surgery and the progression of the occlusive process in patients with peripheral vascular disease. Radiology 124:343–348, 1977.

68. Tillgren C, Stenson S, Lund F: Obliterative arterial disease of the lower limb studied by means of repeated femoral arteriography. An attempt to evaluate the effect of long-term anticoagulant therapy. Acta Radiol Diagn 1:1161–1178, 1963.

69. O'Mara CS, Flinn WR, Neiman HL, et al: Correlation of foot arterial anatomy with early tibial bypass patency. Surgery 89:743–752, 1981.

70. Kinnison ML, Kadir S: Long superficial femoral artery occlusion: Observations that influence patient selection criteria for angioplasty. Cardiovasc Intervent Radiol 7:102–103, 1984.

71. Crummy AB, Rankin RS, Turnipseed WD, et al: Biplane arteriography in ischemia of the lower extremity. Radiology 126:111–115, 1978.

72. Juergens JL: Thromboangiitis obliterans. In Juergens JL, Spittell JA Jr, Fairbairn JF II (eds): Peripheral Vascular Diseases. Philadelphia, WB Saunders, 1980, pp. 469–491.

73. Haimovici H: Peripheral arterial embolism. A study of 330 unselected cases of embolism of the extremities. Angiology 1:20–45, 1950.

74. Darling RC, Austen WG, Linton RR: Arterial embolism. Surg Gynecol Obstet 124:106–114, 1967.

75. Williams GM, Harrington D, Burdick J, et al: Mural thrombus of the aorta: An important, frequently neglected cause of large peripheral emboli. Ann Surg 194:737–744, 1981.

76. Thompson T, Evans W: Paradoxical embolism. Q J Med 23:135–150, 1930.

77. Crane C: Atherothrombotic embolism to lower extremities in arteriosclerosis. Arch Surg 94:96–101, 1967.

78. Lord JW, Rossi G, Daliana M, et al: Unsuspected abdominal aortic aneurysms as the cause of peripheral arterial occlusive disease. Ann Surg 177:767–771, 1973.

79. Edwards EA, Tilney N, Lindquist RR: Causes of peripheral embolism and their significance. JAMA 196:119–124, 1966.

80. Krag DN, Stansel HC Jr: Popliteal cyst producing complete arterial occlusion. A case report. J Bone Joint Surg 64-A:1369–1370, 1982.

81. Dardik H, Dardik I, Sprayregen S, et al: Asymmetrical nonocclusive ischemia of the lower extremities. JAMA 227:1417–1419, 1974.

82. Maurizi CP, Barker AE, Trueheart RE: Atheromatous emboli. A post-mortem study with special reference to the lower extremities. Arch Pathol 86:528–534, 1968.

83. Kempczinski RF: Lower extremity arterial emboli from ulcerating atherosclerotic plaques. JAMA 241:807–810, 1979.

84. Anderson WR, Richards AM: Evaluation of lower extremity muscle biopsies in the diagnosis of atheroembolism. Arch Pathol 86:535–541, 1968.

85. Karmody AM, Powers SR, Monaco VJ, et al: "Blue toe syndrome." An indication for limb salvage surgery. Arch Surg 111:1263–1268, 1976.

86. Case Records of the Massachusetts General Hospital: Case 33–1974. N Engl J Med 291:406–412, 1974.

87. Babb RR, Alarcon-Segovia D, Fairbairn JF II: Erytheromalalgia. Review of 51 cases. Circulation 29:136–141, 1964.

88. Little JM, Goodman AH: Cystic adventitial disease of the popliteal artery. Br J Surg 57:708–713, 1970.

89. McArdle B: Myopathy due to a defect in muscle glycogen breakdown. Clin Sci 10:13–33, 1951.

90. Bjordal RI: Intermittent venous claudication. A report of two cases. Acta Chir Scand 136:641–645, 1970.

91. Rich NM, Collins GJ, McDonald PT: Popliteal vascular entrapment. Its increasing interest. Arch Surg 114:1377–1384, 1979.

92. Cannon JA: Intermittent claudication. What it is and isn't. Cal Med 102:301–305, 1965.

93. Mufson I: Intermittent limping—intermittent claudication. Their differential diagnosis. Ann Intern Med 14:2240–2245, 1941.

94. Verbiest J: A radicular syndrome from developmental narrowing of the lumbar vertebral canal. J Bone Joint Surg 36B:230–237, 1954.

95. Coffman JD: Intermittent claudication and rest pain. Physiological concepts and therapeutic approaches. Prog Cardiovasc Dis 32:53–72, 1979.

96. Morris GC Jr, Beall AC Jr, Roof WR, et al: Surgical experience with 220 acute arterial injuries in civilian practice. Am J Surg 99:775–781, 1960.

97. Drapanas T, Hewitt RL, Weichert RF III, et al: Civilian vascular injuries: a critical appraisal of three decades of management. Ann Surg 172:351–360, 1970.

98. Shuck JM, Omer GE Jr, Lewis CE Jr: Arterial obstruction due to intimal disruption in extremity fractures. J Trauma 12:481–489, 1972.

99. Makin GS, Howard JM, Green RL: Arterial injuries complicating fractures or dislocations: The necessity for a more aggressive approach. Surgery 59:203–209, 1966.

100. Snyder LL, Binet EF, Thompson BW: False aneurysm with arteriovenous fistula of the anterior tibial artery following fracture of the fibula. Radiology 143:405–406, 1982.

101. McDonald EJ Jr, Goodman PC, Winestock DP: The

clinical indications for arteriography in trauma to the extremity. Radiology 116:45–47, 1975.

102. Spencer AD: The reliability of signs of peripheral vascular injury. Surg Obstet Gynecol 114:490–494, 1962.

103. Saletta JD, Freearck RJ: Occult vascular injuries of the extremities. J Occup Med 12:304–307, 1970.

104. Snyder WH III, Thal ER, Bridges RA, et al: The validity of normal arteriography in penetrating trauma. Arch Surg 113:424–428, 1978.

105. Kreipke DL, Holden RW, Wass JL: Two angiographic signs of pseudoaneurysms: systolic jet and diastolic washout. Radiology 144:79–82, 1982.

106. Todd GJ, Bregman D, Voorhees AB, et al: Vascular complications associated with percutaneous intraaortic balloon pumping. Arch Surg 118:963–964, 1983.

107. Foster JH, Carter JW, Graham CP, et al: Arterial injuries secondary to the use of the Fogarty catheter. Ann Surg 171:971–978, 1970.

108. Milnor WR: Regional circulations. In Mountcastle VB (ed): Medical Physiology. New York, CV Mosby, 1974, pp. 944–945.

109. Hertzman AB: Vasomotor regulation of cutaneous circulation. Physiol Rev 39:280–306, 1959.

110. Kontos HA, Richardson DW, Patterson JL Jr: Effects of hypercapnia on human forearm vessels. Am J Physiol 212:1070–1080, 1967.

111. Athanasoulis CA: Upper gastrointestinal bleeding of arteriocapillary origin. In Athanasoulis CA, Pfister RC, Greene R, et al (eds): Interventional Radiology. Philadelphia, WB Saunders, 1982, pp. 55–89.

112. Bagby RJ, Cooper RD: Angiography in ergotism. Report of two cases and review of the literature. AJR 116:179–186, 1972.

113. Fedotin MS, Hartman C: Ergotamine poisoning producing renal arterial spasm. N Engl J Med 283:518–520, 1970.

114. Richter AM, Banker VP: Carotid ergotism. A complication of migraine therapy. Radiology 106:339–340, 1973.

115. Berman JK, Brown HM, Foster RT, et al: Massive resection of the intestine. JAMA 135:918–919, 1947.

116. Cranley JJ, Krause RJ, Strasser ES, et al: Impending gangrene of four extremities secondary to ergotism. N Engl J Med 269:727–729, 1963.

117. Sutton D, Preston BJ: Angiography in peripheral ischaemia due to ergotism. Report of two cases. Br J Radiol 43:776–780, 1970.

118. O'Dell CW Jr, Davis GB, Johnson AD, et al: Sodium nitroprusside in the treatment of ergotism. Radiology 124:73–74, 1977.

119. Henry LG, Blackwood JS, Conley JE, et al: Ergotism. Arch Surg 110:929–932, 1975.

120. Kramer RA, Hecker SP, Lewis BI: Ergotism: Report of a case studied angiographically. Radiology 84:308–311, 1965.

121. Furey NL, Schmid FR, Kwaan HC, et al: Arterial thrombosis in scleroderma. Br J Dermatol 93:683–693, 1975.

122. Bollinger A, Vogt B, Veragut U, et al: Ischaemisches Syndrom der unteren Extremitaeten hervorgerufen durch Spasmen der Muskulaeren Verteilerarterien. Schw Med Wochenschr 97:693–698, 1967.

123. Hegglin R: Differentialdiagnose innerer Krankheiten, 12th Ed. Stuttgart, Georg Thieme Verlag, 1972, pp. 782–783.

124. Roy P: Peripheral angiography in ischemic arterial disease of the limbs. Radiol Clin North Am 5:467–496, 1967.

125. Kadir S, Athanasoulis CA: Peripheral vasospastic disorders: Management with intraarterial infusion of vasodilatory drugs. In Athanasoulis CA, Pfister RC, Greene R, et al (eds): Interventional Radiology. Philadelphia, WB Saunders, 1982, pp. 343–354.

126. Tice DA, Clauss RH, Keirle AM, et al: Congenital arteriovenous fistulae of the extremities. Observations concerning treatment. Arch Surg 86:460–465, 1963.

127. Adler SC, Wexler L, Castellino RA: Angiography of lower extremity soft tissue arteriovenous fistulas. J Can Assoc Radiol 23:207–213, 1972.

128. Gomes AS, Busuttil RW, Baker JD, et al: Congenital arteriovenous malformations. The role of transcatheter arterial embolization. Arch Surg 118:817–825, 1983.

129. Kadir S, Ernst CB, Hamper U, et al: Management of vascular soft tissue neoplasms using transcatheter embolization and surgical excision. Am J Surg 146:409–412, 1983.

130. Kornmann JE: Die Haemangiome. Uebersicht der Literatur sowie eigene pathologisch-anatomische untersuchungen. Zentralbl Chir 40:1427–1428, 1913.

131. Watson WL, McCarthy WD: Blood and lymph vessel tumors. A report of 1056 cases. Surg Gynecol Obstet 71:569–588, 1940.

132. Levin DC, Gordon DH, McSweeney J: Arteriography of peripheral hemangiomas. Radiology 121:625–630, 1976.

133. Lindenauer SM: The Klippel-Trenaunay syndrome. Varicosity, hypertrophy and hemangioma with no arteriovenous fistula. Ann Surg 162:303–314, 1965.

134. Mueller JHA, Schmidt KH: Angiographische Befunde beim Klippel-Trenaunay-Weber-Syndrom. Fortsch Roentgenstr 110:540–552, 1969.

135. Phillips GN, Gordon DH, Martin EC, et al: The Klippel-Trenaunay-syndrome. Clinical and radiological aspects. Radiology 128:429–434, 1978.

136. Ghahremani GG, Kangarloo H, Volberg F, et al: Diffuse cavernous hemangioma of the colon in the Klippel-Trenaunay syndrome. Radiology 118:673–678, 1976.

137. Atkins HJB, Key JA: A case of myxomatous tumor arising in the adventitia of the left external iliac artery. Br J Surg 34:426–427, 1947.

138. Powis SJA, Morrissey DM, Jones EL: Cystic degeneration of the popliteal artery. Surgery 67:891–894, 1970.

139. Haid SP, Conn J Jr, Bergan JJ: Cystic adventitial disease of the popliteal artery. Arch Surg 101:765–770, 1970.

140. Bunker SR, Lauten GJ, Hutton JE Jr: Cystic adventitial disease of the popliteal artery. AJR 136:1209–1212, 1981.

141. Alder W, Zwicker H: Zur Diagnose der zystischen Adventitiadegeneration. Fortschr Roentgenstr 126:331–334, 1977.

142. Ishikawa K, Mishima Y, Kobayashi S: Cystic adventitial disease of the popliteal artery. Angiology 12:357–366, 1961.

143. Flanigan DP, Burnham SJ, Goodreau JJ, et al: Summary of cases of adventitial cystic disease of the popliteal artery. Ann Surg 189:165–175, 1979.

144. Richardson JD, Polk HC Jr: Adventitial cystic disease of the popliteal artery. Arch Surg 116:478–479, 1981.
145. Gibson MHL, Mills JG, Johnson GE, et al: Popliteal entrapment syndrome. Ann Surg 185:341–348, 1977.
146. Insua JA, Young JR, Humphries AW: Popliteal artery entrapment syndrome. Arch Surg 101:771–775, 1970.
147. Baker WH, Stoney RJ: Acquired popliteal artery entrapment syndrome. Arch Surg 105:780–781, 1972.
148. Biemans RGM, Van Bockel JH: Popliteal artery entrapment syndrome. Surg Gynecol Obstet 144:604–609, 1977.
149. Antinori CH, Donaldson MH, Sussman SJ, et al: Common femoral artery entrapment in an infant. JAMA 249:1326–1327, 1983.

# Arteriographic Evaluation After Aortic, Iliac, and Peripheral Vascular Bypass Surgery

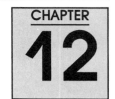

The most commonly used prosthetic materials for reconstruction of larger vessels are woven or knitted Dacron grafts. Knitted Dacron grafts are commonly used in aorto-iliac and aorto-femoral reconstruction, whereas woven grafts are used for thoracic aortic replacement. Another type, the polytetrafluoroethylene (eg, Goretex) graft, is used for extra-anatomical and femoro-popliteal bypass grafts. Autogenous saphenous vein is the most durable substitute for smaller arteries and is widely used for femoro-popliteal and femoro-infrapopliteal reconstruction.[1] Occasionally, glutaraldehyde-treated human umbilical cord vein grafts are used for femoro-popliteal reconstruction. Because of their propensity for aneurysm formation, bovine grafts are no longer used as arterial substitutes.[1]

Late complications of vascular surgery may result from defective healing, deterioration of the arterial substitute, or progression of disease in the host vessels.[2] Such complications may result in the development of anastomotic aneurysm, vascular-enteric fistula, anastomotic stenosis, infection, and graft or graft-limb thrombosis. The overall incidence of late complications after abdominal aortic reconstruction is about 9%.[3] Thrombosis accounts for approximately half these complications. For some types of complications, eg, infection and retroperitoneal hemorrhage, computed tomography (CT) and ultrasonography provide an excellent means of diagnosis.[4, 5] However, arteriography is required for the evaluation of most other complications and for the determination of graft patency.

In the management of peripheral vascular disease, the goals of arterial reconstruction are restoration of function of the affected limb, alleviation of symptoms, and limb salvage. Objective, noninvasive methods for the assessment of success of the operation are palpation of the arterial or graft pulse, transcutaneous Doppler ultrasonography, recording of flow velocity wave forms, and measurement of the systolic pressure by means of occlusive cuffs and the calculation of the systolic pressure index. Such evaluation is indicated as a routine procedure for the detection of new lesions and hemodynamic failures, ie, patent graft as determined by Doppler ultrasonography but lack of hemodynamic improvement or relief of symptoms.

For peripheral vascular surgery, arteriography is required to confirm the clinical and noninvasive laboratory diagnosis and to provide a preoperative "road map" for corrective surgery. In general, arteriography is indicated if the physical examination or noninvasive laboratory data suggest the development of new stenotic lesions or a graft complication, eg, for evaluation of (1) a decrease in the systolic pressure index by greater than 0.20, (2) a hemodynamically failed graft, (3) a suspected graft or graft-limb occlusion, or (4) an anastomotic aneurysm.

## THORACIC AORTA

Prosthetic grafts are used for the replacement of the diseased thoracic aorta. In the ascending aorta, either a tube or a composite graft (ascending aorta and aortic valve prosthesis) is used. After placement of the graft, the native aorta is wrapped and sutured around it. This provides hemostasis by means of tamponade if postoperative bleeding should occur.

Thoracic aortography is indicated for the assessment of late operative complications and to evaluate progression of the disease. Although CT provides a method for the follow-up of such patients, there are several limiting factors that may compromise its usefulness.[6] Other methods of evaluation are digital subtraction angiography (DSA) and magnetic resonance imaging (MRI).

Late complications of thoracic aortic surgery that may require arteriography are[6-10] (Figs. 12–1 and 12–2):

1. Suture dehiscence at the proximal or distal anastomosis: Suture dehiscence around an aortic valve prosthesis may result in aortic valvar insufficiency or in paravalvar aortic

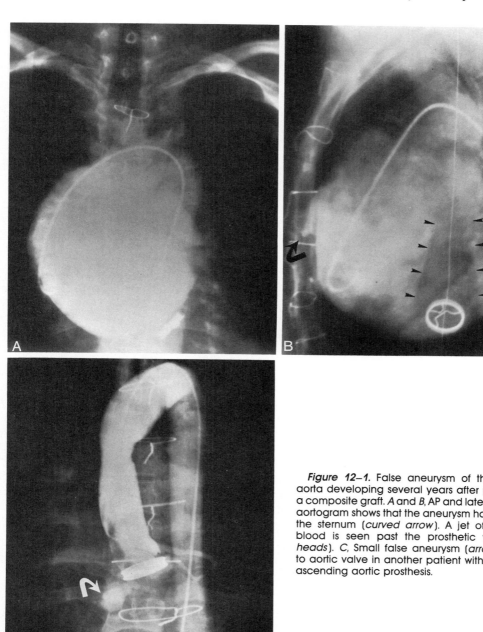

*Figure 12–1.* False aneurysm of the ascending aorta developing several years after placement of a composite graft. *A* and *B*, AP and lateral ascending aortogram shows that the aneurysm has eroded into the sternum (*curved arrow*). A jet of unopacified blood is seen past the prosthetic valve (*arrowheads*). *C*, Small false aneurysm (*arrow*) adjacent to aortic valve in another patient with a composite ascending aortic prosthesis.

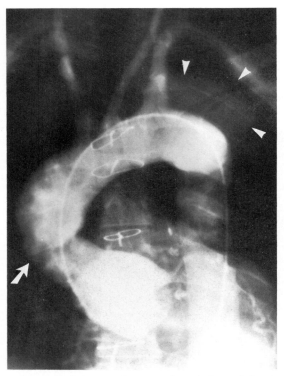

*Figure 12–2.* Composite ascending aortic graft. Arrow points to the distal anastomosis. The patient was studied because of symptoms of recurrent dissection. Although a second channel is not opacified, a large soft tissue shadow is present at the distal arch (*arrowheads*), indicating a redissection.

**TABLE 12–1.** Aortogram for the Evaluation of Thoracic Aortic Grafts

| | |
|---|---|
| Approach | Femoral artery |
| Catheter: | 5–7 Fr pigtail |
|   Position | Proximal ascending aorta |
| Guide wire | 0.035 inch J |
| Contrast medium | 76% diatrizoate meglumine sodium* |
| Injection rate/volume | 25–30 ml/sec, total 50–60 ml |
| Films: | 13 films per projection |
|   Filming | 3 per second for 9 films |
| | 1 per second for 4 films |
|   Projection | a. Biplane AP/lateral *or* |
| | b. LAO 45° |

*20% concentration for DSA.

cated for the evaluation of (a) a suspected new dissection, (b) extension of the previous dissection, or (c) aneurysm formation.

After repair of a dissection, opacification of the false channel per se may be a normal postoperative finding. In one series, it was observed in 85% of patients and half of these patients were asymptomatic.[9]

The following arteriographic methods may be used for the evaluation of the thoracic aorta (Table 12–1): (1) intravenous DSA, (2) intraarterial DSA, or (3) standard transfemoral aortography.

## AXILLO-FEMORAL GRAFTS

The axillo-femoral graft is an extra-anatomical bypass graft extending from the axillary artery to the femoral arteries (Fig. 12–3). It is usually performed in high operative risk patients or patients in whom anatomical reconstruction is not possible (eg, due to infection).

Arteriography may be required for the evaluation of the following problems:[11–13]

1. Suspected graft or graft-limb occlusion (Fig. 12–4).

2. Assessment of inflow disease or progression of outflow disease.

3. Anastomotic aneurysm.

4. Thrombosis of the axillary artery.

5. Ischemia of the distal donor extremity: This may be due to either a steal phenomenon or thromboembolism.

Arteriography of axillo-femoral bypass grafts can be performed by the following methods:

1. Intravenous DSA.

2. Catheterization of the donor vessel: This

insufficiency if the dehiscence causes a communication with the left ventricle.[7] Communication of the left ventricle with the perigraft space may lead to a characteristic angiographic finding: collapse (or compression) of the ascending aortic graft during ventricular systole.[7a]

2. Leakage around the suture with the formation of a hematoma around the graft: Leakage of a small volume of contrast medium, with opacification of a small pocket between the graft and the surrounding native aorta, has also been observed in asymptomatic individuals.[8] Such leakage may not be demonstrated on cut films and is best seen on cineangiography,[7] CT,[8] and intraarterial DSA.

3. False aneurysm formation.

4. In addition to the formation of an aneurysm, restenosis or aortic dissection may occur in patients with a previously repaired coarctation.

5. Finally, in patients operated upon for aortic dissection, arteriography may be indi-

**TABLE 12–2.** Subclavian Arteriography for Evaluation of Axillo-Femoral Grafts

| | |
|---|---|
| Approach | Opposite axillary artery |
| Catheter: | 5–7 Fr sidewinder II |
|    Position | Proximal subclavian artery |
| Guide wire | 0.035 inch J LLT |
| Contrast medium | 60% diatrizoate meglumine sodium* |
| Injection rate/volume | 8 ml/sec, total 24 ml |
| Films: | 6 films |
|    Filming | 1 film per second |
|    Projection | AP |

*20% concentration for DSA.

method is used for evaluation of the proximal anastomosis or selective catheterization of the graft. The donor vessel can be catheterized from either the contralateral axillary artery approach or a high brachial artery puncture from the ipsilateral side. From the contralateral axillary artery approach, a sidewinder II catheter is used to catheterize the donor subclavian artery to evaluate the proximal graft anastomosis (Table 12–2). From this approach, catheterization of the graft is difficult. Catheterization of the graft is accomplished through a high brachial artery puncture from the ipsilateral side, using either a cobra C1 or a single curve catheter (Table 12–3).

3. Direct graft puncture: This approach is best suited for the evaluation of the distal graft anastomosis and for assessment of the

**TABLE 12–3.** Catheterization of Axillo-Femoral Graft for Evaluation of Femoral Anastomosis and Distal Vessels

| | |
|---|---|
| Approach | Ipsilateral axillary artery |
| Catheter: | Single curve or cobra C1 (end and side holes) |
|    Position | Proximal graft |
| Guide wire | 0.035 inch J LLT |
| Contrast medium | 76% diatrizoate meglumine sodium* |
| Injection rate/volume | 6 ml/sec, total 24–50* ml |
| Films/filming† | a. 6 films at 1 film per second (for distal anastomosis) |
| | b. long leg changer/stepping table top‡ |
|    Projections | AP |
| | Oblique pelvis |

*20% concentration for DSA.
†Time delay between contrast injection and filming being assessed by hand test injection.
‡For vessels distal to the femoral anastomosis.

status of the runoff vessels. In our own experience, percutaneous graft puncture has been without complications. The graft is punctured percutaneously, in an antegrade fashion, where it crosses the lower rib cage. A short 5 Fr multiple hole straight catheter can be inserted over a movable core J guide wire. We prefer to use the Amplatz needle for graft puncture. The sheath is easily inserted into the graft without the aid of a

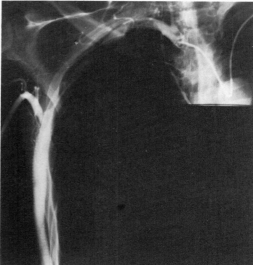
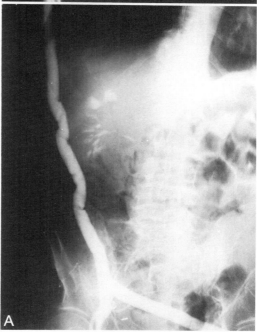

**Figure 12–3.** Normal axillo-femoral bypass graft. *A,* Conventional arteriogram from the left axillary artery approach using a long film changer. This study required a single contrast injection.

*Illustration continued on following page*

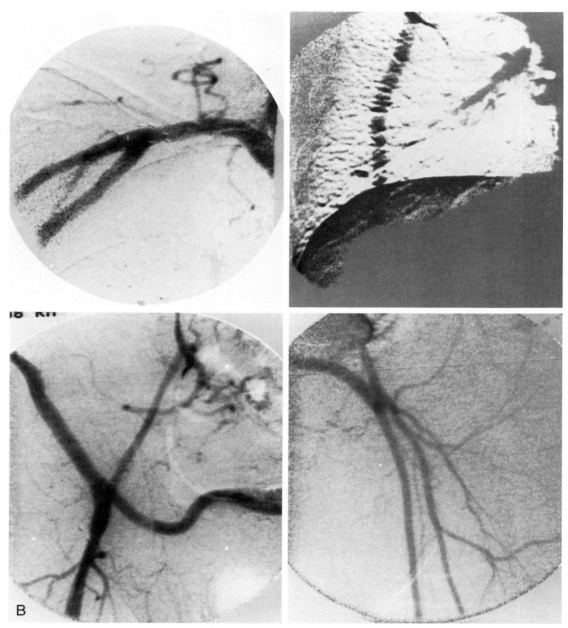

***Figure 12–3 Continued. B,*** Intravenous DSA in another patient with a normal axillo-femoral bypass graft. This study necessitated four contrast injections (each 20 ml/sec for 30 ml) in the vena cava. It shows the proximal anastomosis, the graft as it crosses the rib cage, and the right and left distal anastomoses.

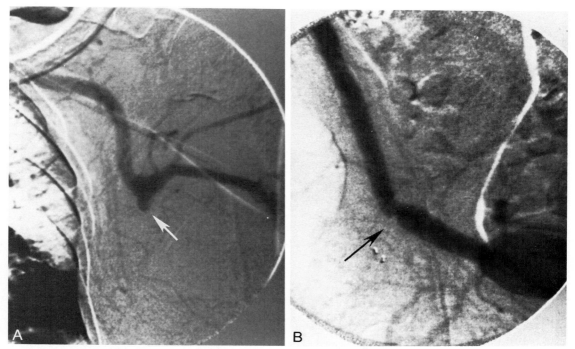

*Figure 12–4.* Complications of axillo-femoral bypass grafts. *A,* Intravenous DSA shows an occluded left axillo-femoral bypass graft (*arrow*). *B,* Intravenous DSA in another patient shows occlusion of the right limb of a right axillo-femoral bypass graft (*arrow*).

guide wire and can be used for contrast injection. The contrast injection and filming programs listed in Table 12–3 are used.

Complete arteriographic evaluation includes assessment of the proximal and distal anastomoses and the inflow and outflow vessels. We prefer to use a combination of intravenous DSA for the donor vessel and proximal anastomosis and a direct graft puncture with antegrade arteriography (DSA or cut film) for evaluating the distal anastomosis and run-off vessels. In some patients the entire examination can be performed with intravenous DSA. This latter method is particularly helpful for evaluating the pelvic and thigh vessels in patients with occluded axillo-femoral bypass grafts (since the central contrast injection opacifies all possible collaterals).

For the intraarterial studies, films are obtained by using either the stepping table, the long film changer, or multiple stationary runs.

## FEMORO-FEMORAL GRAFTS

Such extra-anatomical grafts are used to bypass a unilateral iliac artery occlusion. The long-term patency of such grafts depends upon the severity of disease involving the donor iliac artery and the recipient vessels. In one study, donor vessel disease was the single most important factor contributing to graft failure[14] (Figs. 12–5 and 12–6).

Complications of femoro-femoral bypass grafts and graft failure are usually due to progression of disease or to unrecognized donor iliac artery disease. Complications may be manifested as:

1. Graft thrombosis (Fig. 12–5).

2. Femoral steal phenomenon:[15] This refers to the development of ischemic symptoms in the previously asymptomatic donor limb and is usually a manifestation of stenosis in the donor iliac artery.

3. Hemodynamic graft failure (Fig. 12–6): This is due to severe donor iliac artery disease. Hemodynamic graft failure can also manifest with reversal of blood flow in the graft. Such blood flow reversal is readily detected by Doppler ultrasonography.

4. Anastomotic aneurysm (Fig. 12–7). It is frequently associated with a stenosis of the distal anastomosis and has also been observed after femoro-popliteal saphenous vein grafts (referred to as a "spoon bowl" deformity).[15a]

5. Anastomotic stenoses.

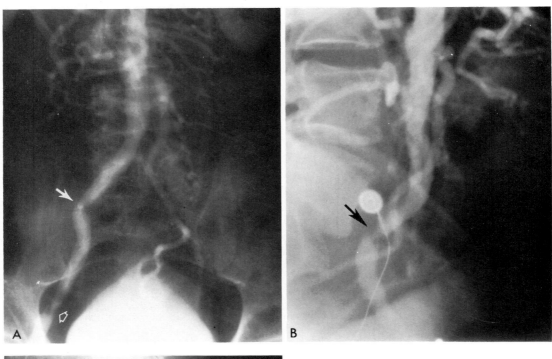

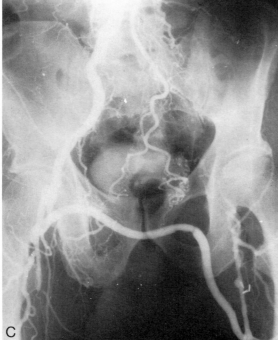

Figure 12–5. Failed femoro-femoral bypass graft due to significant inflow disease. A, AP pelvic arteriogram perfomed via the left axillary artery approach shows two areas of stenosis in the right iliac artery (arrows). The graft is occluded. B, Lateral pelvic arteriogram shows the severity of the proximal stenosis, which was not apparent from the AP arteriogram (arrow). C, AP pelvic arteriogram after angioplasty of the stenoses and thrombectomy of the graft. (A and B From Kadir S et al: Selected Techniques in Interventional Radiology. Philadelphia, WB Saunders, 1982.)

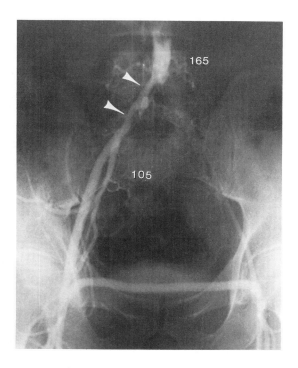

**Figure 12–6.** Hemodynamically failed graft. A graft pulse was not palpable. AP pelvic arteriogram shows a patent femoro-femoral bypass graft. Two areas of stenosis are seen in the donor common iliac artery (*arrowheads*). There was a resting pressure gradient of 60 mm Hg. The stenoses were managed by balloon angioplasty.

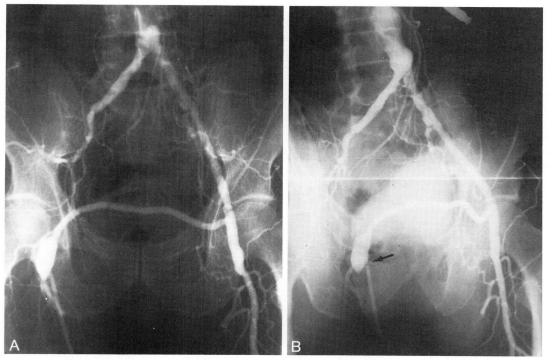

**Figure 12–7.** Anastomotic aneurysm following a femoro-femoral bypass graft for occlusion of the right external iliac artery. *A,* AP pelvic arteriogram shows an anastomotic aneurysm on the right side. The arterial anastomosis is obscured by the aneurysm. *B,* Left posterior oblique arteriogram reveals a severe stenosis at the anastomosis with the superficial femoral artery (*arrow*).

**TABLE 12–4.** Lower Aortic and Pelvic Arteriogram

| | |
|---|---|
| Approach | Femoral, axillary artery, graft puncture, translumbar |
| Catheter: | 5 or 6 Fr pigtail, TLA needle/ sheath |
|    Position | Lower abdominal aorta proximal to graft anastomosis |
| Guide wire | 0.035 inch J LLT<br>*or*<br>0.035 inch high torque |
| Contrast medium* | 76% diatrizoate meglumine sodium† |
| Injection rate/volume | 6–10 ml/sec, total 40 ml |
| Films:<br>   Filming | 10 films<br>2 per second for 4 films<br>1 per second for 6 films |
|    Projection | a. AP/lateral (aorta)<br>b. AP and oblique pelvis |

*20% concentration for DSA.
†Add 2 mg of lidocaine per ml of contrast medium.

Arteriography of femoro-femoral bypass grafts can be performed via (Table 12–4): (1) intravenous DSA, (2) the axillary artery approach, (3) donor femoral artery puncture, (4) translumbar aortography, or (5) direct graft puncture. The last approach is rarely necessary.

From the axillary and femoral artery approaches, a 5 Fr pigtail catheter is placed in the distal abdominal aorta, and AP and oblique arteriograms are performed to evaluate the donor iliac artery and the graft anastomoses. If an iliac artery stenosis is demonstrated, it is evaluated for hemodynamic significance by measurement of an intraarterial pressure gradient at rest and after injection of a vasodilator to simulate exercise.

## AORTO-ILIAC AND AORTO-FEMORAL RECONSTRUCTION

The cumulative 5 year patency of aorto-iliac and aorto-femoral bypass grafts is 93% and 88%, respectively.[16] Complications of such grafts are infrequent and are most often due to progression of vascular disease and rarely to technical factors such as a tight anastomosis or fibrosis at the anastomosis. Complications may be manifested as:

1. Graft limb thrombosis (Fig. 12–8).
2. Anastomotic stenosis (Fig. 12–9).
3. Anastomotic aneurysms (Figs. 12–10 and 12–11).
4. Vascular-enteric fistula (see Chapter 14).

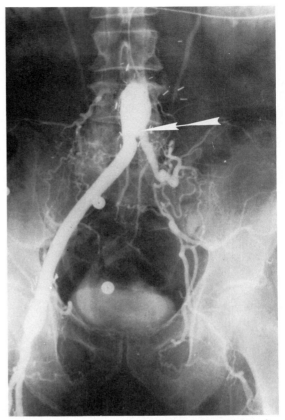

***Figure 12–8.*** Translumbar aortogram shows an aorto-femoral bypass graft with occlusion of the left limb of the graft (*arrow*).

Arteriography for the evaluation of such vascular prostheses can be performed via (Table 12–4): (1) a high translumbar aortic puncture, (2) the axillary artery approach, (3) femoral artery or direct graft puncture in the groin, or (4) intravenous DSA.

**Technique for Arterial Graft Puncture** (Table 12–5). The presence of scar tissue around the graft and the delicate neointima in the graft dictate extreme caution during the puncture of prosthetic arterial grafts. The

**TABLE 12–5.** Guidelines for Safe Catheterization of Synthetic Arterial Grafts

2–3 mm skin incision
Spread subcutaneous scar tissue
Predilatation of tract
Movable core or LLT J guide wire
Teflon or reinforced polyurethane catheters
Removal of pigtail catheter over J guide wire
Minimal catheter or guide wire manipulation
Catheter introducer sheath*

*If multiple catheter exchanges are anticipated or if catheters with softer materials, eg, polyethylene, are used.

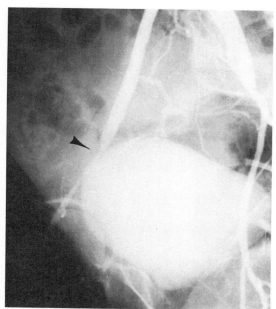

*Figure 12–9.* Anastomotic stenosis at the iliac anastomosis of an aorto-iliac bypass graft (*arrowhead*). There was a 35 mm Hg resting pressure gradient across the lesion.

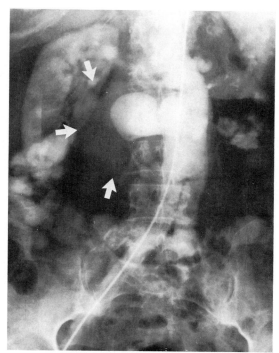

*Figure 12–11.* Anastomotic aneurysm with contained rupture. AP aortogram shows an anastomotic aortic aneurysm. A large soft tissue density surrounds the aneurysm (*arrows*). At operation a ruptured aneurysm was found.

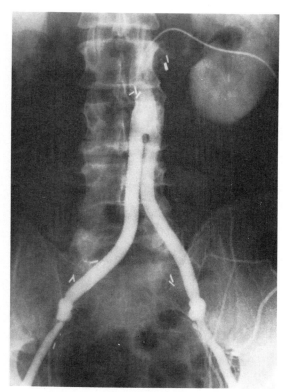

*Figure 12–10.* Translumbar aortogram shows an aorto-iliac graft with the typical corrugations of the prosthetic material. Small aneurysms are present at both iliac anastomoses. In addition, there is a stenosis at the right iliac anastomosis.

presence of scar tissue and the graft material result in a higher resistance to the passage of catheters. Thus, for aortography or lower extremity arteriography, we have found the Teflon or polyurethrane nylon (Mallinckrodt, St. Louis, Missouri) pigtail catheters to be the safest and the easiest to use. For all other types of catheter materials, when multiple catheter exchanges are anticipated, and for selective arteriography, a catheter introducer sheath should be used. The latter should also be used if the peri-graft scar tissue is unusually tough (to prevent damage to the catheter tip and catheter tip separation at the time of catheter removal).

An adequate skin incision (2 to 3 mm) and careful spreading of the subcutaneous scar tissue (with a mosquito clamp) are necessary for atraumatic catheterization. A metal or a sheath needle (Amplatz) may be used. With the metal needle, a soft-tipped J guide wire (movable core or LLT) is used for catheter insertion. With the J tip in the suprarenal aorta, the needle tract is dilated with 5 or 6 Fr Teflon dilators prior to insertion of a 5 or 6 Fr Teflon pigtail catheter. In unusually tough scars, tract dilation with a larger Teflon dilator (one Fr size larger than the catheter) may be necessary for atraumatic catheter insertion. In our experience, this has not resulted in excessive bleeding. Tract dilatation is not necessary if a catheter introducer sheath is to be used.

At the time of catheter removal, a soft-tipped J guide wire should be inserted through the catheter to straighten out the pigtail. The presence of such a guide wire does not prevent bond separation or stretching of soft catheters when these are used without an introducer sheath. The only purpose it serves is to prevent the relatively stiff catheter tip from damaging the delicate neointima.

## FEMORO-POPLITEAL GRAFTS

Autogenous saphenous vein grafts are widely used as arterial substitutes in the lower extremity (Fig. 12–12). Exposure of the vein to arterial pressure and blood flow re-

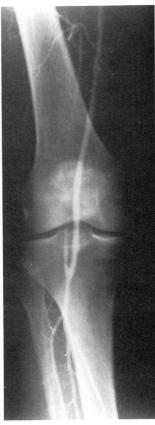

*Figure 12–12.* Femoral arteriogram shows a normal distal femoro-popliteal bypass graft anastomosis.

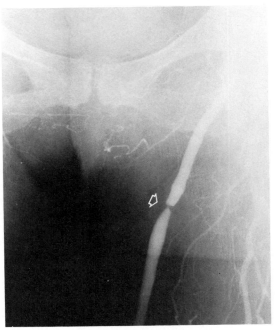

*Figure 12–13.* Intimal proliferation at the site of a saphenous vein valve causing a hemodynamically significant stenosis (*arrow*).

sults in several changes in the vein. Histologically and angiographically, these may be manifested as:[17]

1. Intimal thickening.
2. Atherosclerosis: This is found in 80% of veins implanted for longer than 2 years.
3. Fibrosis at the site of a vein valve or due to vascular clamp trauma (Fig. 12–13).
4. Anastomotic stenosis (Fig. 12–14).
5. Anastomotic aneurysm (Fig. 12–15).

Early graft failures are most often due to technical problems such as a tight anastomosis or residual clot, or a poor runoff. The routine use of intraoperative arteriography has contributed significantly towards reducing the number of early failures due to technical problems.[18] Late failures are most often caused by progression of distal disease.

Approximately 25% of graft failures are due to a tight anastomosis or fibrosis at the site of a vein valve.[19] It is important to recognize these causes of graft failure early, before graft thrombosis occurs, since such patients can be successfully managed by operation or nonoperatively by percutaneous transluminal angioplasty (Fig. 12–16).[20, 21]

Femoro-popliteal bypass grafts can be studied by intravenous DSA or standard lower extremity arteriography. Oblique arteriography of the pelvis is necessary to visu-

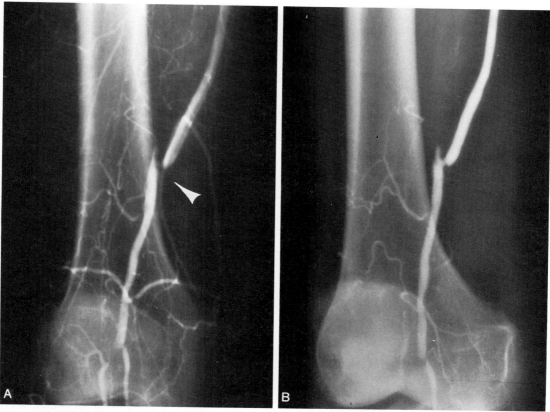

***Figure 12–14.*** Anastomotic stenosis. *A,* Severe stenosis at the distal anastomosis of a femoro-popliteal bypass graft (*arrowhead*) to an isolated popliteal artery segment. *B,* Arteriogram following angioplasty.

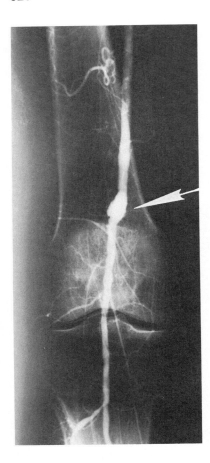

*Figure 12–15.* Anastomotic aneurysm after a femoro-popliteal bypass graft (*arrow*).

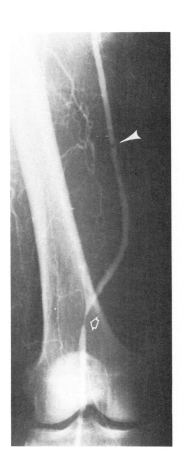

*Figure 12–16.* Hemodynamically failed femoro-popliteal bypass graft. Femoral arteriogram shows a saphenous vein valve (*arrowhead*) and a severe distal anastomotic stenosis (*open arrow*). Both lesions were treated by angioplasty.

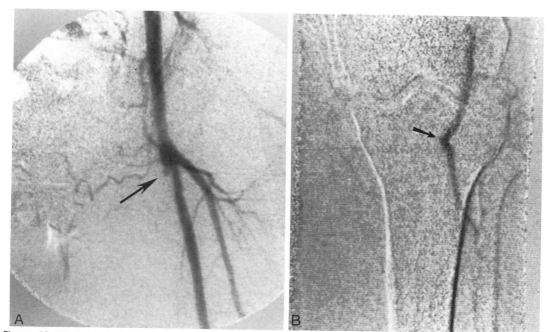

*Figure 12–17.* Occluded femoro-popliteal bypass graft. *A,* Intravenous DSA of the left femoral artery shows the stump of the occluded graft (*arrow*). *B,* Intravenous DSA of the distal leg shows reconstitution of the popliteal artery. Arrow points to the site of the distal graft anastomosis.

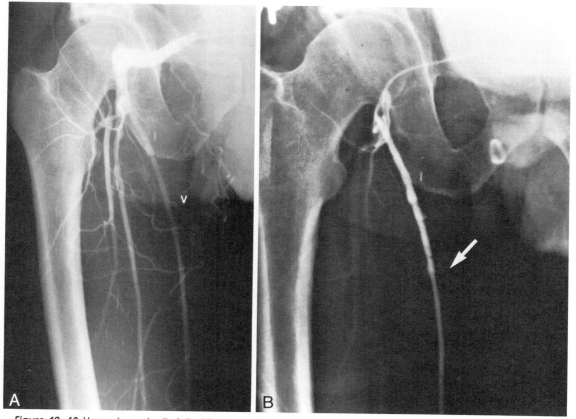

*Figure 12–18.* Hemodynamically failed in-situ saphenous vein bypass graft. *A,* Right leg arteriogram via puncture of a femoro-femoral graft shows an in-situ saphenous vein graft and an arteriovenous fistula. V = saphenous vein branch that was left unligated. *B,* Selective arteriogram of the saphenous vein graft after successful balloon embolization. Arrow points to the 1 mm silicone balloon.

321

alize the proximal anastomosis. Patients with suspected graft failure can also be evaluated by intravenous DSA on an outpatient basis. Such a study provides sufficient information with respect to graft patency, and in some patients the runoff vessels can also be evaluated (Fig. 12–17).

Saphenous vein graft puncture is safe and may become necessary if percutaneous transluminal angioplasty of a vein graft stenosis is to be performed.[21, 22]

In-situ saphenous vein grafts can be evaluated in the same way as reversed saphenous vein or synthetic femoro-popliteal grafts. Although in-situ vein grafts are technically more difficult to perform, they offer several advantages: (1) less trauma and damage to the saphenous vein, and thus increased durability, and (2) anatomically compatible anastomoses. Complications associated with such grafts are similar to those seen with reversed saphenous vein grafts (ie, anastomotic stenoses and fibrosis at the site of valves). In addition, hemodynamic graft failure may occur as a result of arteriovenous shunting through a saphenous vein branch that was overlooked and not ligated during surgery (Fig. 12–18). Such arteriovenous communications can also be managed by interventional radiological techniques and do not require reoperation.

## REFERENCES

1. Thompson JE, Garrett WV: Peripheral arterial surgery. N Engl J Med 302:491–503, 1980.
2. Szilagyi DE, Elliott JP, Smith RF, et al: Secondary arterial repair. The management of late failures in reconstructive arterial surgery. Arch Surg 110:485–493, 1975.
3. Thompson WM, Johnsrude IS, Jackson DC, et al: Late complications of abdominal aortic reconstructive surgery: Roentgen evaluation. Ann Surg 185:326–334, 1977.
4. Brown OW, Stanson AW, Pairolero PC, et al: Computerized tomography following abdominal aortic surgery. Surgery 91:716–722, 1982.
5. Gooding GAW, Herzog KA, Hedgcock MW, et al: B mode ultrasonography of prosthetic vascular grafts. Radiology 127:763–766, 1978.
6. Godwin JD, Turley K, Herfkens RJ, et al: Computed tomography for follow up of chronic dissections. Radiology 139:655–660, 1981.
7. Nath PH, Zollikofer C, Castaneda-Zuniga WR, et al: Radiological evaluation of composite aortic grafts. Radiology 131:43–51, 1979.
7a. Tadavarthy SM, Castaneda-Zuniga WR, Amplatz K, et al: Systolic collapse of an ascending aortic graft: an angiographic sign of perigraft hematoma communicating with the left ventricle. AJR 138:353–354, 1982.
8. Jacobs NM, Godwin JD, Wolfe WG, et al: Evaluation of the grafted ascending aorta with computed tomography. Radiology 145:749–753, 1982.
9. Guthaner DF, Miller CM, Silverman JF, et al: Fate of the false lumen following surgical repair of aortic dissections: an angiographic study. Radiology 133:1–8, 1979.
10. Clark RA, Colley DP, Siedlecki E: Late complications at repair site of operated coarctation of aorta. AJR 133: 1071–1075, 1979.
11. Bandyk DF, Thiele BL, Radke HM: Upper-extremity emboli secondary to axillofemoral graft thrombosis. Arch Surg 116:393–395, 1981.
12. Kempczinski R, Penn I: Upper extremity complications of axillofemoral grafts. Am J Surg 136:209–211, 1978.
13. Kerstein MD, Stansel HC Jr: Ischemia and subsequent amputation of the upper extremity following axillo-femoral bypass. Angiology 25:305–308, 1974.
14. Flanigan DP, Pratt DG, Goodreau JJ, et al: Hemodynamic and angiographic guidelines in selection of patients for femorofemoral bypass. Arch Surg 113:1257–1262, 1978.
15. Trimble IR, Stonesifer GL Jr, Wilgis EFS, et al: Criteria for femoro-femoral bypass from clinical and hemodynamic studies. Ann Surg 175:985–993, 1972.
15a. Root JA, Giustra PE: "Spoon bowl" deformity of proximal femoral bypass vein graft. A cause of late graft failure on four occasions. Arch Surg 112:166–169, 1977.
16. Brewster DC, Darling RC: Optimal methods for aortoiliac reconstruction. Surgery 84:739–748, 1978.
17. Szilagyi DE, Elliott JP, Hageman JH, et al: Biologic fate of autogenous vein implants as arterial substitutes: clinical, angiographic and histopathologic observations in femoro-popliteal operations for atherosclerosis. Ann Surg 178:232–246, 1973.
18. Liebman PR, Menozian JO, Mannick JA, et al: Intraoperative arteriography in femoropopliteal and femorotibial bypass grafts. Arch Surg 116:1019–1021, 1981.
19. Yao JST, O'Mara CS, Flinn WR, et al: Postoperative evaluation of graft failure. In Bernhard VM, Towne JB (eds): Complications in Vascular Surgery. New York, Grune & Stratton, 1980, pp. 1–19.
20. O'Mara CS, Flinn WR, Johnson ND, et al: Recognition and surgical management of patent but hemodynamically failed arterial grafts. Ann Surg 193:467–476, 1981.
21. Kadir S, Smith GW, White RI, et al: Percutaneous transluminal angioplasty as an adjunct to the surgical management of peripheral vascular disease. Ann Surg 195:786–795, 1982.
22. Zajko AB, McLean GK, Freiman DB, et al: Percutaneous puncture of venous bypass grafts for transluminal angioplasty. AJR 137:799–802, 1981.

# Neoplasms and Neoplasm-like Conditions of the Extremities, Shoulders, and Pelvis

 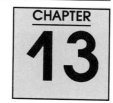
In this chapter, the discussion will focus upon the general angiographic criteria used for the evaluation of neoplasms, followed by a discussion of the angiography of neoplasms and neoplasm-like conditions involving the extremities, shoulders, and pelvis. Visceral neoplasms will be discussed in the appropriate chapters. Since a detailed review of individual tumors is clearly beyond the scope of this book, the interested reader is referred to the references listed at the end of this chapter.

## GENERAL ANGIOGRAPHIC CRITERIA FOR EVALUATION OF NEOPLASMS

Most of the individual angiographic signs used for identification of neoplasms are nonspecific, since they are also observed in association with nonneoplastic conditions. The vascular changes may involve large and small vessels and appear to be related to tumor growth characteristics, tumor size, and stage of disease. Such changes are due to alterations of the pre-existing blood vessels and/or to the formation of neovascular channels (Table 13–1).[1, 2]

**Alteration of Vascular Course** (Fig. 13–1; see also Figs. 13–14 and 13–15). Alteration in the normal course of a vessel may be in the form of bowing or stretching around a mass lesion or an abrupt change in direction. Whereas the former is a nonspecific sign and may be observed in association with both benign and malignant lesions, the latter is seen in association with malignancy. Occasionally, bowing and stretching of otherwise normal vasculature may be the only indication of the presence of a mass.

**Alteration in Lumen Diameter** (Figs. 13–2 to 13–4). Segmental vascular encasement or

invasion by a neoplasm may lead to either a narrowing of the lumen or an occlusion. The narrowing may be serrated, irregular, or smooth and concentric. In larger visceral arteries, the last may simulate atherosclerotic narrowing. Occasionally, the vessels may appear beaded or pleated as a result of a fibrotic reaction. Abrupt, beaklike vascular occlusion is indicative of the presence of a malignancy.[3] Angiographic demonstration of such occlusion may be facilitated by the use of pharmacologic enhancement techniques. Demonstration of venous occlusion may necessitate venography.

**TABLE 13–1.** Summary of Vascular Changes Associated with Neoplasms

*Alteration of Course*:
  Displacement
  Abrupt change in direction

*Alteration in Lumen Diameter*:
  Encasement
  Dilatation
  Aneurysm formation
  Absence of normal tapering
  Occlusion

*Alteration in Blood Flow*:
  Accelerated circulation time
  Arteriovenous shunting
  Parasitization
  Demonstration of venous collaterals
  Enlarged draining veins
  Tortuous draining veins
  Venous invasion, extension, or occlusion
  Abnormal orientation of draining veins

*Neovascularity*:
  Absence of normal tapering
  Irregular, unpredictable course
  Branches occasionally larger than parent vessel
  Tumor "stain"
  Vascular lakes
  Aneurysm formation

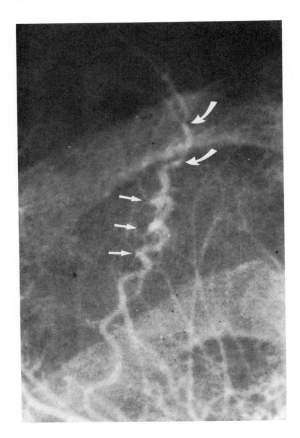

*Figure 13–1.* Abrupt alteration in arterial course due to a neoplasm. The hepatic artery branches show an abrupt change in direction (*straight arrows*) in a patient with hepatoma. Focal encasement is also present (*curved arrows*).

*Figure 13–2.* Drawing illustrating alterations in vascular lumen due to neoplastic encasement and invasion: smooth encasement (*A*); encasement and alteration of course (*B*); invasion (*C*); abrupt change in course (*D*).

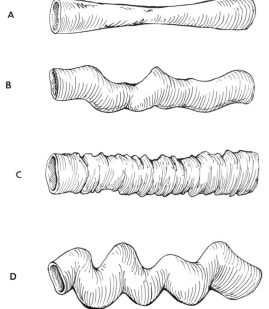

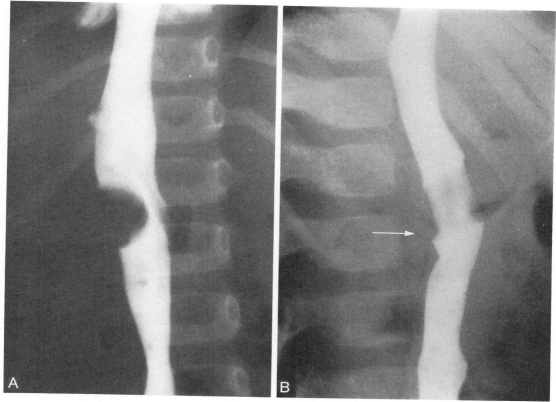

*Figure 13–3. A* and *B,* Alteration in lumen diameter due to invasion by neoplasm. AP and lateral inferior vena cavagram in a child with a Wilms' tumor of the right kidney shows a nodular intraluminal defect. The margins are shelflike, which is characteristic of neoplastic invasion. In addition, there is anterior displacement of the inferior vena cava due to lymphadenopathy (*arrow*).

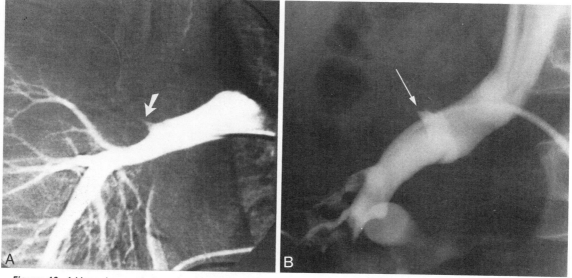

*Figure 13–4.* Vascular occlusion due to neoplasm. *A,* AP pulmonary arteriogram in a patient with squamous cell carcinoma of the lung. There is encasement and occlusion of the artery to the upper lobe (*arrow*). *B,* AP right renal venogram in a patient with renal cell carcinoma. There is amputation of the upper pole renal veins due to encasement by the tumor (*arrow*).

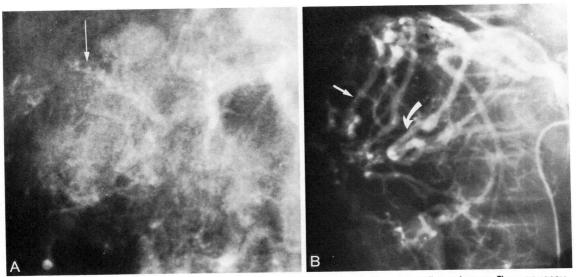

**Figure 13–5.** Neovascularity. *A*, Diffuse, fine neovascularity in a patient with renal cell carcinoma. The neovasculature shows an unpredictable criss-cross course. Abrupt change in course is also seen (*arrow*). *B*, Coarse neovasculature in a patient with a hepatic cell carcinoma. There is absence of the progressive tapering and branching seen in normal vessels (*straight arrow*). Instead, distal enlargement of tumor vessels is seen (*curved arrow*).

Vessels supplying neoplasms often show an absence of the normal arborization and progressive tapering that are characteristic of normal vasculature. Focal areas of vascular dilatation and occasionally aneurysm formation may be seen in both benign and malignant neoplasms.

**Neovascularity** (Fig. 13–5). Neovasculature is usually associated with an increase in the number of vessels within a tumor. This neovascularity may consist of small, fine vasculature or coarse vessels. Typically, tumor vessels are irregular, do not follow a normal predetermined course, show abrupt changes in course, and do not demonstrate progressive caliber reduction. In addition, the pattern of normal arborization is absent.

Tumor neovascularity may be extremely fine and thus may be barely visible on arteriography. Neovascularity may also be seen in nonmalignant processes such as inflammatory lesions, postoperative conditions, benign tumors, reparative or reactive neovascularity, and collateral arterial channels in occlusive arterial diseases.[1, 4]

**Parasitization** (Fig. 13–6). Fast growing, highly vascular tumors may attract blood supply from neighboring arterial sources. This parasitization is almost always associated with a malignancy. For example, in renal cell carcinoma, parasitization of blood supply has been observed from the retroperitoneal and visceral arteries.

**Tumor "Stain"** (Fig. 13–7; see also Figs. 13–11, 13–14, and 13–20). A transient accumulation of contrast medium within dilated tumor vasculature may be demonstrated as a tumor "stain." This appearance of in-

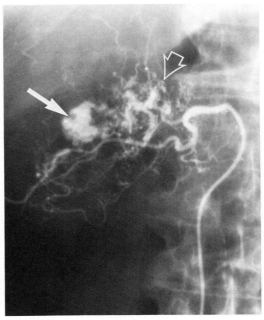

**Figure 13–6.** Parasitization. AP lumbar arteriogram in a patient with a large renal cell carcinoma. The tumor has parasitized blood supply from the lumbar artery branches. Tumor vessels (*open arrow*) and a dense tumor stain are present (*arrow*).

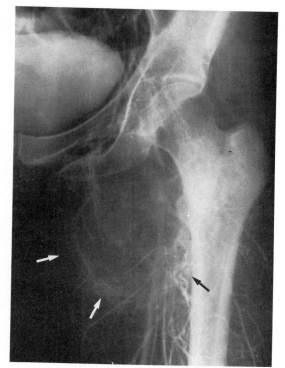

**Figure 13–7.** Rim enhancement. Hypovascular rhabdomyosarcoma with rim enhancement (*arrows*).

tumor bed may result in an increase in the blood flow through a tumor. Arteriographically, this is manifested as early venous opacification that occurs during the late arterial or early parenchymal phase. Large, direct arteriovenous communications may lead to very early and dense venous opacification. In the presence of arteriovenous shunting, the draining veins are usually enlarged, and such neoplasms are usually hypervascular.

The normal course of peripherally located veins is in the direction of blood flow, ie, toward the centrally located major venous channels. Veins draining neoplastic tissues are often tortuous and usually follow a different course. This is often perpendicular to the direction of normal blood flow.[3] Angiographic demonstration of early draining veins may have a bearing on the type of operation to be performed.[8] Early ligation of such veins may prevent tumor embolization and further dissemination.

Invasion of venous structures may lead to venous obstruction and absent venous opacification. In this situation, multiple, enlarged collateral venous channels are opacified. However, the demonstration of such collat-

creased vascularity helps to delineate the tumor from the adjacent uninvolved tissue. Occasionally, a hypervascular zone is seen in the periphery of the tumor or in normal tissue adjacent to it (rim enhancement) while the tumor itself is hypovascular or avascular (central necrosis). Both these signs (tumor stain and rim enhancement) are nonspecific, since they may be seen in association with nonneoplastic conditions.[5] This zone of peripheral hypervascularity is often due to edema and has been termed the reactive tumor zone. Although the hypervascularity leads to overestimation of tumor size by angiography and computed tomography (CT), this portion of the soft tissues must be resected during surgery.[6, 7]

**Vascular Lakes** (Figs. 13–8 and 13–9). Accumulation of contrast medium in poorly defined neoplastic vascular spaces, which persists into the venous phase, is also considered a sign of malignancy.[3] However, this sign alone is not reliable, since it may also be seen in benign conditions such as a hemangioma.

**Alterations in Blood Flow** (Fig. 13–9; see also Figs. 13–13 to 13–15). An abnormal microcirculation due to the presence of multiple abnormal vascular communications in the

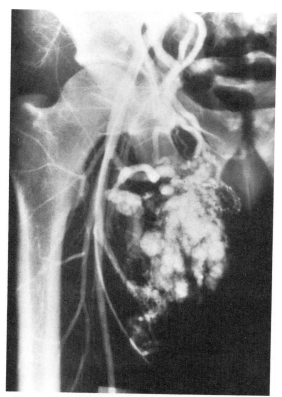

**Figure 13–8.** Vascular lakes. Dilated vascular spaces (lakes) in an intramuscular hemangioma.

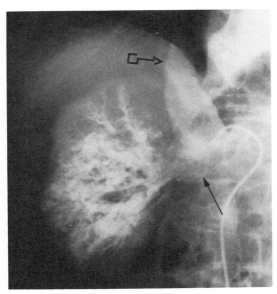

*Figure 13–9.* Tumor-induced alteration in blood flow. Renal arteriogram shows arteriovenous shunting in a renal cell carcinoma. There is early opacification of the inferior vena cava (*hooked arrow*). In addition, tumor growth into the renal vein is seen (*arrow*). Densely opacified vascular lakes are seen within the neoplasm.

eral channels alone is not proof of the presence of venous occlusion.[9]

Venous invasion by tumor may also lead to growth within the draining veins. This is seen most frequently in renal cell carcinoma and occasionally in hepatoma and malignant adrenal neoplasms.

## ARTERIOGRAPHY OF NEOPLASMS OF THE EXTREMITIES, SHOULDERS, AND PELVIS

Arteriography is rarely indicated for the establishment of the diagnosis, localization, or staging of neoplasms of the extremities; this is accomplished by CT scanning. Nevertheless, the value of diagnostic arteriography should not be negated, since it provides complementary information that may not be available by other means.[10]

The indications for angiography are:

1. To demonstrate the relationship of the neoplasm to major vascular structures in order to evaluate the feasibility of resection: This may be of particular importance in proximal extremity and pelvic neoplasms.

2. Occasionally, to define the longitudinal extent of extremity neoplasms.

3. To define tumor vascularity and the vascular supply of hypervascular neoplasms:

This may be an indicator of anticipated intraoperative blood loss.

4. To assess the need for preoperative tumor embolization.

5. For selective catheter placement for intraarterial chemotherapy.

6. For embolization, either preoperatively to reduce tumor size and intraoperative blood loss or as a palliative measure for treatment of pain.

### Arteriography Technique

Initially, a survey arteriogram is performed of the region of interest, eg, a pelvic arteriogram for intrapelvic tumors, a common femoral arteriogram for tumors of the thigh, and a superficial femoral arteriogram for tumors arising distal to the knee. In this fashion, all potential sources of blood supply are evaluated. In most cases, this provides sufficient information with respect to tumor blood supply, venous drainage, vascularity, and extent. Selective arteriography of the major arterial feeders is necessary only if transcatheter intervention is planned or if the information derived from the survey arteriogram is insufficient. For neoplasms arising in the distal extremities, antegrade arteriography is desirable. For small lesions and those with calcification or overlying bone, subtraction films or intraarterial DSA may be required to define the tumor. Catheterization of small branch vessels for diagnostic arteriography may provide misleading results (see later section on Pitfalls in Angiographic Diagnosis). The techniques for selective arteriography and contrast medium injection volume and flow rates have been described in Chapters 9 to 11.

### Arteriographic Findings

Most bone neoplasms derive their blood supply from the adjacent soft tissue vasculature. Occasionally, an enlarged nutrient artery of the involved bone may be demonstrated on arteriography. A tumor is "avascular" only if necrosis has occurred. The arterial blood supply of hypovascular tumors may not be adequately demonstrated on nonenhanced arteriography. However, the use of pharmacological enhancement and film subtraction may enable demonstration of such vasculature.

The arteriographic findings may range from no appreciable abnormality on the arteriogram to marked hypervascularity and extensive vascular parasitization. Table 13–2

**TABLE 13–2.** Angiographic Appearance of Neoplasms and Neoplasm-like Conditions of the Bones and Soft Tissues

| Neoplasm | Vascularity | Tumor Stain | Neovascularity | Remarks | References |
|---|---|---|---|---|---|
| Osteoid osteoma | Hypervascular nidus | + | − | May need film subtraction or DSA | 11 |
| Osteochondroma | Hypovascular | − | − | | 12 |
| Osteoblastoma | Hypo- or hypervascular | + | (+) | | 13 |
| Osteosarcoma | Hypervascular, occasionally hypovascular | + | + | May have sunburst pattern, AV shunt, can be multicentric, Fig. 13–10 | 13–15 |
| | | − | + | | |
| Chondroblastoma | Hypo- or hypervascular | + | (+) | | 16, 16a |
| Enchondroma | Hypovascular | − | − | | |
| Chondromyxoid fibroma | Hypovascular | (+) | (+) | | 16 |
| Chondrosarcoma* | Hypervascular, occasionally hypovascular | + | + | Central necrosis may be present, Fig. 13–11 | 17 |
| Fibrosarcoma* | Very variable, hypo- to hypervascular | + | + | May show AV shunt, Fig. 13–12 | 18–20 |
| Reticulum cell sarcoma | Hypo- to hypervascular | + | + | | |
| Rhabdomyosarcoma | Hypervascular | + | + | | 21 |
| Myxofibrosarcoma | Hypervascular | + | + | | 21 |
| Lipoma | Hypovascular | − | − | Displaced vessels Fig. 13–13 | |
| Liposarcoma | Hypo- to moderately vascular | + | + | | |
| Pigmented villonodular synovitis | Hypervascular | + (synovium) | (+) | Displaced vessels, occasional AV shunt | 16, 22–24 |
| Synovial sarcoma | Hypervascular | + | + | AV shunt | 22–25 |
| Neurogenic tumor | Hypo- to hypervascular | + | + | Fig. 13–14 | 26 |
| Fibrous desmoid | Hypovascular | (+) | (+) | Displaced vessels, Fig. 13–15 | 26a |
| Myositis ossificans | | | | | |
|   Early | Hypervascular | + | − | | 27, 28 |
|   2 weeks–3 months | Hypervascular | + | − | Calcification, Fig. 13–16 | |
|   Healed | Minimally increased to normal | − | − | Calcification | |
| Giant cell tumor | Hypervascular, hypovascular (10%) | + | + | May have AV shunt, Fig. 13–18 | 29, 30 |
| Aneurysmal bone cyst | Hypervascular | + | + | May have AV shunt | 31, 32 |
| Adamantinoma | Hypo- to hypervascular | (+) | (+) | | |
| Hemangioendothelioma | Hypervascular | + | + | May have AV shunt | 16, 33 |
| Paget's disease of bone | Hypervascular | + | + | May have AV shunt | 34 |
| Ewing's sarcoma | Hypovascular, occasionally hypervascular | + | + | Occasionally AV shunt, Fig. 10–58, Chapter 10 | 16, 34 |
| Malignant fibrous histiocytoma | Hypervascular | + | + | AV shunt, pooling | 35 |
| Solitary myeloma | Hypervascular, occasionally hypovascular | + | + | Nonhomogeneous stain (early veins) | 16, 36 |
| Metastases | Usually similar to primary | | | | 16 |
|   GI tumors, renal, thyroid | Very vascular | + | + | Figure 13–17 | |
|   Melanoma | Hyper- to hypovascular | + | | | |

*Vascularity correlates with malignant potential.

*Key:* + = present, − = absent, (+) = occasionally present.

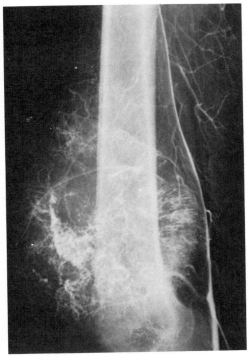

**Figure 13–10.** Osteosarcoma of the distal femur. The tumor is hypervascular and the neovasculature shows a sunburst pattern. There is posterior displacement of the popliteal artery by the tumor mass. (Courtesy of Dr. CA Athanasoulis.)

lists the salient angiographic features of some of the more frequent bone and soft tissue neoplasms.

## Pharmacoangiography

Pharmacological techniques for enhancement of tumor visualization have been an important part of the arteriographic evaluation of bone and soft tissue neoplasms.[11, 37–39] However, our experience and that of several other authors show that, in most instances, pharmacologically enhanced arteriograms provide little additional information compared with nonenhanced arteriography using a high volume, high flow technique.[40, 41] In general, vasoconstrictors appear to provide more information than vasodilators with respect to definition of the tumor and the tumor vessels.[40] The drugs used most frequently for the evaluation of extremity neoplasms are tolazoline (Priscoline, Ciba Pharmaceuticals) and angiotensin (Hypertensin, Ciba Pharmaceuticals). Epinephrine is the most frequently used vasoconstrictor for the evaluation of visceral neoplasms.

The concept of pharmacoangiography is based upon the inability of neoplastic vessels to constrict after an appropriate stimulus. This concept cannot be used for differentiating benign from malignant tissue, because of the variable response of these tissues.

Newly formed tumor vasculature lacks contractile elements, which makes it unresponsive to a vasoconstrictor stimulus. Similarly, inflammatory and hemangiomatous vessels may also be devoid of contractile elements, making them unresponsive to vasoconstrictors.[42, 43] On the other hand, some tumor vessels (especially some slow growing tumors) may also constrict in response to vasoconstricting stimuli.[44, 45]

**Tolazoline.** The vasodilatory effect of this drug is directly upon the vascular smooth muscle.

*Dosage:* 25 mg of tolazoline diluted in 10 to 15 ml of 5% glucose is injected intraarterially over 10 to 15 seconds immediately before contrast arteriography. The contrast injection rate should be increased by 25 to 50% and the contrast volume by about 25%.

**Angiotensin.** This drug is a vasoconstrictor with direct action upon the smooth muscu-

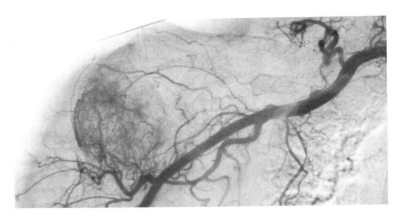

**Figure 13–11.** Chondrosarcoma of the humeral head. Subtraction film from a right subclavian arteriogram shows a hypervascular tumor. (Courtesy of Dr. CA Athanasoulis.)

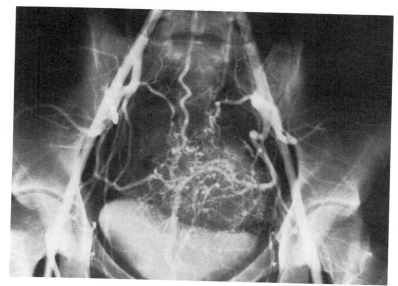

*Figure 13–12.* Fibrosarcoma. AP pelvic arteriogram in a 20 year old woman shows a large hypervascular presacral neoplasm. Tumor blood supply is derived from branches of both the internal iliac and the inferior mesenteric arteries.

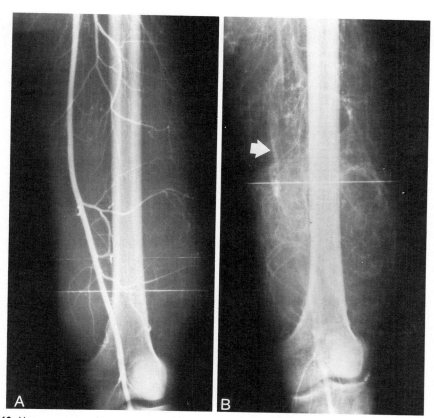

*Figure 13–13.* Liposarcoma of the distal thigh. *A,* The distal branches of the superficial femoral artery are stretched. Several branches have an unusually horizontal course. *B,* Parenchymal phase of the same arteriogram as *A.* Although there is only minimal neovascularity and the tumor is hypovascular, early venous opacification is seen (*arrow*).

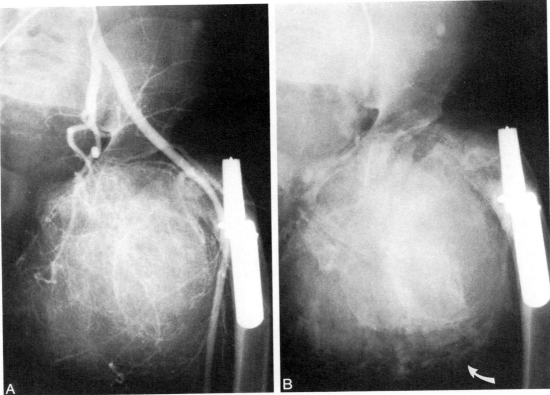

*Figure 13–14.* Schwannoma. *A,* Common iliac arteriogram shows a hypervascular schwannoma of the proximal left thigh. The tumor derives its blood supply from both the internal iliac and branches of the profunda femoris arteries. The SFA is displaced by the mass. *B,* Later frame from the same arteriogram shows a dense tumor stain. On the tumor periphery, abnormally oriented veins (perpendicular to the direction of normal venous flow) are seen (*arrow*).

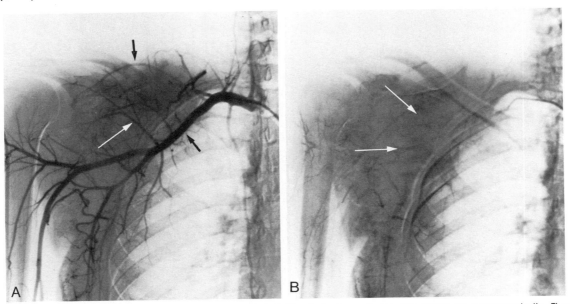

*Figure 13–15.* Desmoid. *A,* The arterial phase of a right subclavian arteriogram shows no neovascularity. The subclavian artery is displaced inferiorly and several of the branches are stretched and bowed around the hypovascular tumor (*arrows*). *B,* A later frame from the same arteriogram shows abnormally oriented (horizontal) veins (*arrows*).

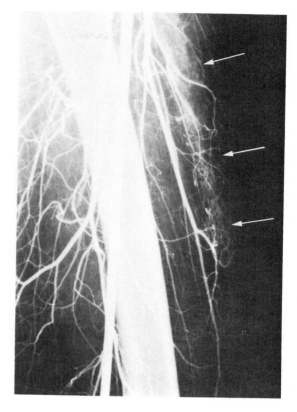

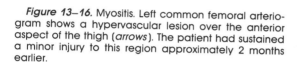

*Figure 13–16.* Myositis. Left common femoral arteriogram shows a hypervascular lesion over the anterior aspect of the thigh (*arrows*). The patient had sustained a minor injury to this region approximately 2 months earlier.

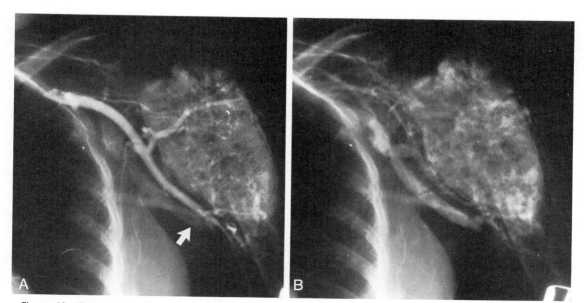

*Figure 13–17.* Hypervascular metastasis from renal cell carcinoma to the left humerus with arteriovenous shunting. *A,* Left axillary arteriogram shows a hypervascular metastasis with early opacification of the axillary vein (*arrow*). *B,* Venous phase of the same arteriogram shows densely opacified, enlarged draining veins.

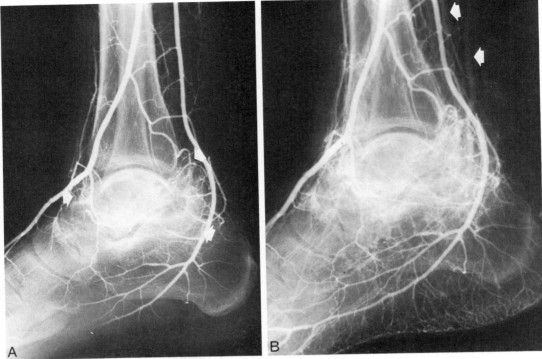

**Figure 13–18.** Giant cell tumor of the talus. Advantages of pharmacoangiography. *A,* Arteriogram without tolazoline shows a slightly vascular tumor extending into the soft tissues (*arrows*). *B,* Repeat arteriogram after intraarterial injection of 25 mg of tolazoline in the distal superficial femoral artery shows significantly improved tumor definition and early venous opacification (*arrows*). (From Kadir S et al: Radiology 133:792–795, 1979. Used with permission.)

lature of the peripheral vessels. At the dosage used for visceral and peripheral angiography, no adverse systemic side effects have been reported.[45, 46]

*Dosage:* 5 to 10 μg of angiotensin diluted with 10 ml of normal saline is injected intraarterially immediately before arteriography. The contrast injection rate should be decreased by approximately 25% and the duration of filming must be prolonged.

**Advantages and Disadvantages of Pharmacological Enhancement.** Some of the benefits that may be derived from the use of pharmacological enhancement include (Fig. 13–18):

1. To overcome proximal vasospasm by intraarterial injection of 25 mg of tolazoline.[40]

2. To improve visualization of skip and satellite lesions.[41]

3. To improve visualization of venous structures.

4. To improve visualization in some poorly vascularized lesions by injection of vasoconstrictors.

The disadvantages are:

1. Vasodilators act nonselectively, causing vasodilatation of normal vasculature around the tumor and thereby tend to obscure the tumor stain (Fig. 13–19). Thus, small tumors may go unrecognized if only tolazoline-enhanced arteriography is used.[40]

2. Although the vasoconstrictive action of angiotensin is more peripheral than that of epinephrine, delivery (to the region of interest) of an appropriate dose for peripheral extremity tumors may pose a problem.[40]

PITFALLS IN DIAGNOSIS

As mentioned earlier, several or all of the angiographic features of malignant neoplasms may also be observed in benign tumors. Similarly, several of these angiographic findings may also occur in nonneoplastic conditions or may be induced iatrogenically. For these reasons, arteriography cannot be used to differentiate between benign and malignant tumors.

Pitfalls in diagnosis include the following (Fig. 13–20):

1. Alteration of course and lumen diameter: Benign, nonneoplastic lesions such as simple cysts, bursal cysts, and hematomas may cause alteration in the course of vessels.

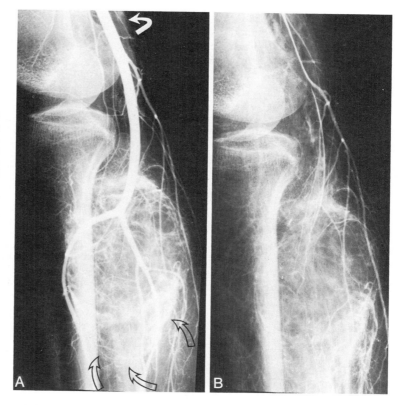

*Figure 13–19.* Giant cell tumor of the proximal fibula. Disadvantages of pharmacological enhancement. *A,* Lateral femoral arteriogram shows a highly vascular tumor with early venous opacification (*curved arrow*). The lower margin of the tumor is well delineated (*open arrows*). *B,* Repeat arteriogram following intraarterial injection of 25 mg of tolazoline. There is nonselective vasodilatation of both normal and tumor vasculature, resulting in poorer definition of the tumor. (From Kadir S et al: Radiology 133:792–795, 1979. Used with permission.)

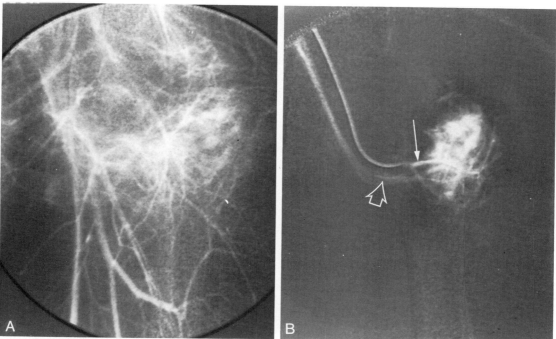

*Figure 13–20.* Early venous opacification due to wedge catheter position. *A,* Common femoral arteriogram (DSA) shows a hypervascular metastasis (from a hepatic cell carcinoma) in the proximal left femur. There is no arteriovenous shunting. *B,* DSA with catheter wedged in a small branch shows early venous opacification (*open arrow*). A dense parenchymal stain is apparent. Persistent arterial opacification is seen as a result of the wedged catheter position, which prevents washout of contrast medium (*arrow*). The normal course of the opacified vein should be compared with the tumor venous drainage demonstrated in Figures 13–14 and 13–17.

Changes in lumen diameter may occur as a result of vascular spasm (catheter or guide wire induced) or an arteriopathy. Beading and pleating due to fibrosis can occasionally be simulated by standing waves.

2. Neovascularity: This finding may also be seen in chronic inflammatory processes.

3. Tumor stain: A large volume of contrast medium injected into a small vessel or a wedge injection of contrast medium may result in dense opacification of normal parenchymal tissue, which may simulate a tumor stain. The arteriogram of an organizing hematoma or a healing fracture may also simulate a tumor stain.[42]

4. Alterations in blood flow: Early venous opacification may also be observed after wedge injection of contrast medium into a small branch or after intraarterial injection of a vasodilator. Therefore, pharmacological enhancement techniques should be used only as an adjunctive measure.[41] The normal venous branches opacified by either wedge injection into small arterial branches or as a result of vasodilator injection almost invariably have a normal course towards the next major vein. In contrast, veins arising from tumors usually demonstrate some tortuosity and often have an anomalous course. Early venous opacification may also be seen after trauma, in organizing hematomas, and in myositis.[47]

5. Arteriogram after recent operation: Arteriography after a recent biopsy or operation may present a misleading picture that may simulate a neoplastic process. Operative trauma and the ongoing reparative process may lead to increased vascularity, distortion, and abrupt termination of vessels.

6. Repeat arteriography following radiation therapy or embolotherapy: The typical vascular pattern of neoplastic tissue may no longer be seen after transcatheter embolization or radiation therapy.[3, 48]

7. Vasodilator-enhanced arteriogram: As noted earlier, dilatation of normal vessels adjacent to a neoplasm may obscure the tumor stain. This most likely reflects the inability of the tumor vessels to respond to the vasodilatory stimulus.

## REFERENCES

1. Viamonte M Jr, Roen S, LePage J: Nonspecificity of abnormal vascularity in the angiographic diagnosis of malignant neoplasms. Radiology 106:59–63, 1973.
2. Kido C, Sasaki T, Kaneko M: Angiography of primary liver cancer. AJR 113:70–81, 1971.
3. Strickland B: The value of arteriography in the diagnosis of bone tumours. Br J Radiol 32:705–713, 1959.
4. Finlayson M, Nayak V: Atypical vascular proliferation in benign soft tissue tumors. Arch Pathol Lab Med 103:224–227, 1979.
5. Thomas ML, Andress MR: Angiographic appearance of an intramuscular hematoma. Acta Radiol Diagn 14:65–68, 1973.
6. Egund N, Ekelund L, Sako M, et al: CT of soft tissue tumors. AJR 137:725–729, 1981.
7. Enneking WF, Spanier SS, Malawer MM: The effect of the anatomic setting on the results of surgical procedures for soft parts sarcoma of the thigh. Cancer 47:1005–1022, 1981.
8. Hudson TM, Haas G, Enneking WF, et al: Angiography in the management of musculoskeletal tumors. Surg Gynecol Obstet 141:11–21, 1975.
9. Goncharenko V, Gerlock AJ, Kadir S, et al: Frequency of venous involvement in hypernephroma. AJR 133:263–265, 1979.
10. Ekelund L, Herrlin K, Rydholm A.: Comparison of computed tomography and angiography in the evaluation of soft tissue tumors of the extremities. Acta Radiol Diagn 23:15–28, 1982.
11. Lateur L, Baert AL: Localization and diagnosis of osteoid osteoma of the carpal area by angiography. Skeletal Radiol 2:75–79, 1977.
12. Laurin S: Angiography of benign bone tumors. Acta Radiol 22:601–607, 1981.
13. Yaghmai I: Angiographic features of osteosarcoma. AJR 129:1073–1081, 1977.
14. Lagergren C, Lindbom A, Soederberg G: The blood vessels of osteogenic sarcomas: Histologic, angiographic and microradiographic studies. Acta Radiol 55:161–176, 1961.
15. Rittenberg GM, Schabel SI, Vujic I, et al: The vascular sunburst appearance of osteosarcoma. A new angiographic finding. Skeletal Radiol 2:243–244, 1978.
16. Yaghmai I: Angiography of Bone and Soft Tissue Lesions. New York, Springer Verlag, 1979.
16a. Hudson TM, Hawkins IF Jr: Radiological evaluation of chondroblastoma. Radiology 139:1–10, 1981.
17. Lagergren C, Lindbom A, Soederberg G: The blood vessels of chondrosarcomas. Acta Radiol 55:321–328, 1961.
18. Dibbelt W: Ueber die Blutgefaesse der Tumoren. Arch Pathol Anat Bakt 8:114–128, 1912.
19. Lagergren C, Lindbom A, Soederberg G: Vascularization of fibromatous and fibrosarcomatous tumors: Histopathologic, microangiographic and angiographic studies. Acta Radiol 53:1–16, 1960.
20. Yaghmai I: Angiographic features of fibromas and fibrosarcomas. Radiology 124:57–64, 1977.
21. Levin DC, Watson RC, Baltaxe HA: Arteriography in diagnosis and management of acquired peripheral soft tissue masses. Radiology 103:53–58, 1972.
22. Lagergren C, Lindbom A: Angiography of peripheral tumors. Radiology 79:371–377, 1962.
23. Probst FP: Extraarticular pigmented villonodular synovitis affecting bone. The role of angiography as an aid in its differentiation from similar bone destroying conditions. Radiologe 13:436–442, 1974.
24. Rosenthal DI, Coleman PK, Schiller AL: Pigmented villonodular synovitis: correlation of angiographic and histologic findings. AJR 135:581–585, 1980.

25. Martel WM, Abell RM: Radiologic evaluation of the soft tissue tumors. A retrospective study. Cancer 32:352–366, 1973.

26. Dunnick NR, Castellino RA: Arteriographic manifestations of ganglioneuromas. Radiology 115:323–328, 1975.

26a. Miller EM, Newton TH: The angiographic features of extraabdominal desmoid tumors. Radiology 132:305–308, 1979.

27. Gronner AT: Muscle necrosis simulating a malignant tumor angiographically. Case report. Radiology 103:309–310, 1972.

28. Yaghmai I: Myositis ossificans: Diagnostic value of arteriography. AJR 128:811–816, 1977.

29. Laurin S: Angiography in giant cell tumors. Radiologe 17:118–123, 1977.

30. Prando A, de Santos LA, Wallace S, et al: Angiography in giant cell bone tumors. Radiology 130:323–331, 1979.

31. Lindbom A, Soederberg G, Spjut HL, et al: Angiography of aneurysmal bone cyst. Acta Radiol 55:12–16, 1961.

32. de Santos LA, Murray JA: The value of arteriography in the managaement of aneurysmal bone cyst. Skeletal Radiol 2:137–141, 1978.

33. Levin DC, Gordon DH, McSweeney J: Arteriography of peripheral hemangiomas. Radiology 121:625–630, 1976.

34. Halpern M, Freiberger RH: Arteriography as a diagnostic procedure in bone disease. Radiol Clin North Am 8:277–288, 1970.

35. Hudson TM, Hawkins IF Jr, Spanier SS, et al: Angiography of malignant fibrous histiocytoma of bone. Radiology 131:9–15, 1979.

36. Laurin S, Akerman M, Kindblom L-G, et al: Angiography in myeloma (plasmacytoma): a correlated angiographic histologic study. Skeletal Radiol 4:8–18, 1979.

37. Hoffman ET, Viamonte M Jr: Pharmacoangiography. CRC Crit Rev Clin Radiol Nucl Med 203–217, 1973.

38. Hawkins IF Jr, Hudson TM: Priscoline in bone and soft tissue angiography. Radiology 110:541–546, 1974.

39. Ekelund L, Lunderquist A: Pharmacoangiography with angiotensin. Radiology 110:533–540, 1974.

40. Lechner G, Powischer G, Waneck R: Diagnostischer Wert der Pharmakoangiographie bei Tumorösen und entzündlichen Knochen und Weichteilprozessen. Ein Bericht über 81 Fälle. Fortschr Roentgenstr 132:68–75, 1980.

41. Kadir S, Athanasoulis CA, Waltman AC: Tolazoline augmented arteriography in the evaluation of bone and soft tissue tumors. Radiology 133:792–795, 1979.

42. Doppman JL, Fried LC, Di Chiro G: Absent vasoconstrictive response of wound vessels to intraarterial vasopressors: angiographic observations. Radiology 93:57–62, 1969.

43. Bartley O, Wickbom I: Angiography in soft tissue hemangiomas. Acta Radiol 51:81–94, 1959.

44. Kligerman, MM, Henel DK: Some aspects of the microcirculation of a transplantable experimental tumor. Radiology 76:810–817, 1961.

45. Kaplan JH, Bookstein JJ: Abdominal visceral pharmacoangiography with angiotensin. Radiology 103:79–83, 1972.

46. Novak D, Weber J: Pharmakoangiographie mit Angiotensin. Fortschr Roentgenstr 124:301–309, 1976.

47. Stener B, Wichbom I: Angiography in three cases of muscle rupture with organizing hematoma. Acta Radiol Diag 4:169–176, 1966.

48. Yamada R, Sato M, Kawabata M, et al: Hepatic artery embolization in 120 patients with unresectable hepatoma. Radiology 148:397–401, 1983.

# VISCERAL ANGIOGRAPHY

## Esophago-Gastrointestinal Angiography

### ARTERIAL ANATOMY

The main sources of blood supply to the gastrointestinal tract are the three major ventral branches of the abdominal aorta, ie, the celiac artery and the superior and inferior mesenteric arteries. There is considerable variation in the origins of some of the branches of these arteries supplying the individual abdominal organs, and knowledge of these variations is important in order to facilitate a complete angiographic evaluation.

### Celiac Artery (Fig. 14–1)

The celiac artery (celiac axis) is a short trunk (1 to 4 cm) that arises from the ventral surface of the aorta, just below the diaphragm, at the level of the lower half of the 12th thoracic vertebra. It may be ventrally oriented (ie, perpendicular to the aorta), or may course craniad (eg, in some obese individuals) or caudally.

In about 65% of individuals, the celiac artery divides into three major branches: the splenic, hepatic, and left gastric arteries. In the remainder, it has either fewer or more branches.[1, 2] Rarely, the celiac artery is congenitally absent.

**Splenic Artery.** This is the largest branch of the celiac artery and is usually very tortuous in adults. Several centimeters from the

splenic hilum it divides into two (occasionally three) end branches, which further subdivide before they enter the splenic parenchyma. The main branches of the splenic artery are the:

1. Pancreatic arteries: These include the dorsal pancreatic (in 40% of individuals this arises from the splenic artery); pancreatica magna, and caudal pancreatic arteries and several smaller arteries to the body and tail of the pancreas.

2. Short gastric arteries.

3. Left gastroepiploic artery: Occasionally, this may arise from the lower end-branch of the splenic artery.

**Common Hepatic Artery** (Fig. 14–2). The common hepatic artery courses to the right; after giving off the gastroduodenal artery, it is called the proper hepatic artery. Its main branches are the:

1. Gastroduodenal artery (GDA): This gives off the superior pancreaticoduodenal arteries and continues as the right gastroepiploic artery along the greater curvature of the stomach.

2. Proper hepatic artery: This gives off the right and left hepatic arteries and occasionally a middle hepatic artery.

3. Supraduodenal artery: This vessel arises from either the GDA or the common or right hepatic artery.

4. Cystic artery: This is usually a branch of the right hepatic artery.

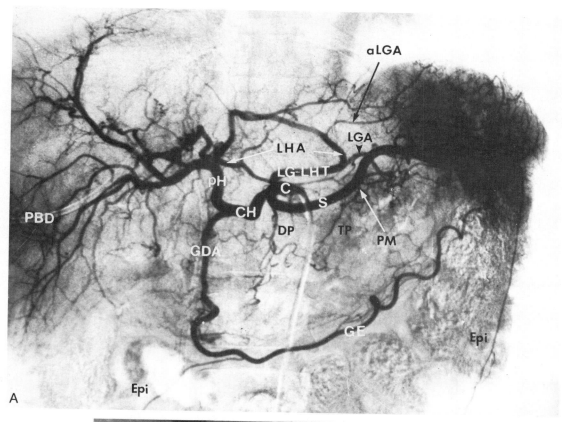

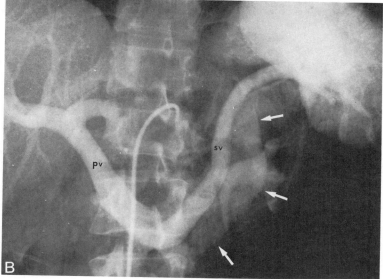

**Figure 14–1.** Normal celiac arteriogram. *A,* Arterial phase. aLGA = accessory left gastric; C = celiac; CH = common hepatic; DP = dorsal pancreatic; Epi = epiploic; GDA = gastroduodenal; GE = right gastroepiploic; LGA = left gastric; LG–LHT = left gastric–left hepatic trunk; LHA = left hepatic; pH = proper hepatic; PM = pancreatica magna; S = splenic; TP = transverse pancreatic arteries; PBD = percutaneous biliary drainage catheter. *B,* Venous phase. pv = portal vein; sv = splenic vein. Arrows point to normal pancreatic blush.

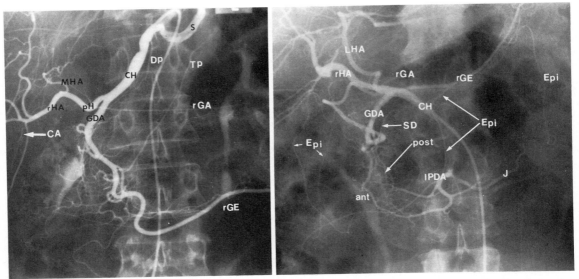

*Figure 14–2. Left* and *right*, Normal common hepatic arteriograms. ant = anterior pancreaticoduodenal arcade; post. = posterior pancreaticoduodenal arcade (also called the retroduodenal artery); CA = cystic; CH = common hepatic; DP = dorsal pancreatic; Epi = epiploic; GDA = gastroduodenal; IPDA = inferior pancreaticoduodenal; J = jejunal; LHA = left hepatic; MHA = middle hepatic; pH = proper hepatic; rGA = right gastric; rGE = right gastroepiploic; rHA = right hepatic; S = splenic; SD = supraduodenal; TP = transverse pancreatic arteries.

**Left Gastric Artery** (Figs. 14–3 and 14–4; see also Fig. 14–30). The left gastric artery (LGA) is a branch of the celiac artery in 90% of individuals.[2] In 2.5% it originates directly from the aorta, and in the remainder it arises from the splenic artery. In most individuals, the LGA orifice is located proximally on the

celiac artery, but in 25% it lies close to the orifices of the splenic and common hepatic arteries, giving rise to a trifurcation.[2] Accessory left gastric arteries from the splenic artery are observed in 6% and from the celiac artery in 2% of individuals.[2] Accessory gastric branches from the left hepatic artery are observed in 14.2% of left hepatic arteriograms.[3]

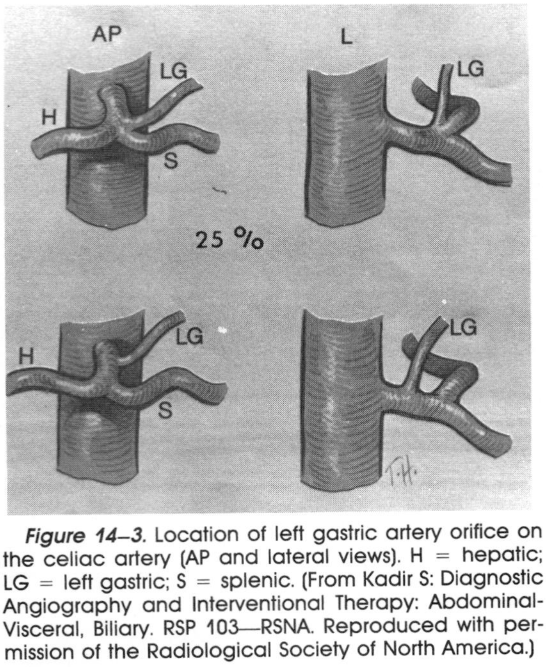

The LGA branches anastomose freely with those of the left and right gastroepiploic and short gastric arteries. The right gastric artery anastomoses with the LGA to form an arcade along the lesser curvature of the stomach. The LGA branches also supply the distal esophagus. The angiographic appearance of the LGA may be variable, depending upon the anatomical position and distention of the stomach.

**Right Gastric Artery** (see Fig. 14–30). This is a small vessel, usually one third the diameter of the LGA. It arises from the proper hepatic artery in 40% of individuals, the left hepatic artery in another 40%, the GDA in 8%, and the right or middle hepatic arteries in about 10% of individuals.[2]

*Figure 14–3. Location of left gastric artery orifice on the celiac artery (AP and lateral views). H = hepatic; LG = left gastric; S = splenic. (From Kadir S: Diagnostic Angiography and Interventional Therapy: Abdominal-Visceral, Biliary. RSP 103—RSNA. Reproduced with permission of the Radiological Society of North America.)*

## Superior Mesenteric Artery (Fig. 14–5)

The superior mesenteric artery (SMA) arises from the ventral surface of the aorta approximately 1 cm below the origin of the

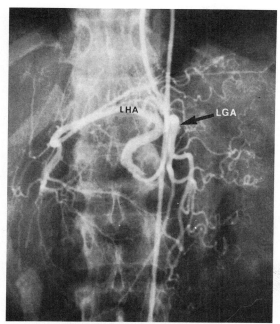

**Figure 14–4.** Left gastric–left hepatic artery trunk. LGA = left gastric artery; LHA = left hepatic artery.

celiac artery, at the level of the upper half of L1. It usually courses in a caudad direction but may have a superiorly oriented or a straight ventral course initially.

Branches of the SMA are the:

**Inferior Pancreaticoduodenal Artery.** This is usually the first branch originating from the right side. Occasionally, it may have a common origin with a jejunal artery. It divides into an anterior and a posterior branch, which anastomose with the corresponding branches of the superior pancreaticoduodenal arteries from the GDA to form the duodenal arcades.

**Jejunal and Ileal Arteries.** These are 10 to 14 in number. Multiple arcade-like anastomoses exist between them. The arcades closest to the small intestine give off the vasa recta.

**Middle Colic Artery.** This is usually a short vessel that divides into a left and a right branch. The former anastomoses with the ascending branch of the left colic artery and the latter with the ascending branch of the right colic artery to form the marginal artery, which runs along the mesenteric border of the colon and gives off the vasa recta to the colon. Occasionally, both branches may have separate origins off the SMA.

**Right Colic Artery.** This arises distal to the middle colic artery. It also divides into an ascending and a descending branch. The former anastomoses with the right branch of the middle colic artery and the latter with the ascending branch of the ileocolic artery.

**Ileocolic Artery.** This is the terminal branch of the SMA. It supplies the cecum, terminal ileum, and appendix.

## Inferior Mesenteric Artery (Fig. 14–6)

The inferior mesenteric artery (IMA) arises from the ventral surface of the aorta at the level of L3 (approximately 3 cm above the aortic bifurcation) and descends to the left. The IMA trunk is usually 3 to 6 cm long, after which it divides into the following branches:

**Left Colic Artery.** This provides the ascending branch, which anastomoses with the left branch of the middle colic artery to form the marginal artery.

**Sigmoid Arteries.** These are usually two to three in number.

**Superior Hemorrhoidal Artery.** Branches from this vessel anastomose with those of the internal iliac arteries.

## Other Arteries

**Marginal Artery (of Drummond).** This vessel runs along the mesenteric border of the colon and is formed by the right and left branches of the middle colic and the left and right colic arteries. It provides the vasa recta to the colon.

**Arc of Riolan.** This is an inconstant anastomotic artery between the middle and left colic arteries.

**Arc of Buehler.** This is a short artery that represents the persistence of the embryologic ventral anastomosis between the celiac artery and the SMA.

**Arc of Barkow** (also called the greater omental arcade). These are omental vessels (artery and vein) running parallel to the gastroepiploic vessels that anastomose with both the left and the right gastroepiploic vessels. The vein serves as an important collateral in splenic vein occlusion.

## Variant Arterial Anatomy[1, 2] (Fig. 14–7)

1. A celiaco-mesenteric trunk (common origin of the celiac artery and SMA) is observed in 0.4% of individuals.

2. In 10% of individuals, a portion of the hepatic blood supply is from the SMA (replaced hepatic artery).

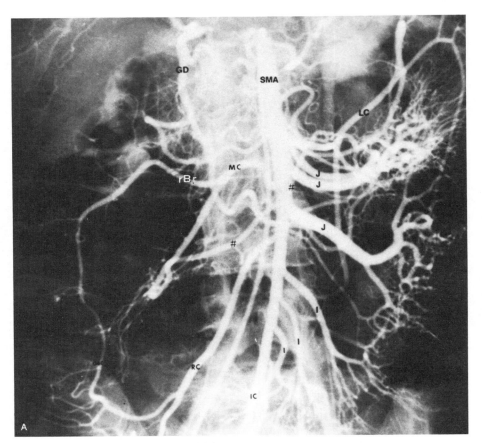

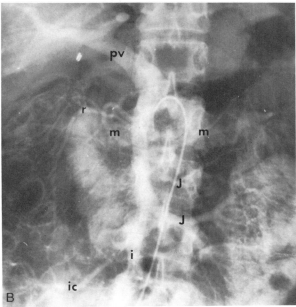

*Figure 14–5.* Normal superior mesenteric arteriogram. *A,* Arterial phase. *B,* venous phase. GD = gastroduodenal artery; I = ileal artery and vein; ic = ileocolic artery and vein; J = jejunal artery and vein; LC = ascending branch of left colic artery; pv = portal vein; m = middle colic vein; MC = middle colic artery; # = left branch of middle colic artery; rBr = right branch of middle colic artery; r = right colic veins; RC = right colic artery; SMA = superior mesenteric artery.

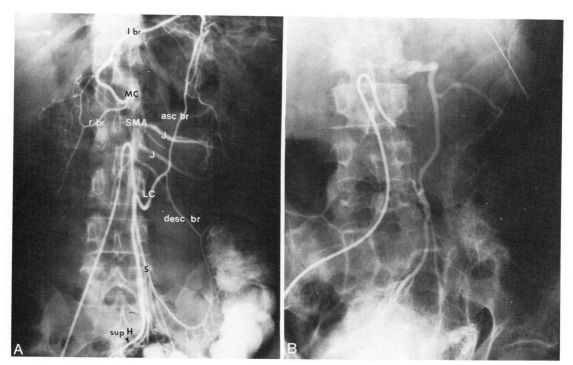

**Figure 14–6.** Normal inferior mesenteric arteriogram. *A*, Arterial phase. *B*, Venous phase. asc br = ascending branch of left colic artery; desc br = descending branch of left colic artery; l br = left branch of middle colic artery; r br = right branch of middle colic artery; LC = left colic; MC = middle colic; J = jejunal; S = sigmoid; sup H = superior hemorrhoidal; SMA = superior mesenteric arteries.

3. The entire hepatic arterial blood supply is from the SMA in 2.5% and from the aorta in 2% of individuals.

4. The LGA arises from the aorta in 2.5% of persons.

5. In 23% of individuals, either a branch of the left hepatic artery or the entire left hepatic artery arises from the LGA. In 4%, the left inferior phrenic artery is a branch of the LGA.

6. An aberrant origin of the splenic artery occurs very infrequently. It may be from the aorta, SMA, LGA, or one of the hepatic arteries.

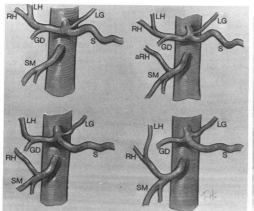

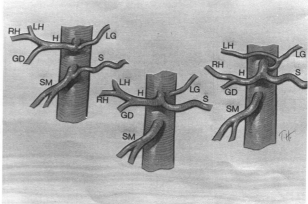

**Figure 14–7.** Variant anatomy of the splanchnic vessels. Hand drawings showing some of the variants. aRH = accessory right hepatic; GD = gastroduodenal; H = common hepatic; LG = left gastric; LH = left hepatic; RH = right hepatic; S = splenic; SM = superior mesenteric arteries. (From Kadir S: Diagnostic Angiography and Interventional Therapy: Abdominal-Visceral, Biliary. RSP 103—RSNA. Reproduced with permission of the Radiological Society of North America.)

7. The inferior phrenic arteries (one or both) may arise from the celiac artery.

8. The dorsal pancreatic artery arises from the celiac artery in 22% of individuals, the splenic artery in 40%, the proximal hepatic artery in about 20%, and the SMA or aorta in 14%.

9. The GDA arises from the celiac artery in 89% of individuals. In the remainder, it originates from a hepatic artery that is replaced to the SMA or aorta.

10. Occasionally, a jejunal branch arises from the celiac artery.


## VENOUS ANATOMY
### (see Figs. 14–1, 14–5, and 14–6)

The venous anatomy generally corresponds to the arterial distribution.

The splenic and superior mesenteric veins join to form the portal vein at the pancreatic head. The splenic vein drains the region supplied by the splenic artery. Venous inflow into the splenic vein comes from the spleen and short gastric, pancreatic, left gastroepiploic, and inferior mesenteric veins.

The inferior mesenteric vein is formed by the left colic, sigmoid (two to three), and superior hemorrhoidal veins. It joins the splenic vein immediately before the junction of the latter with the superior mesenteric vein.

The superior mesenteric vein is formed by the jejunal, ileal, right colic, and middle colic veins. In addition, the right gastroepiploic, pancreatic, and duodenal veins drain into it.

The right and left gastric (coronary) veins drain directly into the portal vein. Venous drainage from the hepatic veins is directly into the inferior vena cava.

**Portosystemic Anastomoses.** Multiple communications exist between the portal and systemic venous systems. These serve as collateral pathways in patients with portal hypertension. Table 14–1 lists the major communications.


## BLOOD SUPPLY OF INDIVIDUAL ORGANS

**Esophagus.** The cervical portion of the esophagus is supplied by branches of the inferior thyroid and subclavian arteries. The mid-esophagus receives its blood supply from the bronchial and intercostal arteries. The distal esophagus is supplied by two

**TABLE 14–1. Porto-Systemic Anastomoses**

Esophageal and gastric cardiac veins → azygos and hemiazygos veins

Esophageal and gastric cardiac veins and left gastric vein → left inferior phrenic vein

Splenic vein → retroperitoneal veins (inferior phrenic, renal, adrenal, and abdominal wall)

Left branch of portal vein → umbilical vein → epigastric veins

Middle colic vein → left colic vein → gonadal vein → left renal vein

Left colic vein → superior hemorrhoidal vein → middle and inferior hemorrhoidal veins → internal pudendal veins → iliac veins

Small mesenteric veins → retroperitoneal veins → inferior vena cava

Intrahepatic portal vein branches → diaphragmatic (phrenic) veins

Portal vein → lumbar, adrenal, and renal veins

unpaired arteries arising from the anterior surface of the distal thoracic aorta (at T6–7 and T7–8). The abdominal segment of the esophagus receives its blood supply via three to four esophageal branches from the left gastric artery. Additional blood supply is from the left inferior phrenic, accessory left hepatic, and celiac arteries and from the aorta directly.

**Stomach.** The gastric blood supply is derived mainly from the branches of the celiac artery, ie, the left and right gastric arteries, left and right gastroepiploic arteries, and short gastric and accessory left gastric arteries from the splenic and left hepatic arteries. In addition, the antrum and pylorus are supplied by branches of the hepatic and/or gastroduodenal artery.

**Duodenum.** The duodenum has a dual blood supply. It receives blood from both the celiac artery and the SMA, ie, it is supplied by the superior pancreaticoduodenal artery (from the GDA) and the inferior pancreaticoduodenal artery (from the SMA).

**Jejunum and Ileum.** The entire small intestine receives its blood supply from the SMA. Occasionally, a jejunal artery may arise from the celiac artery, usually off the dorsal pancreatic artery.

**Colon and Rectum.** The cecum, the ascending colon, and the proximal two thirds of the transverse colon are supplied by the

SMA. The distal transverse colon, descending and sigmoid colon, and upper three fourths of the rectum are supplied by the inferior mesenteric artery. The remainder of the rectum is supplied by the middle and inferior hemorrhoidal arteries from the internal iliac arteries.

## ANGIOGRAPHY

The main indication for arteriography of the esophago-gastrointestinal tract is gastrointestinal bleeding. Other indications include the assessment of continuity of the marginal artery prior to colon interposition for esophageal diseases, evaluation of venous anatomy prior to a meso- or portosystemic shunt, and evaluation of mesenteric ischemia. Arteriography is rarely indicated for the evaluation of alimentary tract tumors.

**Celiac Arteriography.** From the femoral approach, a cobra or sidewinder catheter is used. For catheterization of distal branches and the LGA arising from the distal celiac artery, a cobra catheter in the loop configuration is used (see Chapter 3). The sidewinder catheter is useful only for catheterization of branches arising from the proximal celiac artery or in patients with a short celiac artery. From the axillary approach, a hockey stick–shaped or headhunter catheter is used.

In individuals in whom the LGA originates proximally from the celiac artery, a celiac arteriogram may not opacify this vessel because the catheter tip lies distal to the LGA orifice. Even if the LGA is opacified, the degree of opacification is often insufficient to permit a diagnosis. Thus, if the stomach or distal esophagus is to be evaluated, a selective left gastric arteriogram is essential.

**Splenic Arteriography.** Splenic arteriography can be performed with a cobra or sidewinder catheter. An anteroposterior (AP) arteriogram usually provides sufficient information. Occasionally, a 15 to 20° left anterior oblique (LAO) arteriogram is necessary to uncoil the tortuosity of the splenic artery.

**Superior Mesenteric Arteriography.** For superior mesenteric arteriography either a cobra or a sidewinder catheter is used. A cobra catheter is employed for catheterization of the larger branches (jejunal or ileal). A coaxial system (3 Fr catheter) is used for catheterization of smaller branches. For hepatic arteries arising proximally from the SMA, a sidewinder catheter can be used. In the patients with replaced hepatic arteries arising at some distance from the SMA orifice, the cobra catheter in the loop configuration is used.

**Inferior Mesenteric Arteriography.** The right femoral approach is preferable for the IMA, and either a sidewinder, a cobra, or a visceral hook catheter can be used. For catheterization of the IMA branches, a coaxial system is used.

In general, filming or digital subtraction angiography (DSA) imaging should extend over 20 to 25 seconds. A rapid filming/imaging rate (ie, ≥2/sec) is necessary only for the evaluation of an arteriovenous fistula. For evaluation of the venous phase in patients with portal hypertension or suspected superior mesenteric or splenic vein thrombosis, the imaging sequence is prolonged to 30 seconds.

In most cases, the AP projection is sufficient for arteriography and for the evaluation of the splenic and portal veins. For evaluation of the superior mesenteric vein by cut film angiography, a 15° right posterior oblique (RPO) position is preferred, since this projects the vein off the lumbar spine. For DSA, the AP projection is used, since the gastric air shadow is frequently superimposed upon the portal vein by the RPO projection. During inferior mesenteric arteriography, the rectum should be included on the film/DSA images.

The venous phase can be evaluated by either DSA or conventional cut film angiography using pharmacological enhancement. With DSA, the splenic or superior mesenteric veins can be evaluated by injecting 15 to 20 ml of undiluted contrast medium at 6 to 7 ml/sec. A two-stage imaging program is used: several masks are obtained before contrast medium is injected and subsequently, after an approximately 4 to 6 second delay, images are obtained at 1/sec for a total of 10 to 12 images.

Pharmacological enhancement is not necessary when DSA is used for evaluation of the venous phase. For cut film angiography, 25 mg of tolazoline (Priscoline, Ciba Pharmaceuticals) is injected into the SMA or splenic artery immediately before contrast injection. The rate of contrast injection is increased by about 25 to 33%.

Table 14–2 lists the details for catheterization and imaging of the visceral arteries.

**TABLE 14–2.** Catheterization Materials and Flow Rates for Visceral Angiography

| Study | Catheter | Contrast Medium (%) | Injection Rate/Volume | Filming/Imaging | | |
|-------|----------|---------------------|-----------------------|-----|------|-------------|
| | | | | No. | Rate | Projections |
| Celiac/SMA* | Cobra or sidewinder | 76† | 6–7 ml/sec, 50–60 ml total | 15 | 1.0/sec for 5 0.5/sec for 10 | AP/LAO |
| IMA | Sidewinder or cobra visceral hook | 76† | 3–4 ml/sec, 20–25 ml total | 12 | 1.0/sec for 4 0.5/sec for 8 | AP |
| Splenic* | Cobra or sidewinder | 76 | 5 ml/sec, 30–40 ml total | 12 | 1.0/sec for 4 0.5/sec for 8 | AP/LAO |
| Common hepatic | Cobra or sidewinder | 76 | 5–6 ml/sec, 40 ml total | 12 | 1.0/sec for 5 0.5/sec for 7 | AP |
| LGA | Sidewinder I or cobra in loop | 76 | 3–4 ml/sec, 12–15 ml total | 12 | 1.0/sec for 4 0.5/sec for 8 | AP |
| GDA | Cobra | 76† | 3–4 ml/sec, 12–15 ml total | 12 | 1.0/sec for 4 0.5/sec for 8 | AP/LAO |
| Left hepatic LGA/LHA trunk | Cobra in loop, sidewinder | 76 | 4 ml/sec, 20–25 ml total | 12 | 1.0/sec for 4 0.5/sec for 8 | AP |

*In patients with portal hypertension, the injection rate and volume are increased by 25 to 30% and the duration of filming is prolonged to about 30 seconds (at 0.5/sec and 0.3/sec) for evaluation of the venous phase.
†Add 2 mg of lidocaine per ml of contrast medium.

## ARTERIAL AND VENOUS DISEASES

### Aneurysms

Visceral artery aneurysms are relatively uncommon and are most frequently detected incidentally. In descending order of frequency, they occur in the splenic, hepatic, superior mesenteric, celiac, gastroduodenal/pancreaticoduodenal, gastric/gastroepiploic, and inferior mesenteric arteries.

**Splenic Artery Aneurysms** (Fig. 14–8). The splenic artery is the most frequent location for visceral artery aneurysms. Such aneurysms occur more frequently in women than in men (ratio of 2:1).[4, 5] Eighty-eight per cent of the women with splenic artery aneurysms have had two or more pregnancies.[6] The etiology is medial degeneration with superimposed atherosclerosis. Other causes are congenital, mycotic, following pancreatitis, and traumatic aneurysms. Multiple aneurysms of the extra- and intrasplenic arteries may be seen in patients with portal hypertension.[7]

Specific symptoms are usually absent. Calcification in the aneurysm wall is reported in as many as two thirds of patients.[6] In one report, 20% of the female patients with splenic artery aneurysms also had fibromuscular disease of the renal arteries.[6]

The most frequent complication is aneurysm rupture, which occurs in 6 to 9% of patients.[5–7] In patients who are symptomatic (pain, gastrointestinal bleeding), the mortality from aneurysm rupture may be as high as 76%.[4] Calcified aneurysms also rupture, although less frequently.[6] The risk of aneurysm rupture and associated mortality is higher during pregnancy.[6, 8, 9]

Splenic artery aneurysms (intra- and extrasplenic) can usually be detected on AP arteriography. Occasionally, a renal artery aneurysm or a partially calcified, tortuous splenic artery may simulate a splenic artery aneurysm and may thus necessitate oblique or selective arteriography for differentiation.

**Superior Mesenteric Artery Aneurysms** (Fig. 14–9). Most SMA aneurysms are mycotic, and the SMA is the second most frequent location for mycotic aneurysms (after the aorta).[10, 11] Other causes are congenital, traumatic, and atherosclerotic aneurysms.

SMA aneurysms may involve the main trunk or the branches. The incidence of branch vessel aneurysms is reported at 1.2% of all mesenteric arteriograms.[12] In our own experience, these aneurysms are observed in 5% of such studies.

Complications include aneurysm rupture, which may be intraluminal and thus present as gastrointestinal bleeding, or extraluminal, leading to a mesenteric hematoma.

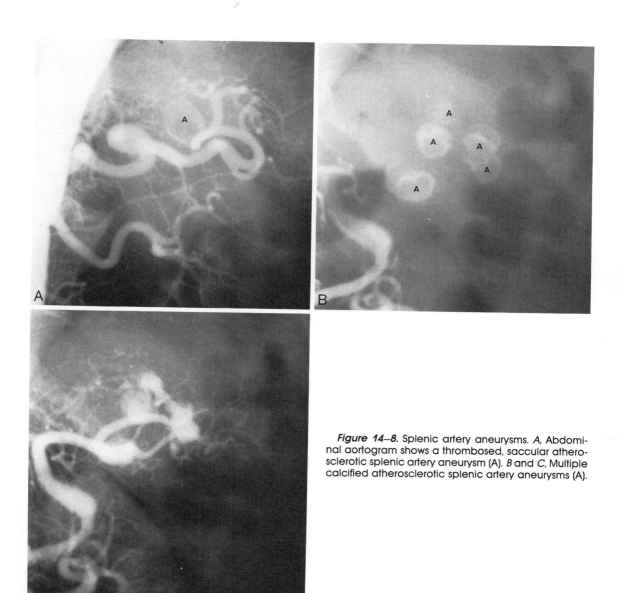

*Figure 14–8.* Splenic artery aneurysms. *A,* Abdominal aortogram shows a thrombosed, saccular atherosclerotic splenic artery aneurysm (A). *B* and *C,* Multiple calcified atherosclerotic splenic artery aneurysms (A).

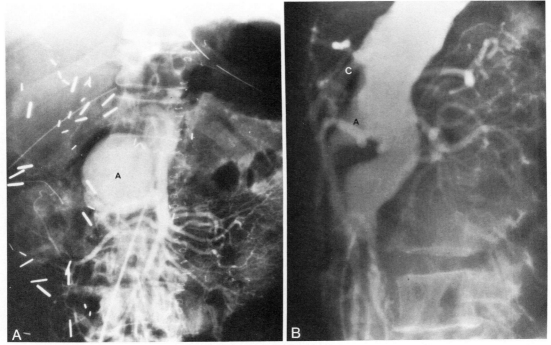

*Figure 14–9.* Superior mesenteric artery aneurysm. *A,* Superior mesenteric arteriogram shows a large saccular aneurysm (A). *B,* Lateral abdominal aortogram shows a fusiform atherosclerotic aneurysm of the proximal SMA (A). C = celiac artery. (From Kadir S, Ernst CB: Current Concepts in Angiographic Management of Gastrointestinal Bleeding. *In* Ravitch MM et al (eds): CURRENT PROBLEMS IN SURGERY. Copyright © 1983 by Year Book Medical Publishers, Inc., Chicago. Used with permission.)

**Gastroduodenal and Pancreaticoduodenal Artery Aneurysms** (Figs. 14–10 and 14–11). Such aneurysms are usually atherosclerotic in origin. They may also occur after pancreatitis or duodenal ulcer disease and in association with occlusion of the celiac artery.[13, 14] Symptoms include abdominal pain and obstructive jaundice, which may simulate a pancreatic neoplasm, and gastrointestinal bleeding. Aneurysm rupture into the gastrointestinal tract occurs in a significant number of patients.[6, 13, 15]

**Other Aneurysms.** Aneurysms of the celiac, gastroepiploic, inferior mesenteric, and left gastric arteries are rare. On the other hand, post-stenotic dilatation of the celiac artery is seen much more frequently and may simulate a true aneurysm (Fig. 14–12). Celiac artery aneurysms are most frequently atherosclerotic.

## Occlusive Arterial Diseases

Because of an efficient collateral system, occlusion of the proximal splanchnic vessels is relatively well tolerated. Symptoms are observed when two of the three major vessels are severely compromised. However, in some patients, even occlusion of two vessels may not be associated with symptoms. On the other hand, mild stenoses may become symptomatic in the presence of a low cardiac output. Thus, the angiographic demonstration of occlusion of a splanchnic artery at its origin or the presence of prominent collateral arterial channels may not by itself be an indicator of the presence of intestinal ischemia.

The symptoms of intestinal angina consist of postprandial abdominal pain; fear of eating because of the pain, leading to anorexia and weight loss; and malabsorption.[16] An epigastric bruit is heard in the majority of patients with celiac or SMA stenosis.[17] Occasionally, occlusion of splanchnic vessels may be simulated by nonocclusive ischemia secondary to cardiac disease. In the latter, there is often no anatomical narrowing of the arterial orifices.

Collateral circulation between the celiac artery and the SMA is established via the gastroduodenal and pancreaticoduodenal arteries. Between the SMA and IMA, the collateral circulation is established via the mar-

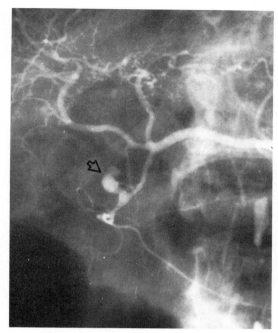

**Figure 14–10.** Aneurysm of the gastroduodenal artery arising adjacent to a peptic duodenal ulcer (*arrow*).

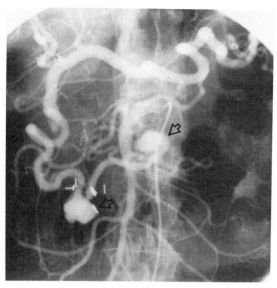

**Figure 14–11.** Aneurysms of the inferior pancreatico-duodenal artery. Superior mesenteric arteriogram shows two large aneurysms (*arrows*). There is retrograde filling of the celiac artery, which is occluded at its origin. (From Kadir S. et al: Cardiovasc Radiol 1:173, 1978. Used with permission.)

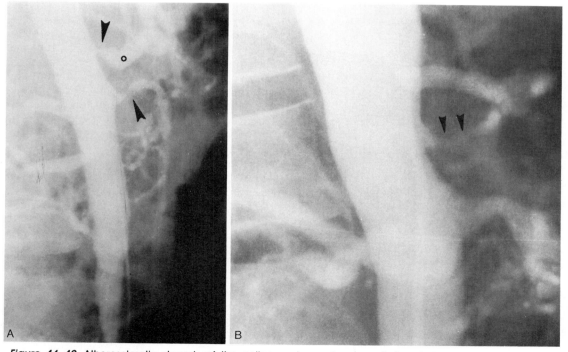

**Figure 14–12.** Atherosclerotic stenosis of the celiac and superior mesenteric arteries. *A,* Lateral abdominal aortogram shows a stenosis of the proximal celiac and superior mesenteric arteries (*arrowheads*). There is post-stenotic dilatation of the celiac artery (o). *B,* Lateral aortogram from another patient shows a smooth stenosis of the celiac artery (*arrowheads*) resembling the neoplastic encasement shown in Figure 14–13.

ginal artery and the arc of Riolan. In addition, the IMA distribution may receive blood from the middle and inferior hemorrhoidal arteries arising from the internal iliac arteries.

**Atherosclerosis.** Atherosclerotic plaque in the abdominal aorta may lead to compromise of the visceral artery orifices. Such stenoses are circumferential and are often associated with post-stenotic dilatation (see Fig. 14–12). This latter finding is observed most frequently in the celiac artery and SMA. Atherosclerosis of the proximal splanchnic arteries can be in the form of a short circumferential, often eccentric, orifice stenosis or an inferior plaque. In contrast, neoplastic encasement is circumferential and usually involves a longer segment of the artery. However, an occasional circumferential atherosclerotic stenosis may simulate encasement by a neoplasm[18] (Fig. 14–13). A similar picture may also be observed in neurofibromatosis.[19]

The stenosis may progress to thrombotic occlusion. The most frequently occluded splanchnic vessel is the IMA, followed by the celiac artery and SMA. On arteriography, an aortic plaque or shallow nubbin is demonstrated (Fig. 14–14). In patients with suspected occlusion, arteriography should be performed promptly in order to facilitate a diagnosis. Noninvasive imaging methods may be extremely misleading in the assess-

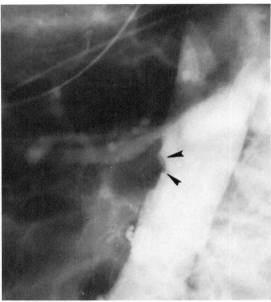

**Figure 14–14.** Thrombotic occlusion of the superior mesenteric artery superimposed upon an atherosclerotic stenosis (*arrowheads*). There is an atherosclerotic stenosis of the proximal celiac artery.

ment of patency because of their inability to detect a thrombus (Fig. 14–15).

Atherosclerosis may also involve the branches of the major splanchnic arteries. On arteriography, this may appear as a smooth or an irregular stenosis or occlusion (Fig. 14–16). Atherosclerotic orifice stenoses and thrombotic occlusions of the splanchnic arteries are evaluated by a lateral abdominal aortogram (see Chapter 10, Fig. 10–20).

**Celiac Artery Compression Syndrome.** Extrinsic compression of the proximal celiac artery by the median arcuate ligament of the diaphragm and/or the celiac neural plexuses and connective tissues is a relatively common arteriographic finding. It occurs most frequently in thin female patients and is usually not associated with symptoms of abdominal angina. However, in some patients with cramplike upper abdominal pain and malabsorption, celiac artery compression has been implicated as the etiology. In some, alleviation of symptoms has been observed after operation, which consisted of widening the diaphragmatic hiatus or resection of the celiac ganglion.[17, 20]

A lateral abdominal aortogram is used to evaluate celiac artery compression. This shows a typical compression of the upper wall of the proximal celiac artery (Fig. 14–17). The compression usually varies with respi-

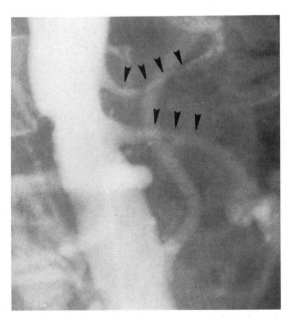

**Figure 14–13.** Neoplastic encasement and stenosis of the proximal celiac and superior mesenteric arteries in a patient with carcinoma of the pancreas (*arrowheads*).

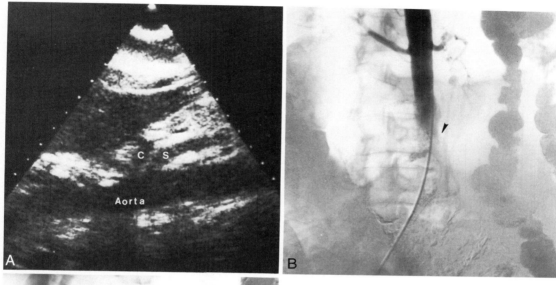

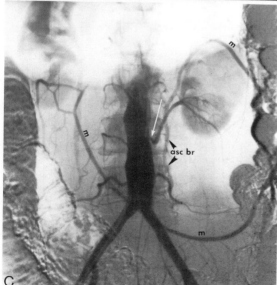

*Figure 14–15.* Intestinal infarction due to thrombotic occlusion of the celiac and superior mesenteric arteries. *A,* Longitudinal sonogram shows the celiac (C) and superior mesenteric (S) arteries. There is no evidence of an occlusion. *B,* RAO abdominal aortogram shows no opacification of the celiac and superior mesenteric arteries. The inferior mesenteric artery is severely stenotic at its orifice (*arrowhead*). *C,* AP aortogram with the catheter in the distal abdominal aorta shows retrograde opacification of SMA branches via the IMA. asc br = ascending branch of the left colic artery; m = marginal artery. There is marked intestinal distention. White arrow points to the orifice stenosis of the accessory left renal artery. *Note:* This demonstrates the inability of ultrasound to detect thrombotic vascular occlusion.

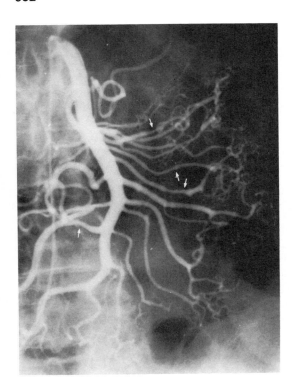

*Figure 14–16.* Small vessel atherosclerosis. Superior mesenteric arteriogram shows atherosclerosis of the branches (*arrows*).

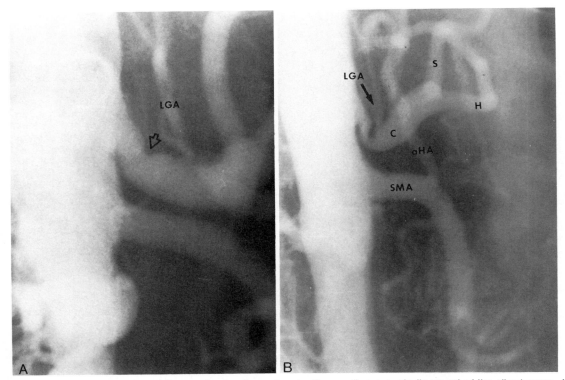

*Figure 14–17.* Compression of the proximal celiac artery by the median arcuate ligament of the diaphragm. *A,* Mild indentation of the celiac artery (*arrow*). *B,* Severe stenosis with post-stenotic dilatation. aHA = accessory right hepatic; C = celiac; H = hepatic; LGA = left gastric; S = splenic; SMA = superior mesenteric arteries.

ration and is most pronounced during expiration.[21] Occasionally the compression is so severe that there is retrograde opacification of the celiac artery branches via enlarged inferior pancreaticoduodenal arteries. On catheterization, the tip of the catheter may not advance past the narrowing during expiration. Relief of the compression during inspiration allows catheterization.

**Dissection.** Aortic dissection may involve the splanchnic arteries, leading to infarction of the affected organs. The most frequent mechanism is compression and occlusion of the orifices by the false channel (see Chapter 8, Fig. 8–34). Rarely, the dissection may extend into the branches (see Chapter 8, Fig. 8–35).

## Embolic Occlusion

Occlusion of the suprarenal aorta or the proximal SMA by an embolus is a surgical emergency. If the occlusion is not treated and leads to ischemic intestinal necrosis, the prognosis is very poor. SMA emboli are considered responsible for acute mesenteric ischemia in up to 50% of cases.[22] In 20% of such cases, multiple vessels are involved.

The most common source of the emboli is the heart (atrial fibrillation, mitral stenosis, recent myocardial infarction). Other sources of emboli are mural thrombus of the aorta, atheromatous material, and paradoxical emboli from the systemic veins.

Clinically, severe, diffuse, often colicky abdominal pain is present. Abdominal tenderness and other physical findings are conspicuously absent.[23, 24] The development of peritoneal signs occurs late and is indicative of intestinal infarction.

The prognosis is determined by the level of vascular occlusion and the delay between onset of symptoms and initiation of definitive treatment. The most frequent sites for lodgment of emboli are the anatomically narrowed segments of normal vessels distal to the origins of major branches.[22] In the SMA, these are the origins of the inferior pancreaticodudenal and middle colic arteries. Smaller emboli are found in the distal branches.

**Arteriography.** Arteriography is required for the diagnosis and contributes significantly towards the decision of the type of therapy required. Large occluding emboli are treated by surgical embolectomy; smaller nonoccluding emboli may be managed conservatively by heparinization in anticipation of sponta-

neous thrombolysis or occasionally by selective infusion of thrombolytic agents.[25] In addition, papaverine may be infused into the SMA to combat vasoconstriction and prevent intestinal necrosis.

The initial study is a biplane aortogram. This is obtained to determine patency of the proximal visceral arteries. Subsequently, a selective (SMA or celiac) arteriogram is performed.

The arteriographic findings include (Fig. 14–18):

1. Abrupt termination of the vessel. A concave or convex meniscus is often seen distal to the origin of a major branch.

2. Stasis of contrast medium proximal to an occlusion if branches are also occluded.

3. Nonoccluding emboli, which are seen as defects in the contrast opacified artery.

4. Vasoconstriction with prolongation of circulation time.[26] This is not observed in all patients.

5. Recanalized vessels. These have smaller and irregular lumina and are indicative of an older process.

PITFALLS IN DIAGNOSIS

1. Pronounced vasoconstriction with prolongation of the circulation time is also observed in nonocclusive mesenteric ischemia and systemic hypotension.

2. Stasis of the contrast medium proximal to an abrupt occlusion of the celiac artery or SMA is also observed in acute catheter-induced arterial dissection (Fig. 14–19).

3. An intraluminal defect simulating an embolus is occasionally seen in intestinal volvulus (see Fig. 14–23).

## Fibromuscular Disease

Extrarenal fibromuscular disease may involve the splanchnic vessels.[6, 27] The splenic, superior mesenteric, and celiac arteries are affected in decreasing order of frequency. On arteriography, a stenosis and the typical beaded aneurysm formation are present (Fig. 14–20).

## Nonocclusive Mesenteric Ischemia

This may be responsible for intestinal ischemia in as many as 50% of patients and carries a very high mortality.[28, 29] Its importance for the cardiovascular radiologist is emphasized by the fact that arteriography is essential not only for establishing the diagnosis but also for initiating the treatment.

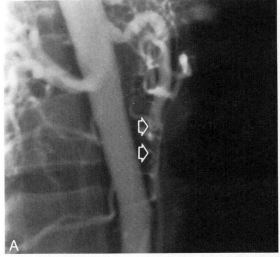

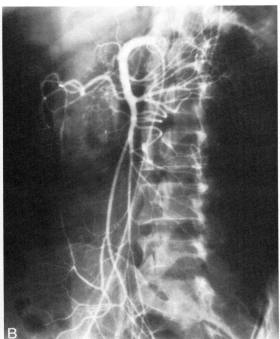

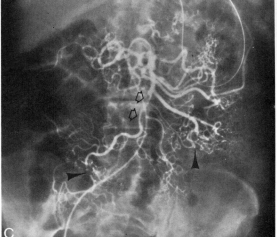

Figure 14–18. Superior mesenteric artery embolus. *A,* Lateral aortogram shows a nonoccluding thrombus in the SMA (*open arrows*). *B,* Superior mesenteric arteriogram obtained a week later shows spontaneous lysis of the embolus. *C,* Superior mesenteric arteriogram from another patient shows a large embolus (*open arrows*), which occludes several jejunal and ileal branches. Arrowheads point to several smaller emboli.

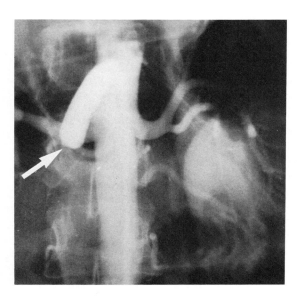

Figure 14–19. Iatrogenic arterial dissection during attempted selective catheterization simulating embolic occlusion. AP aortogram shows an abrupt termination of the superior mesenteric artery (*arrow*).

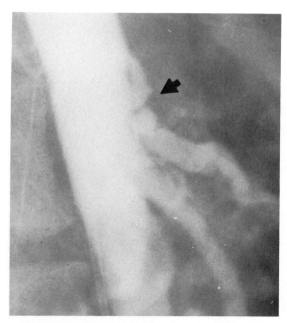

**Figure 14–20.** Fibromuscular disease of the celiac artery. Lateral aortogram shows beading and stenosis of the proximal celiac artery (*arrow*).

The pathophysiology of nonocclusive mesenteric ischemia is an extreme vasoconstriction of the mesenteric vascular bed in response to shock, systemic hypotension or hypovolemia, or decrease in cardiac output. This may be mediated via the renin-angiotensin system.[30] The vasoconstriction persists despite correction of the precipitating event, and, if untreated, results in ischemic necrosis. Clinically, it may not be recognized until intestinal damage has occurred, because the symptomatology of the precipitating event may dominate the picture and the early symptoms of intestinal ischemia may go unrecognized.

Nonocclusive mesenteric ischemia is seen primarily in the elderly patient with heart disease (myocardial infarction, congestive heart failure) or after major surgery. Arteriography is necessary to establish the diagnosis. Radionuclide imaging with technetium pyrophosphate has been tried but does not permit an early diagnosis, since this agent will be taken up only by bowel that is undergoing necrosis.[31] In addition, an intraarterial injection is necessary. Recent studies with intraperitoneally injected xenon-133 appear to be more promising and suggest that this method may provide an early bedside test.[32] With this method, the rate of absorption and washout of the xenon is

measured to provide an indicator of mesenteric perfusion.

**Arteriography.** Emergency arteriography is indicated in patients with suspected mesenteric ischemia in order to establish the diagnosis (vascular occlusion by embolus or nonocclusive ischemia) and to initiate therapy. A biplane abdominal aortogram is obtained to evaluate the splanchnic arteries for proximal occlusion. Subsequently, a selective arteriogram of the SMA must be obtained.

ANGIOGRAPHIC FINDINGS. The angiographic picture in nonocclusive mesenteric ischemia may include[33, 34] (Fig. 14–21):

1. Extreme constriction of the main SMA trunk and mesenteric arterial bed with absent opacification of the smaller mural branches.

2. Poor or absent venous opacification.

3. Reflux of contrast medium into the abdominal aorta despite a slow injection rate, eg, 3 or 4 ml/sec. This is a manifestation of the high mesenteric vascular resistance but is also observed in association with low cardiac output and severe occlusive disease.

4. Focal areas of severe vascular spasm at the origins of the branch vessels.

5. Alternating areas of vasospasm of the main branches causing the arterial lumen to appear irregular.

6. Severe vasospasm leading to vascular occlusion.

7. Intestinal distention with stretching of the branches but without vasoconstriction. This finding is also observed in intestinal volvulus.

PITFALLS IN DIAGNOSIS

None of the angiographic signs is specific for nonocclusive mesenteric ischemia, and only some of the signs may be present in a given patient. Any or all of these angiographic signs may be mimicked by:

1. Intravenous or intraarterial infusion of vasoconstricting drugs, eg, vasopressin.

2. Ergot alkaloids.

3. Systemic hypotension or shock without mesenteric ischemia.

4. Small vessel atherosclerosis or a vasculitis.

After establishing the diagnosis, the catheter is left in the proximal SMA. Papaverine, 60 mg, is slowly injected (over 60 to 90 seconds) into the SMA, followed by an infusion of 1 mg of papaverine/min via a constant infusion pump. The patient is then observed for peritoneal signs. A rapidly injected bolus of papaverine can cause hypotension.

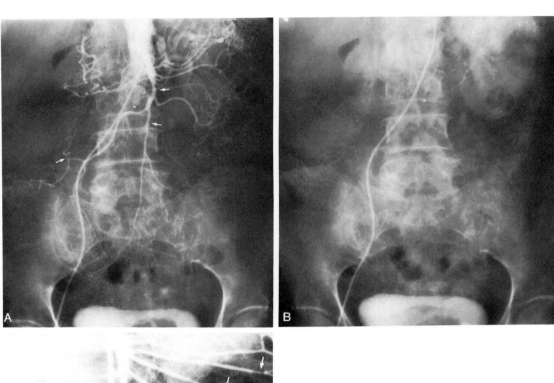

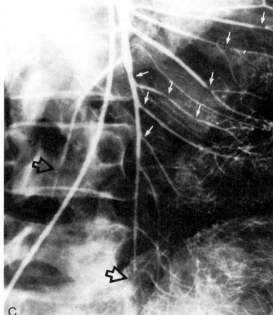

*Figure 14-21.* Nonocclusive mesenteric ischemia. *A,* AP superior mesenteric arteriogram (3 ml/sec). There is reflux of contrast medium into the aorta. Focal areas of arterial narrowing are present (*arrows*). The distal jejunal and several ileal arteries are poorly opacified or occluded. *B,* Late parenchymal phase (about 15 sec). There is persistent arterial and absent venous opacification. *C,* Superior mesenteric arteriogram from another patient shows multiple areas of focal vaso-spasm (*small arrows*) and spastic occlusion (*open arrows*).

## Miscellaneous Disorders

**Arteriovenous Fistula or Malformation.** Congenital or acquired arteriovenous malformations can occur along the intestinal tract. These may be found as isolated congenital or acquired lesions (eg, angiodysplasia or postoperative fistula) or as the manifestation of a hereditary syndrome.[35] Colonic angiomatosis is seen in patients with the Klippel-Trenaunay-Weber syndrome. Patients with the Osler-Weber-Rendu syndrome may also have hemangiomata of the alimentary tract. The most common manifestation of such lesions is gastrointestinal bleeding.

Larger lesions can be detected by selective arteriography, but occasionally magnification arteriography is necessary. Frequently, the congenital lesions are too small or too diffuse and thus escape detection. On arteriography, the arteriovenous fistulae show early venous opacification. Angiomas/hemangiomas are seen as dilated, tortuous vascular spaces (Fig. 14–22).

**Arteritis.** Aortitis of the abdominal aorta (eg, Takayasu's arteritis or abdominal aortic coarctation) may lead to occlusion of the celiac artery or SMA.[36] The IMA is usually spared and enlarged and serves as a collateral (see Chapter 10, Fig. 10–53). Other forms of arteritis (eg, systemic lupus erythematosus, rheumatoid arteritis) may also involve the mesenteric vessels, usually the distal branches.

Thromboangiitis obliterans of the mesenteric vessels can also cause intestinal ischemia.[17] Clinically, these patients have abdominal pain that is often cramplike, bouts of diarrhea, and weight loss. Plain abdominal radiographs may demonstrate segmental intestinal atony.

On arteriography, the main trunks are unaffected. Magnification arteriography of the distal branches may show occlusion of the smaller branches.

**Volvulus.** Intestinal volvulus should be suspected in patients with signs of intestinal ischemia and a history of a recent abdominal operation. The angiographic appearance of intestinal volvulus may be quite typical[37] (Fig. 14–23):

1. Tapering or abrupt termination of mesenteric vessels: This may simulate an embolus.

2. Abnormal course of the mesenteric branches, occasionally demonstrating a whirled arrangement or an abrupt reversal in course.

3. Stretching of arterial branches over distended bowel loops.

4. Marked vasoconstriction and prolonged transit time of the contrast medium, leading to an intense bowel stain.

5. Absent venous opacification.

**Inflammatory Diseases.** Although the evaluation of inflammatory diseases is rarely an indication for splanchnic arteriography, complications (eg, gastrointestinal bleeding) may necessitate arteriography.

Intense hyperemia and early and dense venous opacification are the hallmarks of acute inflammation. Fibrotic changes associated with chronic inflammatory lesions may cause distortion of the vascular architecture. Occasionally, fine neovascularity, which may simulate neoplasia, is seen in regional enteritis.

In active inflammatory bowel diseases or colonic diverticulitis, hyperemia of the bowel wall and early venous opacification are present (Fig. 14–24). The vasa recta are dilated and can be followed to the antimesenteric

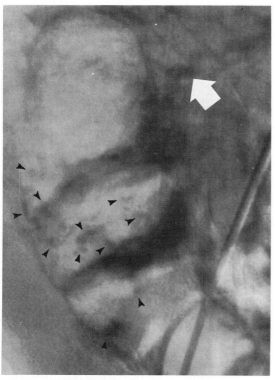

*Figure 14–22.* Colonic angiomatosis. Subtraction film from a superior mesenteric arteriogram in a patient with Klippel-Trenaunay-Weber syndrome shows multiple colonic angiomas (*arrowheads*). Arrow points to the dilated, tortuous right colic vein.

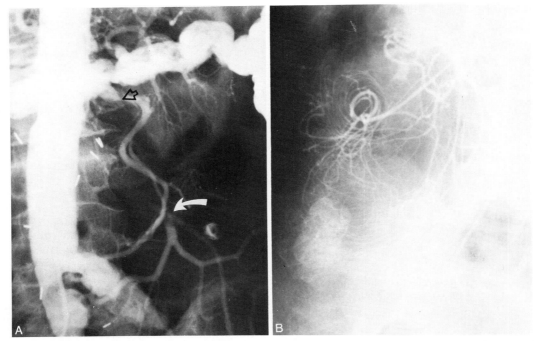

**Figure 14–23.** Intestinal volvulus. *A,* AP aortogram shows a beaklike occlusion of the proximal superior mesenteric artery (*open arrow*). Distally, there is an intraluminal defect that simulates a thrombus (*curved arrow*). *B,* Superior mesenteric arteriogram from another patient shows the typical whirled arrangement of the mesenteric branches. (From Kadir S. et al: Radiology 128:595, 1978. Used with permission.)

border. In the inactive stage, no abnormality may be seen in ulcerative colitis. In regional enteritis and recurrent diverticulitis, focal vascular occlusions or fibrotic distortion may be present.

The arteriographic findings in active inflammatory diseases of the intestine are rather nonspecific. A similar picture has also been observed after multiple cleansing enemas, heavy alcohol consumption, gastrointestinal bleeding (possibly due to prolonged contact of the colonic mucosa with the blood), and wedged contrast injection into a small vessel (eg, the IMA or a branch of the SMA).

**Periarteritis Nodosa.** The mesenteric vessels are affected in 50% of patients with periarteritis nodosa.[38] The kidneys are affected in 85% and the liver in 66% of patients. By contrast, skin and skeletal muscle are affected in only 20% and 39% of individuals, respectively. Symptoms include malaise, low-grade fever, and weight loss. Mesenteric involvement is manifested by abdominal pain, ulcer formation, gastrointestinal bleeding, or, rarely, intestinal infarction.[39]

Arteriography is indicated for establishing the diagnosis and for management of com-

plications (eg, hemorrhage). Selective arteriography should be performed, as it provides the most information.

The arteriographic findings are (Fig. 14–25):

1. Multiple saccular aneurysms of the medium and small branches of the renal, hepatic, and mesenteric arteries: The aneurysms are usually small but may be of varying sizes. The main vessels (eg, SMA trunk) are spared. In contrast, necrotizing angiitis and mycotic aneurysms affect both the large trunks and small vessels.

2. Irregular arterial lumen, also involving the medium and small arteries.

3. A hematoma or hemorrhage may be demonstrated if aneurysm rupture has occurred.

PITFALLS IN DIAGNOSIS

1. Multiple saccular aneurysms may also be seen in necrotizing angiitis from intravascular drug abuse[40] and Wegener's granulomatosis.

2. Multiple intrasplenic arterial aneurysms may be seen in patients with portal hypertension and following splenic trauma (eg, blunt abdominal trauma) or splenoportography.[41]

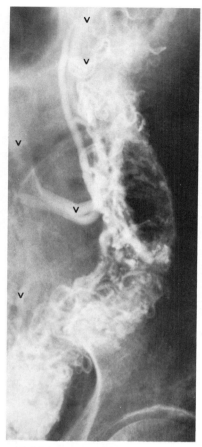

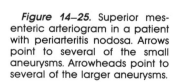

*Figure 14–24.* Inflammatory bowel disease. Late arterial phase of an inferior mesenteric arteriogram in a patient with active ulcerative colitis. There is intense hyperemia of the bowel wall, with visualization of dilated vascular channels extending to the antimesenteric border and early dense venous (v) opacification.

## Venous Diseases

The normal sequence of venous opacification of the mesenteric veins is from left to right: ie, jejunal, then ileal, and finally the colic veins.[42, 43] The normal arteriographic transit time from the beginning of the arterial injection to venous opacification is between 8 seconds (jejunal veins) and 13 seconds (colic veins).[43] Earlier or delayed venous opacification is indicative of disease.

**Early Venous Opacification.** Early venous opacification is seen in arteriovenous fistulae, or malformations, acquired angiodysplasias, inflammatory bowel disease, and neoplasms. Intraarterial injection of vasodilators is also associated with early venous opacification. Early opacification of segmental veins may also be due to selective contrast injection into a branch vessel.

**Delayed Venous Opacification.** This is seen in intestinal strangulation, volvulus, nonocclusive ischemia, and bowel infarction. In all of these conditions, there is usually some degree of mesenteric arterial constriction with prolongation of the arterial phase on the contrast arteriogram.

**Absent Venous Opacification.** This is usually indicative of venous thrombosis but may also be seen in bowel infarction, severe vasoconstriction, and volvulus.[37] In the superior mesenteric circulation, absent venous opacification is associated with attenuation of the arterial channels with prolongation of the arterial phase of the contrast arteriogram. In segmental venous thrombosis, the veins draining the unaffected segments opacify in

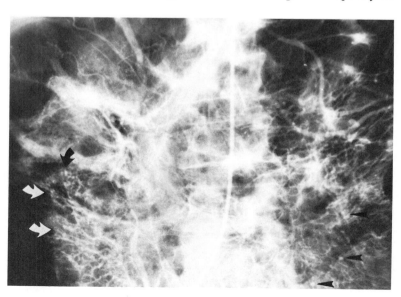

*Figure 14–25.* Superior mesenteric arteriogram in a patient with periarteritis nodosa. Arrows point to several of the small aneurysms. Arrowheads point to several of the larger aneurysms.

a normal fashion. Mesenteric venous thrombosis is seen in extreme hypotension, hematological disorders, hypercoagulable states, abdominal trauma, abdominal sepsis and in individuals taking oral contraceptives.

Occlusion of the superior mesenteric and portal veins can occur following radiation (implantation of radioactive seeds) and due to neoplastic invasion (Fig. 14–26). In these conditions, numerous collateral channels are present.

In splenic vein occlusion, enlargement of the collateral venous channels along the stomach leads to the formation of large gastric varices (Fig. 14–27). Esophageal varices are absent in patients without portal hypertension. The gastroepiploic veins also serve as a collateral. The most frequent cause of splenic vein occlusion is pancreatitis. Other causes are pancreatic or retroperitoneal neoplasms, trauma, or idiopathic splenic vein thrombosis.[44]

Totally absent venous opacification may also result from faulty arteriographic technique (eg, small contrast bolus, too short or too long duration of filming, or inappropriate film exposure parameters). The demonstration of collaterals is a sign of the presence of venous occlusion (or obstruction).

Diseases of the hepatic veins are discussed in Chapter 15.

## GASTROINTESTINAL BLEEDING

Gastrointestinal bleeding accounts for less than 1% of emergency hospital admissions.

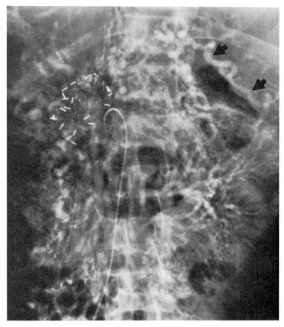

*Figure 14–26.* Mesenteric venous obstruction following local radiation through intraoperatively implanted $^{125}$I seeds in a patient with malignant glucagonoma. Venous phase of the superior mesenteric arteriogram shows occlusion of the superior mesenteric and portal veins. Dilated jejunal and ileal veins and a dilated and tortuous marginal vein are seen (*arrows*).

Despite advances in diagnosis and management, the overall mortality rate has remained approximately 10%.[45] Angiography plays an important role in the diagnosis and management of acute and chronic gastrointestinal bleeding. A careful preangiographic workup is essential for proper application of angio-

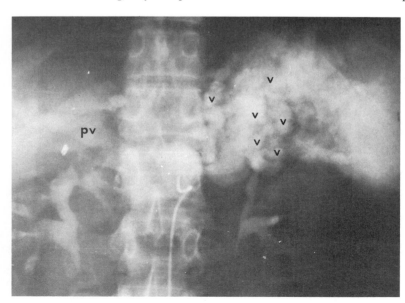

*Figure 14–27.* Splenic vein occlusion following pancreatitis. Venous phase of splenic arteriogram shows large gastric varices. The splenic vein does not opacify. pv = portal vein; v = varices.

graphic techniques. A detailed review of the subject can be found in references 46 to 49.

## Clinical Assessment

Preangiographic evaluation of the patient with acute gastrointestinal bleeding must include (1) assessment of the severity of bleeding; (2) determination of the type of bleeding, ie, arterio-capillary or venous; (3) whether bleeding occurs from the upper or lower gastrointestinal tract; and (4) evaluation of potential predisposing factors (eg, aspirin ingestion, coumarin overdose, disseminated intravascular coagulation).

Since, in the majority of patients, the bleeding can be stopped by conservative non-operative management, such therapy should be tried prior to angiography. At the same time, other means for localization of the source of bleeding (nasogastric tube, endoscopy) should be utilized.

The *nasogastric tube* serves to confirm that the source of bleeding lies proximal to the ligament of Treitz and to assess its severity and response to therapy. Thus, an indwelling nasogastric tube should be in place in all patients with upper gastrointestinal bleeding who are to undergo angiography. In some patients with apparent lower gastrointestinal bleeding (except those with bright red blood per rectum), a diagnostic nasogastric tube serves to identify a source of bleeding proximal to the ligament of Treitz and accelerated passage of blood to the rectum.

In acute bleeding, *endoscopy* prior to arteriography serves to identify patients who do not require arteriography or those who are not likely to respond to transcatheter therapy (eg, patients with variceal bleeding or oropharyngeal, proximal esophageal, or rectal lesions). Endoscopy also serves to guide the angiographic study by providing a "road map."

*Barium examination* should be avoided in acute bleeders. Such studies cannot determine the source of bleeding, and furthermore the presence of barium in the alimentary tract may preclude angiographic detection of a bleeding site.

*Radionuclide studies* have been helpful in some patients, whereas they have been misleading in others.[46] The most commonly used preparations are $^{99m}$technetium sulfur colloid and $^{111}$indium-labeled erythrocytes.

## Arteriography

Arteriography is indicated to (1) localize a source of acute arterial or capillary bleeding, (2) localize a potential source of chronic or intermittent bleeding, and (3) provide trans-catheter therapy.

The accuracy of carefully performed arteriography is about 90% for the localization of upper gastrointestinal bleeding and approximately 50% for lower gastrointestinal bleeding. Accuracy can be maximized by careful preangiographic screening, selection of the optimal timing for arteriography, and utilization of appropriate angiographic studies.[46] It must be borne in mind that only arterial bleeding and capillary bleeding are likely to be detected by angiography and that venous bleeding is rarely demonstrated on the venous phase of a splanchnic arteriogram.

Selective arteriography is performed of the vessel supplying the region from which the bleeding is suspected. Conventional cut film arteriograms are preferable, since the cooperation required for DSA is often not possible in severely ill patients. Films should be obtained over 25 seconds, ie, into the late venous phase. This helps to differentiate between extravasated contrast medium and slow venous wash-out.

For *esophagogastric bleeding*, a left gastric arteriogram is performed. If this is unrevealing, it is followed by a celiac arteriogram to identify a different source for the bleeding. In one series, the left gastric arteriogram demonstrated the gastric bleeding source in 92.6% of patients.[48] In the remainder, the source was in the distribution of the right gastric artery in 2% of patients, the short gastric arteries in 2.7%, and the gastroepiploic arteries in 2.7%.

For *pyloroduodenal bleeding*, a gastroduodenal arteriogram is performed. If the GDA is difficult to catheterize, a common hepatic or a celiac arteriogram should be obtained.

*Small intestinal and colonic bleeding* (up to the mid-transverse colon) is evaluated by superior mesenteric arteriography. The remainder of the colon and the rectum are evaluated by an inferior mesenteric arteriogram. For the distal rectum, an internal iliac arteriogram may be necessary if the IMA injection is unrevealing.

Bleeding from *aorto-enteric fistulae* requires a biplane aortogram. Whenever possible, this should be performed in the prone position in an attempt to demonstrate a false aneurysm or fistulous tract that is located on the anterolateral surface of the aorta.

**Arteriographic Findings.** Active bleeding manifests as contrast extravasation. A source of intermittent or chronic bleeding often shows indirect signs, such as vascular ab-

**TABLE 14–3.** Angiographic Management of Gastrointestinal Bleeding

| Type of Bleeding | Type of Therapy | Success Rate (%) |
|---|---|---|
| Mallory-Weiss tears | Intraarterial vasopressin | 80 |
| | Embolization | 100 |
| Acute hemorrhagic gastritis | Intraarterial vasopressin | 80 |
| Gastric ulcer | Intraarterial vasopressin | 70 |
| | Embolization | |
| Pyloroduodenal ulcer | Intraarterial vasopressin | 50 |
| | Embolization | 90 |
| Small bowel | Intraarterial vasopressin | 70 |
| Colorectal | Intraarterial vasopressin | 90 |
| Variceal | Intravenous vasopressin | 80 |
| | embolization | |

normalities. There are basically four angiographic features that must be searched for in patients with gastrointestinal bleeding:

1. Massive contrast extravasation (see Figs. 14–31, 14–36, and 14–38): This is seen in bleeding from ulcers, aneurysm rupture, diverticula, or trauma. On the arteriogram, extravasation is seen as dense extravascular contrast accumulation that persists past the venous phase. The appearance of extravasation may resemble a vein and has been referred to as a pseudovein (see Figs. 14–28 and 14–38). Contrast extravasation may be a focal or a large formless collection of contrast medium inside or outside the lumen of the bowel. Intraluminal contrast accumulation often outlines the mucosal folds (see Figs. 14–31 A and 14–38). On serial films, a change in configuration is observed and the extravasated contrast medium is propagated with the bowel peristalsis.

2. Punctate contrast extravasation (see Fig. 14–31 C): This is observed in bleeding from mucosal erosions or shallow ulcerations.

3. Hyperemia (hypervascularity) (see Figs. 14–24 and 14–31): This appears as a diffuse increase in opacity of the mucosa during the parenchymal phase of the arteriogram. In most cases, hyperemia is associated with dilatation of the arteries with early and dense opacification of the veins. It is seen in hemorrhagic gastritis and inflammatory diseases. Focal hyperemia of the area surrounding a peptic ulcer is occasionally seen in intermittently bleeding duodenal ulcers (see Fig. 14–34).

4. Demonstration of an arterial aneurysm or arteriovenous malformation (see Figs. 14–10 and 14–35). This provides indirect evidence for the source of bleeding. Similarly, demonstration of a hypervascular mass le-

sion in a patient with clinically manifested gastrointestinal bleeding also provides indirect evidence for the source of bleeding.

**Transcatheter Therapy.** Once the source of bleeding has been identified, transcatheter therapy is available immediately in the form of vasopressin infusion or embolization (Table 14–3). The protocol for vasopressin infusion is shown in Table 14–4.

## Upper Gastrointestinal Bleeding

Bleeding from a source proximal to the ligament of Treitz is defined as upper gastrointestinal bleeding. Frequent causes are listed in Table 14–5.

The source of bleeding is in the distribution

**TABLE 14–4.** Protocol for Intravenous or Intraarterial Vasopressin Infusion

1. Localize bleeding point by arteriography or endoscopy.
2. Start vasopressin infusion: 0.2 U/min for 20–30 minutes (via constant infusion pump).
3. Repeat arteriogram.
4. If bleeding has stopped, continue at this rate for 12–24 hours.
5. If bleeding continues, infuse vasopressin at 0.4 U/min for 20–30 minutes.
6. Repeat arteriogram.
7. If bleeding has stopped, continue vasopressin as follows:
   0.4 U/min for 6–12 hours, then
   0.3 U/min for 6–12 hours, then
   0.2 U/min for 6–12 hours, and finally
   0.1 U/min for another 6–12 hours.
8. Thereafter, infuse 5% dextrose or normal saline at 15–20 ml/hr for 4–6 hours to maintain catheter patency and observe for signs of recurrent bleeding: nasogastric aspirate, central venous pressure, hematocrit, and transfusion requirement.
9. If bleeding has ceased, remove catheter. If bleeding persists after infusion of 0.4 U/min, consider embolization or operation.

**TABLE 14-5.** Sources of Gastrointestinal Bleeding*

| Source | Per Cent |
|---|---|
| *Upper Gastrointestinal Bleeding* | |
| Esophagogastric junction: | |
| Varices | ~ 17 |
| Mallory-Weiss tears | 7–14 |
| Stomach: | |
| Acute hemorrhagic gastritis | 17–27 |
| Gastric ulcer | 10 |
| Pyloroduodenal | 17–25 |
| Other | ~ 14 |
| *Lower Gastrointestinal Bleeding* | |
| Pyloroduodenal | |
| Small intestine: | ~ 30 |
| Tumors | |
| Vascular malformations | |
| Ulcers | |
| Aorto-enteric fistula | |
| Trauma | |
| Diverticula | |
| Inflammatory bowel disease | |
| Visceral artery aneurysms | |
| Colorectal: | 70 |
| Diverticula | |
| Angiodysplasia | |
| Colitis | |
| Tumors | |

*Data from references 13, 46, and 50 to 60.

of the left gastric artery in only half the patients with upper gastrointestinal bleeding, stressing the importance of preangiographic endoscopy as a guide for arteriography. Celiac arteriography alone may not document an esophagogastric bleed because of the anatomical variations of the left gastric artery origin.

In patients with endoscopically documented bleeding, the appropriate vessel is catheterized, ie, left gastric artery for gastric bleeding and gastroduodenal artery for pyloroduodenal bleeding. In patients who have not been endoscoped prior to arteriography or in whom endoscopy was unsuccessful, a celiac arteriogram is performed first. If this is unrevealing, a left gastric arteriogram is performed. If the latter does not detect a bleeding site, it is followed by a gastroduodenal arteriogram.

**Esophagogastric Junction Bleeding** (Figs. 14–28 to 14–30). The most common nonvariceal source of bleeding is the Mallory-Weiss tear. In 77% of patients, such tears are single and are located on the gastric side of the esophagogastric junction.[50, 51] Other less frequent causes are esophagitis, erosions, and ulcers.

Bleeding from Mallory-Weiss tears located on the anterior or lateral walls appears as a linear extravasation. Posterior wall lesions show a focal accumulation of extravasated contrast medium. Occasionally, the actual bleeding site is not demonstrated, instead, a collection of extravasated contrast medium is seen in the gastric folds. Esophagitis appears as diffuse hypervascularity.

**Gastric Bleeding** (Figs. 14–31 and 14–32). Gastric bleeding is most frequently due to acute hemorrhagic gastritis, which, according to some authors, may be responsible for 43% of hospital admissions for upper gastrointes-

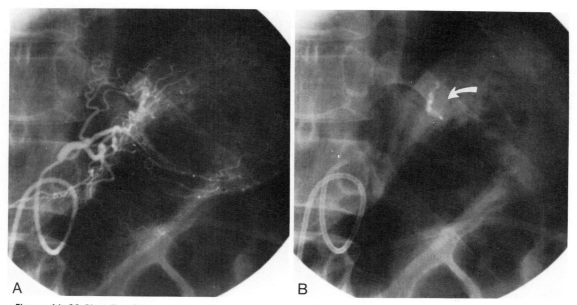

A      B

*Figure 14-28.* Bleeding from a Mallory-Weiss tear. *A*, Early arterial phase of left gastric arteriogram. No contrast extravasation is seen. *B*, Late film from same study shows a focal accumulation of extravasated contrast medium (*arrow*).

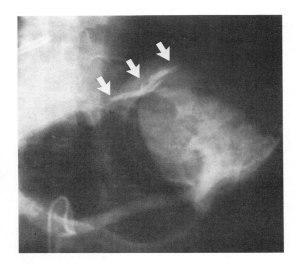

**Figure 14–29.** Bleeding from a Mallory-Weiss tear. Late venous phase of a celiac arteriogram shows a linear accumulation of extravasated contrast medium (*arrows*).

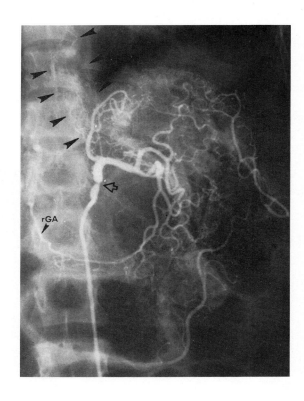

**Figure 14–30.** *Candida* esophagitis. Left gastric arteriogram shows hypervascularity of the distal esophagus (*arrowheads*), and the stomach. There is no contrast extravasation. Bleeding from esophagitis was confirmed by endoscopy. Focal catheter-induced spasm of the left gastric artery is seen (*arrow*). There is retrograde opacification of the right gastric artery (*rGA*).

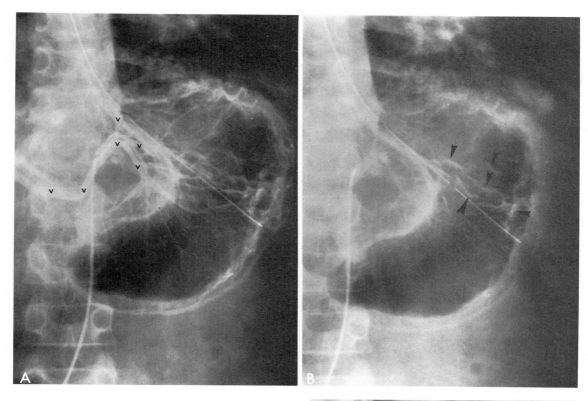

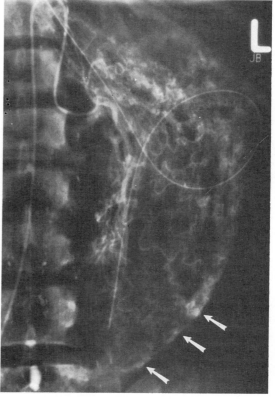

Figure 14–31. Bleeding from hemorrhagic gastritis. A, Early arterial phase of left gastric arteriogram. There is diffuse hyperemia of the stomach with early and intense venous opacification (v). B, Later film from the same arteriogram shows extravasated contrast medium in gastric folds (arrowheads). C, Late arterial phase of left gastric arteriogram from another patient shows punctate contrast extravasation from superficial gastric erosions (arrows). (C, From Kadir S, Ernst CB: Current Concepts in Angiographic Management of Gastrointestinal Bleeding. In Ravitch MM et al (eds): CURRENT RPOBLEMS IN SURGERY. Copyright © 1983 by Year Book Medical Publishers, Inc., Chicago. Used with permission.)

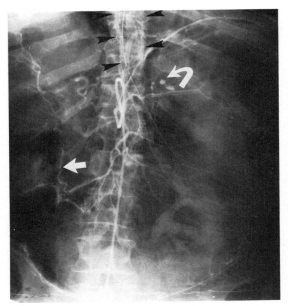

*Figure 14–32.* Gastric ulcer bleeding. Left gastric arteriogram shows contrast extravasation from a high lesser curvature ulcer (*curved arrow*). In addition, there is marked hyperemia of the distal esophagus (*arrowheads*). Marked gastric distention and retrograde opacification of the right gastric (*straight arrow*) and hepatic arteries are also seen.

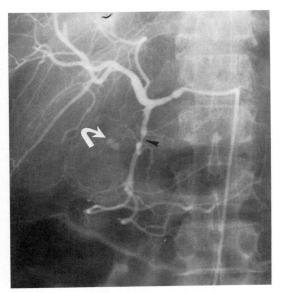

*Figure 14–33.* Duodenal ulcer bleeding. Common hepatic arteriogram shows contrast extravasation from a branch to the gastroduodenal artery (*curved arrow*). Arrowhead points to focal arterial spasm. (From Kadir S et al: Selected Techniques in Interventional Radiology. Philadelphia, WB Saunders, 1982.)

tinal bleeding.[52] Gastric ulcers are responsible for 10% of acute bleeding from the upper gastrointestinal tract.[52, 56]

On arteriography, hemorrhagic gastritis is seen as diffuse hyperemia of the stomach. Occasionally, there is extravasation of contrast medium. Bleeding from peptic ulcers is manifested as contrast extravasation. Bleeding originating from the anterior wall may be easily overlooked unless the stomach is collapsed and the extravasated contrast medium collects in the gastric folds. In the distended stomach, extravasated contrast medium from the anterior wall may appear as a linear collection, usually along the lesser curvature.

Other causes include arteriovenous malformations, aneurysms, and, rarely, gastric neoplasms and diverticula.

**Pyloroduodenal Bleeding** (Figs. 14–33 to 14–35). This may be the source for upper gastrointestinal bleeding in up to 25% of patients. The most frequent etiology is peptic ulcer disease. Other causes are visceral artery aneurysms, vascular malformations, and primary and metastatic neoplasms.[13, 46, 47] Most patients with a pyloroduodenal bleeding source present with upper gastrointestinal bleeding. However, in 10% the initial presentation may be that of lower gastrointestinal bleeding, and the nasogastric aspirate may

not contain blood in 20% of patients with duodenal ulcer bleeding.[57]

On arteriography, active bleeding appears as contrast extravasation. Nonbleeding ulcers

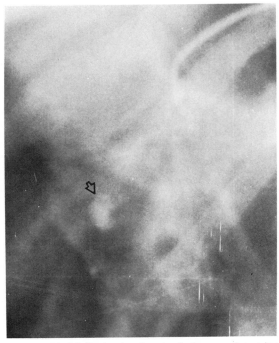

*Figure 14–34.* Gastroduodenal arteriogram shows hyperemia around an intermittently bleeding duodenal ulcer (*arrow*).

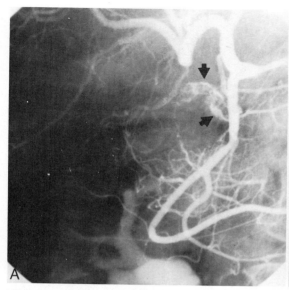
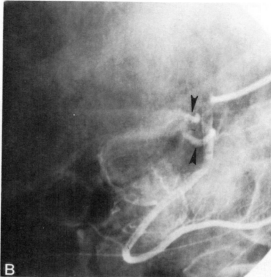

Figure 14–35. Duodenal arteriovenous malformation. *A*, Early arterial phase of a gastroduodenal arteriogram. A focal arteriovenous malformation is seen with early venous opacification (*arrows*). *B*, Late arterial phase from the same arteriogram shows dense opacification of early draining veins (*arrowheads*). (From Kadir S, Ernst CB: Current Concepts in Angiographic Management of Gastrointestinal Bleeding. *In* Ravitch MM et al (eds): CURRENT PROBLEMS IN SURGERY. Copyright © 1983 by Year Book Medical Publishers, Inc., Chicago. Used with permission.)

may appear as focal areas of hyperemia. Occasionally, a false aneurysm is found adjacent to the ulcer (see Fig. 14–10).

## Lower Gastrointestinal Bleeding

Bleeding originating distal to the ligament of Treitz is defined as lower gastrointestinal bleeding. Frequent causes are listed in Table 14–5.

**Small Intestinal Bleeding** (Fig. 14–36). The small intestine is the source of bleeding in 5% of all patients with acute gastrointestinal bleeding and in 30% of those with acute lower gastrointestinal bleeding.[58] The most frequent etiology is a tumor.[59]

On arteriography, contrast extravasation is not demonstrated from tumors or vascular malformations unless there is active bleeding. In patients with arteriovenous malformations, intraoperative localization of the segment of bowel containing the malformation can be facilitated by preoperative placement of a 3 Fr catheter into the vessel supplying the malformation. Such a catheter is placed coaxially through the angiographic catheter. Once the bowel has been exposed during surgery, 1 ml of methylene blue is injected through the 3 Fr catheter to identify the segment of bowel containing the vascular malformation (Fig. 14–37).

**Colorectal Bleeding** (Figs. 14–38 to 14–40). The most frequent cause of acute lower gas-

trointestinal bleeding is diverticular disease. In one series, this was responsible for 70% of such bleeding.[60] In up to 75% of patients with diverticular bleeding, the source lies in the right colon, despite the fact that divertic-

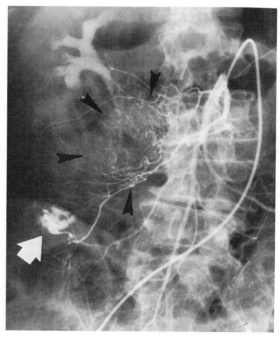

Figure 14–36. Small intestinal bleeding in a patient with lymphoma. Superior mesenteric arteriogram shows contrast extravasation (*white arrow*) and neovasculature (*arrowheads*).

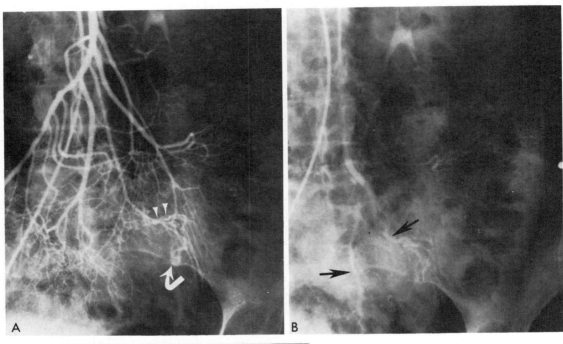

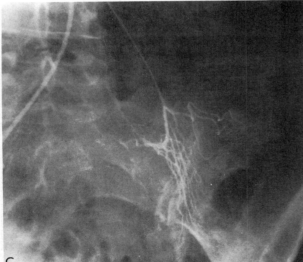

**Figure 14–37.** Jejunal arteriovenous malformations (AVM). *A,* Early arterial phase of a superior mesenteric arteriogram shows an AVM (*curved arrow*) with an early draining vein (*arrowheads*). *B,* Late arterial phase from the same arteriogram shows two densely opacified veins (*arrows*). *C,* Arteriogram of the jejunal branch supplying the AVM (shown in *A*) through coaxially placed 3 Fr catheter for intraoperative methylene blue injection. (From Kadir S et al: Selected Techniques in Interventional Radiology. Philadelphia, WB Saunders, 1982.)

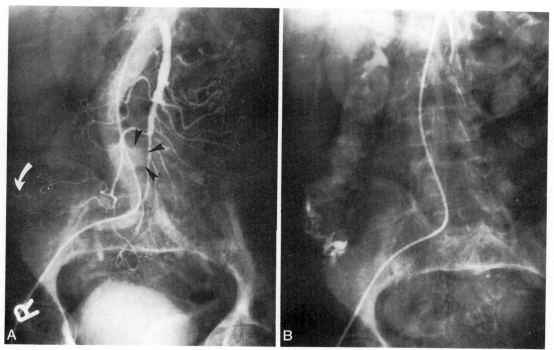

*Figure 14–38.* Bleeding right colonic diverticulum. *A,* Early arterial phase of superior mesenteric arteriogram shows contrast extravasation from the right colon, which appears as a pseudovein (*arrow*). Reflux of contrast medium into the aorta opacifies a mycotic aneurysm (*arrowheads*). *B,* Late venous phase from the same arteriogram shows the contrast extravasation in the right lower quadrant.

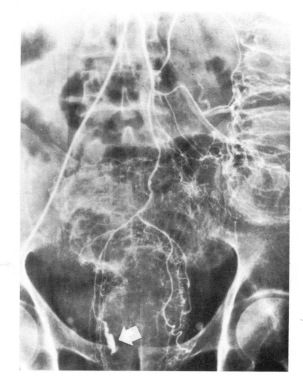

*Figure 14–39.* Rectal bleeding following balloon trauma. Inferior mesenteric arteriogram shows hyperemia of the distal colon and rectum with extravasation of contrast medium from the distal rectum (*arrow*). (From Kadir S et al: Selected Techniques in Interventional Radiology. Philadelphia, WB Saunders, 1982.)

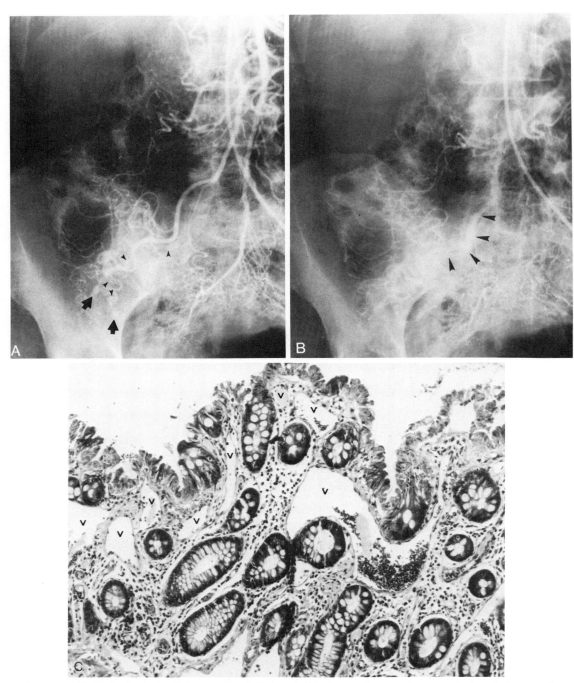

*Figure 14–40.* Angiodysplasia of the cecum. *A,* Early arterial phase of a superior mesenteric arteriogram shows cecal vascular tufts (*arrows*) and early venous opacification (*arrowheads*). *B,* Late arterial phase from the same arteriogram shows a densely opacified ileocolic vein (*arrowheads*). *C,* Histological section through an angiodysplasia shows the dilated submucosal vascular spaces (v). (*C,* From Kadir S, Ernst CB: Current Concepts in Angiographic Management of Gastrointestinal Bleeding. *In* Ravitch MM et al (eds): CURRENT PROBLEMS IN SURGERY. Copyright © 1983 by Year Book Medical Publishers, Inc., Chicago. Used with permission.)

ula occur more frequently in the left colon.[61] Less frequent causes are colitis, neoplasms, angiodysplasia, ulcers, mesenteric varices, and trauma.

**Angiodysplasia** (Fig. 14–40). This may be the cause of chronic intermittent low-grade and occasionally massive bleeding in up to 50% of individuals 55 years of age and older.[62, 63] However, angiographic demonstration of angiodysplasia is not necessarily evidence that it is the source of bleeding. In one review, angiodysplasia was an incidental finding in 15% of nonbleeding patients.[64] Its incidence at autopsy is 2%.[65]

The typical angiographic features of angiodysplasia are: (1) early opacification of the ileocolic vein, (2) dense opacification of this vein persisting late into the venous phase, and (3) demonstration of one or more vascular "tufts" along the antimesenteric border of the cecum or ascending colon.

## Postoperative Bleeding

This may occur in the immediate postoperative period or several days later. Such bleeding may occur at the operation site or remote from it. Bleeding at the operation site may be due to a slipped ligature, incomplete ligation or cauterization, infection, or trauma (either operative or from indwelling tubes or drains).[66] Postoperative bleeding remote from the operative site may occur as a result of stress ulceration.

Bleeding originating from an operation site several months or years after surgery may result from the development of focal abdominal wall varices in patients with or without portal hypertension[46, 67] or a vascular enteric fistula (if major vascular surgery had been performed). Varices may also develop around an ileostomy stoma or around the cutaneous entry site of surgically placed Silastic biliary stents.

## Vascular-Enteric Fistulae (Fig. 14–41)

Vascular-enteric fistulae can occur anywhere from the esophagus to the colon. The duodenum is the most frequently involved gastrointestinal site and is affected in over 80% of cases. Such fistulae are observed after aortic surgery, most frequently following placement of a prosthetic graft, or they may occur spontaneously.[68–70] On aortography, a false aneurysm may be seen at the proximal aortic anastomosis. In the absence of an

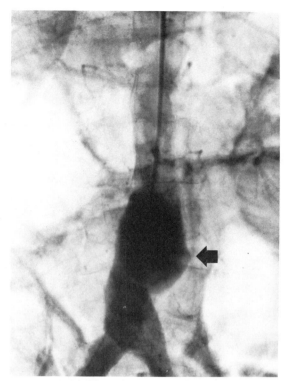

*Figure 14–41.* Aorto-enteric fistula. AP abdominal aortogram shows a beaklike projection at the site of the fistulous communication (*arrow*). (From Kadir S, Ernst CB: Current Concepts in Angiographic Management of Gastrointestinal Bleeding. *In* Ravitch MM et al (eds): CURRENT PROBLEMS IN SURGERY. Copyright © 1983 by Year Book Medical Publishers, Inc., Chicago. Used with permission.)

aneurysm, a nipple-like outpouching may be present. A fistulous tract or actual bleeding is demonstrated infrequently.

## Variceal Bleeding

The most common cause of variceal bleeding is portal hypertension. Bleeding from focal varices at an operative site is rare and has been described in the section on Postoperative Bleeding.

**Variceal Bleeding in Portal Hypertension.** In patients with portal hypertension, varices can develop anywhere along the alimentary tract. However, the most common location is the esophagogastric region.

Esophagogastric varices are responsible for massive bleeding in about 17% of patients with upper gastrointestinal bleeding.[52, 53] However, the presence of varices in the distal esophagus and stomach is not necessarily evidence that these are the source of bleeding. Thus, in up to 60% of patients with portal hypertension, bleeding may be due to hemorrhagic gastritis or an ulcer, even though varices are demonstrated by endoscopy.[71]

Since the diagnosis is made by endoscopy and the treatment of choice is intravenous vasopressin, emergency arteriography is not indicated for the management of such patients unless an emergency shunt is to be performed. (For angiography of patients with portal hypertension, see Chapter 15.)

Focal mesenteric varices may develop at operative sites (eg, ileostomy) in patients with portal hypertension. These may occasionally be responsible for massive bleeding. Local operative revision is often curative.

### Bleeding From Solid Organs

Bleeding into a major duct of the liver or the pancreas may also manifest as gastrointestinal bleeding. The diagnosis and etiology of such bleeding are discussed in Chapter 15.

PITFALLS IN DIAGNOSIS

Some of the pitfalls in the angiographic diagnosis of gastrointestinal bleeding are:

1. Dense opacification of a small vessel seen end-on may simulate an aneurysm or focal contrast extravasation. To confirm or exclude the presence of an aneurysm, the arteriogram should be repeated in a different projection, or a selective arteriogram is obtained of that particular vessel. Extravasated contrast medium persists as a densely opacified area even after the venous phase and exhibits some change in configuration, ie, it spreads.

2. A dense, sustained parenchymal stain of the stressed adrenal gland may be observed on celiac, left gastric, or inferior phrenic arteriography. This can also be mistaken for an area of bleeding (Fig. 14–42).

3. If the stomach is distended, extravasation of contrast medium may not be seen because the contrast medium cannot collect between gastric folds (as it can in the nondistended stomach). Similarly, the presence of blood clots and air may also make it difficult to detect a small extravasation.

4. Hypervascularity (or hyperemia) of a segment of bowel may be iatrogenic as a result of selective contrast injection into a branch vessel, injection of an excessive volume of contrast medium, or the injection of vasodilators. It may also be due to inflammatory bowel disease. Colonic hyperemia is

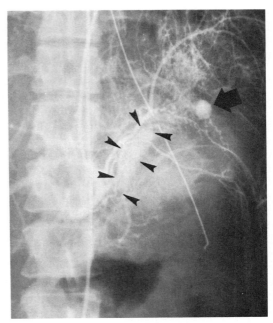

*Figure 14–42.* Stressed adrenal gland in a patient with upper gastrointestinal bleeding following postpartum pancreatitis. Left inferior phrenic arteriogram shows marked hyperemia of the left adrenal gland (*arrowheads*) and a site of bleeding (*arrow*). *Note:* In the absence of the demonstration of such a bleeding site, this adrenal blush could easily be mistaken for a bleed. (Reprinted with permission from Kadir S, Athanasoulis CA: CRC Crit Rev Diag Imag 1979; pp 35–78. Copyright CRC Press, Inc.)

frequently due to prolonged contact of blood with the mucosal surface. Another cause of iatrogenic colonic hyperemia is the use of cleansing enemas.

5. Early venous opacification in the absence of an arteriovenous malformation may be seen in colitis, tumor, selective branch vessel injection, or the use of vasodilators.

6. The angiographic features of some tumors may mimic an arteriovenous malformation and thus make it difficult to differentiate between them. However, with the help of endoscopy and good quality barium studies, a mass lesion can usually be detected.

7. The corpus cavernosum blush may simulate lower rectal bleeding (Fig. 14–43).

### TRAUMA

The evaluation of a hollow viscus injury is not an indication for arteriography. However, a patient with multiple abdominal injuries may undergo abdominal angiography

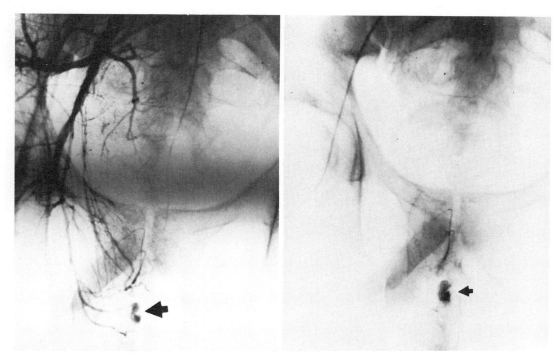

*Figure 14–43.* Subtraction films from an early (*left*) and late (*right*) arterial phase of a right internal iliac arteriogram shows a corpus cavernosum blush (*arrow*) simulating rectal bleeding in a patient with lower gastrointestinal bleeding.

for the assessment of major vessel injury. In such patients, any of the signs of vascular injury that have been discussed previously (see Chapters 8 to 11) may be observed, ie, mural arterial hematoma, vascular occlusion, arterial spasm, traumatic aneurysms, or arteriovenous fistula. In addition, contrast extravasation into the bowel lumen may be noted.

Mesenteric hematoma or mural hematoma of the bowel may also be seen. These manifest as stretching and attenuation of vessels and slowed circulation. Penetrating injuries may result in arteriovenous fistula with dynamic portal hypertension, false aneurysms, or vascular occlusion.

## TUMORS

Angiography is rarely indicated for the evaluation of neoplasms of the esophago-gastrointestinal tract. Most such tumors are detected incidentally during angiography for other causes (eg, gastrointestinal bleeding). Most neoplasms show the general angiographic features described in Chapter 13, ie, neovascularity, encasement and occlusion of vessels, alteration of course, tumor stain, and early venous opacification.

Of the benign neoplasms, adenomatous polyps, villous adenomas, and smooth muscle and neurogenic tumors are usually hypervascular.[72] Hemangiomas may occur anywhere along the gastrointestinal tract, either as isolated lesions or as part of a syndrome (eg, Osler-Weber-Rendu syndrome).

Carcinoid is the second most common tumor of the small bowel. Less than 10% of patients with carcinoid tumor develop the carcinoid syndrome, which is mediated by the release of serotonin and kinins. Carcinoid tumors show relatively typical angiographic features. Although these features can occasionally be mimicked by some other neoplasms (carcinoma) and retractile mesenteritis,[73, 74] their demonstration on arteriography is highly indicative of a carcinoid (Fig. 14–44).

Angiographic features of intestinal carcinoid tumors include:

1. Thickening and foreshortening of the mesentery due to an intense fibrotic reaction.

2. Kinking of small and medium-sized vessels (arteries and veins), which come to lie in a stellate fashion around the tumor.

3. Venous occlusion with demonstration of mesenteric varices.

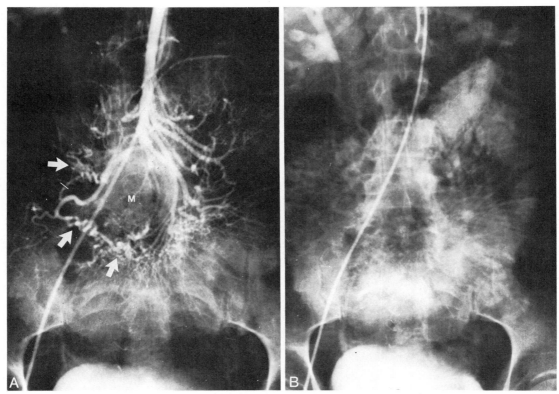

***Figure 14–44.*** Ileal carcinoid. *A*, Superior mesenteric arteriogram shows a mass (M) with draping of mesenteric vessels. Foreshortening of the mesentery has resulted in a "bunched together" appearance of the vessels. Several branches show the typical kinking (*arrows*). *B*, Venous phase of the same arteriogram shows a stellate configuration of the veins. Again, the small intestine appears bunched together in the mid-abdomen.

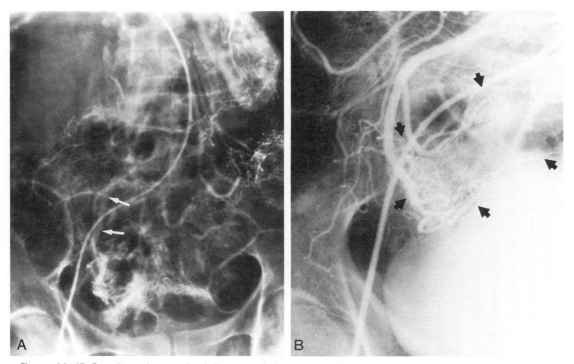

***Figure 14–45.*** Cecal carcinoma simulating an arteriovenous malformation. *A*, Late arterial phase of a superior mesenteric arteriogram shows an early and densely opacified vein (*arrows*). *B*, Early arterial phase from a magnification ileocolic arteriogram shows a hypervascular cecal carcinoma (*arrows*).

4. Encasement of medium-sized vessels and occlusion of smaller vessels.

5. Demonstration of a hypervascular tumor: However, more often the tumor itself is very small and may not be demonstrated by arteriography, but there is an apparent hypervascularity in the region of the fibrotic reaction. This is caused by the fibrotic retraction, because of which numerous blood vessels are brought closer together and thereby simulate hypervascularity.

In malignant tumors, the arteriographically detectable vascular abnormality can be quite variable. Adenocarcinoma can be hypo- or hypervascular. Arterial and venous encasement, neovascularity, and arteriovenous shunting may be seen. The absence of the characteristic angiographic signs does not exclude the presence of a malignant neoplasm.

Metastases can be hypovascular (eg, malignant melanoma) or hypervascular (eg, choriocarcinoma, certain sarcomas). Lymphoma is usually hypovascular but occasionally may be hypervascular. Fine neovascularity may also be demonstrated (see Fig. 14–36).

Pitfalls in angiographic evaluation of gastrointestinal tumors include:

1. Differentiation between inflammatory disease and malignancy is often not possible.

2. Arteriovenous shunting in tumors may simulate an arteriovenous malformation (Fig. 14–45).

## REFERENCES

1. Warwick R, Williams PL: Gray's Anatomy, 35th Brit. Ed. Philadelphia, WB Saunders, 1973, pp. 660–667.
2. Michels NA: Blood Supply and Anatomy of the Upper Abdominal Organs. With a Descriptive Atlas. Philadelphia, JB Lippincott, 1955.
3. Nakamura H, Uchida H, Kuroda C, et al: Accessory left gastric artery arising from left hepatic artery: Angiographic study. AJR 134:529–532, 1980.
4. Owens JC, Coffey RJ: Aneurysm of the splenic artery including a report of 6 additional cases. Int Abstr Surg 97:313–335, 1953.
5. Spitell JA Jr, Fairbairn JF II, Kincaid OW, et al: Aneurysm of the splenic artery. JAMA 175:452–456, 1961.
6. Stanley JC, Thompson NW, Fry WJ: Splanchnic artery aneurysms. Arch Surg 101:689–697, 1970.
7. Boijsen E, Efsing H-O: Aneurysm of the splenic artery. Acta Radiol Diag 8:29–41, 1969.
8. McFarlane JR, Thorbjarnarson B: Rupture of splenic artery aneurysm during pregnancy. Am J Obstet Gynecol 95:1025–1037, 1966.
9. Schug J, Rankin RP: Rupture of a splenic artery aneurysm in pregnancy. Report of a survivor and review of the literature. Obstet Gynecol 25:717–723, 1965.
10. Stengel A, Wolferth CC: Mycotic (bacterial) aneurysms of intravascular origin. Arch Intern Med 31:528–554, 1923.
11. DeBakey ME, Cooley DA: Successful resection of mycotic aneurysms of superior mesenteric artery. Case report and review of literature. Am Surg 17:202–212, 1953.
12. Reuter SR, Fry WJ, Bookstein JJ: Mesenteric artery branch aneurysms. Arch Surg 97:497–499, 1968.
13. Kadir S, Athanasoulis CA, Yune HY, et al: Aneurysms of the pancreaticoduodenal arteries in association with celiac axis occlusion. Cardiovasc Radiol 1:173–177, 1978.
14. Knight RW, Kadir S, White RI: Bleeding transverse pancreatic artery aneurysms: Treatment with transcatheter embolization. Cardiovasc Intervent Radiol 5:37–39, 1982.
15. West JE, Bernhardt H, Bowers RF: Aneurysms of the pancreaticoduodenal artery. Am J Surg 115:835–839, 1968.
16. Szilagyi DE: Discussion to reference 17. Arch Surg 93:31, 1966.
17. Rob C: Surgical diseases of the celiac and mesenteric arteries. Arch Surg 93:21–31, 1966.
18. Jonsson K, Wattsgard C, Genell S: Malignant occlusion of the coeliac axis. Acta Radiol Diag 23:123–125, 1982.
19. Cameron AJ, Pairolero PC, Stanson AW, et al: Abdominal angina and neurofibromatosis. Mayo Clin Proc 57:125–128, 1982.
20. Dunbar JD, Molnar W, Beman FF, et al: Compression of the celiac trunk and abdominal angina. Preliminary report of 15 cases. AJR 95:731–744, 1965.
21. Hegedus V: Stenosis of the celiac artery. Radiologe 13:443–447, 1973.
22. Brandt LJ, Boley SJ: Ischemic intestinal syndromes. Adv Surg 15:1–45, 1981.
23. Zuidema GD, Reed D, Turcotte JG, et al: Superior mesenteric artery embolectomy. Ann Surg 159:548–553, 1964.
24. Price WE, Rohrer GV, Jacobson ED: Editorial. Mesenteric vascular diseases. Gastroenterology 57:599–604, 1969.
25. Vujic I, Stanley T, Gobien R: Treatment of acute embolus of the superior mesenteric artery by topical infusion of streptokinase. Cardiovasc Intervent Radiol 7:94–96, 1984.
26. Aakhus T, Evensen A: Angiography in acute mesenteric arterial insufficiency. Acta Radiol Diag 19:945–954, 1978.
27. Palubinskas AJ, Ripley HR: Fibromuscular hyperplasia in extrarenal arteries. Radiology 82:451–454, 1964.
28. Boley SJ, Sprayregen S, Siegelman SS, et al: Initial results from an aggressive approach to acute mesenteric ischemia. Surgery 82:848–855, 1977.
29. Ottinger LW, Austen WG: A study of 136 patients with mesenteric infarction. Surg Obstet Gynecol 124:251–261, 1967.
30. Bailey RW, Bulkley GB, Levy KF, et al: Pathogenesis of nonocclusive mesenteric ischemia: studies in a porcine model induced by pericardial tamponade. Surg Forum 33:194–196, 1982.
31. Schimmel DH, Moss AA, Hoffer PB: Radionuclide imaging of intestinal infarction in dogs. Invest Radiol 11:277–281, 1976.
32. Gharagozloo F, Bulkley GB, Zuidema GD, et al: The use of intraperitoneal xenon for early diagnosis of acute mesenteric ischemia. Surgery 95:404–410, 1984.

33. Aakhus T, Brabrand G: Angiography in acute superior mesenteric arterial insufficiency. Acta Radiol Diag 6:1–12, 1967.

34. Siegelman SS, Sprayregen S, Boley SJ: Angiographic diagnosis of mesenteric arterial vasoconstriction. Radiology 112:533–542, 1974.

35. Korobkin M, Kantor I, Pollard JJ, et al: Arteriovenous fistula between systemic and portal circulations following partial gastrectomy. Radiology 109:311–314, 1973.

36. Gotsman MS, Beck W, Schirire V: Selective angiography in arteritis of the aorta and its major branches. Radiology 88:232–248, 1967.

37. Kadir S, Athanasoulis CA, Greenfield A: Intestinal volvulus: angiographic findings. Radiology 128:595–599, 1978.

38. Nuzum JW Jr, Nuzum JW Sr: Polyarteritis nodosa: a statistical review of 175 cases from the literature and report of a "typical" case. Arch Intern Med 94:942–955, 1954.

39. Finkbiner RB, Decker JP: Ulceration and perforation of the intestine due to necrotizing arteriolitis. N Engl J Med 268:14–18, 1963.

40. Citron BP, Halpern M, McCarron M, et al: Necrotizing angiitis associated with drug abuse. N Engl J Med 283:1003–1011, 1970.

41. Boijsen E, Efsing H-O: Intrasplenic arterial aneurysms following splenoportal phlebography. Acta Radiol Diag 6:487–496, 1967.

42. Boijsen E, Haertel M: Kontrastmittelpassegezeit im Versorgungsgebiet der Arterial mesenterica superior. Fortschr Roentgenstr 118:491–498, 1973.

43. Scott WW Jr, Harrington DP, Siegelman SS: Functional abnormalities of mesenteric blood flow. A guide to organic disease of the bowel. Gastrointest Radiol 1:367–374, 1977.

44. Muhletaler C, Gerlock AJ, Goncharenco V, et al: Gastric varices secondary to splenic vein occlusion: Radiographic diagnosis and clinical significance. Radiology 132:593–598, 1979.

45. Allan R, Dykes P: A study of the factors influencing mortality rates from gastrointestinal hemorrhage. Q J Med (New Series) 180:533–550, 1976.

46. Kadir S, Ernst CB: Current concepts in angiographic management of gastrointestinal bleeding. Curr Prob Surg 20:287–343, 1983.

47. Kadir S, Kaufman SL, Barth K, et al: Selected Techniques in Interventional Radiology. Philadelphia, WB Saunders, 1982.

48. Athanasoulis CA: Upper gastrointestinal bleeding of arteriocapillary origin. In Athanasoulis CA, Pfister RC, Green R, et al (eds): Interventional Radiology. Philadelphia, WB Saunders, 1982, pp. 55–89.

49. Athanasoulis CA: Lower gastrointestinal bleeding. In Athanasoulis CA, Pfister RC, Green R, et al (eds): Interventional Radiology. Philadelphia, WB Saunders, 1982, pp. 115–148.

50. St. John DJB, Masterton JP, Yoemans ND, et al: The Mallory-Weiss syndrome. Br Med J 1:140–143, 1974.

51. Knauer CM: Mallory-Weiss syndrome. Characterization of 75 Mallory-Weiss lacerations in 528 patients with upper gastrointestinal bleeding. Gastroenterology 71:5–8, 1976.

52. Katz D: Peptic Ulcer. A Medcom Perspective on Progress. Fort Washington, Pa., William H. Rorer, 1971, pp. 34–39.

53. Katon RM, Smith FW: Panendoscopy in the early diagnosis of acute upper gastrointestinal bleeding. Gastroenterology 65:728–734, 1973.

54. Ivey KJ: Acute hemorrhagic gastritis: modern concepts based upon pathogenesis. Gut 12:750–757, 1971.

55. Palmer ED: Hemorrhage from erosive gastritis and its surgical implications. Gastroenterology 36:856–860, 1959.

56. Dorsey JM, Burkhead HC, Bonus RL, et al: Five year study on gastrointestinal bleeding. Surg Gynecol Obstet 120:784–786, 1965.

57. Blackstone MO, Kirsner JB: Establishing the site of gastrointestinal bleeding. Editorial. JAMA 241:599–600, 1972.

58. Briley CA Jr, Jackson DC, Johnsrude IS: Acute gastrointestinal hemorrhage of small bowel origin. Radiology 136:317–319, 1980.

59. Brief DK, Botsford TW: Primary bleeding from the small intestine in adults. The surgical management. JAMA 184:18–22, 1963.

60. Noer RJ, Hamilton JE, Williams DJ, et al: Rectal hemorrhage: Moderate and severe. Ann Surg 155:794–805, 1962.

61. Casarella WJ, Galloway SJ, Taxin RN, et al: Lower gastrointestinal tract hemorrhage. New concepts based on angiography. AJR 121:357–368, 1974.

62. Athanasoulis CA, Galdabini JJ, Waltman AC, et al: Angiodysplasia of the colon. A cause of rectal bleeding. Cardiovasc Radiol 1:3–13, 1978.

63. Baum S, Athanasoulis CA, Waltman AC, et al: Angiodysplasia of the right colon: A cause of gastrointestinal bleeding. AJR 129:789–794, 1977.

64. Kadir S, Athanasoulis CA, Waltman AC, et al: Angiodysplasia of the colon: Incidence and coexistence with other bowel lesions in nonbleeding patients. Abstract. Am Roentgen Ray Society Meeting, March, 1979.

65. Baer JW, Ryan S: Analysis of cecal vasculature in search for vascular malformations. AJR 126:394–405, 1976.

66. Kadir S, Athanasoulis CA: Angiographic diagnosis and control of postoperative bleeding. CRC Crit Rev Diag Imag, 1979, pp. 35–78.

67. Barth V, Koelmel B: Blutende Dünndarmvarizen bei portaler Hypertension als seltene Komplikation nach abdominellen Operationen. Fortschr Roentgenstr 132:219–221, 1980.

68. Case Records of the Massachusetts General Hospital: Case 41–1977. N Engl J Med 297:828–834, 1977.

69. O'Mara C, Williams GM, Ernst CB: Secondary aortoenteric fistula. Am J Surg 124:203–209, 1981.

70. Foster JH, Vetto RM: Aortic intraaneurysmal abscess caused by sigmoid aortic fistula. Am J Surg 104:850–854, 1962.

71. McCray RS, Martin F, Amir-Ahmadi H, et al: Erroneous diagnosis of hemorrhage from esophageal varices. Am J Dig Dis 14:755–760, 1969.

72. Kaude J, Silseth CH, Tylen U: Angiography in myomas of the gastrointestinal tract. Acta Radiol Diag 12:691–704, 1972.

73. Gold RE, Redman HC: Mesenteric fibrosis simulating the angiographic appearance of ileal carcinoid tumor. Radiology 103:85–86, 1972.

74. Case Records of the Massachusetts General Hospital: Case 21–1984. N Engl J Med 310:1374–1381, 1984.

# Angiography of the Liver, Spleen, and Pancreas

The number of diagnostic angiograms performed for diseases of the abdominal organs has decreased quite significantly in recent years. Although the emphasis on visceral angiography as a diagnostic procedure has diminished, it continues to be of importance since it also provides the basis for many interventional procedures. Such procedures are being utilized more frequently and require skillfully performed diagnostic angiography.

Angiography for diagnosis is required only occasionally for the evaluation of diseases of the spleen and pancreas. For most diseases of these organs, computed tomography (CT) and ultrasonography are the primary diagnostic modalities. In addition, because of changing concepts in management, certain problems (eg, splenic trauma) do not necessitate arteriographic evaluation. On the other hand, angiographic evaluation of the liver remains an essential part of the workup of patients with portal hypertension, mass lesions, and vascular diseases.

## ANATOMY

### Segmental Anatomy of the Liver

The right and left lobes of the liver are separated by an oblique fissure that extends from the groove of the inferior vena cava to the gallbladder fossa. The middle hepatic vein lies in this fissure, and no major duct or arterial or portal vein branch traverses it.[1] The right lobe, which makes up approximately 80% of the liver substance, is divided into an anterior and a posterior segment by another oblique fissure. A similar fissure, which corresponds to the plane of the falciform ligament, divides the left lobe into lateral and medial segments. The medial segment of the left lobe includes a part of the quadrate lobe of the liver.[1] The segmental

fissures are traversed by smaller branches of the blood vessels and the biliary ducts.

The hepatic segments are subdivided into superior and inferior subsegments. Each subsegment of the liver is supplied by a hepatic artery and drained by a bile duct. The subsegments of the medial left lobe each have two hepatic arteries and two bile ducts.

Although the caudate lobe is attached to the right lobe of the liver, its blood supply and biliary drainage differ from that of the rest of the liver. It is divided into three segments, usually has two hepatic artery branches, and is drained by three bile ducts.[1]

Histologically, the liver parenchyma is made up of small polyhedral lobules. Each lobule consists of columns of liver cells and sinusoids with a central hepatic venule. The portal triad, which consists of a bile duct, hepatic artery, and portal vein branch, lies between the lobules. The lymphatic channels are also located in the portal triad. The hepatic sinusoids are endothelium-lined vascular spaces that are bathed with arterial and portal venous blood, which drains into the central venule and subsequently into the hepatic veins.

### Anatomy of the Spleen and Pancreas

The normal spleen is a small organ weighing about 150 gm and measuring only 12 cm in length and about 7 cm in width. Accessory spleens (small, encapsulated collections of splenic tissue) occur in approximately 10% of individuals and are usually located in the gastrosplenic ligament and the greater omentum. The configuration of the spleen can be variable. On an abdominal radiograph, fetal lobulation or deep notches may occasionally simulate a left upper quadrant mass or splenic rupture in the traumatized patient.[2]

The pancreas extends from the duodenal loop (head) to the splenic hilus (tail). The body and tail may occupy a relatively hori-

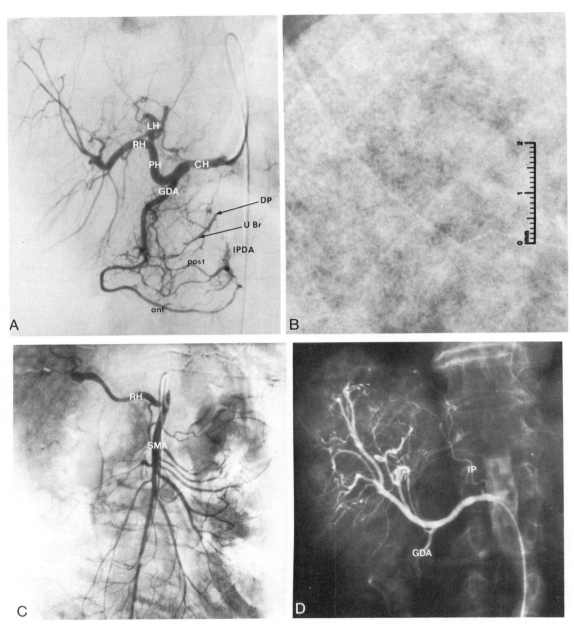

*Figure 15–1.* Normal and variant hepatic arterial anatomy. *A* and *B,* Common hepatic arteriograms. *A,* Normal arterial phase. *B,* Close-up of normal arterial hepatogram. *C* and *D,* Variant hepatic arterial anatomy. *C,* Right hepatic artery arising from the superior mesenteric artery. *D,* Common hepatic artery arising from the aorta. ant = anterior and post = posterior pancreaticoduodenal arcades; CH = common hepatic; DP = dorsal pancreatic; GDA = gastroduodenal; IP = right inferior phrenic; IPDA = inferior pancreaticoduodenal; LH = left hepatic; PH = proper hepatic; RH = right hepatic; SMA = superior mesenteric arteries; U Br = uncinate branch. (*B,* Courtesy of Dr. Vincent P. Chuang. From Chuang VP: Radiology 148:633–639, 1983. Used with permission.)

zontal position or may course obliquely towards the left upper quadrant (see Chapter 14, Fig. 14–1B). The head and neck of the pancreas are closely related to the superior mesenteric vein as it joins the splenic vein to form the portal vein. The body is in intimate contact with the splenic vein.

## Vascular Anatomy

The normal and variant anatomy of the splanchnic arteries and veins and their branches has been described in detail in Chapter 14. The description here will be limited to the vascular anatomy of the organ being discussed.

### Vascular Anatomy of the Liver
(Figs. 15–1 to 15–4; see also Fig. 15–32; and Chapter 14, Figs. 14–1, 14–2, 14–4, and 14–7)

There is considerable variation in the origin of the hepatic arteries. Most commonly, the hepatic arteries originate from the celiac artery. Aberrant, ie, replaced and/or accessory, hepatic arteries are observed in 41.5% of individuals. In 18.5% of individuals, some or all of the hepatic blood supply is from the superior mesenteric artery (SMA) (ie, common hepatic artery off the SMA in 2.5% of persons, right hepatic artery off the SMA in 10%, accessory right hepatic artery off the

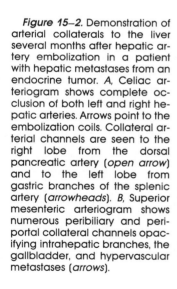

*Figure 15–2.* Demonstration of arterial collaterals to the liver several months after hepatic artery embolization in a patient with hepatic metastases from an endocrine tumor. *A,* Celiac arteriogram shows complete occlusion of both left and right hepatic arteries. Arrows point to the embolization coils. Collateral arterial channels are seen to the right lobe from the dorsal pancreatic artery (*open arrow*) and to the left lobe from gastric branches of the splenic artery (*arrowheads*). *B,* Superior mesenteric arteriogram shows numerous peribiliary and periportal collateral channels opacifying intrahepatic branches, the gallbladder, and hypervascular metastases (*arrows*).

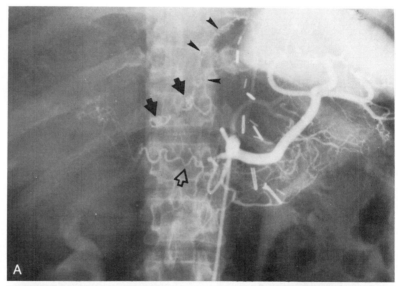

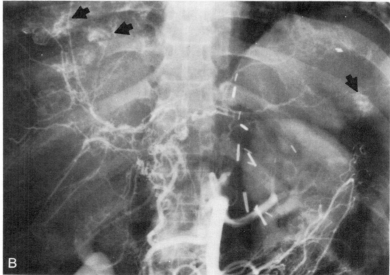

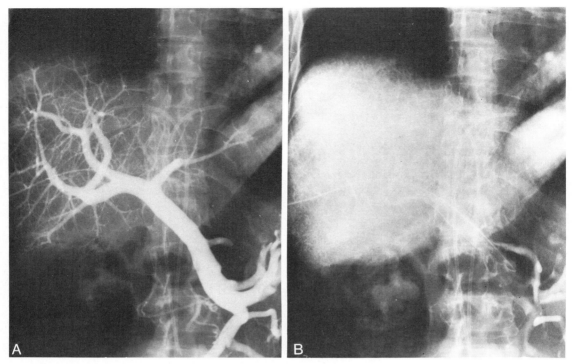

**Figure 15–3.** Normal transhepatic portal venogram. *A*, Vascular phase; *B*, Parenchymal (hepatogram) phase.

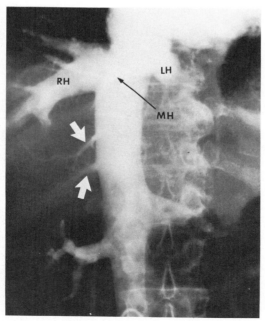

**Figure 15–4.** AP inferior venacavagram shows reflux of contrast medium into hepatic and renal veins. Several smaller hepatic veins draining directly into the inferior vena cava are also opacified (*arrows*). LH = left hepatic; MH = middle hepatic; and RH = right hepatic veins.

SMA in 6%). In 23% of individuals, a part of or the entire left hepatic blood supply is from the left gastric artery. The cystic artery is usually a branch of the right hepatic artery. It may also originate from the common, left, or middle hepatic artery or the gastroduodenal artery. Occasionally, there are two cystic arteries.

Occasionally, the right hepatic artery makes a characteristic caterpillar loop (see Fig. 15–16). It divides into an anterior and a posterior segmental artery, corresponding to the segments of the right hepatic lobe. In 87% of individuals, it passes behind the common hepatic duct.[1] An anterior location of this vessel or its branches can be responsible for ductal obstruction.[3] The left hepatic artery also divides into two major branches corresponding to the two segments. In 25% of individuals, the segmental arteries arise separately from the common hepatic artery.[1]

The artery that supplies the medial segment of the left lobe is also called the middle hepatic artery. The artery to the caudate lobe usually comes from the right hepatic artery.

The hepatic artery branches are essentially end arteries. Anastomoses between them are observed mainly in the extrahepatic segments and in the liver capsule.[1, 4] Extrahepatic anastomoses are observed in 25% of dissections.[1] They are seen more frequently in patients with hepatic artery occlusion, in which they serve as collateral channels and can also be demonstrated by arteriography.[4] Such collateral pathways include (Fig. 15–2; see also Fig. 15–16):

1. Normally occurring variants, ie, accessory and replaced hepatic arteries.

2. The gastroepiploic, short gastric, and gastroduodenal arteries.

3. The left and right gastric arteries.

4. The pancreaticoduodenal, choledochal, esophageal, and diaphragmatic arteries.

The branching pattern of the portal vein in the liver, which is similar to that of the hepatic artery, is dichotomous, with progressive decrease in caliber of the branches. These branches do not anastomose with one another. The portal vein approximately is 8 cm long and is formed by the confluence of the splenic and superior mesenteric veins. It lies retroduodenal, behind the hepatic artery (Fig. 15–3).

In 2% of individuals, the portal vein lies anterior to an aberrant hepatic artery.[1] Anomalies of the portal vein are extremely uncommon. A preduodenal portal vein is usually associated with congenital abnormalities of the cardiovascular system or biliary or intestinal tract. Congenital absence of the portal vein is also rare.[5] In such individuals, the mesenteric and splenic veins drain into the systemic venous system either directly or via the renal or azygos veins.

At the porta hepatis, the portal vein lies between the hepatic artery and the common hepatic duct. It divides into a larger right and a smaller left branch before entering the liver. The ligamentum teres (fibrous cord of the obliterated umbilical vein) and the ligamentum venosum (fibrous cord of the obliterated ductus venosus) join the left branch of the portal vein.

Hepatic venous drainage occurs via three main hepatic veins (Fig. 15–4). Several smaller veins drain into the inferior vena cava. Branches of the hepatic veins communicate extensively with one another. The hepatic veins do not have valves, and their distribution is nonsegmental, unlike that of the portal veins.

**Right Hepatic Vein.** This lies in the plane separating the anterior and posterior segments of the right hepatic lobe. It drains the posterior and a large portion of the anterior segment of the right lobe.

**Middle Hepatic Vein.** This vein lies in the plane separating the left and right lobes. It drains a portion of the right lobe and the medial segment of the left lobe.

**Left Hepatic Vein.** This lies in the segmental fissure of the left lobe and drains the lateral segment and superior portion of the medial segment of the left lobe. The middle and left hepatic veins frequently form a common trunk before entering the inferior vena cava. The veins from the *caudate lobe* (two to three small veins) drain directly into the inferior vena cava.

Lymphatic drainage of the liver is either via the deep chain to the porta hepatis and into the cisterna chyli or along the hepatic veins to the paracaval lymph nodes.[6]

### Vascular Anatomy of the Spleen
(Figs. 15–5 and 15–6)

The splenic artery is the largest branch of the celiac artery and arises together with the left gastric and hepatic arteries in 82% of individuals.[1] Occasionally, it may originate directly from the aorta, from the SMA, or from the hepatic arteries. Rarely, it is duplicated.

In children and young adults, the splenic artery either is straight or has a gently undulating course. With increasing age, the

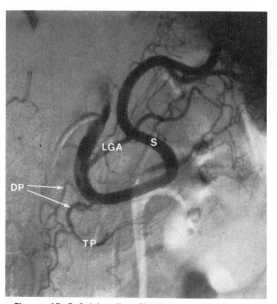

**Figure 15–5.** Subtraction film from a splenic arteriogram shows the normal pancreatic arterial anatomy. The dorsal pancreatic artery is duplicated. For abbreviations, see legend for Figure 15–6.

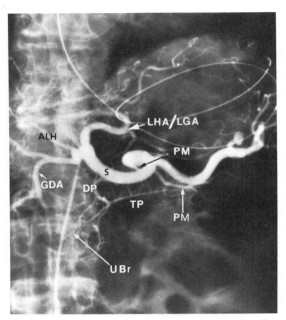

*Figure 15–6.* Celiac arteriogram demonstrating the normal pancreatic arteries. ALH = accessory left hepatic; DP = dorsal pancreatic; GDA = gastroduodenal; LGA = left gastric; LHA/LGA = left hepatic/left gastric trunk; PM = pancreatica magna; S = splenic artery; TP = transverse pancreatic artery; U Br = uncinate branch.

tortuosity increases. In the vast majority of individuals (>90%) it lies suprapancreatic and is retropancreatic in only 8% of individuals.[1]

At the splenic hilus, the splenic artery divides into two (80% of persons) or three branches, which further subdivide several times before entering the spleen. Multiple extrasplenic anastomoses exist between these branches. The intrasplenic vessels are considered end arteries with only a few peripheral anastomoses.

The splenic vein runs along the pancreas and joins the superior mesenteric vein behind the pancreatic head. The lymphatic drainage from the spleen is mainly into the pancreaticosplenic lymph nodes, which are located along the splenic artery and in the gastrosplenic ligament.

### Vascular Anatomy of the Pancreas

(Figs. 15–1, 15–5, 15–6; see also Chapter 14, Fig. 14–2)

The pancreas is supplied by a vast vascular network originating from both the celiac artery and the SMA. This network often serves as a collateral route to the liver or spleen in the event of occlusion of the proximal hepatic or splenic arteries.

The pancreatic head receives its blood supply from the pancreaticoduodenal arcades. The larger anterior arcade lies anterior to and the posterior arcade lies behind the pancreas. The blood supply to the uncinate process and the neck comes from the dorsal pancreatic artery.

The body and tail of the pancreas are supplied by branches of the splenic artery. In addition to the larger branches described below, there are between two and eight small vessels that arise from the splenic artery as it courses along the body and tail. The major arteries supplying the pancreas are the:

1. Dorsal pancreatic artery: This originates from the proximal splenic artery in 40% of individuals, proximal hepatic artery in about 20%, celiac artery in 22%, and SMA in about 14%.[1] It divides into three branches, ie, the transverse pancreatic artery and branches to the head and uncinate process.

2. Transverse pancreatic artery: This vessel lies over the dorsal aspect of the gland. Occasionally, it may originate from the gastroduodenal artery. Its branches anastomose freely with those of the pancreatica magna and epiploic vessels from the transverse mesocolon.

3. Arteria pancreatica magna: This is the largest branch of the distal splenic artery and is located over the body of the pancreas.

4. Caudal pancreatic artery: This is the largest of the pancreatic vessels supplying the tail. It usually arises from the splenic artery and occasionally from the left gastroepiploic artery.

Venous drainage via the pancreatic veins goes into the splenic vein and through the pancreaticoduodenal veins into the superior mesenteric and portal veins. Lymphatic drainage from the pancreas is into the pancreaticosplenic lymph nodes and along the pancreaticoduodenal and superior mesenteric vessels.

## PHYSIOLOGY AND PATHOPHYSIOLOGY OF THE HEPATIC CIRCULATION

The liver has a dual blood supply, similar to that of the lungs. Under normal circumstances only 20 to 30% of the hepatic blood flow is derived from the hepatic arteries and the remainder comes from the portal vein. Venous drainage is via the hepatic veins, which drain directly into the inferior vena cava.

Normal individuals have hepatopetal portal blood flow. In the parenchymal phase of the portogram, uniform sinusoidal filling results in a homogeneous hepatogram. The normal portal blood flow is approximately 1200 ml/min with a flow velocity between 16 and 25 cm/sec.[7] In portal hypertension, there is hepatofugal flow, and depending upon severity of the hypertension, flow may be bidirectional or completely hepatofugal. In the latter, a portal hepatogram is absent.

In the hepatic sinusoids, blood flows from the hepatic arterioles and portal vein branches into the central venule because of the higher arterial and portal pressures. In addition, sphincters, which regulate blood flow, are present in the sinusoids. Together with the presinusoidal arterioportal anastomoses, these sphincters are responsible for the ratio of arterial and portal venous blood in the sinusoids.

In the normal liver, proximal hepatic artery occlusion is well tolerated because of the portal venous flow and collateral circulation. Anatomical studies confirm the absence of intrahepatic arterial communications between the lobes.[1] Extrahepatic and capsular anastomoses between branches of the hepatic arteries contribute to the collateral supply across major fissures.

Direct communications do not exist between branches of the portal vein. On the other hand, the hepatic vein branches anastomose freely with one another. Although direct arterioportal communications exist, arterioportal shunting is not observed in normal individuals. Such communications are via[1, 8–10] (1) the hepatic sinusoids, (2) the peribiliary arterial plexuses and portal venules, (3) the vasa vasorum of the portal vein branches, and (4) direct presinusoidal anastomoses between hepatic artery and portal vein branches.

Alterations in the intrahepatic pressure balance in patients with hepatic cirrhosis and portal hypertension lead to changes in the flow dynamics and are responsible for arterioportal shunting, which is observed in many patients with hepatic cirrhosis (see Fig. 15–25).[11, 12] Following a portosystemic shunt, the hepatic blood flow decreases but arterioportal shunting occurs more frequently.[13, 14] Postoperatively, arterioportal shunting will not be detected unless hepatic arteriography is performed. In most patients, the postoperative study for evaluation of a shunt consists of either a splenic or a superior mesenteric arteriogram, and hepatic arteriography is usually not necessary.

Other conditions in which arterioportal shunting has been observed are the Budd-Chiari syndrome, highly vascular benign lesions (eg, some hemangiomas), malignant neoplasms (hepatoma, metastases), systemic shock, regenerating hepatic nodules, schistosomiasis, and trauma.[15–19]

Because it occurs in so many clinical conditions, arterioportal shunting cannot be considered a specific finding. Moreover, technical factors during arteriography (prolonged contrast injection, reflux of contrast medium into the splenic artery during hepatic arteriography, and portal venous opacification via the duodenal veins) may occasionally simulate arterioportal shunting. Similarly, injection of pharmacological agents (eg, angiotensin) into the hepatic artery enhances arterioportal shunting.[20]

## ANGIOGRAPHY

### Angiography of the Liver

The main indications for hepatic angiography are:

1. The evaluation of portal hypertension.
2. Hepatic trauma.
3. Hemobilia.
4. Hepatic metastases: in preparation for operation or the placement of a chemotherapy infusion pump or transcatheter embolization.
5. Arteriography may be required to establish the diagnosis of a primary hepatic tumor, eg, isodense hepatoma that cannot be detected by CT,[21] focal nodular hyperplasia, adenoma, or hemangioma. Arteriography may also be indicated for the evaluation and management of complications associated with highly vascular tumors such as spontaneous hemorrhage in hepatoma or hepatic adenoma.
6. The evaluation of vascular diseases.
7. The differentiation between hepatic and extrahepatic masses (Fig. 15–7).
8. In addition, interventional angiographic procedures such as transcatheter embolization find application in the management of some hepatic diseases.[22–24]

**Hepatic Arteriography.** Celiac arteriography is used as a survey arteriogram to evaluate arterial anatomy and extent of diseases (unless this has accurately been deter-

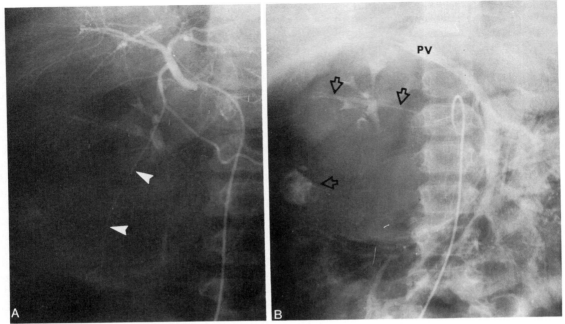

*Figure 15–7.* The utilization of angiography for differentiation between hepatic and extrahepatic masses. CT and ultrasonography were able to distinguish this retroperitoneal mass from a hepatic lesion. *A,* Hepatic arteriogram shows craniad displacement of intrahepatic branches and stretching of the superior pancreaticoduodenal artery (*arrowheads*). *B,* Venous phase of the superior mesenteric arteriogram shows a well-defined portal hepatogram and displacement of the superior mesenteric and portal veins (PV) by an avascular mass. Arrows point to the rudimentary skeletal parts of the fetus in fetu. Reprinted with permission of Georg Thieme Verlag, Stuttgart. (From Kadir S: Fortschr Roentgenstr 134:449–452, 1981.)

mined by CT). From the femoral approach, a sidewinder or cobra catheter is used, and in most instances an AP arteriogram is sufficient. From the axillary approach, a hockey stick–shaped or headhunter catheter is utilized.

Selective hepatic arteriography provides better arterial detail because of selective delivery of a higher volume of contrast medium and a smaller field size (reduced scatter radiation). For common hepatic arteriography, both the sidewinder and the cobra catheters can be used. For catheterization of the proper or left hepatic arteries, a cobra catheter is usually necessary. The cobra catheter is also used for catheterization of the left hepatic artery arising from the left gastric artery and for catheterization of the segmental branches (using the loop technique). Hepatic arteries arising from the SMA are catheterized with a sidewinder or cobra catheter in the loop configuration. In general, an AP hepatic arteriogram is sufficient. For the evaluation of segmental disease, an ipsilateral posterior oblique arteriogram is performed. (See Chapter 14, Table 14–2, for the injection and filming rates for visceral arteriography.)

In the normal individual, the fifth to sixth order hepatic artery branches can be identified on the hepatic arteriogram. The course of the vessels is straight or gently undulating, and they can usually be followed to the liver periphery. The arterial hepatogram is relatively homogeneous and can usually be differentiated from the portal and the mixed hepatogram (the latter following celiac arteriography).[25]

**Infusion Hepatic Arteriography.** Infusion hepatic arteriography (2 to 3 ml/sec, total 60 ml) has been employed for the detection of hypovascular lesions. However, such lesions can now be detected accurately with CT.

**Arterial Dynamic CT Scanning.** Another method for the detection of small or hypovascular lesions is intraarterial dynamic CT scanning: The arterial catheter is left in the hepatic artery after conventional or digital subtraction arteriography, and the patient is taken for CT scanning. Two different techniques can be used, both of which provide comparable information.

1. With the first technique, 60 to 80 ml of 30% contrast medium is injected through the arterial catheter at 6 ml/sec. Using the dy-

namic scanning program with automatic table increments, 8 mm scans are obtained through the region of interest at 10 second intervals after a 0 to 2 second delay (following contrast injection).

2. With the second technique, each scan is obtained after injection of a small bolus of contrast medium. Approximately 10 ml of 30% contrast medium is injected at 3 to 4 ml/sec. An 8 mm thick section is obtained about 10 seconds after the contrast injection is begun.

We have found arterial dynamic CT to be far superior to conventional CT and arteriography for the determination of resectability of hepatoma and metastases and for the detection of smaller, relatively hypovascular lesions in hepatic segments that appeared to be normal on other studies. A similar technique has also been used for the localization of hypovascular pancreatic tumors.[25a]

## Angiography of the Spleen

There are only a few indications for angiography of the spleen other than the workup of patients with portal hypertension. These are evaluation of vascular diseases and gastrointestinal bleeding and differentiation of accessory spleens from vascular pancreatic masses. Diagnostic arteriography for splenic trauma is being performed infrequently. In our experience, diagnostic splenic angiography (other than for portal hypertension) is most often a part of an interventional procedure, ie, therapeutic embolization in patients with hypersplenism or splenic trauma,[26] or preoperatively to reduce intraoperative blood loss during splenectomy.

For catheterization of the proximal splenic artery from the femoral approach, a sidewinder or cobra catheter is used. If the distal splenic artery is to be catheterized for embolization, a cobra catheter is used. From the axillary approach, a hockey stick–shaped or headhunter catheter is preferred. In most instances, an AP arteriogram provides sufficient information. However, a right posterior oblique (RPO) projection is used for the evaluation of a tortuous splenic artery. Oblique projections may also be necessary for the evaluation of other splenic abnormalities.

## Angiography of the Pancreas

The main indications for angiography of the pancreas are the localization of endocrine tumors and the diagnosis and management

of hemorrhage.[27] Occasionally, angiographic evaluation of a small pancreatic carcinoma is indicated to determine involvement of the vascular structures for assessment of resectability.

The type of angiographic evaluation is determined by the indications for the study. For neoplasms, especially pancreatic carcinoma, both the arterial and the venous phase must be evaluated. Survey celiac and superior mesenteric arteriograms are performed initially to determine the arterial supply to the pancreas, assess the degree of vascular involvement, and detect liver metastases. The last may require selective hepatic arteriography. Selective pancreatic arteriography is necessary only for the localization of vascular tumors, vascular diseases, or hemorrhage. For this purpose, the different sections of the pancreas must be evaluated. (The type of catheter used for selective catheterization is indicated in parenthesis.)

Pancreatic head:

1. Gastroduodenal artery (cobra).
2. Dorsal pancreatic artery (cobra, dorsal pancreatic curve; see Chapter 3, Fig. 3–17).
3. Inferior pancreaticoduodenal artery or SMA (cobra, cobra in loop configuration, sidewinder).

Neck and body:

1. Dorsal pancreatic artery (cobra, dorsal pancreatic curve; see Chapter 3, Fig. 3–17).
2. Splenic artery (sidewinder, cobra).

Tail:

1. Splenic artery (sidewinder, cobra).

For the dorsal pancreatic artery, contrast medium is injected at 2 to 3 ml/sec for a total 9 to 12 ml. Films are obtained at one per second for six films and one every other second for another six films. For the inferior pancreaticoduodenal arteriogram, the contrast injection and filming are the same as for the gastroduodenal artery (see Chapter 14, Table 14–2; see Table 14–2 also for the details of angiography of the other visceral arteries.)

For endocrine-active tumors, oblique arteriography is often necessary in addition to the AP study. Evaluation of the venous phase of the splenic and superior mesenteric arteriograms is essential. The superior mesenteric vein is best evaluated in the RPO projection, in which it does not overlie the spine.

## Evaluation of the Portal Venous System

Methods for the evaluation of the portal system are arterial portography, percutaneous transhepatic or transjugular portal vein catheterization, percutaneous spleno-portography, percutaneous hepatography, hepatic wedge venography, and umbilical vein catheterization.

## Arterial Portography

The indications for arterial portography are the evaluation of (1) mesenteric, splenic, and portal veins for patency prior to a shunt procedure, (2) portal dynamics (hepatopetal

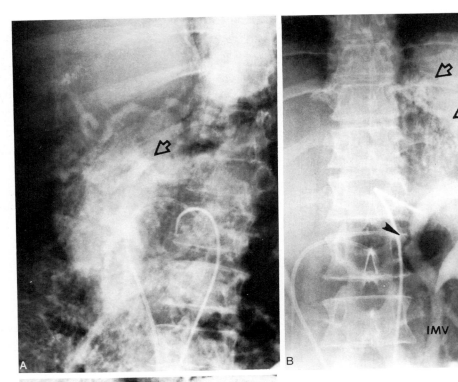

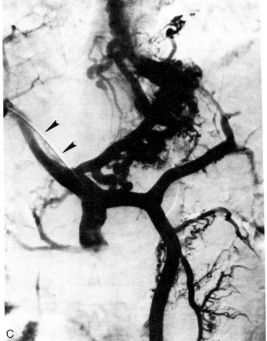

Figure 15–8. Pseudothrombus in the portal vein in a patient with portal hypertension. A, The intrahepatic branches of the portal vein are opacified on the venous phase of the superior mesenteric arteriogram performed in the RPO projection, but the main portal vein and the superior mesenteric vein are not opacified. Numerous tortuous mesenteric veins are seen. In addition, large paragastric varices are opacified (arrow). B, Venous phase of the splenic arteriogram shows an apparent occlusion of the splenic vein (arrowhead) with hepatofugal flow into the inferior mesenteric vein (IMV) and opacification of small gastric varices (arrows). C, Subtraction film from the transhepatic portogram shows a patent portal vein. Only a short segment of the superior mesenteric vein is patent. The size and number of gastroesophageal varices seen on this study are much greater than on the splenic arterial portogram. There is a focal area of narrowing of the portal vein (arrowheads). At operation, this was due to a chronic inflammation.

versus hepatofugal blood flow), (3) shunt patency after surgery, and (4) occasionally for the documentation of gastric and mesenteric varices.

Superior mesenteric or splenic arteriography is used most frequently. If the spleen is very large or absent (ie, following transcatheter ablation or splenectomy), the SMA or left gastric artery is injected for arterial portography. A high volume left gastric arteriogram (approximately 30 ml injected at 6 to 8 ml/sec; filming up to 25 seconds) often provides superior opacification of gastroesophageal varices.[28] The results are even better when this technique is used in conjunction with intraarterial digital subtraction angiography (DSA).

Intraarterial DSA can also be used for SMA or splenic arterial portography. The limitations of DSA for arterial portography are discussed in Chapter 7. For conventional arteriography, the superior mesenteric vein is evaluated in a 15° RPO projection, and pharmacoangiography (25 mg of tolazoline given intraarterially) may be used to enhance venous opacification. For DSA, an AP projection is used.

PITFALLS OF ARTERIAL PORTOGRAPHY

1. Pseudothrombus: Inflow of unopacified blood from the other large tributary of the portal vein (ie, splenic vein inflow on superior mesenteric arterial portography and vice versa) may simulate occlusion or a thrombus.

For clarification, the venous phase of the other artery is evaluated, or splenoportography or transhepatic portography is performed (Figs. 15–8 and 15–9).

2. Absent or poor splenic vein opacification on the venous phase of the splenic arteriogram, suggesting splenic vein occlusion (see Fig. 15–10): This occurs most frequently in the presence of splenomegaly. Either a high volume splenic arteriogram (60 to 70 ml), DSA, splenoportography, or transhepatic portography is performed to assess splenic vein patency. In one series, the splenic vein was not demonstrated on the venous phase of the conventional splenic arteriogram in 6.4% of patients, but was found to be patent at operation.[29]

3. Inadequate opacification: If the entire portal system is inadequately opacified, this may be due to excessive contrast dilution, hepatofugal flow, or spontaneous portosystemic shunting.

4. Failure to demonstrate varices: Occasionally both superior mesenteric and splenic arteriograms may be necessary for the demonstration of varices.

### Percutaneous Transhepatic Portography and Portal Vein Catheterization

The indications for this procedure are:

1. To establish the patency of the portal vein and evaluate the anatomy of the splenic

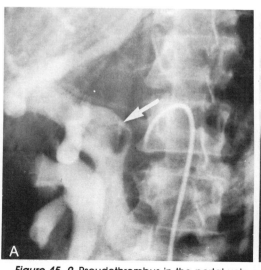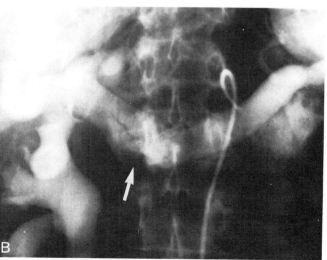

*Figure 15–9.* Pseudothrombus in the portal vein caused by inflow of unopacified blood. *A,* Venous phase of the superior mesenteric arteriogram shows an unopacified area in the portal vein, which simulates a thrombous (*arrow*). This is caused by inflow of unopacified blood from the splenic vein at the junction of the superior mesenteric and splenic veins. *B,* Venous phase of the splenic arteriogram shows a patent splenic vein. Again a defect is present at the inflow of the superior mesenteric vein (*arrow*).

**TABLE 15–1.** Percutaneous Transhepatic Portography and Splenoportography

| Procedure | Catheter/Needle | Injection Rate (ml/sec)/Total | Filming—AP Projection (films/sec) |
|---|---|---|---|
| Transhepatic portogram | Portal vein needle | 12–15/40–60 | 2/sec for 6 films<br>1/sec for 4 films |
| Splenoportogram | Portal vein needle<br>20 Gauge | 6–14/40–50* | Every other sec for 6 films<br>Every third sec for 8 films |
| High dose splenoportogram[30] | Portal vein needle<br>20 Gauge | 6–14/80–100 | Filming over 60 sec |

*Very large spleens require higher volumes (approximately 60–70 ml).

and superior mesenteric veins if arterial portography or splenoportography does not provide satisfactory results.

2. To measure portal pressure and assess portal hemodynamics.

3. For embolization of esophagogastric varices.

4. For venous sampling for the localization of endocrine tumors. For details see references 30a and 31.

5. For autologous islet cell transplantation.

This procedure is contraindicated in patients with severe ascites or hypervascular liver lesions (neoplasms, hemangioma) and in the presence of abnormal clotting parameters (platelet count <100,000 cells/mm³; prothrombin time >33% over control). In patients with ascites and abnormal clotting parameters, the transjugular approach can be used.

**Technique.** With the patient in the supine position, the right arm is tucked under the head. Excursions of the hemidiaphragm are observed fluoroscopically for localization of the lowest point of the costophrenic sulcus to avoid inadvertent puncture of the pleural space. Local anesthetic is infiltrated in the skin and subcutaneous tissues and at the liver capsule during suspended respiration.

Although it is not necessary in the majority of cases, ultrasonographic localization or ultrasound-guided puncture of the portal vein may be used.

Using the portal vein needle (see Chapter 2, Fig. 2–4), the mid-portion of the liver is entered in the mid-axillary line, during suspended respiration (most often in shallow inspiration). An attempt is made to cannulate a larger right hepatic branch of the portal vein close to the porta hepatis. Puncture of the extrahepatic segments of the portal vein must be avoided to prevent hemorrhage.

The trocar is removed, and gentle suction is applied with a 10 ml syringe as the catheter is withdrawn slowly. When blood is aspir-ated, 1 to 2 ml of contrast medium is injected to localize the position (ie, hepatic or portal vein). If the catheter tip is in a portal vein branch, a J-LTT or a high torque guide wire is inserted to advance the catheter into the main portal vein. The portal pressure is measured, and the catheter is further advanced into the splenic or superior mesenteric vein for contrast injection or venous sampling (Table 15–1).

Upon completion of the study, the catheter is withdrawn to about 2 cm from the liver edge. One or two large (5 × 5 mm) plugs of Gelfoam are carefully deposited in the tract as the catheter is withdrawn from the liver. If undiluted contrast medium (60%) is used to deliver the Gelfoam plugs, stasis of the contrast column in the tract helps to verify success of the embolization. Alternatively, blood clot may be embolized or the catheter gradually withdrawn over several hours.[31] In uncomplicated procedures, bed rest is prescribed for 2 to 4 hours.

In the normal individual, there is hepatopetal flow with prompt washout of contrast medium. The intrahepatic portal vein branches are well opacified and a homogeneous hepatogram is present (see Fig. 15–3). The hepatic veins are rarely demonstrated.

If only portal pressure measurements and dynamics are to be evaluated or the portal vein patency determined, a 22 gauge Chiba needle can be used.

Complications associated with percutaneous transhepatic portal vein catheterization are:

1. Hemorrhage: This can be in the form of intrahepatic (hematoma) or peritoneal bleeding or hemobilia. Embolization of the tract has significantly reduced the incidence of peritoneal hemorrhage.

2. Traumatic hepatic artery aneurysm or arterioportal fistula.

3. Hemo- bilio- or pneumothorax. The last is due to a high puncture.

4. Infection: Sepsis or hepatic abscess.

5. Portal vein thrombosis.

6. Inadvertent puncture of the intestine.[31]

With this method, the portal system can be opacified in 93% of patients with portal hypertension.[32] The incidence of complications is high in patients undergoing embolization of varices.[33] It is much lower in patients undergoing diagnostic portal vein catheterization. Although the overall incidence of complications in transhepatic portal vein catheterization may be slightly higher than that observed after percutaneous splenoportography, the diagnostic yield is greater (ie, demonstration of patency of the portal vein in hepatofugal flow and visualization of portosystemic collaterals).[32]

### Percutaneous Splenoportography

Percutaneous transsplenic portography is a relatively simple method for the evaluation of the portal venous system. In our experience, it is indicated:

1. When arterial portography does not provide sufficient information (ie, cannot establish patency of the portal vein).

2. For direct portal pressure measurement by measuring the splenic pulp pressure, which correlates with the portal pressure.

3. For suspected splenic vein occlusion and evaluation of portosystemic or portoportal anastomoses in such patients.

4. If transhepatic portography is contraindicated.

This procedure is contraindicated in patients with abnormal coagulation parameters (platelet count <100,000 cells/mm³; prothrombin time >33% over control), a known splenic mass, contrast allergy, splenic arteriovenous fistula, ascites, or infectious splenomegaly or when the patient is uncooperative. Massive splenomegaly is a relative contraindication. With the aid of DSA, a small needle (20 gauge or even 22 gauge) and hand injection of contrast medium can be used and provides satisfactory opacification.

**Technique.** With the patient in the supine position and the left arm tucked under the head, the spleen is localized by percussion and palpation. Indelible ink may be used to outline the margins. The skin and subcutaneous tissues are infiltrated with a local anesthetic. Percutaneous puncture should be performed in the posterior axillary line at the point of maximal splenic dullness. This is usually between the eighth and ninth ribs. In the presence of splenomegaly, a subcostal approach can also be used.

A portal vein needle (see Chapter 2, Fig. 2–4) or a 20 gauge needle is used. A 22 gauge needle may be used in conjunction with digital subtraction imaging. Under fluoroscopic guidance and during suspended respiration, the needle is inserted at about a 45° angle, pointing towards the dome of the diaphragm. After piercing the splenic capsule, the needle is advanced for 3 to 4 cm. Once the needle is in place, only shallow respirations are permitted. The trocar or stylet is removed, and the intrasplenic position is confirmed by aspiration of blood and by the injection of 2 to 3 ml of contrast medium. The needle hub is connected to a water manometer or pressure transducer for the measurement of the splenic pulp pressure. Contrast splenoportography is performed after the pressure has been measured (Table 15–1). Catheter or needle manipulations should be carried out only during suspended respiration.

Upon completion of the study, the catheter or needle is removed and bed rest is prescribed for 24 hours. Vital signs and the abdomen (for guarding) are monitored for 6 to 8 hours.

A satisfactory study can be obtained in up to 90% of patients.[34, 35] In normal individuals, only the splenic and portal veins are opacified. Other branches may opacify, but only transiently. Inflow of nonopacified blood from the superior mesenteric vein can be seen diluting the contrast column in the portal vein. The left branch of the portal vein is often poorly opacified owing to its anterior location. The contrast medium reaches the porta hepatis in about 3 to 4 seconds, and a hepatogram is seen at approximately 5 seconds.

In the abnormal splenoportogram, multiple tributaries and/or collaterals are opacifed (Fig. 15–10). In addition, there is hepatofugal flow with slow washout and a prolonged hepatogram.

Complications of splenoportography include:

1. Inadvertent puncture of other organs, ie, kidney, colon, stomach, or lung (pneumothorax).

2. Hemorrhage: Intrasplenic hematoma or rarely splenic rupture may occur. Some bleeding is common after splenoportography, and blood loss of up to 300 ml has been reported.[34, 35]

3. Contrast extravasation: Inappropriate catheter position (close to the capsule) or a high contrast injection rate (catheter recoil)

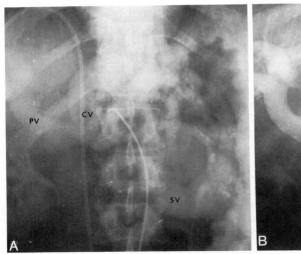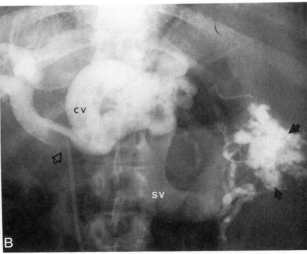

*Figure 15–10.* Splenoportography. *A,* Venous phase of splenic arteriogram shows a markedly enlarged spleen, enlarged coronary vein (CV), gastric varices, and patent portal vein (FV). Patency of the distal splenic vein (SV) is not determined with certainty. *B,* Splenoportogram shows a markedly enlarged but patent splenic vein. The open arrow points to inflow of unopacified blood from the superior mesenteric vein. Solid arrows point to parenchymal stain from the contrast injection.

may result in extrasplenic or subcapsular injection of contrast medium. This is usually without consequences, other than transient pain.

4. Intrasplenic arterial aneurysms and arteriovenous fistula.[36]

PITFALLS IN INTERPRETATION. The most important limitation of splenoportography is the failure to demonstrate a patent splenic or portal vein. Reversal of blood flow in the portal system may simulate splenic or portal vein occlusion.[37] This occurs because the high portal pressure and hepatofugal blood flow prevent hepatopetal flow of contrast medium.

## Hepatic Venography (Fig. 15–11; see also Fig. 15–4)

The indications for hepatic vein catheterization are:

1. Measurement of hepatic wedge pressures in patients with portal hypertension.

2. Hepatic wedge venography for the evaluation of the sinusoid pattern and demonstration of flow reversal in the portal vein.

3. Retrograde opacification of the portal vein.

4. Detection of hepatic vein thrombosis.

5. Estimation of hepatic blood flow or for the study of hepatic metabolism.

**Technique.** There are several methods by means of which the hepatic veins can be opacified.

1. Inferior venacavography with the Val-

salva maneuver to reflux contrast medium into the hepatic veins.

2. Catheterization of the hepatic veins for wedge or free venography.

3. Balloon occlusion venography. Either the femoral or the cubital vein approach can be used. In our experience, the cubital approach has provided a faster and easier method and access to many more hepatic veins than the femoral approach.[38]

4. In addition to the catheterization techniques, percutaneous transhepatic skinny needle (22 gauge) puncture may be used for the evaluation of the hepatic veins if other methods are unsuccessful.

For hepatic wedge pressure measurement and venography, an end hole angiographic or balloon occlusion catheter is used. The same catheter can be used for free hepatic venography. Alternatively, a multiple hole catheter is used for free hepatic venography.

From the cubital vein approach, a hockey stick–shaped (multipurpose) end hole catheter is used. Catheter passage through the right atrium is accomplished with the aid of a J guide wire. From the femoral approach, a straight catheter (with the aid of a tip deflector) or a cobra catheter is used.

**Hepatic Wedge Venography** (see also Chapter 5, Pressure Measurements and Hemodynamics). The catheter is advanced into a wedge position and pressure is recorded. Absence of a wave form confirms a wedge position. Subsequent to the pressure

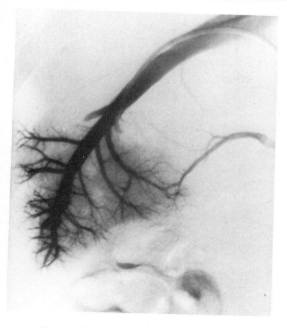
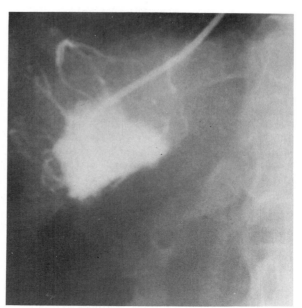

*Figure 15–11.* Normal hepatic venograms. *A,* Free hepatic venogram. *B,* Wedge hepatic injection. (*A,* From Miller F et al: Radiology 115:313–317, 1975. Used with permission.)

recording, catheter position is confirmed by contrast injection (approximately 1 ml). Wedge venography is then performed either with hand injection or preferably using a power injection (2 ml/sec for a total of 6 ml). Films are obtained in the AP projection at one per second for a total of eight films. Conventional radiographs are used, since they provide better resolution for assessment of the sinusoidal pattern.

In the normal individual, several hepatic veins are opacified. If the injection is forceful, portal vein branches may also opacify. The flow in the portal vein is always hepatopetal with a fast washout. Depending upon the force of the injection, the sinusoids may not be discernible because of an intense parenchymal stain (forceful injection), or a granular but confluent and homogeneous sinusoidal pattern is observed.

In the abnormal liver, the wedge injection demonstrates an inhomogeneous opacification of the sinusoids. This sinusoidal inhomogeneity varies with severity of the liver disease. In addition, there is opacification of the portal vein. Flow in the portal vein may be hepatopetal or hepatofugal, depending upon the severity of the portal hypertension (see Table 15–5).

**Free Hepatic Venography.** After completion of the hepatic wedge pressure measure-ment and venography, the catheter is withdrawn into a larger hepatic vein. Venography can be performed by hand or by power injection of contrast medium (8 to 10 ml/sec for a total of 24 ml). Films are obtained at two films per second for six films and one film per second for two additional films.

Alternatively, the balloon occlusion technique may be used for venography (Swan or Berman wedge balloon catheter). The balloon catheter is inflated in the main hepatic vein, 10 to 15 ml of contrast medium is injected to opacify the balloon occluded hepatic vein, and a single film is obtained, following which the balloon is deflated. Such balloon catheters can also be used to measure occlusion pressures, which have been correlated with hepatic wedge pressures.[39]

In the normal liver, the free hepatic venogram shows symmetrical arborization of the hepatic vein branches and up to the fifth order branches are visualized (Fig. 15–11). There is usually some sinusoidal opacification under normal circumstances. In cirrhosis, distortion is present and fewer branches are visualized.

**Complications of Hepatic Venography.** Complications of hepatic wedge venography include:

1. Intrahepatic hematoma and focal hemorrhagic infarcts.[40]

2. Perforation of the liver with subcapsular injection of contrast medium. This is usually without consequences (Fig. 15–12).

### Percutaneous Transhepatic Hepatography

With this technique a skinny needle is used to inject 10 to 15 ml of contrast medium into the liver parenchyma to assess hepatic venous physiology.[41, 42] In the normal liver, there is a dense parenchymal stain and multiple hepatic veins are opacified. Occasionally, a portal vein branch may be visualized with hepatopetal flow. The main portal vein is never opacified. In portal hypertension, the portal vein branches fill preferentially and hepatofugal flow is observed with opacification of the main portal vein. In addition, some hepatic veins are also opacified.

### Umbilical Vein Catheterization

This procedure requires surgical exposure of the umbilical vein. It provides an alternative method for studying the portal circulation in patients with coagulation defects, splenectomy, or massive ascites. In addition,

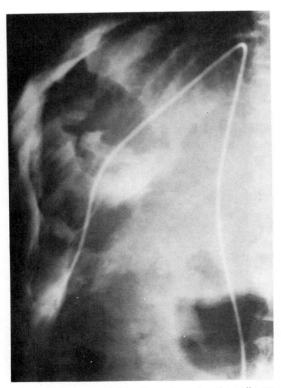

**Figure 15–12.** Complication of wedge hepatic venography. There is subcapsular extravasation of contrast medium. (Courtesy of Dr. CA Athanasoulis.)

the umbilical vein has been used as a shunt and for the infusion of drugs.[43, 44]

### Evaluation of Hepatic Lymphatics

Hepatic lymphatics can be evaluated (although not consistently) by intraparenchymal injection of contrast medium. Lymphatic channels are frequently opacified during percutaneous transhepatic cholangiography in patients with obstructive jaundice and ascites.

## DISEASES OF THE BLOOD VESSELS

### Aneurysms

**Hepatic Artery Aneurysms.** Arteriography is indicated for (1) localization of the aneurysm (because of variability of hepatic arterial anatomy in preparation for operation, and (2) transcatheter embolization.

Earlier reports indicated that mycotic and atherosclerotic hepatic artery aneurysms occurred more frequently than traumatic aneurysms.[45] Other infrequent causes are iatrogenic aneurysms, ie, focal arterial trauma due to catheter and guide wire manipulation and infusion of chemotherapeutic agents.[46, 47] In our own experience, hepatic trauma is now the most common cause of hepatic aneurysms. This is in part due to the increased use of percutaneous biliary drainage and operative placement of transhepatic Silastic stents for benign and malignant disease.[48] Whereas atherosclerotic aneurysms are mostly single, mycotic and occasionally traumatic aneurysms can be multiple. The most common locations for hepatic artery aneurysms are the common hepatic artery (about 65%), right hepatic artery (about 30%), and left hepatic artery or both hepatic arteries (about 4%)[45, 49] (Fig. 15–13).

Traumatic aneurysms following transhepatic biliary drainage procedures or operatively placed Silastic biliary drainage catheters are intrahepatic and most frequently involve the right hepatic artery or its branches. The most likely reason is that such procedures are performed more frequently on the right hepatic ducts (see also later section on Trauma).

Spontaneous occlusion of a hepatic artery aneurysm is observed occasionally. However, the most frequent complication and the presenting symptom in the majority of patients is aneurysm rupture, which has a high

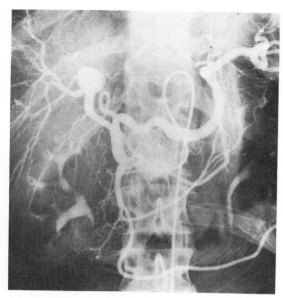

*Figure 15–13.* Mycotic hepatic artery aneurysm. Common hepatic arteriogram shows an aneurysm of the right hepatic artery. The splenic artery arises from the proper hepatic artery.

associated mortality. The classic triad of abdominal pain, jaundice, and gastrointestinal bleeding is present in only one third of patients.

On the plain radiographs, a rimlike calcification may be present and is occasionally misdiagnosed as cholelithiasis. Whereas extrahepatic aneurysms require operation, intrahepatic aneurysms are managed by transcatheter embolization.[24]

Multiple aneurysms are seen in polyarteritis nodosa and necrotizing angiitis.[50, 51] In the former, the liver is involved in two thirds of patients, and hepatic arteriography can be used to confirm the diagnosis. Spontaneous regression of such aneurysms may occur occasionally.[52] More frequently, they rupture spontaneously and cause subcapsular hematoma formation.[53] On arteriography, multiple saccular and fusiform aneurysms are seen in the smaller branches of the hepatic arteries (Fig. 15–14).

**Splenic and Pancreatic Artery Aneurysms.** Aneurysms of the splenic artery are discussed in Chapter 14. Aneurysms of the intrasplenic branches may be due to trauma, portal hypertension, or arteritis or may be mycotic.[36, 51]

Aneurysms of the pancreatic arteries are most frequently due to pancreatitis. Approximately 10% of patients with chronic pancreatitis have pseudoaneurysms of the visceral arteries.[54–56] The pancreatic arteries are also affected in 35% of patients with polyarteritis nodosa (see Fig. 15–14).[51] Arteriography is indicated for the evaluation of hemorrhage, which is the most frequent complication.[27, 55, 56]

## Atherosclerosis (see Fig. 15–16)

Atherosclerosis may affect the hepatic or splenic arteries or the smaller parenchymal branches. On arteriography, atherosclerosis

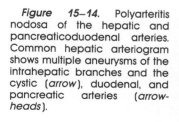

*Figure 15–14.* Polyarteritis nodosa of the hepatic and pancreaticoduodenal arteries. Common hepatic arteriogram shows multiple aneurysms of the intrahepatic branches and the cystic (*arrow*), duodenal, and pancreatic arteries (*arrowheads*).

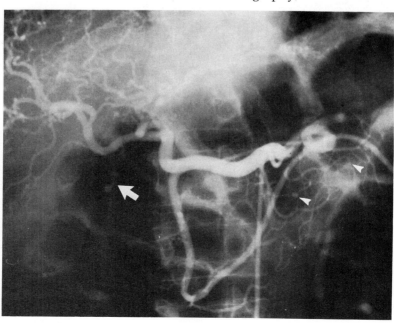

of the larger vessels is manifested as a diffuse abnormality similar to that seen in the extremity vessels (diffusely irregular and stenotic lumen) or focal smooth stenoses and occasionally as occlusion. Enlarged collateral channels may be demonstrated in severe stenosis or occlusion. A smooth stenosis of the splenic artery simulating atherosclerosis is also observed in pancreatitis. Fibromuscular disease of the hepatic or splenic arteries is rare.[57]

Other causes of visceral artery occlusion include operative ligation, inflammation (eg, abscess, pancreatitis), radiation, malignancy, and trauma.

PITFALLS IN DIAGNOSIS

The primary diagnostic pitfall is pseudoocclusion. In patients with severe portal hypertension or diaphragmatic compression of the celiac artery, the gastroduodenal artery is enlarged and opacifies the intrahepatic arteries during an SMA injection. In several such patients, we have observed a beaklike pseudoocclusion of the common hepatic artery without inflow of unopacified blood. The celiac arteriogram in such patients shows a patent common hepatic artery and in some patients there is a stenosis of the proximal celiac artery (Fig. 15–15).

## Arteriovenous Fistula (See also section on Trauma)

Most arteriovenous fistulae are traumatic; others are congenital or postoperative.[58, 59] In the liver, most fistulae are arterioportal. Congenital or acquired fistulae between the hepatic artery and hepatic vein are rare.[60] A diffuse arteriocapillary abnormality with arteriovenous shunting is seen in hereditary telangiectasia of the liver and pancreas.[61] Congenital hepatic vein–portal vein fistula has also been observed.[62] Pancreatic arteriovenous fistulae, which are also rare, can be the cause of massive hemorrhage.[55]

## Embolic Occlusion (Fig. 15–16)

Embolic occlusion of the celiac artery branches is rare. The most common source for the emboli is the heart. On arteriography, a typical intraluminal defect is seen in nonoccluding emboli, whereas larger emboli cause complete occlusion. Arterial spasm may also be present. Collateral circulation is established within a short period of time and may be demonstrated by arteriography.[63, 64]

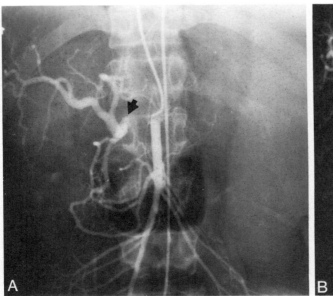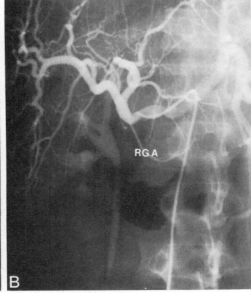

*Figure 15–15.* Pseudo-occlusion of the hepatic artery in a patient with portal hypertension. *A,* Superior mesenteric arteriogram shows an enlarged gastroduodenal artery with apparent occlusion of the common hepatic artery (*arrow*). B, Hepatic arteriogram shows that the common hepatic artery is patent, but there is absence of reflux into the gastroduodenal artery. RGA = right gastric artery.

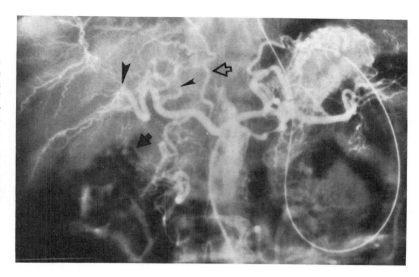

*Figure 15–16.* Thromboembolic occlusion of the hepatic artery. Celiac arteriogram shows embolic occlusion of the right and left hepatic arteries (*arrowheads*). Intrahepatic branches are opacified via collaterals, which include the pancreaticoduodenal arteries (*arrow*) and enlarged right inferior phrenic artery (*open arrow*). Atherosclerotic stenosis of the proximal splenic artery is present.

## Miscellaneous Arteriographic Findings

Splaying and stretching of the intrahepatic branches is a nonspecific finding and may be observed in the absence of a mass lesion. It is seen in diseases that cause hepatomegaly, eg, passive congestion due to right heart failure and other causes of hepatic outflow obstruction (Budd-Chiari syndrome), hepatitis, granulomatous infiltration of the liver, biliary tract obstruction, Caroli's disease, polycystic disease of the liver, and fatty infiltration. Extreme slowing of hepatic arterial flow with decreased peripheral perfusion has been observed after halothane anesthesia.[65]

### INFLAMMATORY DISEASES

Angiography is rarely performed for the diagnosis of inflammatory diseases of the liver, spleen, or pancreas. Vascular complications of such diseases (eg, hemorrhage) are the most frequent indication for angiography. The following is a brief discussion of the angiographic appearance of some of these diseases to familiarize the reader with their appearance and thus facilitate their recognition and aid in the differential diagnosis.

**Abscess** (Fig. 15–17). Hepatic abscesses may be hyper- or hypovascular. In the latter, there is displacement of the vessels during the arterial and venous phases. In the hepatogram phase, the abscess appears as an avascular lesion. Occasionally, there is rim enhancement. An abscess often cannot be differentiated from a cyst or hypovascular

tumor. Such an abscess may simulate a hematoma in both the spleen and the liver.[66]

If the abscess is hypervascular, the arteriogram may show dilated, irregular vessels and occasionally arteriovenous shunting. On the hepatogram phase, amebic liver abscess also appears as a lucent area with occasional rim enhancement. On the arterial phase, there is stretching and thinning of hepatic artery branches.[67]

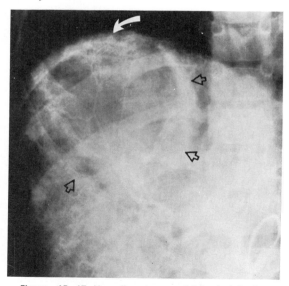

*Figure 15–17.* Hepatic abscess. Mid-arterial phase from a common hepatic arteriogram shows some hypervascularity at the dome of the liver (*white arrow*). A relatively hypovascular mass is seen in the region of the hepatic abscess, with stretching of hepatic artery branches and rim enhancement (*open arrows*). The latter is most prominent at the medial aspect of the abscess.

**Cholecystitis.** In normal individuals, the gallbladder is opacified as a thin-walled, oval-shaped structure on the parenchymal phase of the hepatic or celiac arteriogram (see Fig. 15–50B). In patients with acute cholecystitis, the gallbladder stain is hypervascular with an irregular and patchy accumulation of contrast medium. The chronically inflamed gallbladder is poorly opacified.

**Cysts.** On arteriography, most cysts are hypovascular. They cause vascular displacement and are often best seen during the parenchymal phase. The angiographic appearance of hydatid disease (ie, hypo- or hypervascular) varies with the activity of the disease.[68, 69] Occasionally, rim enhancement is present. Other lesions that are hypovascular and mimic cysts are pseudocysts, abscesses, hematoma, lymphoma, and cystic neoplasms.

**Hepatitis.** In acute hepatitis, the arteriogram shows stretching and splaying of the intrahepatic branches with slowed arterial washout. The vascular outlines may be indistinct. The hepatogram is intense and inhomogeneous. In chronic hepatitis, no abnormality may be seen other than hepatomegaly.[70]

**Pancreatitis.** The angiographic picture of acute pancreatitis is nonspecific. In most instances, the angiogram is normal, ie, the gland is not hypervascular and no venous abnormality is present. There may be some increase in caliber of both large and small hepatic and pancreatic arteries, suggesting hypervascularity. Arterial displacement due to swelling of the gland is observed occasionally, but it is nonspecific, since alteration in the course of vessels also occurs during respiration.

In recurrent pancreatitis, several abnormalities may be observed: (1) focal fibrotic arterial stenoses, often resulting in an irregular appearance of the arterial lumen; (2) hypervascularity of the gland; (3) intense parenchymal staining and early venous opacification; (4) occlusion of the splenic vein; and (5) formation of pseudoaneurysms.[71]

In chronic pancreatitis, there is often an intense fibrotic reaction that leads to vascular stenoses and occlusions. Smooth narrowing of the splenic artery may simulate neoplastic encasement (Fig. 15–18) or an atherosclerotic plaque. Unlike the splenic artery of other patients with atherosclerosis, that in patients with chronic pancreatitis is often not tortuous. Vascular displacement is not seen in the absence of a pseudocyst.

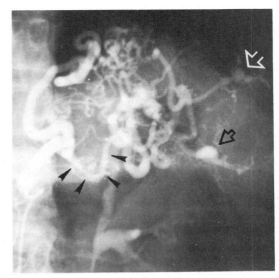

*Figure 15–18.* Smooth stenosis of the proximal splenic artery due to pancreatitis (*arrowheads*). The left gastric artery is markedly enlarged and intrasplenic arterial aneurysms are visualized (*arrows*). The splenic vein was occluded.

Pseudoaneurysm formation in patients with chronic pancreatitis is due to arterial wall necrosis as a result of autodigestion by trypsin.[72] The most frequent location for such pseudoaneurysms is the splenic artery (approximately 50%), followed by the pancreatico- and gastroduodenal arteries and the smaller arteries of the pancreas.[55] Such aneurysms are observed in approximately 10% of patients with chronic pancreatitis.[54–56] They can enlarge rapidly and may be responsible for massive hemorrhage[27, 55, 56] (Fig. 15–19).

**Pseudocysts.** Pancreatic pseudocysts are most frequently due to trauma or pancreatitis. Hemorrhage is reported in 41% of patients with pseudocysts of the pancreas and is mostly due to a pseudoaneurysm.[73] This association has led some authors to suggest that angiography be performed in all patients with pancreatic pseudocysts to detect pseudoaneurysms, which can be multiple and small enough to escape detection by other means.[74]

On arteriography, pseudocysts are avascular and cause vascular displacement (Fig. 15–19). Pseudocysts that communicate with pseudoaneurysms may demonstrate intermittent (ie, systolic) opacification with contrast medium, similar to that observed with false aneurysms in the groin[55] (see Chapter 11, Fig. 11–41).

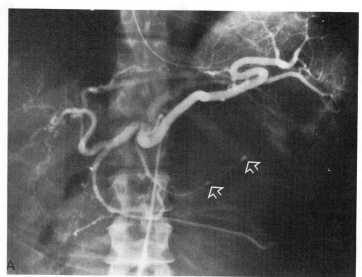

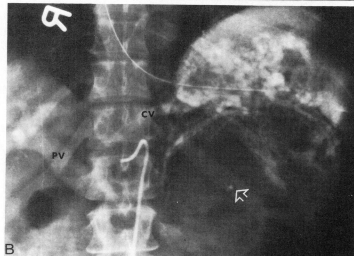

*Figure 15–19.* Aneurysms of the transverse pancreatic artery in a patient with pancreatitis. *A,* Celiac arteriogram shows two small aneurysms of the transverse pancreatic artery (*arrows*). *B,* Venous phase from the same study shows gastric fundal varices and splenic vein occlusion. Retained contrast medium is seen in one of the aneurysms (*arrow*). CV = coronary vein; PV = portal vein. *C,* Transverse pancreatic arteriogram obtained several days later shows that the distal aneurysm has enlarged markedly. Arrow points to the proximal aneurysm. (From Knight RW et al: Cardiovasc Intervent Radiol 5:37–39, 1982. Used with permission.)

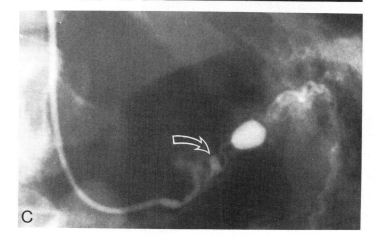

## PORTAL HYPERTENSION

Portal hypertension may be classified into presinusoidal and intrahepatic[75] or pre-, intra-, and posthepatic. Table 15–2 lists the etiology of the different types of portal hypertension. The most common cause of portal hypertension is hepatic cirrhosis, and its most frequent clinical manifestation is gastrointestinal bleeding (from varices, gastritis, or peptic ulcer disease). Approximately one third of patients with hepatic cirrhosis develop portal hypertension.

In normal individuals, 70 to 80% of hepatic blood comes through the portal system and the remainder via the hepatic artery. In patients with portal hypertension, the ratio of portal:hepatic artery blood flow is altered. A decrease in portal inflow is compensated by an increase in hepatic artery inflow. The greatest increase in hepatic artery inflow is observed in patients with complete reversal of portal blood flow and extrahepatic portal vein obstruction.

**TABLE 15–2. Classification of Portal Hypertension***

| |
|---|
| **Presinusoidal** |
| *Extrahepatic* |
|   Portal vein obstruction |
|     Neonatal sepsis |
|     Portal phlebitis |
|     Neoplastic invasion |
|     Lymphadenopathy |
|     Bland thrombus |
|     Trauma |
|     Pancreatitis, pseudocyst |
|   Arterioportal fistula |
|     Traumatic, neoplastic |
|   Splenic vein occlusion |
|   Superior mesenteric vein occlusion |
| *Intrahepatic* |
|   Congenital hepatic fibrosis |
|   Chronic malaria |
|   Felty's syndrome |
|   Idiopathic noncirrhotic fibrosis |
|   Myelofibrosis |
|   Primary biliary cirrhosis |
|   Reticuloendothelioses |
|   Sarcoid liver disease |
|   Schistosomias |
|   Toxic fibrosis |
|     Arsenic, copper |
|     PVC vapors |
|   Wilson's disease |
| **Intrahepatic (Sinusoidal)** |
|   Cirrhosis |
|   Sclerosing cholangitis |
| **Posthepatic (Postsinusoidal)** |
|   Hepatic vein occlusion |
|     (see Table 15–6) |

*Data from references 75 to 79.

## Angiography

The indications for angiography in portal hypertension are:

1. Assessment of the severity of portal hypertension by measurement of portal pressures and venography.

2. Differentiation between the types of portal hypertension and determination of etiology.

3. Assessment of patency of the superior mesenteric, splenic, and portal veins prior to a shunt procedure. This also determines the type of procedure that can be performed.

4. Evaluation of portal dynamics, ie, hepatopetal versus hepatofugal blood flow, and demonstration of varices.

5. Evaluation of the liver for neoplasms: Hepatoma is discovered as an incidental finding in 4.5% of patients with cirrhosis.[29]

6. Postoperative evaluation for shunt patency and dynamics, ie, pressure gradient across an anastomosis.

7. Transcatheter therapy, ie, embolization of varices, angioplasty of shunt stenoses.

8. Diagnosis and treatment of nonvariceal bleeding.

The angiographic study is tailored to provide the information that is required:

*Arterial portography* (either superior mesenteric or splenic) is used to evaluate the superior mesenteric or splenic veins, portal vein, and portal dynamics. If a splenorenal shunt is to be performed, anatomy and patency of the left renal vein is documented by venography (hand injection of contrast medium and a spot film). In addition, a catheter is left in the renal vein at the time of the splenic arteriogram to assess proximity of the splenic and renal veins. An anomalous course (retroaortic, circumaortic) must also be documented.

*Hepatic wedge pressure* (HWP) measurement and *wedge venography* are used to assess severity and in certain cases to differentiate between types of portal hypertension (for HWP measurement technique, see Chapter 5). Hepatic wedge venography provides an excellent method for demonstration of reversal of portal blood flow and estimation of hepatopetal blood flow.

*Hepatic arteriography* serves to detect neoplasms, and the appearance of the hepatic arteries, together with hemodynamic and other angiographic data, helps to differentiate between the types of portal hypertension.

If further questions need to be answered,

splenoportography or transhepatic portography may be performed. Varices are usually demonstrated on the venous phase of the superior mesenteric or splenic arteriograms. For improved visualization of esophagogastric varices, a high volume left gastric arteriogram is obtained (preferably with DSA).

**Correlation Between Hemodynamics and Angiographic Appearance for Assessment of Type and Severity of Portal Hypertension.** The normal portal pressure is only 2 to 3 mm Hg above the inferior vena cava (IVC) pressure. In portal hypertension, the pressure usually does not exceed 33 mm Hg.[80, 81] Rarely, we have measured pressures up to 40 mm Hg. Higher portal pressure is decompressed through portosystemic collaterals and by regulation of splanchnic inflow.

The HWP, which is normally less than 10 mm Hg, corresponds to the portal pressure in patients with cirrhosis. In addition, the HWP has been correlated with the severity of the disease, and differences between direct portal pressure measurement and HWP have been less than 4 mm Hg.[82] In presinusoidal portal vein obstruction and in the presence of portosystemic anastomoses, the corrected sinusoidal pressure (CSP) does not reflect the portal pressure. The CSP does not correlate with size of varices or the risk of hemorrhage. However, larger varices have a greater likelihood for hemorrhage.

The splenic pulp pressure, which is normally about 8 mm Hg (range 3 to 17 mm Hg), has also been correlated with the severity of the portal hypertension.[83] However, the wide range of normal pressures limits its usefulness. False high pressures may be recorded if the needle/catheter tip lies in close proximity to a splenic artery branch.

Table 15–3 shows the correlation between the angiographic and hemodynamic data and the type of portal hypertension. Table 15–4 shows the relationship between the CSP, the

**TABLE 15–3.** Portal Hypertension: Angiographic and Hemodynamic Evaluation

| Type | HWP | HV | PV | HA |
|------|-----|-----|-----|-----|
| Presinusoidal | NL | NL | ABN | NL |
| Sinusoidal | ↑ | ABN | NL[1*] | ABN |
| Postsinusoidal | ↑ | ABN | NL[2*] | NL[2] |

HWP = hepatic wedge pressure.
HA = angiographic appearance of the hepatic artery.
HV = angiographic appearance of the hepatic vein.
PV = angiographic appearance of the portal veins.
NL = normal; ABN = abnormal.
* = abnormal flow pattern.
1 = see Table 15–5.
2 = stretched and splayed; no intrinsic abnormality.

**TABLE 15–4.** Portal Hypertension: Correlation Between Corrected Sinusoidal Pressure (CSP), Hepatic Venography, and Severity of Liver Cirrhosis

| Severity of Cirrhosis | CSP (mm Hg) | Hepatic Vein Branch Visualization |
|------|-----|-----|
| Normal | <5 | Fifth order |
| Mild | 6–10 | Fourth order |
| Moderate | 11–15 | Second to third order |
| Severe | >16 | Zero to first order |

appearance of the hepatic veins on venography, and the severity of portal hypertension in cirrhosis. This correlation cannot be used once therapy is begun, since the healing process leads to perivascular fibrosis, cicatrization, and occlusion of the hepatic vein branches.

PITFALLS IN THE INTERPRETATION OF HWP AND CSP

1. False low HWP readings can be obtained by improperly wedged catheters.

2. False high HWP readings may be obtained if contrast medium is injected prior to the pressure recording. This is due to vasospasm and hematoma formation associated with wedge injection of contrast medium.

3. False high CSP readings may be obtained if the right atrial pressure is used as the zero point in patients with ascites.[80] In this situation, the high intraabdominal pressure is subtracted from a low reference pressure. For an accurate reading, the IVC or the hepatic veins should be used as the zero point. In severe ascites, the IVC is compressed at the hepatic segment and the caval and hepatic wedge pressures are elevated. Following paracentesis, there is relief of the obstruction, the caval and wedge pressures fall (the latter by as much as one third), and the augmentation of venous return results in an increase in the cardiac output.[84]

4. Normal wedge pressures may be measured in patients with nonhepatogenic ascites, ie, tuberculous, fungal, or chylous ascites or peritoneal carcinomatosis.[80]

5. When a high hepatic vein pressure is recorded, the right atrial pressure should also be measured to exclude suprahepatic obstruction, ie, constrictive pericarditis or congestive heart failure. In addition, the proximal IVC should be evaluated for the presence of a web.

### Prehepatic (Presinusoidal) Portal Hypertension

This may be due to an abnormality of the extra- or intrahepatic branches of the portal vein or a tributary of the portal system (Fig. 15–20). Table 15–2 lists the different causes.

*Extrahepatic portal vein obstruction* may be in the form of extrinsic compression (tumor, periportal lymphadenopathy, fibrosis, pseudocyst) or occlusion (thrombosis due to infection, oral contraceptives, coagulopathy, invasion by neoplasm, pancreatitis). In obstruction without occlusion, some hepatopetal flow may be preserved. The degree of hepatofugal flow depends upon the severity of obstruction. In portal vein occlusion, portal blood flow is via portosystemic and portoportal collaterals. These are best demonstrated on the venous phase of the superior mesenteric arteriogram. Collaterals in extrahepatic portal vein obstruction may be via:

1. Splenic → short gastric and coronary veins → portal vein.

2. Splenic → gastroepiploic → portal vein.

3. Splenic → omental vein (arc of Barkow) → portal vein.

4. Pancreaticoduodenal and cystic veins → hilar portal veins.

Other portosystemic collaterals are listed in Table 14–1, Chapter 14.

Liver function remains normal in the absence of associated liver disease. The HWP does not correspond to the portal pressure proximal to the obstruction.

In *intrahepatic presinusoidal occlusion*, the obstruction is in the portal venules (Fig. 15–20B). A number of diseases may cause this type of portal hypertension (see Table 15–2). The HWP is normal or only slightly elevated because of the presinusoidal location of the obstruction or the presence of normal anastomoses.[80] Intrahepatic portal vein obstruction is also best seen on the venous phase of the superior mesenteric arteriogram. This may show hepatofugal flow with opacification of portosystemic shunts and a patent extrahepatic portal vein or the so-called cavernous transformation of the portal vein.

*Splenic vein occlusion* results in segmental portal hypertension (Fig. 15–21). The portal pressure is normal, whereas the splenic pulp pressure is elevated. In proximal (close to the splenic hilum) splenic vein obstruction, blood flow is via the gastric and omental collaterals, which results in gastric fundal varices. In distal (close to its junction with the superior mesenteric vein) splenic vein occlusion, the inferior mesenteric vein also serves as a collateral. In addition, spontaneous splenorenal and splenoretroperitoneal collaterals may be present. Esophageal varices are usually absent and splenomegaly is present in only half the patients.[85, 86] Rarely, gastric varices may be localized to the body of the stomach.[87] Concomitant esophageal varices (other than focal distal esophageal varices) usually indicate the presence of another more hepatopetal obstruction or a high flow state (arterioportal fistula). The size of the spleen does

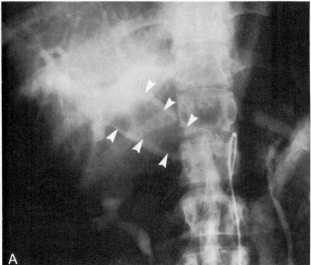
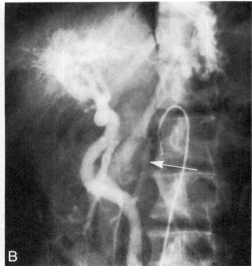

*Figure 15–20.* Presinusoidal portal hypertension. *A,* Portal vein thrombosis. Venous phase of a superior mesenteric arteriogram shows a thrombus in the portal vein (*arrowheads*). B, Congenital hepatic fibrosis. Venous phase of a superior mesenteric arteriogram shows distortion and attenuation of intrahepatic portal vein branches with a normal-caliber extrahepatic portal vein. There is hepatofugal flow with visualization of the coronary vein (*arrow*) and gastroesophageal varices.

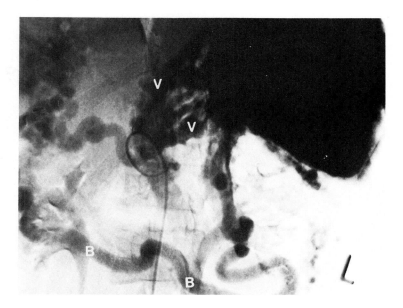

*Figure 15–21.* Splenic vein occlusion with gastric varices (V) in a patient with a malignant islet cell tumor. Collateral venous drainage is seen via the arc of Barkow (B). In addition, there is cavernous transformation of the portal vein.

not correlate with the degree of portal pressure elevation, and splenomegaly is more prominent in children.

Splenic vein occlusion and the collateral flow are best demonstrated on the venous phase of the splenic arteriogram. The portal and superior mesenteric veins are normal. In 6.4% of patients, a patent splenic vein may also not be demonstrated by this method.[29] Causes of splenic vein occlusion include pancreatitis, pseudocyst, tumor, trauma, operative ligation, radiation, or complications of umbilical vein catheterization. In the last, gastric and esophageal varices have been observed.[88]

*Superior mesenteric vein occlusion,* due to pancreatitis, tumor, trauma, or radiation, also causes segmental hypertension in the mesenteric venous bed with development of mesenteric varices (see Chapter 14, Fig. 14–26).

*Dynamic portal hypertension* is due to an arteriovenous communication in the intra- or extrahepatic portal venous bed. Such communications may be congenital or acquired. The congenital type, which is rare, may be due to arterioportal or arteriovenous (SMV, splenic vein) fistula or hemangiomatosis.[89, 90] The acquired type is most frequently a traumatic arterioportal fistula from penetrating abdominal injury, liver biopsy, splenoportography, percutaneous transhepatic biliary drainage, or operative placement of biliary stents.[91] An infrequent cause is rupture of a visceral artery aneurysm.[92]

Clinical manifestations are gastrointestinal bleeding and ascites. Arteriography of the

vessel supplying the region in which the abnormality is suspected is usually diagnostic. There is prompt and dense opacification of the draining vein. The portal vein is usually dilated, and hepatofugal flow is observed (Fig. 15–22). On transhepatic portography or splenoportography, the venous limb of the fistula may not opacify owing to the higher arterial pressure transmitted through the arteriovenous communication.

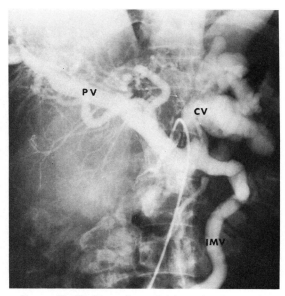

*Figure 15–22.* Dynamic portal hypertension caused by a hepatic artery to portal vein fistula. Hepatic arteriogram shows dense opacification of the portal vein with hepatofugal flow. CV = coronary vein and gastric varices; IMV = inferior mesenteric vein; PV = portal vein.

**TABLE 15–5. Summary of Angiographic Findings in Hepatic Cirrhosis**

| Stage | Liver Size | Hepatic Arteries | | Hepatic Venography | | Portal Veins | | Portosystemic Collaterals |
|---|---|---|---|---|---|---|---|---|
| | | Appearance | Flow | Free | Wedge | Appearance | Flow | |
| Early (Stage 1) | Normal, enlarged in fatty infiltration | Normal or stretched intrahepatic branches; normal hepatogram | Slightly delayed arterial filling and emptying; GDA opacified | 3rd–4th order branches, narrowed; sinusoidal filling but irregular | Slightly inhomogeneous sinusoidal pattern; no PV opacification | Normal, prompt homogeneous hepatogram | Normal | Absent |
| Moderate (Stage 2) | Small | CHA enlarged; intrahepatic: parallel tracking or "tram track" appearance; ↑vascularity; poor peripheral hepatogram | Increased; GDA not opacified | 2nd–3rd order branches, "pruned tree" appearance; irregular HV margins; sinusoidal filling absent or irregular | Inhomogeneous sinusoidal pattern; preferential PV opacification; slow hepatopetal washout; HV also opacifies | Some tortuosity; normal branching; delayed patchy hepatogram | Bidirectional | Present |
| Advanced (Stage 3) | Very small | Corkscrew intrahepatic branches; dense hepatogram | Markedly increased; PV opacification on venous phase | 1st order branches, "bare tree" appearance; irregular HV margins; no sinusoidal filling | Coarse or patchy sinusoidal pattern; PV opacified with hepatofugal flow; HV not opacified | Distorted changing caliber; delayed or absent hepatogram | Bidirectional or hepatofugal | Present |

GDA = gastroduodenal artery; CHA = common hepatic artery; PV = portal vein; HV = hepatic vein.

Although spontaneous closure is observed occasionally, the treatment of choice for intrahepatic fistulae is transhepatic embolization. Extrahepatic and mesenteric arteriovenous fistulae may require operative closure.

### Intrahepatic (Sinusoidal) Portal Hypertension

Cirrhosis is the most common cause of intrahepatic portal hypertension. Histologically, the abnormality involves the portal zones, sinusoids, and hepatic venules. There is fibrosis with obliteration of the hepatic venous outflow. The angiographic picture varies with the stage of the disease. Table 15–5 provides a summary of the angiographic findings in cirrhosis.

In *early cirrhosis*, portal perfusion is maintained, and in the absence of fatty infiltration and hepatomegaly, the arteriogram may be normal. On hepatic venography, only the fourth order branches are seen (Fig. 15–23).

In *moderate cirrhosis*, the intrahepatic resistance increases, resulting in some reversal of portal flow, which leads to the development of portosystemic collaterals and compensatory increase in hepatic arterial flow (Fig.

15–24). Splenomegaly and increased hepatic and splenic blood flow with enlargement of the splenic and common hepatic arteries are seen, and intrasplenic arterial aneurysms may be present. On the common hepatic arteriogram, the gastroduodenal artery is not opacified or is only partially opacified because of reversal of flow in this vessel. On the superior mesenteric arteriogram, this artery opacifies via the inferior pancreaticoduodenal arteries, and there is contrast opacification of the intrahepatic branches. This ''hepatic steal'' reflects the increased arterial demand of the liver to compensate for decreased portal inflow.

In moderate cirrhosis, the hepatic venogram shows only the second or third order branches (Fig. 15–24). Dilatation of the hepatic artery with reversal of portal venous flow has also been observed in patients with alcoholic hepatitis.[93]

In *advanced cirrhosis*, there is a typical corkscrew appearance of the intrahepatic arteries as a result of a shrunken liver. The extrahepatic segments enlarge in response to increased arterial flow. The intrahepatic arteries do not enlarge in patients with

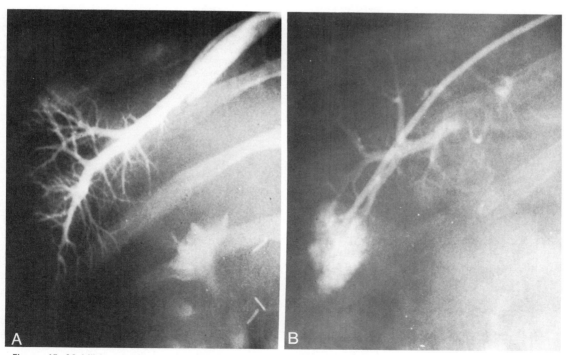

*Figure 15–23.* Mild portal hypertension. *A*, Free hepatic venogram. The general appearance is that of a normal study except that only the fourth-order branches are visualized. *B*, Wedge hepatic venogram. The sinusoidal pattern is mildly nonhomogeneous. The portal vein branch is opacified with hepatopetal washout. (*A*, From Kadir S: Diagnostic Angiography and Interventional Therapy: Abdomino-Visceral, Biliary. RSP 103–RSNA. Reproduced with permission of the Radiological Society of North America.)

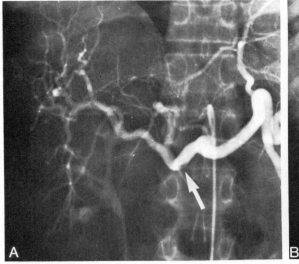

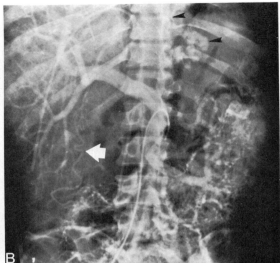

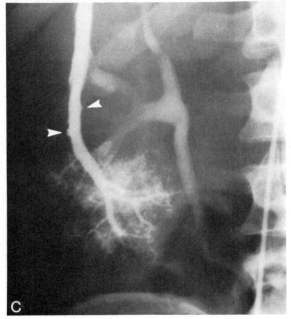

*Figure 15–24.* Moderate portal hypertension. *A,* Celiac arteriogram shows mild tortuosity of the hepatic artery branches (compare with Fig. 15–1A). There is reversal of blood flow in the gastroduodenal artery. Arrow points to inflow of unopacified blood. *B,* Arterial portogram (venous phase of superior mesenteric arteriogram) shows normal portal vein branches. There is hepatofugal flow and gastric and esophageal varices are opacified (*arrowheads*). In addition, a dilated paraumbilical vein is seen (*arrow*). *C,* Free hepatic venogram. There is a relatively abrupt change in caliber of the branches. Only second- and occasionally third-order branches can be identified. The sinusoidal filling is irregular and patchy. Several of the hepatic vein branches are amputated (*arrowheads*).

uncomplicated cirrhosis. Enlargement of these arteries is observed in patients developing a hepatoma.[94] Because of the high intrahepatic resistance, portal flow is reversed and spontaneous portosystemic shunts are present (Fig. 15–25). In addition, arterioportal shunting may be observed on hepatic arteriography. Thrombosis of the portal vein is a rare complication of advanced cirrhosis and is observed in 0.6% of cirrhotics.[94a]

In general, the portal hepatogram and the direction of portal blood flow correspond to the severity of hypertension. In moderate cirrhosis, the portal hepatogram is delayed and prolonged and is absent towards the liver periphery. In advanced cirrhosis, the hepatogram may be totally absent. Patients with hepatocellular failure have a dense hepatogram.[94] Tumors and regenerating nodules may cause an inhomogeneous hepatogram. A technetium sulfur colloid scan helps to differentiate between regenerating nodules and neoplasms.

Esophagogastric varices are demonstrated by transhepatic portography in 78% of patients with portal hypertension due to hepatic cirrhosis.[96] Using this method, a patent

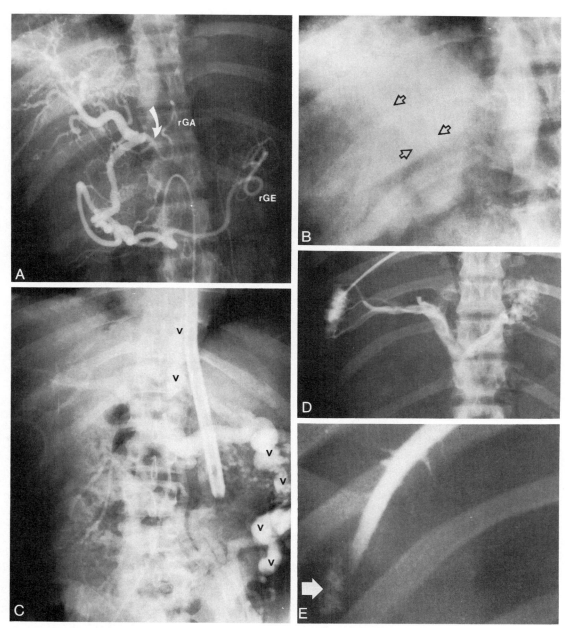

*Figure 15–25.* Severe portal hypertension. *A,* Inferior pancreaticoduodenal arteriogram shows a markedly enlarged inferior pancreaticoduodenal artery with opacification of the hepatic artery. There is tortuosity of the hepatic artery branches, which also appear pruned and crowded. The liver is small. A beaklike obstruction of the common hepatic artery is present (*arrow*). Inflow from the celiac artery is not seen. rGA = right gastric; rGE = right gastroepiploic arteries. *B,* Late arterial phase from a hepatic arteriogram shows portal vein opacification (*arrows*). *C,* Arterial portogram (venous phase of superior mesenteric arteriogram) from another patient. There is poor opacification and attenuation of the intrahepatic portal vein branches, and portal blood flow is mainly hepatofugal. Esophageal and large colonic varices (V) are opacified. *D,* Wedge hepatic venogram. There is portal vein opacification with hepatofugal flow and visualization of gastric varices. The hepatic veins do not opacify. The sinusoidal pattern is nonhomogeneous. *E,* Free hepatic venogram from the same patient. Only markedly attenuated first-order branches are opacified. There is no sinusoidal opacification. A marked discrepancy between the caliber of the main hepatic vein and the opacified branches is seen. Arrow points to residual intraparenchymal contrast material from the preceding wedge venogram.

umbilical vein was demonstrated in 26% of patients, which is a much higher incidence than was previously reported (ie, 9%).[97]

### Posthepatic (Postsinusoidal) Hypertension

Obstruction of hepatic venous outflow or Budd-Chiari syndrome may be caused by thrombosis or, less frequently, by obstruction without thrombosis (Table 15–6). The most common etiology is hepatic vein thrombosis in patients with polycythemia vera (one third of patients). Other frequent causes are venous extension of renal cell carcinoma and IVC webs.

Women are affected more frequently than men, and the clinical presentation is mostly that of an insidious onset of intractable ascites and hepatomegaly without derangement of liver function. If untreated, compromise of liver function occurs. Occasionally, the onset is sudden, leading to shock and hepatic failure. Lower extremity venous pressures are elevated, and the IVC may be occluded.[101]

The diagnosis is established by hepatic venography and inferior venacavography. Occlusion of the smaller intrahepatic hepatic vein branches may be diagnosed only by liver biopsy.[104, 105] Angiographic evaluation consists of hepatic venography and inferior venacavography, hepatic arteriography to exclude a tumor, and the superior mesenteric arteriogram to evaluate the portal vein and portal blood flow.

The angiographic findings are characteristic (Fig. 15–26). The hepatic venogram shows absence of a main hepatic vein. Instead a spider web–like appearance of the collateral and recanalized veins is present. The inferior venacavogram may show obstruction of the hepatic segment. This may be due to either compression from an enlarged liver and ascites, or occlusion by thrombus or tumor.

The hepatic arteriogram shows hepatomegaly with stretching and draping of the intrahepatic branches. True neovascularity is not seen in the absence of a neoplasm. The hepatogram is inhomogeneous. Inhomogeneity may be in the form of a fine mottling with a prolonged, intense hepatogram or may be seen as large lakes of sinusoidal contrast accumulation.[105] The latter has been reported in a patient on oral contraceptives and most likely represents an exaggerated form of peliosis hepatis.

The portal vein may opacify on the venous phase of the hepatic arteriogram. Portal vein flow is bidirectional or hepatofugal and is best demonstrated by percutaneous transhepatic hepatography.[106] The radionuclide scan may be normal or may show a slightly diminished uptake.

PITFALLS IN DIAGNOSIS

1. Inability to catheterize hepatic veins and absent hepatic venous opacification may also be observed in advanced cirrhosis.[107]

2. The hypervascular lesions seen in the liver[105] must be differentiated from hemangiomas or metastases (from carcinoid or islet cell, renal cell, or thyroid carcinoma).

3. Vena caval obstruction at the diaphragmatic hiatus can also occur after a Valsalva maneuver and may simulate a web or may be due to massive ascites and hepatomegaly.

### Idiopathic Portal Hypertension

Idiopathic noncirrhotic portal hypertension is manifested by splenomegaly, anemia, varices, and gastrointestinal bleeding. The disease is much more common in the Orient.[108] Liver function is unimpaired and the hepatic and extrahepatic portal veins are patent, but the HWP may be elevated slightly. The disease is most likely caused by occlusion of the smaller intrahepatic portal vein branches.[109] Clinically, it may mimic cirrhosis.

Some angiographic features that can distinguish idiopathic portal hypertension from that due to cirrhosis have been reported.[108] The peripheral portal vein branches are poorly opacified on the portal hepatogram. The number of smaller branches is diminished, and there is an irregular branching pattern, distortion, and occlusion. Apparent anastomoses are observed between peripheral portal vein branches, and there is visualization of enlarged intrahepatic paraportal collaterals.

**TABLE 15–6.** Etiology of the Budd-Chiari Syndrome*

| Thrombotic Occlusion | Nonthrombotic occlusion |
|---|---|
| Bland thrombus | Constrictive pericarditis |
|   Polycythemia vera | IVC membrane/diaphragm |
|   Paraoxysmal noctur- | Right heart failure |
|     nal hemoglobinuria | Right atrial tumor |
|   Pregnancy | Tumor growth in IVC or |
|   Sickle cell anemia |   hepatic veins |
| Oral contraceptives |     Renal cell carcinoma |
| Phlebitis |     Hepatic cell carcinoma |
| Tumor |     Adrenal carcinoma |

*Includes data from references 81 and 98 to 103.

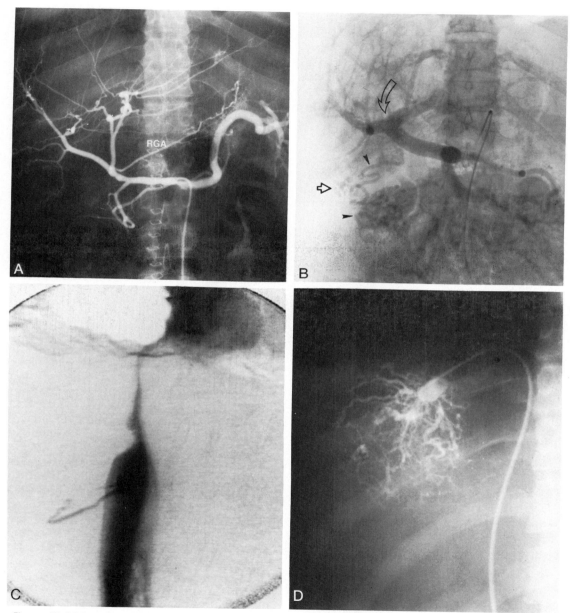

*Figure 15–26.* Budd-Chiari syndrome. *A,* Celiac arteriogram shows stretching and attenuation of the intrahepatic branches. An unusually prominent right gastric artery (RGA) is seen. *B,* Arterial portogram shows splaying of the portal bifurcation (*curved arrow*), stretching of the portal vein branches, and hepatofugal flow through paraumbilical veins (*arrowheads*). Calculi are present in the gallbladder (*straight arrow*). *C,* AP image from a digital subtraction inferior venacavagram shows narrowing of the hepatic segment of the inferior vena cava. *D,* Balloon occlusion hepatic venogram. The normal hepatic venous architecture is absent. The typical "spidery" appearance of the hepatic veins is seen.

### Obstructive Jaundice

Patients with acute biliary obstruction have an increase in hepatic arterial blood flow. Hepatomegaly results in stretching of arterial and portal vein branches. Initially, the resistance is presinusoidal, but with the development of biliary cirrhosis there is also intrahepatic resistance with progressive decrease in hepatic artery perfusion and development of portosystemic shunts.[110, 111] Histological examinations have demonstrated thrombi in portal vein branches.[110]

### Cavernous Transformation of the Portal Vein

This term is misleading and refers to multiple tortuous venous channels that are seen in place of the portal vein in patients with portal vein occlusion. These represent enlarged paraportal collateral channels (eg, choledochal veins) and a partially recanalized portal vein that drain into a network of portal branches at the porta hepatis (Fig. 15–27; see also Fig. 15–21).

### Cruveilhier–von Baumgarten Syndrome (Disease)

A recanalized umbilical vein that serves as a portosystemic collateral in patients with portal hypertension is also known as Cruveilhier–von Baumgarten syndrome (Fig. 15–28). The umbilical vein may remain patent in children with hypoplasia of the portal system in the absence of portal hypertension. This is also known as Cruveilhier–von Baumgarten disease.[112, 113] In the latter, a characteristic paraumbilical venous hum may be heard.

With the aid of transhepatic portography, a patent umbilical vein has been demonstrated in 26% of patients with portal hypertension.[96] However, some authors refute the existence of such recanalized umbilical veins and suggest that these represent enlarged paraumbilical veins.[113a] Our angiographic data indicate that umbilical vein recanalization does occur in some patients with portal hypertension, whereas in most other patients, enlarged paraumbilical veins are demonstrated. The umbilical vein has a characteristic course (see Fig. 15–28). The paraumbilical veins are much smaller and are usually very tortuous.

### The Portal System Following Portosystemic Shunt

The most frequently used shunts are portacaval, mesocaval, proximal, and distal (Warren) splenorenal shunts.[114] More recently, the mesoatrial shunt has been used in patients with IVC abnormalities.[115]

Postoperative evaluation is indicated for assessment of shunt patency in patients with recurrent symptoms, for obtaining hemodynamic data (ie, measurement of pressure gradients and assessment of portal hemodynamics), and for the management of complications (angioplasty of the shunt anastomosis) and recurrent gastrointestinal bleeding.[116, 117]

For the evaluation of shunt patency and portal dynamics, a superior mesenteric arteriogram (for portacaval, mesocaval, and mesoatrial shunts) or a splenic arteriogram (for splenorenal shunts) is performed (Figs. 15–29 and 15–30). Either arterial DSA or cut film arteriography (enhanced with tolazoline) can be used. For anatomical studies in patent but stenotic shunts, contrast injection may have to be performed proximal to the anastomosis after catheterization of the shunt.

For the measurement of pressure gradients in mesocaval, portacaval, and splenorenal shunts, a cobra catheter is used to catheterize the shunt. The pressure gradient is measured across the anastomosis, and contrast angiography is then performed. The volume and

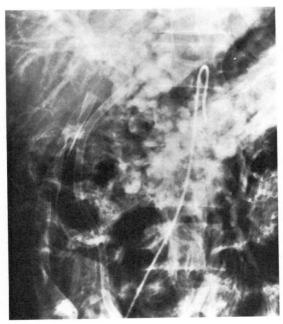

**Figure 15–27.** Cavernous transformation of the portal vein. Venous phase of the superior mesenteric arteriogram shows dilated and tortuous collaterals entering the porta hepatis. The portal vein is occluded. The intrahepatic portal vein branches are normal.

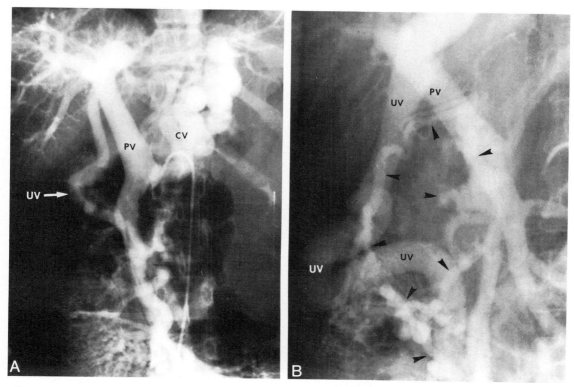

**Figure 15–28.** Cruveilhier–von Baumgarten syndrome. *A,* Venous phase of the superior mesenteric arteriogram shows a patent umbilical vein (UV) in a patient with portal hypertension. CV = coronary vein; PV = portal vein. *B,* Venous phase of an RPO superior mesenteric arteriogram in another patient with portal hypertension. There is a large umbilical vein (UV), which has a diameter similar to that of the portal vein (PV). In addition, dilated parumbilical veins are opacified (*arrowheads*).

**Figure 15–29.** Normal splenorenal shunt seen on the venous phase of a digital subtraction celiac arteriogram. IVC = inferior vena cava; S = shunt.

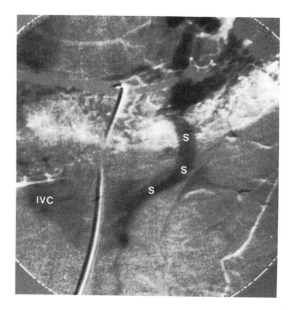

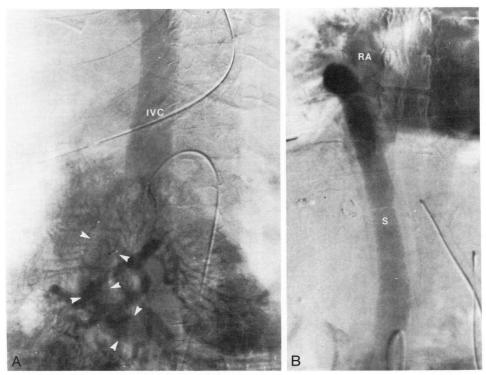

*Figure 15–30.* Portosystemic shunts. Subtraction films from the venous phase of the superior mesenteric arteriograms from two different patients show: *A,* Normal mesocaval shunt (*arrowheads*). *B,* Normal mesoatrial shunt. IVC = inferior vena cava; RA = right atrium; S = shunt.

rate of contrast injection are determined by the size and location of the shunt. In general, 20 to 25 ml is injected at 4 or 5 ml/sec. Films are obtained in the AP projection at two per second for 3 seconds and one per second for another six seconds (total of 12 films). Additional projections may be required to define stenoses.

For mesoatrial shunts, either the femoral or the cubital vein approach can be used. The latter is preferred. From the femoral approach, a cobra catheter is advanced through the right atrium into the shunt and further into the superior mesenteric vein over a J LLT guide wire. From the cubital vein approach, a headhunter or multipurpose catheter is used. Contrast injection and filming are similar to that for the other shunts.

## TRAUMA

### Hepatic Trauma

Blunt or penetrating hepatic trauma (the latter including injuries occurring during operation and percutaneous biliary drainage) can lead to a number of minor or serious abnormalities, many of which can be diagnosed and some also treated by angiographic techniques.

The liver is injured in up to 10% of patients with blunt abdominal trauma.[118] Specific signs of hepatic injury are often absent. The severity of injury and the proximity to the liver of other injured organs provide clues for the presence of hepatic injury (eg, elevation of right hemidiaphragm, pleural effusion, rib fractures).

The clinical manifestations of blunt injury may occur several days or weeks after the traumatic event. Such symptoms may be due to pseudoaneurysms and hemobilia, arteriovenous fistulae, venous obstruction, or infected hematomas.

Angiography is indicated for the diagnosis and often for the management of both blunt and penetrating injuries to the liver. Selective hepatic arteriography should be performed in the AP projection. If an abnormality is poorly seen or if no abnormality is detected, oblique views should be obtained. If the hepatic artery cannot be catheterized, a good quality celiac arteriogram may demonstrate the pathology. In severe blunt abdominal injury, an inferior venacavagram should also be performed to detect caval injury.

The angiographic findings may be divided into two categories: (1) minor parenchymal and small vessel injuries (eg, hematomas and contusions that do not require specific treatment) and (2) major parenchymal trauma (liver fracture, fragmentation) and vascular injuries. Major parenchymal injury usually requires immediate surgery, and preoperative arteriography is rarely indicated.

### Minor Injuries

**Hematomas** (Fig. 15–31). Subcapsular hematomas are usually due to superficial lacerations after blunt injury but may also occur after penetrating injury (and also after percutaneous liver biopsy). Arteriography shows an avascular mass with crowding of the peripheral branches and compression of the liver parenchyma. The margin of the compressed liver is often concave. The hematoma is best demonstrated in the hepatogram phase and often only in the oblique projection.

Intraparenchymal hematomas, which may also be due to blunt or penetrating injury (including percutaneous cholangiography or

drainage and needle biopsy), appear as avascular masses that displace (ie, by stretching, draping) the arterial and portal venous branches. Infected hematomas may show some vascularity and rim enhancement. Perihepatic hematomas displace the liver without distorting the liver margin.

PITFALLS IN DIAGNOSIS

1. Spontaneous or trauma-induced hematoma from hypervascular liver masses (eg, adenoma) cannot always be differentiated from hematoma in a normal liver.

2. Absence of a hepatogram in the region supplied by a small accessory hepatic artery may simulate a hematoma. However, there is no associated vascular abnormality such as crowding or displacement (Fig. 15–32).

**Contusion.** Hepatic contusion may be seen with or without associated laceration. On arteriography, this injury has a relatively characteristic appearance; ie, there is inhomogeneous hypervascularity with focal areas of contrast extravasation from lacerated small vessels. In this setting, a focal area of hypovascularity is suggestive of a hematoma. Hepatic contusion may also be seen in association with major vessel injury.

### Major Injuries

**Laceration.** Arterial laceration is seen either as contrast extravasation, if studied soon after the traumatic episode, or as arterial occlusion or false aneurysm. The portal and hepatic veins and the hepatic segment of the IVC may also be injured in severe blunt abdominal trauma.[119] Venous injuries are usually not studied by angiography because patients with such trauma are severely injured and require immediate surgery. The mortality associated with venous injury is very high. The portal vein may also be injured during an operation.[120]

**False Aneurysms** (Figs. 15–33 and 15–34). These usually manifest several days or weeks after the trauma. A frequent clinical presentation is right upper quadrant pain, transient or intermittent jaundice, and hemobilia. Although CT and ultrasonography may detect an occasional larger aneurysm, angiography is diagnostic.[121] The aneurysm or aneurysms are demonstrated on hepatic or celiac arteriography. In patients with hemobilia, contrast extravasation into the bile ducts may also be observed.

**Arterioportal/Arteriovenous Fistula** (Fig. 15–35; see also Fig. 15–22). Penetrating and occasionally blunt abdominal trauma may result in an arterioportal or rarely an arteriovenous fistula. In our own experience, the

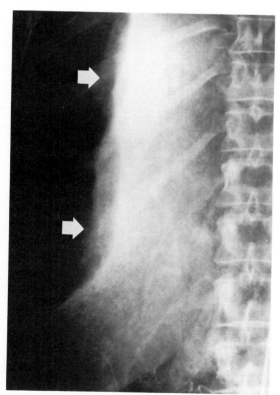

**Figure 15–31.** Subcapsular hepatic hematoma. Parenchymal phase from a hepatic arteriogram shows compression of the lateral margin of the liver by a subcapsular hematoma (*arrows*).

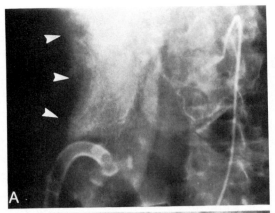

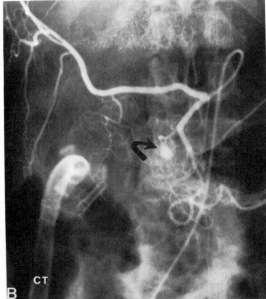

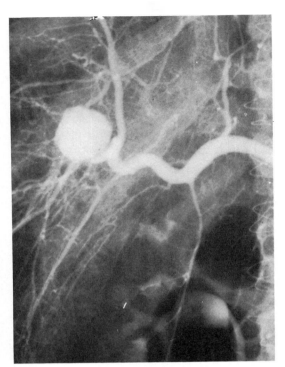

**Figure 15–33.** Blunt hepatic trauma. Right hepatic arteriogram shows an intrahepatic aneurysm. (From Kadir S et al: Radiology 134:335–339, 1980. Used with permission.)

**Figure 15–32.** Accessory right hepatic artery simulating hepatic hematoma. *A,* Parenchymal phase of common hepatic arteriogram shows a concave defect in the hepatogram at the lateral margin of the liver (*arrowheads*). *B,* Arteriogram of the accessory right hepatic artery shows vessels supplying the lateral portion of the liver which was unopacified on the common hepatic arteriogram. There is an aneurysm of a pancreaticoduodenal artery branch (*arrow*). CT = cholecystostomy tube.

most common cause of arterioportal fistulae is hepatobiliary surgery; less frequent causes are percutaneous transhepatic biliary drainage, penetrating abdominal trauma, and occasionally liver biopsy. Such fistulae usually involve centrally located hepatic artery branches and occasionally a peripheral branch.

## Other Injuries

Other manifestations of hepatic trauma are major vessel occlusion, hemobilia, and trau-

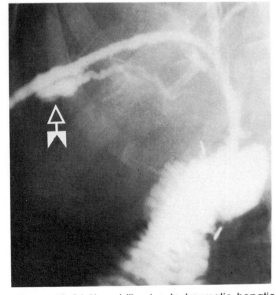

**Figure 15–34.** Hemobilia due to traumatic hepatic artery aneurysm following percutaneous transhepatic biliary drainage. Cholangiogram opacifies the peripherally located aneurysm (*arrow*). Bleeding was successfully controlled by insertion of a 9 Fr catheter introducer sheath for tamponade.

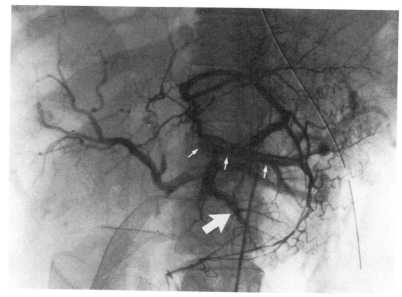

*Figure 15–35.* Operative hepatic trauma causing an arterioportal fistula. Arteriogram of the left hepatic/left gastric trunk shows a fistula (*arrow*) with portal vein opacification (*small arrows*). There is also some contrast reflux into the right hepatic and splenic arteries.

matic bile cysts. The last appear as avascular masses on arteriography.

**Hemobilia** (see Fig. 15–34). Percutaneous transhepatic biliary drainage is by far the most frequent cause of bleeding into the biliary tract. However, in the majority of patients, the bleeding is transient and subsides on conservative management. The etiology is a transient portal or hepatic vein to bile duct fistula that closes spontaneously. Hemobilia requiring interventional therapy is most frequently due to the development of a false aneurysm following biliary tract surgery. Other causes of hemobilia are blunt or penetrating trauma, percutaneous needle biopsy, and rupture of a hepatic or pancreaticoduodenal artery aneurysm.[122, 123]

## Splenic Trauma

The spleen is the most frequently injured intraabdominal organ in patients with blunt abdominal trauma. Although there are several signs that may suggest splenic trauma (rib fracture; renal, gastric, or colonic displacement; elevation of the left hemidiaphragm), none of them is specific. Splenic injury can also be detected by radionuclide scanning, ultrasonography, and CT, and most patients with minor trauma do not require angiography.

Current concepts of management call for a conservative approach because of the risk of overwhelming sepsis in splenectomized patients.[124] Angiography for either diagnosis or transcatheter therapy is performed only in a few patients.[26, 27] A splenic arteriogram is obtained in the AP projection. Oblique views are often necessary to detect or confirm the presence of an abnormality. Films are obtained over 20 to 25 seconds.

Splenic injury may manifest immediately after trauma or may become apparent several days or weeks later (delayed rupture). The angiographic findings may be subtle and vary with the severity of the injury.[125]

**Hematoma/Laceration** (Fig. 15–36). Splenic hematoma may be intra- or extracapsular. The former may be subcapsular or intraparenchymal. Larger hematomas usually represent a significant vascular injury.

The subcapsular hematoma causes compression and displacement of the normal splenic parenchyma. The spleen may be enlarged and the intrasplenic vessels stretched. On angiography, the parenchymal phase is very dense, and there may be early venous opacification, which simulates an arteriovenous fistula. The capsular vessels are draped around the hematoma. The margin between the hematoma and the compressed splenic parenchyma is fuzzy but may be sharp when viewed in profile.

The extrasplenic hematoma displaces the spleen. The parenchymal phase is usually not dense; the spleen does not appear compressed and is of normal size (unless enlarged owing to an underlying abnormality). Wedge-shaped avascular areas due to laceration or vascular occlusion may be present.

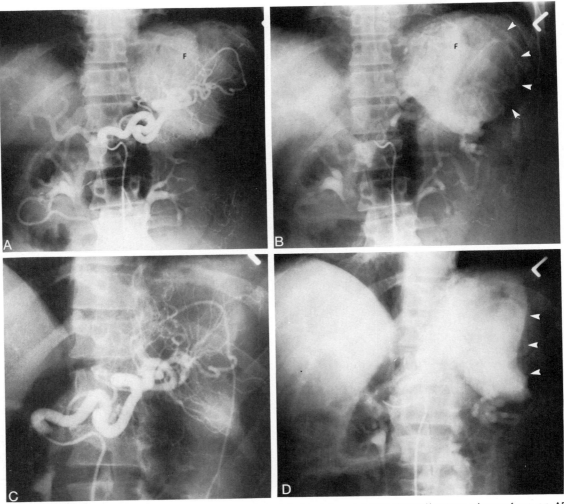

**Figure 15–36.** Subcapsular splenic hematoma. *A* and *B*, Arterial and parenchymal/venous phases from an AP splenic arteriogram show stretching of some lateral branches. A hypovascular area is seen over the lateral aspect of the spleen during the parenchymal phase (*arrowheads*). The splenic vein is occluded and gastric varices are seen. The latter were due to a pancreatic pseudocyst. F = gastric fundus. *C* and *D*, Arterial and parenchymal phases from a splenic arteriogram in the left anterior oblique projection. The subcapsular hematoma is better defined. The typical concave compression defect is seen during the parenchymal phase (*arrowheads*).

**Rupture/Fragmentation** (Fig. 15–37). Splenic rupture is a manifestation of severe injury. Vascular occlusion with resultant wedge-shaped infarcts or hypo- or avascular areas (hematomas) may be seen. One or more sites of contrast extravasation may also be present. Occasionally, there is arteriovenous shunting. The smaller splenic artery branches are splayed around the hypo- or avascular areas, and the parenchymal phase is inhomogeneous because of the presence of hematomas.

Fragmentation refers to injury resulting in the breakup of the spleen into two or more parts. Large avascular areas are seen during the parenchymal phase of the splenic arteri-ogram, and there is poor definition of the splenic outline in these regions. The overall spleen size may be normal or enlarged.

Other angiographic manifestations are occlusion of the splenic artery or vein and multiple small intraparenchymal aneurysms. The latter finding has also been called the "starry night" appearance and may involve the entire spleen or only a portion thereof (Fig. 15–38).

PITFALLS IN DIAGNOSIS

1. Wedge-shaped defects can also be due to fetal lobulation or abscess of the spleen.[2] In the former, oblique views and the absence of vascular abnormalities help to establish the diagnosis.

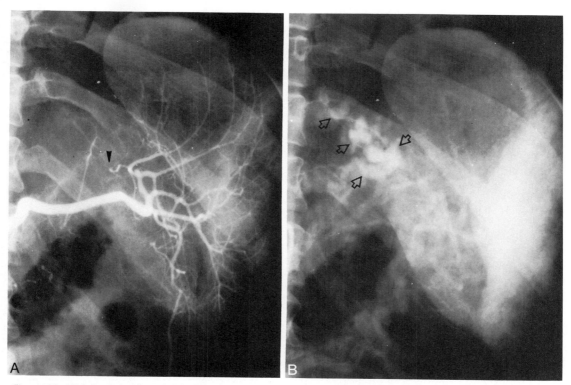

*Figure 15–37.* Splenic trauma. *A,* Arterial phase of a splenic arteriogram shows stretching, bowing, and amputation (*arrowhead*) of splenic branches. *B,* Parenchymal phase shows absent parenchymal stain in the upper portion of the spleen and contrast extravasation (*arrows*). At operation, the spleen was fragmented.

*Figure 15–38.* Splenic trauma. Splenic arteriogram shows multiple areas of focal contrast extravasation. This has also been called the "starry night" appearance.

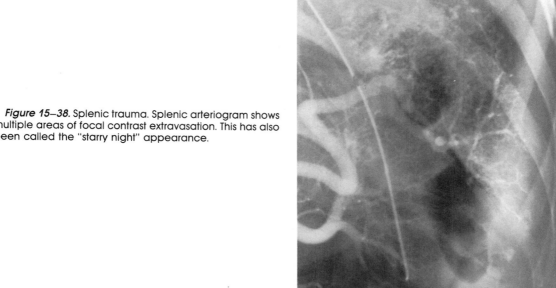

2. Avascular-appearing intrasplenic lesions may also be caused by cysts and by hypovascular metastases (melanoma, lymphoma).

3. Splenic artery occlusion may also be due to posttraumatic torsion of the spleen.[126]

4. Spontaneous subcapsular hematomas also occur in patients with infectious diseases and may be unrelated to the trauma.[127]

### Pancreatic Trauma

Blunt or penetrating trauma to the pancreas is a rare indication for angiography. The study is usually performed for the evaluation of associated injuries to other organs (eg, liver, spleen, or aorta). Contrast extravasation, traumatic aneurysms, or vascular occlusion may be present. Hematomas cause stretching and displacement of vessels.

### TUMORS

#### Hepatic Tumors

Although most circumscribed hepatic tumors, including hemangiomas, are readily identified by CT, some diffuse lesions may go undetected. Angiography plays a complementary role in evaluation and is indicated to establish or confirm the diagnosis in primary hepatic tumors and to provide a preoperative vascular "road map." In addition, transcatheter therapy has been used successfully in some tumors (eg, giant hemangiomas, hepatomas, and endocrine-active metastases).[22, 23, 128]

Angiography also plays an important role in the diagnosis, differential diagnosis, and management of iatrogenic hepatic tumors induced by medications or exposure to toxic agents (Table 15–7). Table 15–8 lists the salient angiographic features of the more common hepatic tumors.

#### Hormone-Related Hepatic Tumors

**Adenoma** (Figs. 15–39 and 15–40). The benign liver cell adenoma, which had been a rare tumor occurring most frequently (>90%) in women of child-bearing age, is observed with much greater frequency since the use of oral contraceptives has become widespread.[129] It develops in an otherwise healthy liver, is encapsulated, and is composed of normal hepatocytes. This tumor is usually a solitary lesion, although multiple adenomas

**TABLE 15–7. Iatrogenic Liver Tumors Induced by Drugs or Toxic Agents**

| Tumor | Drug/Agent | Reference |
|---|---|---|
| Adenoma | Oral contraceptives | 129 |
| Focal nodular hyperplasia | Oral contraceptives | 129 |
| Angiosarcoma | Oral contraceptives Androgenic-anabolic steroids Substituted hydrazines (isoniazid) Vinyl chloride, arsenic, Thorotrast | 130–133 |
| Hepatoblastoma | Oral contraceptives | 134 |
| Hepatoma | Oral contraceptives Diethylstilbestrol Androgenic-anabolic steroids | 135–137 |

have also been observed. It may be pedunculated in approximately 10% of patients. Benign liver cell adenoma may develop after several months to years of oral contraceptive intake or may manifest after the contraceptives have been discontinued.

Symptoms may be absent (ie, the tumor is discovered incidentally at angiography or laparotomy); the patient may have right upper quadrant pain; or a hepatic mass may be palpated during a routine physical examination. Occasionally, spontaneous hemorrhage resulting in a subcapsular hematoma or free intraperitoneal rupture may be the initial symptom (Fig. 15–40). The latter may be massive and can be fatal.[138] Because of the risk of hemorrhage, the treatment of choice is resection, although regression of the tumor may occur after discontinuation of oral contraceptives.[139]

On angiography, the lesion is usually round, hypervascular, and well circumscribed[140] (see Table 15–8). The hepatic arteries are enlarged and displaced by the tumor, so that the feeding arteries often lie at the tumor periphery and give off numerous branches to the lesion. Areas of hemorrhage and focal necrosis may be present and appear as hypo- or avascular regions. Some tumors are hypovascular but demonstrate fine neovascularity. Adenomas complicated by subcapsular hemorrhage may be difficult to localize, and the arteriogram may show only the subcapsular hematoma. The risk of hemorrhage is higher in tumors associated with the use of oral contraceptives than in those arising spontaneously.[129]

**TABLE 15–8. Hepatic Tumors: Angiographic Appearance and Differential Diagnosis***

| Tumor | Feeding Size | Artery Location | Neo-vascularity | Contrast Pooling (Lakes) | Tumor Stain | A-V Shunt | Veins | Tc-Sulfur Colloid Uptake | Gallium Uptake |
|---|---|---|---|---|---|---|---|---|---|
| Adenoma | ↑ | Peripheral | + | - | + (- in some) | Occasional | Displaced | ↓ | N |
| Focal nodular hyperplasia | ↑ | Peripheral (large tumors); central (small tumors) | Occasional | - | + | Rarely | Displaced | N in 1/3, or ↓, or ↑ | N |
| Regenerating nodule | N | Central | - | - | - | Very rarely | Displaced, stretched | N | N |
| Hemangioma | N or ↑ | Peripheral (in cavernous) | - | + ≥30 sec | - | Giant heman-gioma of infancy; Hemangio-endothelioma | Unaffected | ↓ | |
| Hepatoma | ↑ | Peripheral or diffuse | + | + | + - (if necrotic) | + | Invaded | ↓ | N or ↑ |
| Hepatoblastoma | ↑ | Peripheral or diffuse | + | + | + | Rare | Displaced | ↓ | ↑ |
| Cholangiocarci-noma | N or ↑ | Occlusions, encasement | + | - | + (~60%) | - | Occlusion, encasement | ↓ | N or ↑ |
| Angiosarcoma | N | Displaced | - | + | Rimlike, - (if necrotic) | - | Displaced | ↓ | |
| Hypervascular metastases | N or ↑ | Displaced | + | + | + | - | Displaced, encased, occluded | ↓ | N or ↑ |
| Hypovascular metastases | N | Displaced | + | - | Rimlike or absent | - | Displaced, encased, occluded | ↓ | N or ↑ |

↓ = decreased; ↑ = increased; N = normal; + = present; - = absent.
*Includes data from references 140 to 143.

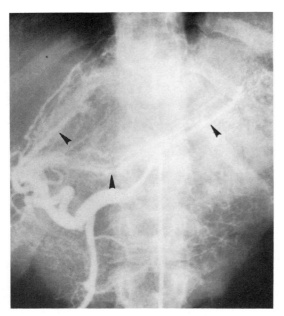

*Figure 15–39.* Adenoma. Common hepatic arteriogram shows a large adenoma in the left lobe of the liver. Diffuse neovascularity is present and the hepatic artery branches supplying the tumor are enlarged (*arrowheads*).

**Focal Nodular Hyperplasia** (Figs. 15–41 and 15–42). Focal nodular hyperplasia (FNH) is a benign, nonencapsulated hepatic tumor. It occurs most frequently in women of childbearing age but has also been observed in

men and children in association with other lesions.[129, 144] The increased incidence of such tumors has been linked to the use of oral contraceptives.[129] Typically, FNH is a solitary subcapsular or pedunculated mass. Multiple lesions are observed in approximately 20% of patients. Clinically, FNH is frequently discovered as an incidental asymptomatic mass. Spontaneous hemorrhage is rare. The tumor usually regresses upon discontinuation of the oral contraceptives.

Histologically, FNH has a characteristic appearance. There is a central fibrous core with radiating fibrous septa, which divide it into pseudolobules. This gives it the typical "spoke wheel" appearance occasionally seen on arteriography.

On arteriography, FNH appears as a well-circumscribed, hypervascular mass. In large tumors, the hepatic artery is enlarged and is located at the tumor periphery. Numerous tortuous vascular channels are present, which represent hypertrophied normal vasculature. In smaller tumors, the hepatic artery enters the tumor centrally and often divides in a spoke wheel pattern. In the parenchymal phase, there is a fine granular appearance and lucent septa are seen. Arteriovenous shunting is observed rarely.

**Regenerating Hepatic Nodules** (Fig. 15–43). These are most frequently seen in hepatic cirrhosis and following hepatic resec-

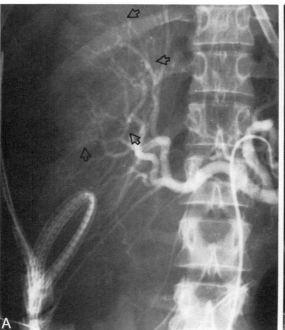

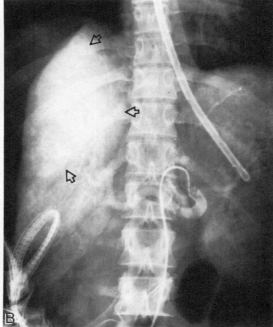

*Figure 15–40.* Hepatic adenoma presenting as a subcapsular hematoma. *A,* Arterial phase of the hepatic arteriogram shows abnormal vasculature over the lateral aspect of the liver (*arrows*). Some hepatic artery branches appear compressed and displaced medially. *B,* Parenchymal phase from the same arteriogram shows a subcapsular hematoma and an area of intense parenchymal staining (*arrows*).

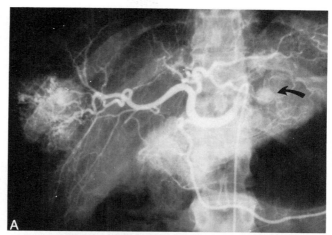

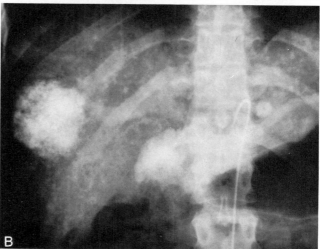

**Figure 15–41.** Multiple focal nodular hyperplasia lesions and peliosis hepatis. Arterial (*A*) and parenchymal (*B*) phase of a common hepatic arteriogram shows hypervascular masses in the right, quadrate, and left (*arrow*) hepatic lobes. Multiple small homogeneously opacified accumulations of contrast medium (peliosis) are also visualized. The hepatic artery branch leading to the larger right hepatic lesion is enlarged and tortuous. *C,* The gastroduodenal arteriogram is normal. *Note:* Initially, the lesion in the quadrate lobe was considered to be a mass in the head of the pancreas supplied by branches of the gastroduodenal artery. The gastroduodenal arteriogram excluded this possibility, and a normal pancreas was found at operation.

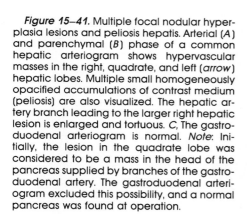

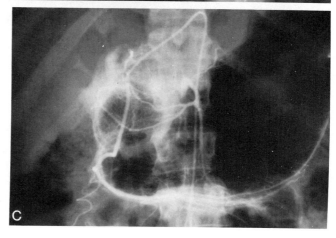

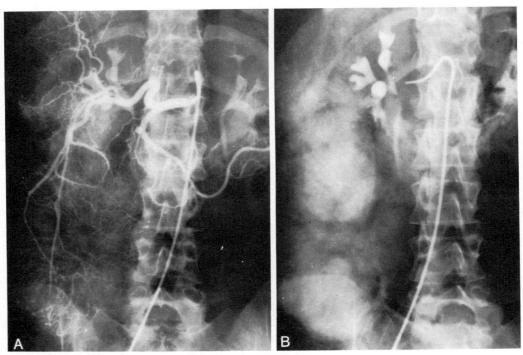

*Figure 15–42.* Focal nodular hyperplasia. *A,* Arterial phase of a common hepatic arteriogram shows an enlarged liver. A large mass with fine neovascularity and a suggestion of radial distribution of the vessels is seen. *B,* Parenchymal phase from the same arteriogram shows lucent septa.

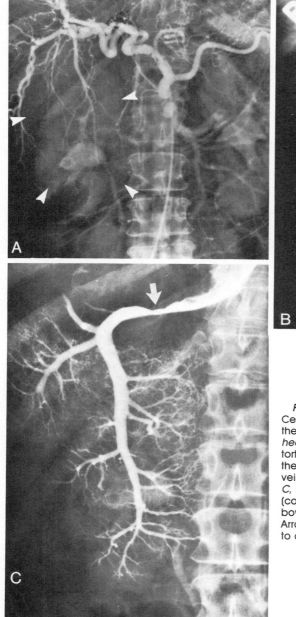

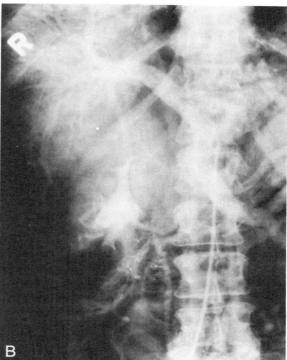

*Figure 15–43.* Macroregenerating hepatic nodules. *A,* Celiac arteriogram shows a relative paucity of vessels in the lower portion of the right lobe of the liver (*arrowheads*). The vessels are stretched, in comparison with the tortuous vessels of the cirrhotic liver in the remainder of the organ. *B,* Arterial portogram shows paucity of portal vein branches in the region of the regenerating nodule. *C,* Hepatic venogram shows distortion of the branches (compare with Figure 15–11). Several branches are bowed and others show an abrupt change in course. Arrow points to narrowing of the main hepatic vein due to compression by a nodule.

tion. They may become quite large and on angiography they appear as isodense or hypovascular masses. There is no neovascularity. The hepatic artery branches are of normal caliber and are centrally located in the nodule, but are stretched if the nodules are large. The portal vein branches are displaced around the mass, and the hepatic veins are distorted.

**Peliosis Hepatis** (Fig. 15–44; see also Fig. 15–41). This refers to a benign intrahepatic vascular disorder of questionable clinical significance. It is discussed in this section because of its frequent association with benign and malignant tumors, especially with those that are hormonally induced. Histologically, there are endothelial-lined, blood-filled vascular spaces that are in communication with the hepatic sinusoids. In addition, the sinusoids themselves are dilated. Rupture of such cystic-dilated spaces, leading to intraperitoneal hemorrhage, is very rare.[145]

Although the exact etiology remains unclear, peliosis hepatis may represent a manifestation of the vasodilatory response of the central venule to sex hormones.[146, 147] It has also been observed in the absence of hepatic tumors, in women taking oral contraceptives, in patients on steroid medications, and in patients with chronic infections, diabetes mellitus, or chronic renal failure.[138, 146–148]

On arteriography, peliosis hepatis has a characteristic appearance. During the parenchymal phase of the hepatic arteriogram, multiple round collections of contrast medium are seen. These may vary in size from several millimeters to 1.5 cm and are scattered throughout the liver. Rarely, larger collections may be seen.[105] The contrast persists during the early venous phase. There is no mass effect or early venous opacification. The lesions do not opacify on the portal phase or during hepatic venography. Hepatic wedge, hepatic venous, and intrasplenic pressures are normal if other hepatic disease does not coexist.[148]

On angiography, peliosis hepatis can be misdiagnosed as hypervascular metastases or cavernous hemangiomas. Peliosis can be differentiated from these lesions by its following characteristics:

1. Absence of feeding arteries or draining veins.

2. Homogeneous collection of contrast medium and absence of nodularity.

3. Contrast accumulation is not as dense as in cavernous hemangiomas.

PITFALLS IN DIAGNOSIS

1. Hypovascular tumors: In most cases, angiography can help in differentiating between adenoma and hepatoma. This may not be possible if the hepatoma is hypovascular. Regenerating nodules are also hypovascular or isodense with the liver.

2. The arteriographic picture of adenoma and FNH can be very similar and differentiation is often not possible.

Because of the absence of Kupffer's cells, adenomas and hepatomas do not take up sulfur colloid, whereas FNH and regenerating nodules contain Kupffer's cells and take up the tracer. In some patients with FNH and regenerating nodules, the sulfur colloid uptake is diminished. In order for the radio-

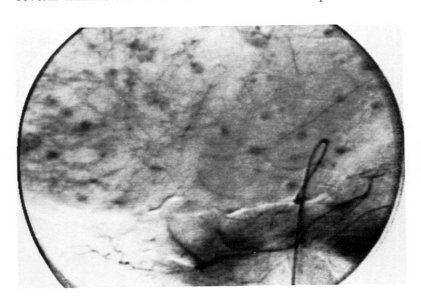

*Figure 15–44.* Peliosis hepatis. Parenchymal phase of a digital subtraction hepatic arteriogram shows multiple focal accumulations of contrast medium.

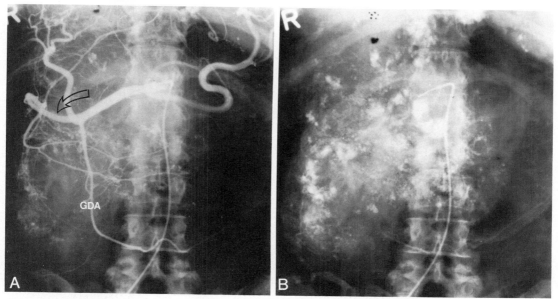

**Figure 15–45.** Giant capillary hemangioma of the left hepatic lobe. *A,* Arterial phase of the celiac arteriogram shows distortion of the normal anatomy with a markedly enlarged left hepatic artery, which is displaced to the right (*arrow*), supplying a massively enlarged left lobe. GDA = gastroduodenal artery. *B,* Parenchymal phase from the same arteriogram shows a nonhomogeneous accumulation of contrast medium. Several small hemangiomas are also present in the right lobe.

nuclide study to be helpful, the tumor must be at least 2 cm in size.

### Hemangiomas

This is the most common benign hepatic tumor and is rarely symptomatic. Most frequently, it is an incidental finding at angiography.

**Capillary Hemangiomas.** These lesions are usually small and asymptomatic. Rarely, they become very large and present as an upper abdominal mass (Fig. 15–45). On the arteriogram, the feeding artery may be enlarged in even smaller lesions. This branches haphazardly into a tangle of capillaries. In the parenchymal phase, there is an inhomogeneous stain. Arteriovenous shunting is absent.

**Cavernous Hemangiomas.** Histologically, the cavernous hemangioma consists of thin-walled, endothelium-lined, septated vascular spaces. Occasionally, these fibrous septa calcify, and very rarely a phlebolith may be present.[149, 150] Cavernous hemangioma occurs most frequently in multiparous women. An increase in size may occur during pregnancy. The tumor is usually single, small, and asymptomatic. Occasionally, multiple or large hemangiomas are observed. Symptoms are usually due to their large size and are only occasionally caused by spontaneous rupture or platelet sequestration and thrombocytopenia.[150–152] The latter is more common in infants.

Cavernous hemangiomas can be diagnosed by CT.[153] On the arteriogram, they have a very characteristic appearance (Fig. 15–46). The feeding vessels are usually not dilated unless the tumor is very large. In the late arterial and parenchymal phases, there is dense opacification (from the periphery) of well-circumscribed, dilated, irregular, nodular-appearing vascular spaces. Smaller lesions appear crescent shaped. The contrast medium in the vascular spaces persists late into the venous phase. The lesions do not opacify via the portal veins.

**Giant Hemangioma of Infancy.** This lesion is seen in the newborn or in small infants. Clinically, there is hepatomegaly in an otherwise asymptomatic infant or high output cardiac failure due to the presence of a large arteriovenous shunt in the tumor. In the former, the lesions involute within the first years of life. In hemangiomas associated with congestive heart failure, an abdominal bruit and cardiac murmurs may be present, and cutaneous hemangiomas are observed frequently.[154] Treatment with steroids or transcatheter embolization has been successful.

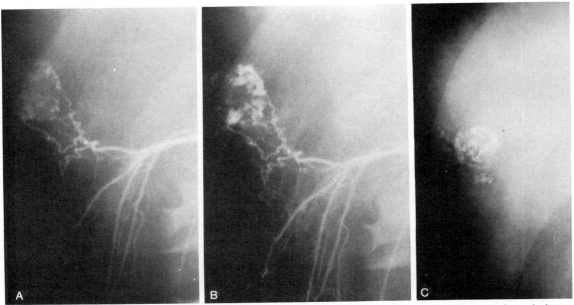

*Figure 15–46.* Cavernous hemangioma. *A,* Early and *B,* late arterial phase of hepatic arteriogram shows tortuous but nonenlarged branches supplying the hemangioma. A dense peripheral stain is present. *C,* Late venous phase shows a persistent, dense stain characteristic of a cavernous hemangioma.

In tumors without arteriovenous shunting, the hepatic artery is usually not enlarged. The parenchymal phase is characterized by a mottled appearance with demonstration of multiple vascular lakes (Fig. 15–47). In tumors with arteriovenous shunting, the hepatic artery and the supraceliac aorta are enlarged. Neovascularity, vascular lakes, and arteriovenous (hepatic vein) shunting are demonstrated.

Occasionally, if the lesion is diffuse, differentiation from hepatoma may be difficult because of the presence of bizarre vascularity and vascular lakes. On the other hand, in hepatoblastoma, congestive heart failure has not been reported and arteriovenous shunting occurs infrequently.

**Hemangioendotheliomas.** These lesions are also seen in children and may present with hepatomegaly and congestive heart failure. Histologically, there are thick-walled, endothelium-lined vascular spaces that are occasionally calcified.[155] The feeding arteries are enlarged and tortuous, and do not taper. The tumor is hypervascular, the tumor stain is inhomogeneous, and vascular lakes are present. In contrast to cavernous hemangiomas, the contrast medium clears rapidly from these vascular lakes.[155] Neovasculature is usually absent, but arteriovenous shunting is present.

**Hereditary Hemorrhagic Telangiectasia.** Hepatic lesions may be observed in patients with this disease. The hepatic artery is enlarged, and arteriovenous and arterioportal shunting may be observed. The liver may be diffusely involved.[61]

PITFALLS IN DIAGNOSIS

1. Capillary hemangiomas may be mistaken for hypervascular metastases. In the latter, the feeding vessels do not taper.[150] The branching pattern in metastases is also irregular, but the clearance of the contrast medium is faster than in hemangiomas.

2. Large cavernous hemangiomas may be difficult to differentiate from hepatoma. Some distinguishing features of hemangiomas are normal-sized feeding vessels (occasionally these may also be enlarged), normal branching pattern, and prolonged, dense opacification of the cavernous vascular spaces (>30 seconds).

3. Hemangioendotheliomas cannot be distinguished from hemangioendotheliosarcoma on the basis of the arteriogram.

*Malignant Hepatic Tumors*

**Cholangiocarcinoma.** After hepatoma, this is the second most common malignant primary hepatic tumor. It accounts for approximately one third of all malignancies originating in the liver. Cholangiocarcinoma occurs

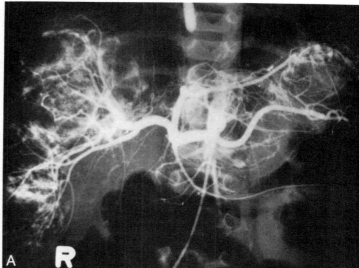

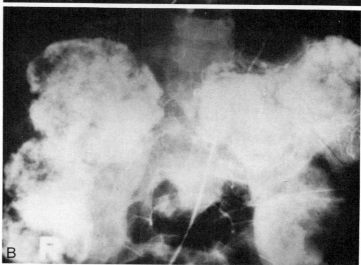

*Figure 15–47.* Giant hemangioma of infancy. *A,* Early arterial phase of celiac arteriogram shows enlargement of the hepatic artery and branches. *B,* Parenchymal phase of the same arteriogram shows a large cavernous hemangioma involving both the left and the right lobes. (Courtesy of Dr. CA Athanasoulis.)

most frequently in males in the fifth to seventh decades.

Angiographically, it is quite similar to the anaplastic hepatoma. Cholangiocarcinoma is essentially a hypovascular tumor that shows vascular encasement, occlusion, and displacement of primarily the intrahepatic branches (Fig. 15–48). These changes involve both the hepatic artery and the portal vein. Neovascularity is present in about half the patients, and the tumor stain is either absent or very poor. Frequent locations for the tumor are the distal left and right and proximal common hepatic ducts; tumors at these sites lead to obstructive jaundice without gallbladder dilatation. On the hepatogram phase, dilated intrahepatic ducts are seen as negative defects.

**Hepatoblastoma.** This is the third most common abdominal tumor in children. It occurs primarily in children less than 3 years of age and is most frequently located in the right lobe of the liver. The symptoms are those of an upper abdominal mass and are occasionally due to endocrine-active substances produced in the tumor (eg, precocious puberty).[142]

On arteriography, the supraceliac aorta and the hepatic artery are enlarged (Fig. 15–49). The tumor is hypervascular and shows marked neovascularity and a dense stain. Vascular lakes may also be present. Avascular areas within the tumor are indicative of necrosis. Arteriovenous shunting is not characteristic of this lesion.

Inferior venacavography should be per-

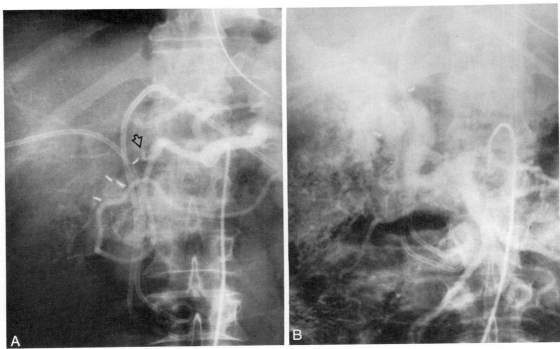

**Figure 15–48.** Cholangiocarcinoma. *A*, Celiac arteriogram shows encasement and occlusion of the right hepatic artery (*arrow*). B, Venous phase of the superior mesenteric arteriogram shows cavernous transformation of the portal vein. Enlarged, tortuous collaterals are present in the porta hepatis. The main portal vein and the left branch of the portal vein are occluded. Surgical clips are from a staging exploratory laparotomy. Bilateral percutaneous biliary drainage catheters were placed for obstructive jaundice.

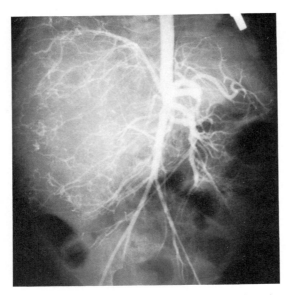

**Figure 15–49.** Hepatoblastoma. Abdominal aortogram shows an enlarged right hepatic artery draped over a large mass. The aorta above the celiac artery is also enlarged. There is extensive neovascularity. In addition, there is catheter-induced spasm of the left external iliac artery. (Courtesy of Dr. P Stanley. From Stanley P: Pediatric Angiography. Baltimore, Williams & Wilkins, 1982. Used with permission.)

formed in all children suspected of having malignant hepatic masses. Demonstration of caval involvement is indicative of unresectability.

**Hepatoma (Hepatic Cell Carcinoma)** (Figs. 15–50 to 15–52; see also Chapter 6, Fig. 6–2, and Chapter 13, Fig. 13–5). Hepatoma, which is the most common primary malignant tumor of the liver, is a highly malignant neoplasm with a poor prognosis. It occurs more frequently in Orientals and is observed in all age groups (older children and adults).[141, 156, 157] The male to female ratio is 5:1. In non-Oriental adults and children, hepatoma occurs most often as a complication of chronic liver disease (eg, cirrhosis).

Symptoms include persistent right upper quadrant pain, fever, weight loss, malaise, hypoglycemia, erythrocytosis, hepatomegaly, and ascites. Endocrine-active substances produced by the tumor may lead to virilization, gynecomastia, and hypercalcemia. Serum alpha-fetoprotein levels are elevated in the majority of patients.

Plain radiographs of the abdomen may demonstrate tumor calcification. The

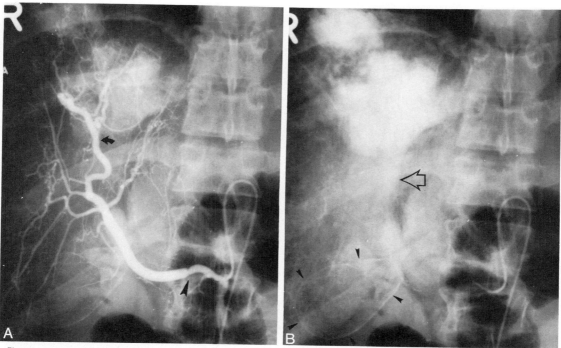

*Figure 15–50.* Multicentric hepatic cell carcinoma with arterioportal shunting in a teen-aged male patient. *A,* Arteriogram of the right hepatic artery arising from the superior mesenteric artery shows hypervascular tumor nodules. Hepatic artery branches supplying the tumor are enlarged (*arrow*). Arrowhead points to catheter-induced spasm of the hepatic artery. *B,* Parenchymal phase from the same arteriogram shows a dense tumor stain and opacification of the portal vein (*arrow*). Arrowheads point to the normal gallbladder wall blush. Several tumor nodules were also present in the left lobe of the liver.

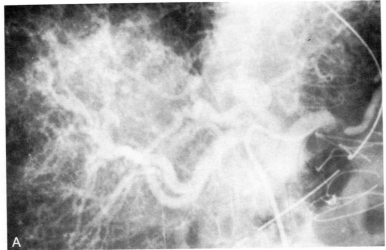

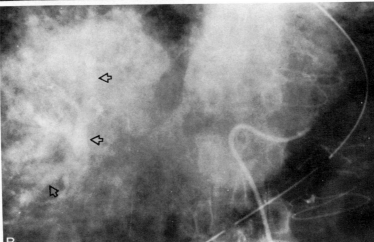

*Figure 15–51.* Diffuse hepatic cell carcinoma. *A,* Arterial phase from a common hepatic arteriogram shows marked enlargement of the hepatic arteries, early opacification of portal vein branches, and diffuse neovascularity. *B,* Parenchymal phase shows arterioportal shunting. Arrows point to the intrahepatic portal vein branches.

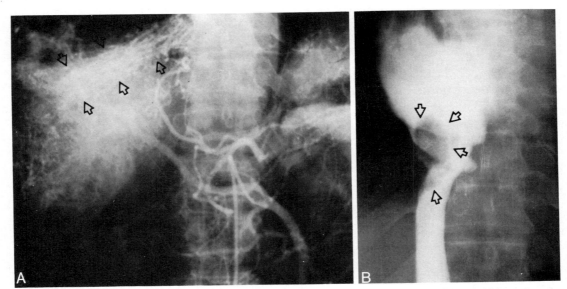

*Figure 15–52.* Hepatic venous extension of hepatic cell carcinoma. *A,* Arteriogram of the right hepatic artery arising from the superior mesenteric artery. There is a hypervascular hepatic cell carcinoma involving almost the entire shrunken liver. Streaky, irregular vessels are seen in the hepatic vein, extending toward the right atrium (*arrow*). *B,* Inferior venacavagram shows tumor extending into the inferior vena cava and right atrium (*arrows*).

99mtechnetium sulfur colloid scan shows decreased uptake, whereas the 67gallium citrate scan shows increased gallium uptake.

Arteriography is indicated for (1) the evaluation of blood supply to the tumor (vascular road map), (2) assessment of the extent of the lesion, (3) palliative embolization, and (4) occasionally for establishing the diagnosis in lesions that are not diagnosed by other means, eg, are isodense with the liver. Conventional arteriography, DSA, and intraarterial dynamic CT and occasionally inferior venacavography and hepatic venography are performed as part of the tumor workup.

Hepatomas may be solitary, multicentric, or diffuse. The solitary type involves the right lobe most frequently. In addition, solitary hepatomas may be well differentiated or anaplastic. In the former, the typical arteriographic features are enlarged arterial feeders, coarse neovascularity, vascular lakes, dense tumor stain, and arterioportal shunting. The abnormal vessels may also appear stretched around an area of necrosis. Uninvolved segments of the liver show the typical corkscrew vessels seen in cirrhosis. In the anaplastic type, there is vascular encasement, displacement, and fine neovascularity. The tumor stain is less dense and poorly defined. Enlargement of the arterial feeders and arteriovenous shunting are seen infrequently. Occasionally, the tumor may be totally hypovascular.

Portal venous invasion and/or occlusion is seen in 73 to 100% of hepatomas.[158–160] The hepatic veins are involved infrequently. The tumor often grows into the hepatic veins and inferior vena cava, leading to the Budd-Chiari syndrome (Fig. 15–52), and occasionally it grows into the bile ducts (Fig. 15–53). Intravenous growth of the tumor is demonstrated on the late arterial and venous phases of the hepatic arteriogram as parallel vascular streaks.[160]

**Metastases** (Figs. 15–54 to 15–56). Metastases are by far the most common malignant lesions of the liver. They may be solitary or multiple and may demonstrate hypo-, moderate, or hypervascularity. Most liver metastases are detectable by CT and rarely require angiography for diagnosis.

The main indications for angiography of liver metastases are:[23, 161, 162]

1. Delineation of vascular anatomy for placement of chemotherapy catheters or resection of solitary lesions.

2. Assessment of resectability of a solitary metastasis.

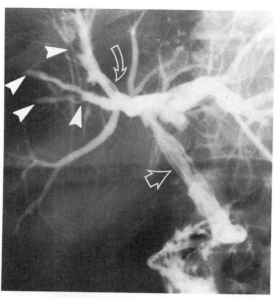

**Figure 15–53.** Hepatic cell carcinoma growing into the biliary ducts. Cholangiogram shows tumor encasement and occlusion of the right hepatic branches (*arrowheads*) and tumor growth into the right hepatic and common bile ducts (*open arrows*).

3. Palliative embolization or chemotherapy in metastases from endocrine-active tumors.

4. Demonstration of occult metastases not detected by other means.

Selective hepatic arteriography is usually necessary for the detection of hypovascular metastases. Hypervascular lesions may also be demonstrated on the celiac arteriogram. In addition, the infusion hepatic arteriogram, pharmacoangiography, or arterial dynamic CT scanning may be used to facilitate detection of hypovascular lesions and to improve visualization of moderately vascular lesions.[163]

Before placement of chemotherapy catheters for use with the implantable pump, a diagnostic arteriogram is performed from the femoral approach. If the infusion catheter is to be placed past the gastroduodenal artery, this vessel is embolized. From the left axillary approach, a 6.3 Fr H-1 catheter is then placed in the vessel to be infused.

The angiographic picture depends upon the size and histology of the metastasis. The vascularity ranges from hypo- to hypervascular (Table 15–9). In large hypovascular lesions, there is vascular displacement, and the lesion is best demonstrated on the parenchymal phase. Tumor vessels may be seen after pharmacological enhancement. The moderate and hypervascular metastases

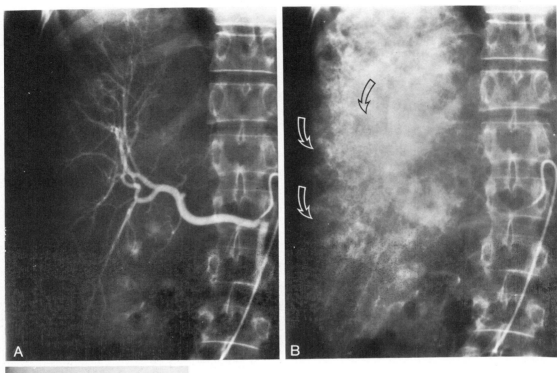

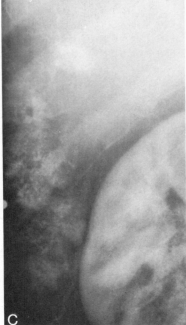

*Figure 15–54.* Hypervascular hepatic metastases. *A,* Right hepatic arteriogram in a patient with metastatic sigmoid carcinoma shows some distortion and stretching of the branches. Fine neovascularity is seen, especially in the upper portion of the right lobe. *B,* Parenchymal phase from the same arteriogram shows diffuse metastases. Several lesions show central hypovascularity suggesting necrosis (*arrows*). C, Hypervascular metastases from renal cell carcinoma. Note similarity to Figure 15–46.

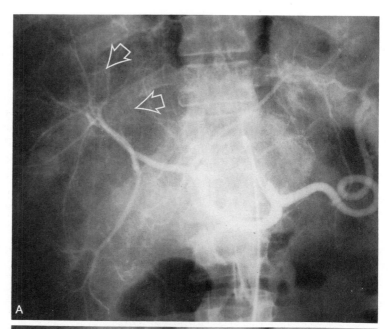

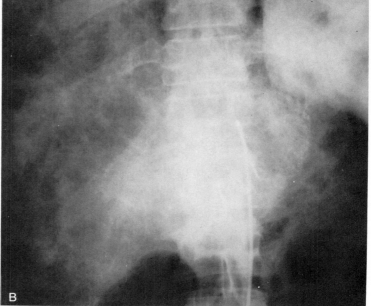

*Figure 15–55.* Hypovascular hepatic metastases from colonic carcinoma. *A,* Celiac arteriogram shows stretching and distortion of hepatic artery branches. Fine neovascularity is seen in some areas (*arrows*). B, Parenchymal phase from the same study shows hypovascular areas corresponding to the metastatic foci.

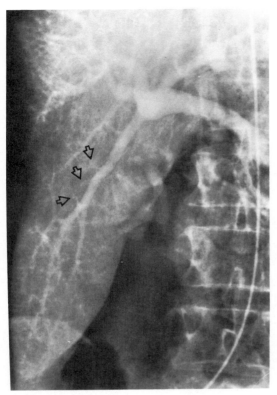

*Figure 15–56.* Amputation of portal vein branches by metastatic colonic carcinoma in a patient with a large solitary metastasis in the right lobe. Venous phase of celiac arteriogram shows several of the portal vein branches in this region are amputated (*arrows*).

show neovascularity and a variable tumor stain. On the late arterial phase, intravenous tumor casts may be demonstrated.[164]

Although venous studies are rarely performed for the evaluation of hepatic metastases, these may demonstrate an abnormality in a large number of patients. Amputation or encasement of portal vein branches is characteristic of hepatic metastases (Fig. 15–56). In addition, the portal vein branches can be stretched and displaced. Although a portion of the blood supply to hepatic metastases is via the portal venous system, the metastases do not opacify on the portal hepatogram.

Retrograde hepatic venography may dem-

onstrate an abnormality in up to 60% of patients with liver metastases.[165] The abnormal findings include: encasement, displacement, and occlusions of the hepatic veins. During the parenchymal phase of the hepatic venogram, the lesions do not opacify and may be demonstrated as negative defects.

PITFALLS IN DIAGNOSIS

1. The irregular encasement of hepatic artery branches, typical of neoplastic encasement, is also seen in amyloidosis.[166] Occasionally, diffuse atherosclerosis may also simulate neoplastic encasement.

2. Diffuse hepatic enlargement with splaying and displacement of hepatic artery branches without encasement are also seen in lymphoma.[167] Occasionally, neovascularity may also be present.

3. Amputation of portal vein branches is typical for liver metastases but may also be seen in arterioportal fistula.

## Tumors of the Spleen

Splenic tumors are rare, and there are few indications for diagnostic splenic arteriography. Cysts, adenomas, and hemangiomas have been studied by arteriography.[90, 168] Calcified splenic cysts have occasionally been misdiagnosed as aneurysms (see Fig. 15–63). One of the most frequent malignant tumors of the spleen is lymphoma; however, angiography does not play a role in the assessment of this disease. Of the metastatic lesions, melanoma is seen as a solitary lesion or as multiple metastases. In both cases, it is hypovascular. Sarcoidosis also shows multiple defects, which may be indistinguishable from metastases (Fig. 15–57).

## Tumors of the Pancreas

### Adenoma

Pancreatic adenomas are rare tumors and are most frequently located in the tail. Two different types are identified: microcystic adenoma and mucinous cystadenoma.[169]

**TABLE 15–9. Hepatic Metastases: Angiographic Appearance**

| Hypervascular | Hyper- or Hypovascular | Hypovascular |
|---|---|---|
| Carcinoid | Cholangiocarcinoma | Esophageal carcinoma |
| Choriocarcinoma | Cholecystocarcinoma | Bronchogenic carcinoma |
| Cystadenocarcinoma | Gastrointestinal carcinomas | Pancreatic carcinoma |
| Islet cell carcinomas | Malignant melanoma | |
| Renal cell carcinoma | | |
| Thyroid carcinoma | | |
| Uterine cancers | | |

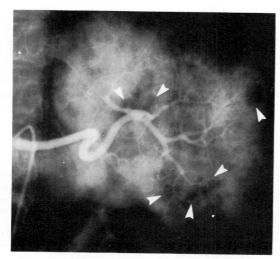

*Figure 15–57.* Sarcoidosis of the spleen. Mid-arterial phase of a splenic arteriogram shows a nonhomogeneous splenic parenchymogram with multiple nodular hypovascular sarcoid granulomas (*arrowheads*).

**Microcystic Adenoma.** This is a benign, lobulated tumor composed of multiple small (1 to 2 mm) cysts. It occurs most frequently in women (ratio of 4.5:1), with the age of onset between 30 and 80 years. The overall tumor size can be large (up to 25 cm).[169] Amorphous calcifications are seen occasionally. On arteriography, the tumor is hypervascular with dilated feeding arteries, dense tumor blush, and densely opacified veins. Neovascularity is present, but vascular encasement does not occur. The splenic vein may be occluded by compression, and arteriovenous shunting is observed occasionally.

**Mucinous Cystadenoma.** This is a thick-walled, uni- or multilocular, potentially malignant tumor composed of large cystic spaces. It is seen in women in an 8.6:1 ratio.[169] This tumor can also become quite large and may demonstrate mural calcification. On arteriography, it is usually hypovascular with sparse neovascularity. Vascular encasement and splenic vein occlusion may be present. Angiographically, the benign tumor cannot be differentiated from its malignant counterpart.

### Adenocarcinoma

This is a highly malignant, poorly vascularized, infiltrating tumor arising from the ductal epithelium of the pancreas. It occurs more frequently in males (ratio of 2:1), with the mean age of onset about 55 years. In the majority of patients (>75%), the tumor is located in the head of the pancreas. The second most frequent location is the body of the pancreas.

The role of arteriography in the management of pancreatic cancer has changed since the introduction of CT and endoscopic retrograde cholangiopancreatography (ERCP). Arteriography is rarely indicated for diagnosis because the lesions are readily diagnosed by CT. The indications for arteriography are:

1. To assess resectability of small tumors.
2. Rarely, to establish the diagnosis if CT is equivocal.
3. To provide a vascular "road map" in certain individuals.

Carcinoma of the pancreas can be diagnosed by arteriography in close to 90% of patients.[170] Angiographic evaluation should include:

1. Splenic arteriography: To evaluate the splenic artery and vein and the pancreatic arteries.
2. Common hepatic or gastroduodenal arteriography: To evaluate the pancreatic head and the liver for metastatic foci.
3. Dorsal pancreatic arteriography: To evaluate the pancreatic vessels if the diagnosis is uncertain.
4. Superior mesenteric arteriography: To evaluate the superior mesenteric artery and vein.

The angiographic findings are (Figs. 15–58 and 15–59; see also Chapter 14, Fig. 14–13):

*Arterial encasement:* This may be smooth or serrated in larger arteries. Small arteries appear serpiginous owing to fibrotic distortion and/or encasement.

*Arterial occlusion:* Large (SMA, celiac artery branches) and small (pancreatic) arteries may be involved.

*Venous encasement or occlusion:* Lesions of the head of the pancreas may encase or occlude the superior mesenteric and distal splenic veins. Lesions of the body and tail affect the splenic vein. Splenomegaly may be present and collateral venous channels are demonstrated.

*Neovascularity:* This is seen in approximately 50% of patients.

Vascular displacement is usually absent because of the infiltrative nature of the tumor. Similarly, a tumor blush and arteriovenous shunting are not seen.

Although angiographic findings can detect the presence of pancreatic carcinoma in close to 90% of patients,[170] these findings may be simulated by a host of other diseases, including carcinomas of the distal common bile duct, duodenum, ampulla, or stomach; pancreatitis; peripancreatic metastases; penetrating gastric and antral ulcers; previous surgery; and arteritis.

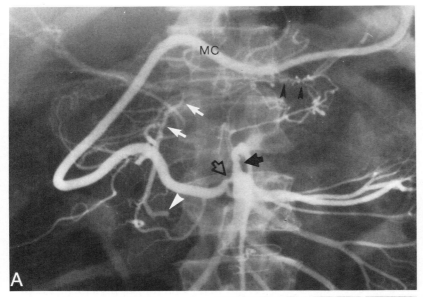

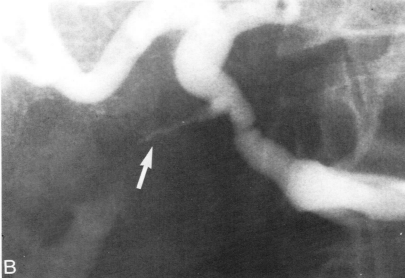

*Figure 15–58.* Carcinoma of the pancreas. *A,* Superior mesenteric arteriogram shows invasion of the proximal superior mesenteric artery, which appears serrated (*closed arrow*) and smooth encasement of the proximal middle colic (MC) artery (*open arrow*). The posterior pancreaticoduodenal artery is occluded (*white arrowhead*). The gastroduodenal artery is also serrated, owing to neoplastic invasion (*white arrows*). Several smaller pancreatic branches appear serpiginous (*black arrowheads*). The middle colic artery is enlarged and serves as a collateral. *B,* Close-up of the celiac arteriogram from another patient shows neoplastic invasion of the common hepatic artery and encasement and occlusion of the gastroduodenal artery (*arrow*).

PITFALLS IN DIAGNOSIS

1. Arterial and venous occlusion (especially splenic) and occasionally smooth arterial narrowing due to fibrosis are also seen in pancreatitis (see Fig. 15–18).

2. Smooth or irregular arterial stenosis may also be due to atherosclerosis. The splenic vein is normal in these patients.

3. Hypervascularity of the pancreas is suggestive of recurrent pancreatitis.

### Islet Cell Tumors

The majority of the islet cell population consists of beta cells. There are at least six different types of islet cell tumors, five of which are endocrine active (Table 15–10). Insulin- and gastrin-producing tumors are the most common types. Islet cell tumors may occur as an isolated abnormality or as part of a multiple endocrine neoplasia (MEN) syndrome (Table 15–11). In descending order of frequency, the tumors most frequently associated with the MEN syndromes are gastrinomas, insulinomas, and VIPomas.

The angiographic picture varies with the type and size of the lesion. The roles of angiography and CT are complementary, since smaller tumors may not be detected by

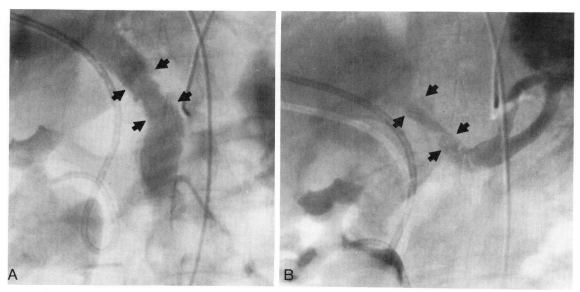

*Figure 15–59.* Carcinoma of the pancreas. Angiogram was obtained to assess resectability. A percutaneous biliary drainage catheter is in place. *A,* Subtraction film from the venous phase of the superior mesenteric arteriogram shows invasion of the portal vein (*arrows*). *B,* Subtraction film from the venous phase of the splenic arteriogram also shows portal vein invasion (*arrows*). Here, the narrowing appears more severe because of unopacified venous inflow from the superior mesenteric vein.

CT, which is the primary method of evaluation. Since most islet cell tumors are hypervascular, the majority of lesions can be localized or diagnosed by angiography. When applied appropriately, the accuracy of angiography for the localization of such tumors is close to 90%.[171, 173] Tumors not detected by CT or arteriography alone can be localized by arterial dynamic CT scanning.

There are no definite angiographic features that permit determination of malignancy of endocrine active pancreatic tumors, except by the demonstration of hepatic metastases. Larger tumors have a greater likelihood of malignancy. Tumor calcification, demonstrated by plain radiographs or tomography, occurs infrequently and has been reported in gastrinoma and insulinoma.[178] When present, it is highly indicative of malignancy.

The indications for angiography are:

1. Localization and occasionally diagnosis of islet cell tumors.

2. Transcatheter ablation of functioning tumors.[179]

Initially, a survey celiac arteriogram is performed. This usually detects the larger hypervascular lesions. If the celiac arteriogram is unrevealing, selective arteriography is performed of the following arteries: splenic, hepatic, gastroduodenal, dorsal pancreatic, and

**TABLE 15–10.** Pancreatic Islet Cell Neoplasms and the Endocrine Syndromes

| Syndrome | Islet Cell Type | Active Hormone | Usual Tumor Size | Most Common Location | Malignancy (%) | References |
|---|---|---|---|---|---|---|
| Zollinger-Ellison (gastrinoma) | Alpha | Gastrin | Up to 10 cm | 50% solitary, head/tail; 10% diffuse, hyperplasia; rarely ectopic | ~60 | 171, 172 |
| Insulinoma | Beta | Insulin | 1–2 cm | Head=body=tail; <10% multiple, 2–5% ectopic | 5–10 | 173, 174 |
| Glucagonoma | Alpha | Glucagon | ≥5 cm | Body/tail | ~80 | 175 |
| VIPoma (WDHA) | Delta | Vasoactive intestinal polypeptide | ≥5 cm or hyperplasia | Body/tail | ~60 | 176 |
| Somatostatinoma | Delta | Somatostatin | ≥4 cm | Head | ~90 | 177 |
| Nonfunctioning | Alpha or beta | None | ≥6 cm | Head | ~25 | 186, 187 |

**TABLE 15–11.** Syndromes of Multiple Endocrine Neoplasias

| Type I | Type II | Type III |
|---|---|---|
| | *Constant Features* | |
| Pituitary adenoma | Medullary carcinoma of thyroid | Medullary carcinoma of thyroid |
| Parathyroid adenoma or hyperplasia | Pheochromocytomas | Pheochromocytomas |
| Pancreatic islet cell tumor | Parathyroid hyperplasia | Mucosal neuromas |
| | | Ganglioneuromatosis coli |
| | | Neurofibromas |
| | | Marfanoid habitus |
| | *Inconstant Features* | |
| Bronchial/intestinal carcinoid | Adrenal cortical hyperplasia | |
| Thyroid adenoma | | |
| Adrenal cortical tumor | | |
| Lipomas | | |
| Thymomas | | |

inferior pancreaticoduodenal (or superior mesenteric) arteries. Oblique views and film subtraction (if DSA is not used) contribute significantly towards the diagnostic accuracy of arteriographic studies. If the arteriograms are nonrevealing, percutaneous transhepatic venous sampling of the pancreatic and peripancreatic veins is performed.[180, 181]

Most islet cell tumors are hypervascular (eg, 90% of glucagonomas, 66% of insulinomas).[175, 182] The degree of vascularity, completeness of the angiographic study, and tumor size determine whether the tumor can be localized by this method. Lesions smaller than 1.0 cm may not be detected. Gastric distention with air, selective arteriography of the pancreas, and oblique views are essential to detect smaller lesions. Filming in the 70 to 75 kVp range enhances angiographic definition.[173] Although pharmacoangiography may

not be helpful in some cases,[173] it serves as a useful adjunct when selective arteriography of the pancreatic vessels is not possible.

The angiographic appearance of the different types of islet cell tumors is similar and does not permit separation of the different types. Larger tumors may be seen on the celiac arteriogram (Figs. 15–60 to 15–62). Smaller tumors require selective arteriography. Typically, islet cell tumors are round and relatively well defined. Irregular tumor vessels are more likely to be demonstrated in larger lesions. Frequently, there is displacement and a characteristic bowing of slightly enlarged pancreatic arteries around a tumor. The tumor stain varies with the vascularity of the lesion. Some tumors have dilated vascular spaces, and enlarged draining veins may be observed.[171]

Hypovascular neoplasms also demonstrate

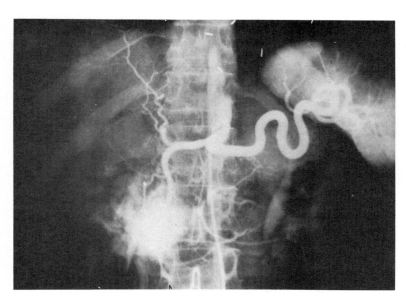

*Figure 15–60.* Gastrinoma. Celiac arteriogram shows an enlarged gastroduodenal artery and an intensely staining tumor in the head of the pancreas.

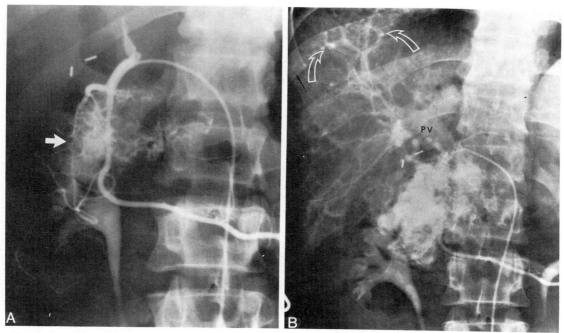

**Figure 15–61.** Malignant glucagonoma. *A,* Gastroduodenal arteriogram shows neovasculature in the pancreatic head. The anterior pancreaticoduodenal (*arrow*) and the gastroduodenal arteries are encased. *B,* Late arterial phase of common hepatic arteriogram shows an intense tumor stain and early portal vein (PV) opacification. Several metastatic foci are seen in the liver (*arrows*).

vascular displacement and bowing along the periphery of the tumor. Some hypovascular lesions may be demonstrated as negative defects on the pancreatogram phase.[175]

**Gastrinoma.** These may occur as single or multiple adenomas in conjunction with the Zollinger-Ellison syndrome (multiple peptic ulcers, gastric hypersecretion, hyperacidity, and occasionally hypoacidity, diarrhea, and gastrointestinal bleeding) or as part of a MEN syndrome. Males are affected more frequently than females, but there is no age predilection. Eight per cent of the tumors occur in patients less than 20 years of age.[172] Most gastrinomas are malignant, with local and distant metastases. Only about one third of the tumors are detected by CT,[183] whereas arteriography is successful in localizing a tumor in 88% of cases.[184]

**Insulinoma.** These lesions are seen more frequently in women, with the average age of manifestation in the fifth decade. Symptoms include hypoglycemia with the fasting glucose <40 mg/dl and elevated insulin levels (>30 μU/ml). Occasionally, the hypoglycemia may present as a psychiatric or seizure disorder. The lesions can be very small and may not be detected by CT. In general, malignant tumors are larger and are more likely

to be calcified.[178] The accuracy of angiography in detecting insulinomas is about 90%.[171, 185]

**Glucagonoma.** This is a rare, slow growing, mostly malignant tumor that occurs

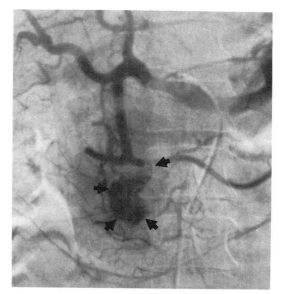

**Figure 15–62.** Insulinoma. Subtraction film from a celiac arteriogram shows a hypervascular mass in the head of the pancreas (*arrows*). The gastroduodenal artery is enlarged.

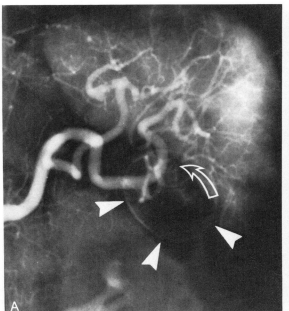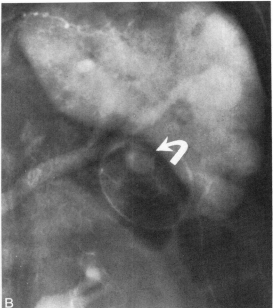

*Figure 15–63.* Accessory spleen simulating a tumor nodule in the tail of the pancreas. *A,* Early arterial phase of a splenic arteriogram shows a calcified splenic cyst (*arrowheads*). This was misdiagnosed as a splenic artery aneurysm on CT. A hilar branch of the splenic artery supplies the accessory spleen (*open arrow*). *B,* Parenchymal phase from the same arteriogram shows the accessory spleen (*arrow*).

more commonly in women. There is no age predilection. The clinical picture is characteristic: typical skin rash (necrolytic erythema migrans), diabetes, diarrhea, anemia, and glossitis. Blood glucagon levels are significantly elevated (normal, <100 pg/ml). The tumors are hypervascular and can be detected by angiography in most patients.

**VIPoma (WDHA Syndrome, Pancreatic Cholera).** This is characterized by secretory *Watery Diarrhea, Hypokalemia,* and *Achlorhydria* (WDHA). The syndrome is produced by an adenoma (VIPoma) or hyperplasia of the islet cells secreting the vasoactive intestinal peptide (VIP) that is held responsible for the clinical syndrome. A similar peptide is also secreted by other neoplasms, ie, bronchogenic carcinoma, medullary thyroid carcinoma, and adrenal pheochromocytoma.[176] Most VIPomas are hypervascular and thus lend themselves to arteriographic localization.

**Somatostatinoma.** This lesion is characterized by diabetes, cholelithiasis, and dyspepsia. Symptoms are caused by the suppressive actions of the hormone somatostatin upon the pancreatic islets, anterior pituitary, gastrointestinal mucosa, thyroid follicles, and the renal juxtaglomerular apparatus.[177]

**Nonfunctioning Islet Cell Tumors.** Endocrine-inactive tumors (usually alpha or beta cell) account for approximately one third of all islet cell tumors.[186] Most of these tumors are asymptomatic. Symptoms are usually indicative of a large tumor and underlying malignancy and include a mass, gastric outlet obstruction, jaundice, or gastrointestinal bleeding. More recent studies suggest that some of these tumors may produce polypeptides that do not manifest with clinical syndromes.[187]

Nonfunctioning islet cell tumors are usually large, which permits detection by CT. On arteriography, they cannot be distinguished from functioning tumors.

PITFALLS IN DIAGNOSIS

1. "Tumor stain": Contrast injection into smaller pancreatic branches may result in an intense parenchymal blush or stain of normal tissue. This has been mistaken for a tumor stain.[171]

2. Hypervascular nodule: Several other abnormalities in and around the pancreas may simulate a hypervascular islet cell tumor. These include an accessory spleen, a hyperplastic lymph node, chronic pancreatitis, and cystadenoma.[188]

3. Accessory spleens can usually be iden-

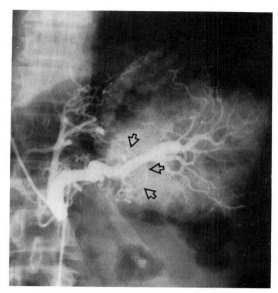

*Figure 15–64.* Spurious abnormality of the pancreatic vessels simulating a mass. Splenic arteriogram in a 28 year old man with symptoms of an endocrine active tumor shows bowing of several branches in the distal body of the pancreas (*arrows*). A CT scan performed prior to arteriography also suggested the presence of a mass in this region. At operation, no tumor was found and histological study of the distal pancreas showed normal islet cells.

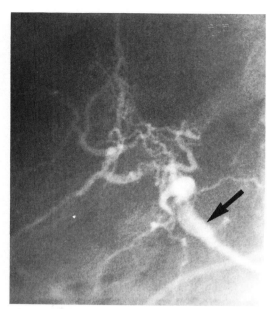

*Figure 15–65.* Arterial changes following intraarterial chemotherapy for metastatic sigmoid carcinoma. (same patient as Figure 15–54, *A* and *B*). Hepatic arteriogram shows a marked decrease in the number of intrahepatic branches opacified and increased tortuosity. The latter probably represent recanalized vessels and/or collaterals. A focal fusiform aneurysm of the hepatic artery is seen (*arrow*). Location of the aneurysm at the catheter tip suggests that it is traumatic.

tified with the aid of pharmacoangiography (normal splenic tissue responds with vasoconstriction following epinephrine or vasopressin) or by arteriography of the distal splenic artery. Vascular supply to the hypervascular nodule from hilar branches of the splenic artery indicates that the nodule is an accessory spleen (Fig. 15–63). Spurious vascular displacement and bowing may simulate a mass in the body and tail of the pancreas (Fig. 15–64).

4. A hypervascular hepatic lesion in an enlarged right lobe or the quadrate lobe may simulate a mass in the head of the pancreas on common hepatic arteriography. The situation can be clarified by proper hepatic or gastroduodenal arteriography (see Fig. 15–41).

5. No tumor found by arteriography. An arterial dynamic CT scan may detect lesions that are less vascular or smaller than 1 cm.

## Arterial Changes After Intraarterial Chemotherapy

With an increasingly aggressive approach for the management of metastatic liver disease, percutaneously or operatively placed arterial chemotherapy infusion catheters are being used more frequently. Arterial changes observed after intraarterial chemotherapy are (Fig. 15–65):[46]

1. Occlusion of the main hepatic artery and intrahepatic branches.

2. Aneurysm formation.

3. Stenoses.

## REFERENCES

1. Michels NA: Blood Supply and Anatomy of the Upper Abdominal Organs. With a Descriptive Atlas. Philadelphia, JB Lippincott, 1955.
2. Madayag M, Bosniak MA, Beranbaum E, et al: Renal and suprarenal pseudotumors caused by variations of the spleen. Radiology 105:43–47, 1972.
3. Luttwak EM, Schwartz A: Jaundice due to obstruction of the common duct by an aberrant artery: Demonstration of celiac anomaly by translumbar aortography and simultaneous choledochogram. Ann Surg 153:134–137, 1961.
4. Redman HC, Reuter SR: Arterial collaterals in the liver hilus. Radiology 94:575–579, 1970.
5. Marois D, Van Heerden JA, Carpenter HA, et al: Congenital absence of the portal vein. Mayo Clin Proc 54:55–59, 1979.

6. Clain D, McNulty J: A radiological study of the lymphatics of the liver. Br J Radiol 41:662–668, 1968.

7. Sovak M, Soulen RL, Reichle FA: Blood flow in the human portal vein. A cineradiographic method using particulate contrast medium. Radiology 99:531–536, 1971.

8. Mitra SK: The terminal distribution of the hepatic artery with special reference to arterioportal anastomoses. J Anat 100:651–663, 1966.

9. McCuskey RS: A dynamic and static study of hepatic arterioles and hepatic sphincters. Am J Anat 119:455–471, 1966.

10. Cho KJ, Lunderquist A: The peribiliary vascular plexus. The microvascular architecture of the bile duct in the rabbit and in clinical cases. Radiology 147:357–364, 1983.

11. Warren WD, Fomon JJ, Viamonte M, et al: Spontaneous reversal of portal venous blood flow in cirrhosis. Surg Gynecol Obstet 126:315–323, 1968.

12. Foster DN, Herlinger H, Miloszewski KJA, et al: Hepatofugal portal blood flow in hepatic cirrhosis. Ann Surg 187:179–182, 1978.

13. Warren WD, Muller WH Jr: A clarification of some hemodynamic changes in cirrhosis and their surgical significance. Ann Surg 150:413–427, 1959.

14. Redeker AG, Kunelis CT, Yamamoto S, et al: Assessment of portal and hepatic hemodynamics after side to side portocaval shunt in patients with cirrhosis. J Clin Invest 43:1464–1471, 1964.

15. Pollard JJ, Nebesar RA: Altered hemodynamics in the Budd-Chiari syndrome demonstrated by selective splenic angiography. Radiology 89:235–243, 1967.

16. Itzchak Y, Adar R, Bogokowski H, et al: Intrahepatic arterial portal communications: angiographic study. AJR 121:384–387, 1974.

17. Okuda K, Moriyama M, Yasumoto M, et al: Roentgenologic demonstration of spontaneous reversal of portal blood flow in cirrhosis and primary carcinoma of the liver. AJR 119:419–428, 1973.

18. Farrell R, Steinman A, Green WH: Arteriovenous shunting in a regenerating liver simulating hepatoma. Report of a case. Radiology 102:279–280, 1972.

19. Sniderman KW, Sos TA: Hepatic schistosomiasis: A case with intrahepatic shunting and extrahepatic portal vein occlusion. AJR 130:365–367, 1978.

20. Bookstein JJ, Cho KJ, Davis GB, et al: Arterioportal communications: Observations and hypotheses concerning transsinusoidal and transvasal types. Radiology 142:581–590, 1982.

21. Kunstlinger F, Federle MP, Moss A, et al: Computed tomography of hepatocellular carcinoma. AJR 134:431–437, 1980.

22. Magid D, Fishman EK, Kadir S, et al: CT evaluation of therapeutic embolization of hepatic hemangiomas. J Comput Assist Tomogr 7:1007–1011, 1983.

23. Carrasco CH, Chuang V, Wallace S: Apudomas metastatic to the liver: Treatment by hepatic artery embolization. Radiology 149:79–83, 1983.

24. Kadir S, Athanasoulis CA, Ring EJ, et al: Transcatheter embolization of intrahepatic arterial aneurysms. Radiology 134:335–339, 1980.

25. Chuang VP: Hepatic tumor angiography: A subject review. Radiology 148:633–639, 1983.

25a. Fink IJ, Krudy AG, Shawker TH, et al: Demonstration of an angiographically hypovascular insu-

26. linoma with intraarterial dynamic CT. AJR 144:555–556, 1985.

26. Sclafani SJA: Role of angiographic hemostasis in salvage of the injured spleen. Radiology 141:645–650, 1981.

27. Knight RW, Kadir S, White RI: Embolization of bleeding transverse pancreatic artery aneurysms. Cardiovasc Intervent Radiol 5:37–39, 1982.

28. Reuter SR, Atkin TW: High dose left gastric arteriography for demonstration of esophageal varices. Radiology 105:573–578, 1972.

29. Levine E: Preoperative angiographic assessment of portal venous hypertension. S Afr Med J 52:103–107, 1977.

30. McNulty JG: High dose percutaneous transsplenic portal venography. Br J Radiol 41:55–58, 1968.

30a. Lunderquist A, Tylén U: Phlebography of pancreatic veins. Radiologe 15:198–202, 1975.

31. Burcharth F: Percutaneous transhepatic portography: I. Technique and application. AJR 132:177–182, 1979.

32. Burcharth F, Nielbo N, Anderson B: Percutaneous transhepatic portography: II. Comparison with splenoportography in portal hypertension. AJR 132:183–185, 1979.

33. Bengmark S, Borjesson B, Hoevels J, et al: Obliteration of esophageal varices by PTP: A follow up of 43 patients. Ann Surg 190:549–554, 1979.

34. Bergstrand I, Ekman C-A: Percutaneous lieno-portal venography. Technique and complications. Acta Radiol Diagn 47:269–279, 1957.

35. DeWeese MS, Figley MM, Fry WJ, et al: Clinical appraisal of percutaneous splenoportography. Arch Surg 75:423–435, 1957.

36. Boijsen E, Efsing H-O: Intrasplenic arterial aneurysms following splenoportal phlebography. Acta Radiol Diagn 6:487–496, 1967.

37. Burchell AR, Moreno AH, Panke WF, et al: Some limitations of splenic portography: Incidence, hemodynamics and surgical implications of the non-visualized portal vein. Ann Surg 162:981–995, 1965.

38. Kadir S: Percutaneous antecubital vein approach for hepatic and renal vein catheterization. AJR 139:825–827, 1982.

39. Groszmann RJ, Glickman M, Blei AT, et al: Wedged and free hepatic venous pressure measured with a balloon catheter. Gastroenterology 76:253–258, 1979.

40. Castenada-Zuniga WR, Jauregui H, Rysavy JA, et al: Complications of wedge hepatic venography. Radiology 126:53–56, 1978.

41. Moreno AH, Ruzicka FF, Rousselot LM: Functional hepatography. Radiology 81:65–79, 1963.

42. Ramsey GC, Britton RC: Intraparenchymal angiography in the diagnosis of hepatic veno-occlusive diseases. Radiology 90:716–726, 1968.

43. Kessler RE, Tice DA, Zimmon DS: Value, complications, and limitations of umbilical vein catheterization. Surg Gynecol Obstet 136:529–535, 1973.

44. Malt RA, Corry RJ, Chavez-Peon F: Umbilical vein cannulation in portal system disease. N Engl J Med 279:930–932, 1968.

45. Guida PM, Moore SW: Aneurysm of the hepatic artery. Report of 5 cases with a brief review of the previously reported cases. Surgery 60:299–310, 1966.

46. Forsberg L, Hafstrom L, Lunderquist A, et al: Arterial changes during treatment with intrahepatic

arterial infusions of 5-fluorouracil. Radiology 126:49–52, 1978.

47. Long JA, Krudy AG, Cramer H, et al: False aneurysm formation following arteriographic intimal dissection: serial studies in two patients. Radiology 135:323–326, 1980.

48. Cameron JL, Broe P, Zuidema GD: Proximal bile duct tumors. Surgical management with Silastic transhepatic biliary stents. Ann Surg 196:412–419, 1982.

49. Bolt RD: Diseases of hepatic blood vessels. In Bockus HL (ed): Gastroenterology, 3rd Ed. Philadelphia, WB Saunders, 1976, pp. 471–491.

50. Citron BP, Halpern M, McCarron M, et al: Necrotizing angiitis associated with drug abuse. N Engl J Med 283:1003–1011, 1970.

51. Nuzum JW Jr, Nuzum JW Sr: Polyarteritis nodosa: Statistical review of 175 cases from the literature and report of a "typical" case. Arch Intern Med 94:942–955, 1954.

52. Robins JM, Bookstein JJ: Regressing aneurysms in polyarteritis nodosa. A report of 3 cases. Radiology 104:39–42, 1972.

53. Ayers AB, Fitchett DH: Hepatic hematoma in polyarteritis nodosa. Br J Radiol 49:184–185, 1976.

54. White AF, Baum S, Buranasiri S: Aneurysms secondary to pancreatitis. AJR 127:393–396, 1976.

55. Walter JF, Chuang VP, Bookstein JJ, et al: Angiography of massive hemorrhage secondary to pancreatic disease. Radiology 124:337–342, 1977.

56. Harris RD, Anderson JE, Coel MN: Aneurysms of the small pancreatic arteries. A cause of upper abdominal pain and intestinal bleeding. Radiology 115:17–20, 1975.

57. Palubinskas AJ, Ripley HR: Fibromuscular hyperplasia in extrarenal arteries. Radiology 82:451–455, 1964.

58. Falappa P, Galofaro G, Cotroneo AR, et al: Portosystemic arteriovenous fistulas. Gastrointest Radiol 5:137–141, 1980.

59. Korobkin M, Kantor I, Pollard JJ, et al: Arteriovenous fistula between systemic and portal circulations following partial gastrectomy. Radiology 109:311–314, 1973.

60. Martin LW, Benzing G, Kaplan S: Congenital intrahepatic arteriovenous fistula: report of a successfully treated case. Ann Surg 161:209–212, 1965.

61. Nyman U: Angiography in hereditary hemorrhagic telangiectasia. Acta Radiol Diag 18:581–592, 1977.

62. Charnsangavej C, Soo CS, Bernadino ME, et al: Portal-hepatic venous malformation: Ultrasound, computed tomography and angiographic findings. Cardiovasc Intervent Radiol 6:109–111, 1983.

63. Koehler RE, Korobkin M, Lewis F: Arteriographic demonstration of collateral arterial supply to the liver after hepatic artery ligation. Radiology 117:49–54, 1975.

64. Bengmark S, Rosengren K: Angiographic study of the collateral circulation to the liver after ligation of the hepatic artery in man. Am J Surg 119:620–624, 1970.

65. Berger PE, Culham JAG, Fitz CR, et al: Slowing of hepatic blood flow by halothane: angiographic manifestations. Radiology 118:303–306, 1976.

66. Jacobs RP, Shanser JD, Lawson DL, et al: Angiography of splenic abscesses. AJR 122:419–424, 1974.

67. Viana RL: Selective arteriography in the diagnosis and evaluation of amebic abscesses of the liver. Am J Dig Dis 20:632–638, 1975.

68. Garti I, Deutsch V: The angiographic diagnosis of echinococcosis of the liver and spleen. Clin Radiol 22:466–471, 1971.

69. Baltaxe HA, Flemming RJ: The angiographic appearance of hydatid disease. Radiology 97:599–604, 1970.

70. Roesch J, Keller FS: Angiography in the diagnosis and therapy of diffuse hepatocellular disease. Radiologe 20:334–342, 1980.

71. Boijsen E, Tylen U: Vascular changes in chronic pancreatitis. Acta Radiol Diagn 12:34–48, 1972.

72. Rich AR, Duff GL: Experimental and pathological studies on the pathogenesis of acute hemorrhagic pancreatitis. Bull Johns Hopkins Hosp 58:212–259, 1936.

73. Erb WH, Grimes EL: Pseudocysts of the pancreas. A report of 17 cases. Am J Surg 100:30–37, 1960.

74. Levin DC, Eisenberg H, Wilson, R: Arteriography in evaluation of pancreatic pseudocysts. AJR 129:243–248, 1977.

75. Sherlock S: Progress report: Portal circulation and portal hypertension. Gut 19:70–83, 1978.

76. Garcia-Palmieri MR, Marcial-Rojas RA: Portal hypertension due to schistosomiasis mansoni. Am J Med 27:811–816, 1959.

77. Kerr, DNS, Harrison CV, Sherlock S, et al: Congenital hepatic fibrosis. Q J Med 30:91–117, 1961.

78. Shaldon S, Sherlock S: Portal hypertension in the myeloproliferative syndrome and the reticuloses. Am J Med 32:758–764, 1962.

79. Taylor WJ, Jackson FC, Jensen WN: Wilson's disease, portal hypertension and intrahepatic vascular obstruction. N Engl J Med 260:1160–1164, 1959.

80. Reynolds TB, Ito S, Iwatsuki S: Measurement of portal pressure and its clinical application. Am J Med 49:649–657, 1970.

81. Moreno AH, Burchell AR, Rousselot LM, et al: Portal blood flow in cirrhosis of the liver. J Clin Invest 46:436–445, 1967.

82. Viallet A, Joly J-G, Marleau D, et al: Comparison of free portal venous pressure and wedged hepatic venous pressure in patients with cirrhosis of the liver. Gastroenterology 59:372–375, 1970.

83. Atkinson M, Sherlock S: Intrasplenic pressure as an index of portal venous pressure. Lancet 1:1325–1327, 1954.

84. Knauer CM, Lowe HM: Hemodynamics in the cirrhotic patient during paracentesis. N Engl J Med 276:191–196, 1967.

85. Cho KJ, Martel W: Recognition of splenic vein occlusion. AJR 131:439–443, 1978.

86. Itzchak Y, Glickman MG: Splenic vein thrombosis in patients with a normal size spleen. Invest Radiol 12:158–163, 1977.

87. Sos T, Meyers MA, Baltaxe HA: Nonfundic gastric varices. Radiology 105:579–580, 1972.

88. Vos LMJ, Potocky V, Broeker FHL, et al: Splenic vein thrombosis and oesophageal varices: a late complication of umbilical vein catheterization. Ann Surg 180:152–156, 1974.

89. Madding GF, Smith WL, Hershberger LR: Hepatoportal arteriovenous fistula. JAMA 156:593–596, 1954.

90. Pitlik S, Cohen L, Hadar H, et al: Portal hypertension and esophageal varices in hemangiomatosis of the spleen. Gastroenterology 72:937–940, 1977.

91. Chait A, Margulies M: Splenic arteriovenous fistula following percutaneous splenoportography. Radiology 87:518–520, 1966.

92. Stone HH, Jordan WD, Acker JJ, et al: Portal arteriovenous fistulas. Review and case report. Am J Surg 109:191–196, 1965.

93. Rouke JA, Bosniak MA, Ferris EJ: Hepatic angiography in "alcoholic hepatis." Radiology 91:290–296, 1968.

94. Kreel L, Gitlin N, Sherlock S: Hepatic artery angiography in portal hypertension. Am J Med 48:618–623, 1970.

94a. Okuda K, Ohnishi K, Kimura K, et al: Incidence of portal vein thrombosis in liver cirrhosis. An angiographic study in 708 patients. Gastroenterology 89:279–286, 1985.

95. Restrepto JE, Warren WD: Total liver blood flow after portacaval shunts, hepatic artery ligation and 70% hepatectomy. Ann Surg 156:719–726, 1962.

96. Aagaard J, Jensen LI, Soerensen TI, et al: Recanalized umbilical vein in portal hypertension. AJR 139:1107–1109, 1982.

97. Burchell AR, Panke WF, Moreno AH, et al: The patent umbilical vein in portal hypertension. Surg Obstet Gynecol 130:77–86, 1970.

98. Parker RGF: Occlusion of the hepatic veins in man. Medicine 38:369–402, 1959.

99. Feingold ML, Litwak RL, Geller SS, et al: Budd-Chiari syndrome caused by a right atrial tumor. Arch Intern Med 127:292–295, 1971.

100. Okulski TA, Soulen RL: Renal cell carcinoma presenting as the Budd-Chiari syndrome. AJR 128:140–142, 1977.

101. Takeuchi J, Takada A, Hasumura Y, et al: Budd-Chiari syndrome associated obstruction of the inferior vena cava. A report of 7 cases. Am J Med 51:11–20, 1971.

102. Simson IW: Membranous obstruction of the inferior vena cava and hepatocellular carcinoma in South Africa. Gastroenterology 82:171–178, 1982.

103. LaLonde G, Theoret G, Daloze P, et al: Inferior vena cava stenosis and Budd-Chiari syndrome in a woman taking oral contraceptives. Gastroenterology 82:1452–1456, 1982.

104. Hanelin LG, Uszler JM, Sommer DG: Liver scan "hot spot" in hepatic venoocclusive disease. Radiology 117:637–638, 1975.

105. Hungerford GD, Hamlyn AN, Lunzer MR, et al: Pseudometastases in the liver: a presentation of the Budd-Chiari syndrome. Radiology 120:627–628, 1976.

106. Galloway S, Casarella WJ, Price JB: Unilobar venoocclusive disease of the liver. Angiographic demonstration of intrahepatic competition simulating hepatoma. AJR 119:89–94, 1973.

107. Smith GW, Westgaard T, Bjorn-Hansen R: Hepatic venous angiography in the evaluation of cirrhosis of the liver. Ann Surg 173:469–480, 1971.

108. Futagawa S, Fukazawa M, Horisawa M, et al: Portographic liver changes in idiopathic non-cirrhotic portal hypertension. AJR 134:917–923, 1980.

109. Marleau D, Villeneuve JP, Huet PM, et al: Non-cirrhotic portal hypertension: Radiology and hemodynamic evaluation of 4 cases by combined hepatic and umbilicoportal catheterization. (Abstract.) Gastroenterology 67:813, 1974.

110. Reuter SR, Chuang VP: The location of increased resistance to portal blood flow in obstructive jaundice. Invest Radiol 11:54–59, 1976.

111. Aronsen KF, Norden JG, Nosslin B, et al: Vascular changes within the liver in biliary obstruction. Acta Chir Scand 135:505–510, 1969.

112. Kuershner HD, Schroeder J: Das Cruveilhier von Baumgarten Syndrom. Fortschr Roentgenstr 125:81–82, 1976.

113. Hanganutz M: Sur la cirrhose de Cruveilhier-Baumgarten. Presse Med 30:732–734, 1922.

113a. Lafortune M, Constantin A, Breton G, et al: The recanalized umbilical vein in portal hypertension. AJR 144:549–553, 1985.

114. Malt RA: Portasystemic venous shunts. N Engl J Med 295:24–29, 1976; 295:80–86, 1976.

115. Cameron JL, Maddrey WC: Mesoatrial shunt: A new treatment for the Budd-Chiari syndrome. Ann Surg 187:402–405, 1978.

116. Kadir S, Athanasoulis CA: Angiographic diagnosis and control of postoperative bleeding. CRC Crit Rev Diagn Imag 35–78, 1979.

117. Cope C: Balloon dilatation of closed mesocaval shunts. AJR 135:989–993, 1980.

118. McCort JJ: Rupture or laceration of the liver by nonpenetrating trauma. Radiology 78:49–57, 1962.

119. Misra B, Wagner R, Boneval H: Injuries of hepatic veins and retrohepatic vena cava. Am Surg 49:55–60, 1983.

120. Tchirkow P, Sliver SC: Injury to the portal vein. A hazard during common bile duct exploration. Arch Surg 113:745–747, 1978.

121. Foley WD, Berland LL, Lawson TL, et al: Computed tomography in the demonstration of hepatic pseudoaneurysm with hemobilia. J Comp Assist Tomogr 4:863–865, 1980.

122. Seltzer RA, Rossiter SB, Cooperman LR, et al: Hemobilia following needle biopsy of the liver. AJR 127:1035–1036, 1976.

123. Kadir S, Athanasoulis CA, Yune HY, et al: Aneurysms of the pancreaticoduodenal arteries in association with celiac axis occlusion. Cardiovasc Radiol 1:173–178, 1978.

124. Zucker K, Browns K, Rossman D, et al: Non-operative management of splenic trauma. Conservative or radical treatment. Arch Surg 119:400–402, 1984.

125. Fisher RG, Foucar K, Estrada R, et al: Splenic rupture in blunt trauma. RCNA 19:141–165, 1981.

126. Rosenthall L, Lisbona R, Banerjee K: A nucleographic and radio-angiographic study of a patient with torsion of the spleen. Radiology 110:427–428, 1974.

127. Patel JM, Rizzolo E, Hinshaw JR: Spontaneous subcapsular splenic hematoma as the only clinical manifestation of infectious mononucleosis. JAMA 247:3243–3244, 1982.

128. Yamada R, Sato M, Kawabata M, et al: Hepatic artery embolization in 120 patients with unresectable hepatoma. Radiology 148:397–401, 1983.

129. Vana J, Murphy GP, Aronoff BL, et al: Primary liver tumors and oral contraceptives. Results of a survey. JAMA 238:2154–2158, 1977.

130. Monroe PS, Riddell RH, Siegler M, et al: Hepatic angiosarcoma. Possible relationship to longterm oral contraceptive ingestion. JAMA 246:64–65, 1981.

131. Whelan JG Jr, Creech JL, Tamburro CH: Angiographic and radionuclide characteristics of hepatic angiosarcoma found in vinylchloride workers. Radiology 118:549–557, 1976.

132. Falk H, Popper H, Thomas LB, et al: Hepatic angiosarcoma associated with androgenic anabolic steroids. Lancet 2:1120–1123, 1979.

133. Daneshmend TK, Bradfield JWB: Letter. Lancet 2:1249, 1979.

134. Meyer P, Livolsi VA, Cornog JL: Letter. Lancet 2:1387, 1974.

135. Bernstein MS, Hunter RL, Yachnin S: Hepatoma and peliosis hepatis developing in a patient with Fanconi's anemia. N Engl J Med 284:1135–1136, 1971.

136. Brooks JJ: Hepatoma associated with diethylstilbestrol therapy for prostatic carcinoma. J Urol 128:1044–1045, 1982.

137. Johnson FL, Feager JR, Lerner KG, et al: Association of androgenic anabolic steroid therapy with development of hepatocellular carcinoma. Lancet 2:1273–1276, 1972.

138. Constostavlos DL: Benign hepatomas and oral contraceptives. Lancet 2:1200, 1973.

139. Penkava RR, Rothenberg J: Spontaneous resolution of oral contraceptive–associated liver tumor. J Comput Assist Tomogr 5:102–103, 1981.

140. Kerlin P, Davis GL, McGill DB, et al: Hepatic adenoma and focal nodular hyperplasia: clinical, pathologic and radiologic features. Gastroenterology 84:994–1002, 1983.

141. Kido C, Sasaki T, Kaneko M: Angiography of primary liver cancer. AJR 113:70–81, 1971.

142. Fredens M: Angiography in primary hepatic tumours in children. Acta Radiol Diagn 8:193–200, 1969.

143. Walter JF, Bookstein JJ, Bouffard EV: Newer angiographic observations in cholangiocarcinoma. Radiology 118:19–23, 1976.

144. Markowitz RI, Harcke HT, Ritchie WGM, et al: Focal nodular hyperplasia of the liver in a child with sickle cell anemia. AJR 134:594–597, 1980.

145. Bagheri SA, Boyer JL: Peliosis hepatis associated with androgenic anabolic steroid therapy. A severe form of hepatic injury. Ann Intern Med 81:610–618, 1974.

146. Sherlock S: Hepatic adenomas and oral contraceptives. Gut 16:753–756, 1975.

147. Yanoff M, Rawson AJ: Peliosis hepatis. An anatomic study with demonstration of two varieties. Arch Pathol 77:159–165, 1964.

148. Poulsen H, Winkler K: Liver disease with periportal sinusoidal dilatation. (Abstract.) Digestion 8:441–442, 1973.

149. Plachta A: Calcified cavernous hemangioma of the liver. Review of the literature and report of 13 cases. Radiology 79:783–788, 1962.

150. McLoughlin MJ: Angiography in cavernous hemangioma of the liver. AJR 113:50–55, 1971.

151. Sewell JH, Weiss K: Spontaneous rupture of hemangioma of liver. A review of the literature and presentation of illustrative case. Arch Surg 83:729–733, 1961.

152. Cooper WH, Martin JF: Hemangioma of the liver with thrombocytopenia. AJR 88:751–755, 1962.

153. Barnett PH, Zerhouni EA, White RI, et al: Computed tomography in the diagnosis of cavernous hemangioma of the liver. AJR 134:439–447, 1980.

154. Slovis TL, Berdon WE, Haller JO, et al: Hemangiomas of the liver in infants. Review of diagnosis, treatment and course. AJR 123:791–801, 1975.

155. Moss AA, Clark RE, Palubinskas AJ, et al: Angiographic appearance of benign and malignant hepatic tumors in infants and children. AJR 113:61–69, 1971.

156. Yu C: Primary carcinoma of the liver (hepatoma): Its diagnosis by selective celiac arteriography. AJR 99:142–149, 1967.

157. Lim RC Jr, Bongard FS: Hepatocellular carcinoma: Changing concepts in diagnosis and management. Arch Surg 119:637–642, 1984.

158. Roche A, Schmit P, Medina F, et al: The value of a portal study in determining the etiology of hepatic masses in the adult. Radiology 143:387–393, 1982.

159. Okuda K, Jinnouchi S, Nagasaki Y, et al: Angiographic demonstration of growth of hepatocellular carcinoma in the hepatic vein and inferior vena cava. Radiology 124:33–36, 1977.

160. Okuda K, Musha H, Yoshida T, et al: Demonstration of growing casts of hepatocellular carcinoma in the portal vein by celiac angiography. The thread and streaks sign. Radiology 117:303–309, 1975.

161. Passariello R, Simonetti G, Rossi P, et al: Tomografia computerizzata e angiografia nelle metastasi epatiche. Radiol Med 66:597–600, 1980.

162. Allison DJ, Modlin IM, Jenkins WJ: Treatment of carcinoid liver metastases by hepatic artery embolization. Lancet 2:1323–1325, 1977.

163. Kaude J, Jensen R, Wirtanen GW: Slow injection hepatic angiography. A comparison with a high injection rate. Acta Radiol Diagn 14:700–712, 1973.

164. Heaston DK, Chuang VP, Wallace S, et al: Metastatic hepatic neoplasms. Angiographic features of portal vein involvement. AJR 136:897–900, 1981.

165. Meves M, Apitzsch DE: Die Lebervenenangiographie zum Nachweis von intrahepatischen Tumoren. Fortschr Roentgenstr 125:247–251, 1976.

166. Yaghoobian J, Pinck RL, Naidich J, et al: Angiographic findings in liver amyloidosis. Radiology 136:332, 1980.

167. Jonsson K, Lunderquist A: Angiography of the liver and spleen in Hodgkin's disease. AJR 121:789–792, 1974.

168. Rösch J: Tumours of the spleen. The value of selective arteriography. Clin Radiol 17:183–190, 1966.

169. Friedman AC, Lichtenstein JE, Dachman AH: Cystic neoplasms of the pancreas. Radiological-pathological correlation. Radiology 149:45–50, 1983.

170. Bookstein JJ, Reuter SR, Martel W: Angiographic evaluation of pancreatic carcinoma. Radiology 93:757–764, 1969.

171. Boijsen E, Samuelsson L: Angiographic diagnosis of tumours arising from the pancreatic islets. Acta Radiol Diagn 10:161–176, 1970.

172. Ellison EH, Wilson SD: The Zollinger-Ellison syndrome: Reappraisal and evaluation of 260 reported cases. Ann Surg 160:512–530, 1964.

173. Clouse ME, Costello P, Legg MA, et al: Subselective angiography in localizing insulinomas of the pancreas. AJR 128:741–746, 1977.

174. Service FJ, Dale AJD, Elveback LR, et al: Insulinoma: clinical and diagnostic features of 60 consecutive cases. Mayo Clin Proc 51:417–429, 1976.

175. Wawrukiewicz AS, Rosch J, Keller FS, et al: Glucagonoma and its angiographic diagnosis. CVIR 5:318–324, 1982.

176. Cooperman AM, DeSanctis D, Winkelman E, et al:

Watery diarrhea syndrome: Two unusual cases and further evidence that VIP is a humoral mediator. Ann Surg 187:325–328, 1978.

177. Krejs GJ, Orci L, Conlon JM, et al: Somatostatinoma syndrome. Biochemical, morphological and clinical features. N Engl J Med 301:285–292, 1979.

178. Imhof H, Frank P: Pancreatic calcifications in malignant islet cell tumors. Radiology 122:333–337, 1977.

179. Moore TJ, Peter LM, Harrington DP, et al: Successful arterial embolization of an insulinoma. JAMA 248:1353–1355, 1982.

180. Roche A, Raisonnier A, Gillon-Savouret M-C: Pancreatic venous sampling and arteriography in localizing insulinomas and gastrinomas. Procedure and results in 55 cases. Radiology 145:621–627, 1982.

181. Ingemansson S, Lunderquist A, Lunderquist I, et al: Portal vein catheterization with radioimmunologic determination of insulin. Surg Gynecol Obstet 141:705–711, 1975.

182. Stefanini P, Carboni M, Patrassi N, et al: Beta islet cell tumors of the pancreas: results of a study on 1067 cases. Surgery 75:597–609, 1974.

183. Damgaard-Peterson K, Stage JG: CT scanning in patients with Zollinger-Ellison syndrome and carcinoid syndrome. Scand J Gastroenterol 14(Suppl 53):117–122, 1979.

184. Gray RK, Rösch J, Grollman JH Jr: Arteriography in the diagnosis of islet cell tumors. Radiology 97:39–44, 1970.

185. Fulton RE, Sheedy PF II, McIlrath DC, et al: Preoperative angiographic localization of insulin producing tumors of the pancreas. AJR 123:367–377, 1975.

186. Fontaine R, Lampert M, Babin S, et al; cited by Boijsen E: Inactive malignant endocrine tumors of the pancreas. Radiologe 15:177–182, 1975.

187. Strodel WE, Vinik AI, Lloyd RV, et al: Pancreatic polypeptide producing tumors. Silent lesions of the pancreas. Arch Surg 119:508–514, 1984.

188. Korobkin MT, Palubinskas AJ, Glickman MG: Pitfalls in arteriography of islet cell tumors of the pancreas. Radiology 100:319–328, 1971.

# Angiography of the Kidneys

## ANATOMY

The kidney is divided into five vascular segments—apical, upper, middle, lower, and posterior—each supplied by a separate branch of the renal artery.[1] There are single renal arteries to the kidneys in about two thirds of individuals.[2, 3] Unilateral multiple renal arteries occur in 32% and bilateral multiple renal arteries in 12% of individuals[2] (Fig. 16–1). Multiple renal arteries entering the hilus are usually of equal caliber, whereas accessory vessels to the poles are smaller than the hilar renal arteries. Although six or seven arteries have been observed, the number of renal arteries infrequently exceeds four. Aberrant renal vascular supply is more likely in patients with malrotated or horseshoe kidneys.[1, 3]

Normally, the renal arteries originate from the lateral or ventrolateral aspect of the abdominal aorta at the level of the first lumbar intervertebral disc space (see Chapter 10, Fig. 10–1). The right renal artery ostium is located close to the ventral surface of the aorta (and occasionally close to the SMA orifice) in over 50% of persons. The orifice of the left renal artery is located close to the ventral surface of the aorta in approximately 25% of individuals.[4] Location of the renal artery orifice close to the posterior surface of the aorta is infrequent and usually involves the left side. The renal arteries lie behind the renal veins, and the orifice of the left renal artery is usually higher than that of the right.

In individuals with multiple renal arteries, the origin of the accessory vessels can be very variable. They usually originate from the infrarenal aorta but may occasionally arise from the lower thoracic aorta or iliac, lumbar, or mesenteric arteries. Such unusual origins are more likely in developmental anomalies of the kidneys.[1, 3]

An independent superior pole renal artery from the aorta is observed in 7% and an independent lower pole artery in 5.5% of individuals.[3] In addition, branches to the upper pole and capsule of the kidney, which may serve as crucial collaterals in occlusive diseases, are provided by the middle adrenal artery.

A short distance from the hilus, the renal artery divides into an anterior and a posterior division. The latter continues to the posterior surface of the kidney to supply the posterior segment, whereas the former further divides into segmental arteries for the remainder of the kidney (Fig. 16–2).

The segmental arteries give rise to the lobar arteries, one for each renal pyramid. These subdivide into interlobar arteries, which divide dichotomously into arcuate arteries at the corticomedullary junction. The arcuate arteries, which give off a number of interlobular arteries to the renal cortex, do not anastomose with one another but also terminate as interlobular arteries. The renal medulla is supplied by the efferent arterioles, derived primarily from the juxtamedullary glomeruli. Some interlobular arteries (and occasionally interlobar or lobar arteries) anastomose with renal capsular vessels derived from renal, adrenal, lumbar, and gonadal arteries (Fig. 16–3; see also Fig. 16–19B).

The interlobular arteries give off afferent arterioles to the glomeruli. The efferent arterioles, which originate from the glomerular capillary plexuses, form the peritubular capillary plexuses around the convoluted tubules.

Branches of the renal arteries are the:

1. Inferior adrenal arteries: These are usually one or more branches to the adrenal gland.

2. Gonadal arteries: These arise from the renal artery in about 20% of individuals.

445

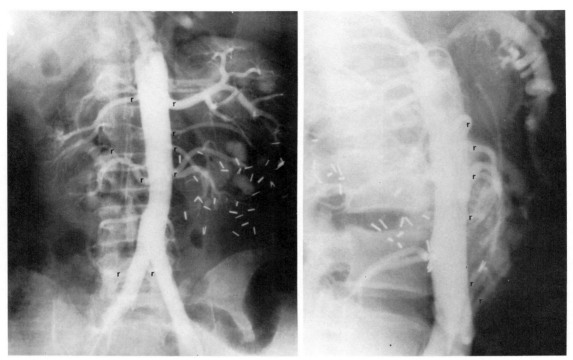

**Figure 16–1.** AP *(left)* and lateral *(right)* abdominal aortogram shows multiple renal arteries in a patient with a horseshoe kidney. Note anterior location of the accessory renal arteries on the lateral aortogram. r = renal artery.

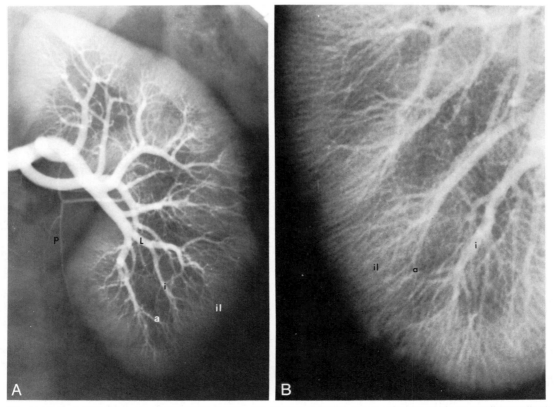

**Figure 16–2.** A, Normal renal arteriogram. B, Closeup of magnification renal arteriogram from another patient. a = arcuate; i = interlobar; il = interlobular; L = lobar; p = pelvic branches.

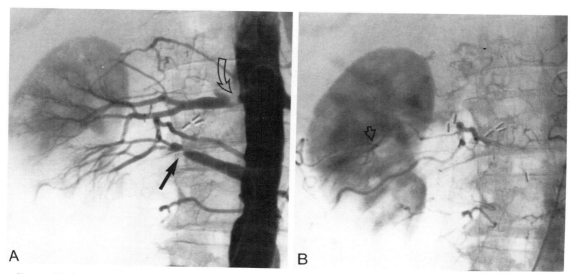

A  B

*Figure 16–3.* Renal collaterals. *A,* Subtraction film from an aortogram shows severe stenosis of the right renal artery (*open arrow*) and distal anastomosis of an aortorenal bypass graft (*solid arrow*). An enlarged lumbar artery is seen above the bypass graft. *B,* Later frame from the same study shows a branch of the lumbar artery anastomosing with a perforating branch of a lobar artery with opacification of intrarenal branches (*open arrow*).

3. Inferior phrenic artery. This vessel may also be a branch of the renal artery. Such an origin occurs more frequently on the right.

The interlobular veins, which course along the interlobular arteries, drain into arcuate veins at the corticomedullary junction (Figs. 16–4 and 16–5). The latter drain into interlobar veins, which join to form the lobar and subsequently the renal veins. Multiple intrarenal venous anastomoses are present.

The *right renal vein* is 2 to 4 cm long and joins the IVC at the level of the lower third of the first lumbar vertebra. Multiple right renal veins occur in 28% of individuals, and rarely a single vein may divide before joining

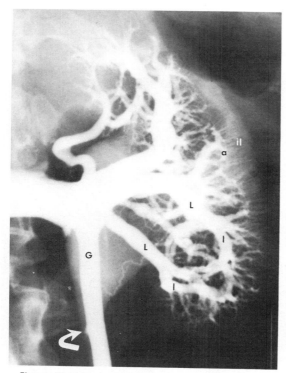

*Figure 16–4.* Normal retrograde renal venogram. The gonadal vein valve is incompetent (*arrow*). a = arcuate; G = gonadal; il = interlobular; l = interlobar; L = lobar veins. (Courtesy of Dr. CA Athanasoulis.)

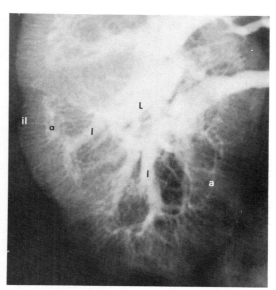

*Figure 16–5.* Retrograde renal venogram showing interlobular veins in a patient with two renal veins. For abbreviations see legend for Figure 16–4.

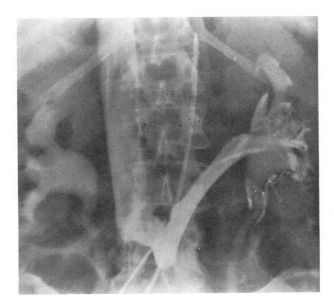

*Figure 16–6.* Retroaortic left renal vein. Retrograde venogram opacifies the left renal vein, which joins the left common iliac vein. (From Kadir S et al: *In* Athanasoulis CA, et al (Eds): Interventional Radiology. Philadelphia, WB Saunders, 1982.)

the IVC.[5] The *left renal vein* is almost three times longer and joins the IVC almost at the right angles, at a slightly higher level than the right renal vein. It passes anterior to the aorta and under the SMA and lies behind the head of the pancreas. The gonadal and the left inferior phrenic/adrenal veins drain into it. The left renal vein communicates with the pancreatic, splenic, ascending lumbar,

and other retroperitoneal veins. Such communications are usually absent on the right side. Renal vein valves are reported in 15% of renal venograms.[5]

The *retroaortic renal vein* refers to a single left renal vein that passes behind the aorta to join the lower IVC or iliac vein (Fig. 16–6). This occurs in 3% of individuals.[6]

A *circumaortic renal vein* refers to a double

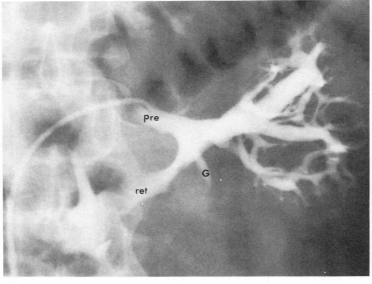

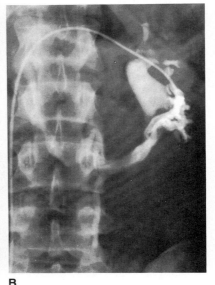

**A**                                                                                     **B**

*Figure 16–7.* Circumaortic left renal vein. *A,* A single vein originates from the renal hilus and subsequently divides into two. There is reflux of contrast medium into the gonadal vein up to the competent valve. G = gonadal vein; pre = preaortic; ret = retroaortic limb. This type occurs in 75% of cases. *B,* Two separate renal veins originate from the kidney. The catheter is in the preaortic limb. (*B* from Kadir S et al: *In* Athanasoulis CA, et al (Eds): Interventional Radiology. Philadelphia, WB Saunders, 1982.)

left renal vein in which the upper (preaortic) limb passes normally to the IVC, while the other, usually smaller, limb passes behind the aorta to join the IVC (or occasionally the iliac vein) at a lower level. This is reported in as many as 17% of individuals.[6] In our own experience with over 300 testicular vein catheterizations, this variant occurs less frequently.

Two types of circumaortic renal veins are observed (Fig. 16–7). In the more common type (75%), there is one renal vein at the renal hilus that bifurcates before reaching the IVC.[7] In the other type, there are two veins originating from the renal hilus. Such vessels serve as a collateral pathway for the lower extremities in the presence of vena caval occlusion. Both veins must be sampled for renin assay in patients with hypertension.

In the presence of a circumaortic renal vein, the gonadal vein joins the retroaortic limb in most cases. The adrenal vein drains into the preaortic limb.

A *horseshoe kidney* is observed in approximately 1 of every 500 to 700 autopsies.[3] It occurs more frequently in males and is usually associated with an aberrant vascular supply. Multiple renal arteries are common (up to six or more) and may originate from the aorta or the mesenteric or iliac arteries[1, 3] (see Fig. 16–1)

Blood supply to the *renal pelvis* and proximal *ureter* is derived mainly from renal artery branches. Arterial supply to the mid- and distal ureter is from the aorta and iliac arteries. The latter serve as an important collateral in renal artery occlusion.

**Gonadal Vessels.** The gonadal arteries originate from the anterior surface of the aorta in approximately 80% of individuals. In the remainder, they arise from the renal artery and occasionally from the adrenal, phrenic, lumbar, or even the iliac artery or SMA[3] (see Chapter 10; Fig. 10–5). Rarely, they may be double. The left gonadal vein drains into the left renal vein about 2 cm from the junction of the latter with the IVC (see Fig. 16–4). The right gonadal vein drains into the IVC at or below the junction of the right renal vein with the IVC. In 8% of individuals, it drains into the right renal vein.[8]

Valves are present in the proximal testicular veins in 54% and in the ovarian veins in 87% of individuals.[9] Incompetent valves occur most frequently in multiparous women.[9] Absent gonadal vein valves are more com-

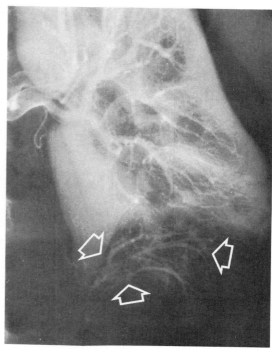

*Figure 16–8.* Intrarenal collaterals. Renal arteriogram in a patient with traumatic occlusion of an accessory lower pole renal artery. The lower pole branches opacify via intrarenal collaterals (*arrows*). (From Kadir S et al: *In* Athanasoulis CA, et al (Eds): Interventional Radiology. Philadelphia, WB Saunders, 1982.)

mon on the left side.[8] Thus, on left renal venography, reflux of contrast medium into the testicular vein (in individuals without a varicocele) occurs less frequently than into the ovarian vein.

**Collateral Circulation to the Kidney.** Although the renal arteries have been considered end arteries, intrarenal anastomoses do exist via the perivascular plexuses of segmental, interlobar, and arcuate arteries[10, 11] (Fig. 16–8; see also Fig. 16–19). Under normal circumstances, these are too small to be demonstrated on arteriography. Main routes of collateral blood supply to the kidney are[10, 12, 13] (Figs. 16–3, 16–8, and 16–9, see also Figs. 16–17 and 16–19):

1. Lumbar, adrenal, and gonadal arteries → peripelvic and periureteric arteries.

2. Subcostal, lumbar, and adrenal arteries → renal capsular arteries.

3. Renal capsular artery → perforating branch of lobar and interlobar arteries.

4. Intrarenal anastomoses via the perivascular plexuses.

5. Anastomotic branch of internal iliac artery → periureteric arteries.

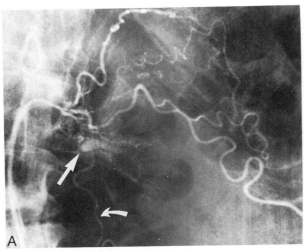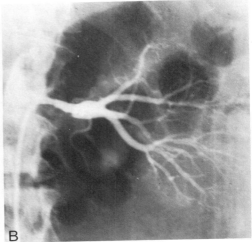

*Figure 16–9.* Renal collaterals. *A,* Opacification of renal artery (*straight arrow*) via subcostal, adrenal, and renal capsular collaterals in a patient with atherosclerotic occlusion of the left renal artery. Curved arrow points to the enlarged ureteral artery. *B,* Arteriogram after percutaneous recanalization, and balloon dilatation. Note absence of thrombosis in the intrarenal branches.

## ANGIOGRAPHY

**Arteriography** (Table 16–1). The most frequent indications for renal arteriography are the evaluation of renovascular hypertension, trauma, and neoplasms and the assessment of potential kidney donors. Both conventional arteriography and intraarterial or intravenous DSA can be used. The former is preferred if small vessel disease or intrarenal abnormalities are to be assessed.

Aortography is essential for the evaluation of hypertension and large neoplasms, ie, to evaluate the renal artery orifices in the former and the vascular supply to the tumor in the latter. Selective arteriography of the renal arteries is necessary for the evaluation of intrarenal disease.

For aortography, the tip of the pigtail catheter is placed at the level of the renal artery orifices, ie, L2. Proximal reflux of contrast medium opacifies the renal arteries satisfactorily. With a higher catheter position, there is opacification of the celiac artery and SMA, which obscures the renal vasculature. For selective arteriography, a single curve (visceral hook), cobra, or sidewinder catheter is used.

The projections used for aortography and selective renal arteriography are determined by the disease process being evaluated. In most cases, an AP arteriogram is performed first. In patients being studied for renovascular hypertension or small hypovascular neoplasms, oblique views are often invaluable.

**Venography and Venous Sampling** (Table 16–2). The main indications for renal vein catheterization are venous sampling for renin determination, diagnosis of renal vein thrombosis, and evaluation of neoplasms.

The renal veins can be catheterized from the femoral or cubital vein approach. From the femoral approach, a C2 cobra catheter with two side holes or a multiple hole straight or pigtail catheter is used with the aid of a tip deflector. From the arm, a multipurpose

**TABLE 16–1. Selective Renal Arteriogram**

| Catheter: | Cobra, sidewinder, visceral hook |
|---|---|
| Position | Proximal renal artery |
| Guide wire | — |
| Contrast medium | 76% diatrizoate meglumine sodium† |
| Injection rate/volume* | 5–6 ml/sec, total 12–15 ml |
| Films: | 10 |
| Rate | 2 per second for 4 films |
| | 1 per second for 6 films |
| Projections | AP |
| | Obliques (LAO/RAO) |
| | (Craniocaudad angulation) |

*In patients with multiple renal arteries, the rate and volume of contrast injected are adjusted according to renal artery size (eg, for smaller arteries: 2–4 ml/sec, total 5–10 ml; ie, contrast medium is injected over 2½ seconds).

†20% concentration for DSA.

**TABLE 16–2. Retrograde Renal Venogram***

| | |
|---|---|
| Catheter: | Cubital approach: end hole occluded NIH type |
| | Femoral approach: pigtail or multiple hole straight |
| Position | Main renal vein |
| Guide wire | Tip-deflecting system for femoral approach |
| Contrast medium | 76% diatrizoate meglumine sodium† |
| Injection rate/volume | 15–18 ml/sec, total 30–36 ml |
| Films: | 10 |
| Rate | 3 per second for 6 films |
| | 1 per second for 4 films |
| Projection | AP |

*Balloon occlusion of renal artery or injection of 8–10 μg epinephrine into the renal artery immediately before venography.

†20% concentration for DSA.

catheter is used, and passage through the right atrium is facilitated by an LLT J guide wire. If the catheter does not advance into a horizontally oriented renal vein, the course of the vein can be altered by deep inspiration in order to facilitate catheterization.

This maneuver is particularly helpful for catheterization of the left renal vein. For venous sampling, we prefer the cobra with side holes (femoral approach) or the multipurpose catheter (cubital vein approach). We have occasionally used the multiple hole straight catheter with the aid of a tip deflector wire. However, this catheter is not suitable for short renal veins, as it may lead to sampling error (tip may lodge in a branch vessel or side hole in the IVC).

During venous sampling for renin, three blood samples are obtained, 10 minutes apart, from each renal vein. Eighteen ml of blood is withdrawn into a syringe containing 2 ml of ededate calcium disodium (Riker Laboratories, Inc., Northridge, California). On the left side, the catheter tip must be beyond the junction of the adrenal and gonadal veins. Immediately after the second sample has been obtained, 20 mg of furosemide (Lasix) is injected intravenously, or the patient is brought into a near-upright position for 10 minutes in an attempt to stimulate renin secretion from the affected kidney. Simultaneous sampling from both renal veins does not offer any advantage over the single catheter technique.

Renal venography can be performed with or without the aid of arterial occlusion (mechanical or pharmacological). During renal venography without arterial occlusion, venous opacification is usually inhomogeneous and incomplete (unless there is renal artery stenosis or occlusion). Epinephrine-assisted renal venography has been the standard. With this method, 8 to 10 μg of epinephrine is diluted with 15 to 20 ml of glucose (5%) and injected slowly into the renal artery (over about 20 seconds) immediately before venography (see Fig. 16–4). This slows the arterial flow and permits an even and complete distribution of the contrast medium injected into the renal veins. However, recent studies indicate that there may be renal toxicity associated with the use of epinephrine.[14]

As an alternative, we have used partial balloon occlusion of the renal artery to slow arterial flow.[15] With this method, a balloon-tipped catheter (5 Fr Swan or Berman wedge balloon catheter or balloon-tipped cobra or sidewinder catheter) is placed in the proximal renal artery. The balloon is test inflated with diluted contrast medium. The volume required to significantly slow (not occlude) renal artery flow is determined. Immediately before renal venography, the balloon is inflated with the predetermined volume of diluted contrast medium and the renal venogram is performed. The balloon is deflated immediately thereafter. Although it may not be necessary to inject an anticoagulant (because the renal flow is not totally obstructed), we have routinely injected 1000 to 2000 units of heparin into the renal artery immediately after balloon inflation.

For venography, multiple hole catheters are necessary to facilitate an even distribution of contrast medium. We prefer to use end hole–occluded catheters, ie, NIH type from the arm and straight catheter with tip occluder from the groin. The pigtail catheter can also be used from the femoral approach. The injection rate and filming program for renal venography are shown in Table 16–2.

## ARTERIAL DISEASES

### The Normally Aging Kidney

Discussion of the angiographic appearance of the kidney in older individuals is important, as this may seem abnormal and simulate renal disease. The angiographic abnormalities seen in the aging renal arteries and kidney most frequently simulate those observed in association with hypertension.

Atherosclerotic stenosis of the renal artery (> 25% of the diameter) was observed in 49% of normotensive individuals in one autopsy study.[16] The proximal third of the renal artery or its orifice was involved in 95.5%. In normotensive patients older than 50 years, renal artery stenosis exceeding 25% of the diameter was present in 64%. On the other hand, the presence of a renal artery stenosis in individuals younger than 50 years was more likely to be associated with hypertension.

In the normal kidney, there is a gradual and progressive tapering of the interlobar and arcuate arteries. Alterations in this normal pattern are observed in normotensive individuals above the age of 40 years. On arteriography, these changes may simulate those observed in longstanding hypertension. Although there is no linear age-related progression, these changes are observed most frequently in older patients (in 12 to 25% of patients between 40 and 69 years and

in 60% of patients older than 70 years).[17] The earliest changes occur in the arcuate arteries. The following may be observed on arteriography[17] (Fig. 16–10):

1. Absence of gradual decrease in diameter of interlobar arteries.

2. Disparity of size between interlobar/arcuate arteries and their branches: The arcuate arteries may appear to terminate abruptly.

3. Increase in tortuosity and atherosclerotic plaques in smaller vessels.

4. Apparent increase in the number of intrarenal vessels: This appearance is caused by a decrease in the renal mass and the failure of the intrarenal vessels to taper normally.

5. Extension of the arcuate arteries to the renal periphery. This occurs as a result of the decrease in cortical tissue.

## Aneurysms

Renal artery aneurysms are observed in approximately 1% of patients undergoing renal arteriography.[18] In the majority of patients, they are detected incidentally at the time of arteriography. Aneurysms occur most frequently in the fourth and fifth decades of life and show no sex predilection.[19] Common causes of renal artery aneurysms are atherosclerosis, fibromuscular dysplasia (FMD), and trauma, as well as congenital or mycotic aneurysms. Multiple aneurysms are most frequently due to FMD, arteritis, or trauma.

Atherosclerotic and congenital aneurysms, which are usually single, may become quite large and involve the main renal artery or its larger branches (anterior or posterior division or segmental arteries) and are often located close to a bifurcation (Fig. 16–11). Curvilinear calcification may be seen on the abdominal radiograph.

Symptoms are nonspecific and most frequently consist of pain or hematuria.[19] Although aneurysm rupture is rare, it may lead to perinephric or retroperitoneal hematoma or the formation of an arteriovenous fistula. Rupture is more likely in aneurysms due to an inflammatory process (eg, polyarteritis nodosa). Other complications include peripheral embolization and thrombosis.[20] Alone, renal artery aneurysms are an infrequent cause of hypertension (unless very large). In most patients with a renal artery aneurysm and hypertension, associated stenoses of the renal arteries are present[20] (Fig. 16–11B) or

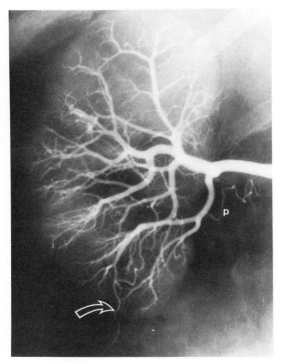

*Figure 16–10.* Angiographic appearance of the normal kidney in the older individual. Only a few interlobular arteries are opacified. There is an apparent increase in the number of intrarenal vessels, abrupt termination of the arcuate arteries, and extension of the arteries to the periphery. A benign cyst is present in the upper pole, resulting in stretching of the branches. Arrow points to a perforating branch. p = pelvic branch.

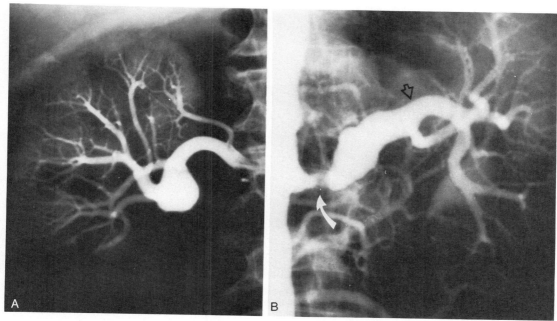

*Figure 16–11.* Atherosclerotic renal artery aneurysms. *A*, Saccular aneurysm arising at the renal artery bifurcation. *B*, Fusiform aneurysm of the main renal artery extending into the branches (*open arrow*). In addition there is a severe proximal renal artery stenosis (*curved arrow*).

there is segmental renal ischemia due to embolization of mural thrombus.

Aneurysms associated with FMD involve the main renal artery and proximal branches (Fig. 16–12*A*). Aneurysms due to arteritis (polyarteritis nodosa, Wegener's granulomatosis, necrotizing angiitis) and most traumatic aneurysms are intrarenal in location. Traumatic aneurysms of the main renal artery are usually due to penetrating trauma (eg, stab or bullet injury) but may also develop as a complication of renal artery angioplasty (see Fig. 16–32). The location of mycotic aneurysms can be variable, but these usually spare the main renal artery (Fig. 16–12*B*).

In polyarteritis nodosa, the kidney is affected in 85% of individuals.[21] Most frequently, the interlobar, arcuate, interlobular, and occasionally the segmental arteries are affected. Some aneurysms may become quite large, while others may rupture, resulting in a perirenal or retroperitoneal hematoma.[22]

**Arteriography.** Arteriography is indicated for:

1. Determination of the etiology and location of the aneurysm.

2. Diagnosis and therapy (embolization) of aneurysms involving branch vessels.[23]

3. Definition of arterial anatomy prior to operative repair.

Although large aneurysms or diffuse disease (eg, polyarteritis nodosa) can be identified on the aortogram, selective arteriography is usually necessary for detailed evaluation. In patients with polyarteritis nodosa, arteriography may be the diagnostic procedure of choice because of the high incidence of renal involvement. Multiple small aneurysms are usually seen, and on the nephrogram phase, peripheral perfusion defects due to cortical infarction may be present (Fig. 16–13).

PITFALLS IN DIAGNOSIS

1. Multiple small aneurysms of the intrarenal arteries are also observed in collagen vascular diseases, cholesterol emboli,[24] inflammatory processes, or following blunt trauma.

2. Spontaneous perirenal or retroperitoneal hemorrhage is most frequently due to renal or retroperitoneal neoplasms. This diagnosis should be considered even if an obvious arterial abnormality is not seen.

## Arteriovenous Malformations and Hemangiomas

Renal arteriovenous malformations are rare congenital lesions that are usually located in the medulla. The most common symptoms

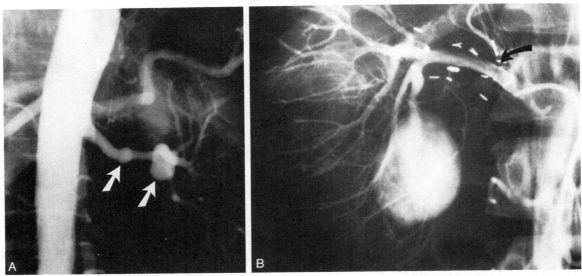

**Figure 16–12.** *A*, Two saccular aneurysms (*arrows*) are present in a patient with medial fibroplasia. A subtle mural abnormality is present in the renal artery segment proximal to the smaller aneurysm. The renal artery segment between the aneurysms is narrowed. *B*, Large mycotic aneurysm in a young drug addict. Arrow points to catheter-induced renal artery spasm.

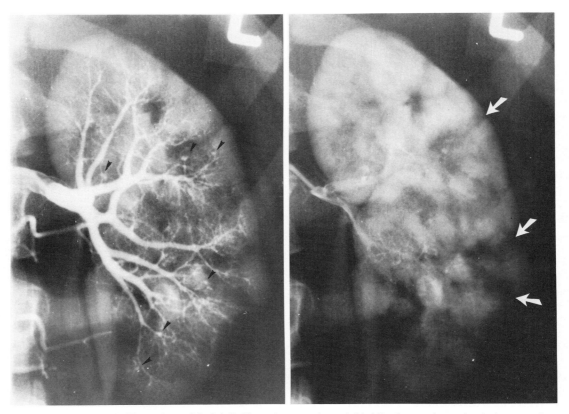

**Figure 16–13.** Polyarteritis nodosa. Arterial (*left*) and parenchymal (*right*) phase of renal arteriogram shows numerous small saccular aneurysms. Arrowheads point to several aneurysms. Cortical perfusion defects are present on the parenchymal phase (*arrows*).

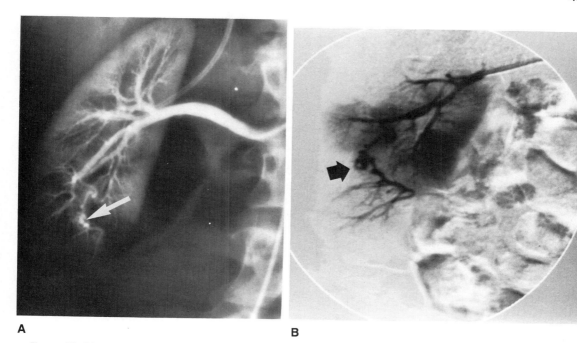

A                                    B

*Figure 16–14.* Arterial malformation. AP right renal arteriogram (*left*) and selective digital subtraction arteriogram of a lower pole branch (*right*) show an arterial malformation (*arrows*) in a teen-aged male with hypertension. There is no arteriovenous shunting. The hypertension was cured following selective embolization.

are hematuria and occasionally hypertension. On arteriography, there are dilated, tortuous vessels with arteriovenous shunting. Small arteriovenous malformations may be indistinguishable from hemangiomas.

Arteriovenous fistulae are usually acquired and most often are posttraumatic (see Figs. 16–32, 16–33, and 16–35). Other causes are congenital, iatrogenic (surgery, biopsy), aneurysm rupture (atherosclerotic or FMD), inflammatory diseases, and neoplasms.[23, 25, 26] Large fistulae may have a significant shunt and can thus lead to congestive heart failure. On arteriography, the feeding artery is enlarged and there is prompt, dense venous opacification. In congenital fistulae, a venous aneurysm (due to increased flow) is observed. Traumatic fistulae often show a false aneurysm at the site of the fistulous communication (see Figs. 16–33 and 16–35).

Hemangiomas of the kidney are also rare lesions. They may be of the capillary or the cavernous type. The most frequent symptoms are gross hematuria and colicky pain. On arteriography, there is a cluster of tortuous vascular spaces and arteriovenous shunting may be observed.[27] In some vascular malformations, diminished cortical perfusion is observed, which occasionally may

be responsible for hypertension (Fig. 16–14). The abnormal vessels do not constrict in response to epinephrine.

## Dissection

The left renal artery is frequently involved in aortic dissection. Spontaneous dissection of the renal artery without aortic dissection is rare. It occurs most frequently in association with FMD and occasionally in atherosclerosis. Men are more commonly affected than women. Posttraumatic renal artery dissection is seen after blunt abdominal trauma or arterial catheterization.[28-30] In spontaneous dissections, symptoms are related to renal ischemia (ie, due to hypertension). The dissection is located in the outer third of the media.

On arteriography, a typical intimal flap may be seen, but, more frequently, the arterial lumen is irregular and widened (sausagelike) as a result of opacification of the false channel (see Fig. 16–22). The dissection may extend into the branches. On the parenchymal phase, cortical hypoperfusion may be observed. Traumatic dissections often lead to arterial occlusion, and an intimal flap may not be demonstrated.

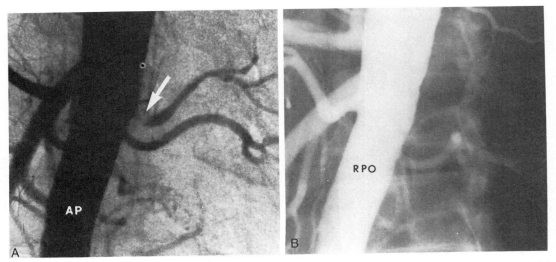

**Figure 16–15.** Progression of renal artery stenosis to occlusion. *A,* AP aortogram shows severe stenosis of the upper left renal artery (*arrow*). *B,* RPO aortogram performed several months later shows complete occlusion of this vessel.

## Embolization and Thrombosis

The most frequent source for renal thromboemboli is the heart. Such emboli usually obstruct the main renal artery or larger branches. The resulting ischemia leads to hypertension and/or compromise of renal function. Embolization into the peripheral renal circulation is observed in renal artery aneurysms. Cholesterol embolization may occur spontaneously or after arterial catheterization. Small intrarenal arterial aneurysms that develop following cholesterol embolization may simulate polyarteritis nodosa.[24]

In severe renal artery stenosis, the development of in situ thrombosis is the natural history of the lesion (Fig. 16–15). The intrarenal vessels usually remain patent and are supplied by collaterals (see Figs. 16–9 and 16–17). The resulting renal ischemia leads to hypertension. If the occlusion is relatively recent, the renal artery can be reopened by balloon angioplasty, or surgical revascularization can be attempted.[31]

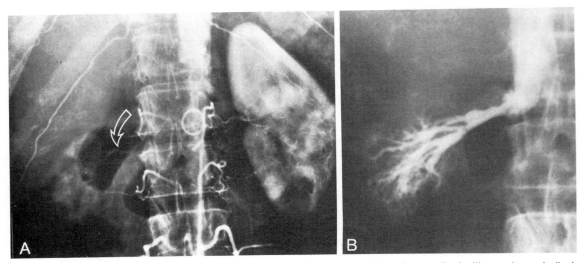

**Figure 16–16.** Shrunken kidney due to longstanding occlusion of renal artery in a patient with poorly controlled hypertension. *A,* Late phase from an abdominal aortogram shows opacification of a diminutive renal artery via collaterals (*open arrow*). *B,* Retrograde renal venogram. There is complete opacification of the intrarenal branches on manual contrast injection because of minimal antegrade blood flow.

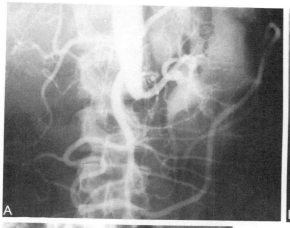
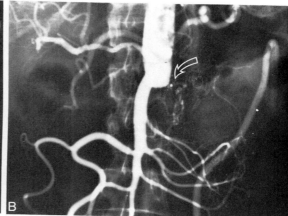
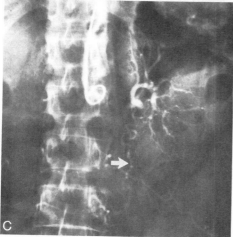

*Figure 16–17.* Retrograde propagation of aortic thrombus leading to renal artery occlusion. *A,* Aortogram via left axillary artery approach shows infrarenal aortic occlusion. The right kidney was removed several years earlier. *B,* Aortogram performed several months later for evaluation of acute renal failure shows thrombotic occlusion of the left renal artery. The middle adrenal artery is enlarged and provides collaterals to the kidney (*arrow*). *C,* Later film from the same study shows opacification of intrarenal branches of the renal artery and pelvic and ureteric collaterals (*arrow*).

Longstanding renal artery occlusion leads to severe shrinkage of the kidney. On arteriography, the intrarenal vessels are opacified during the late phase of the aortogram (Fig. 16–16). Markedly diminished flow in the renal vein permits excellent opacification of the entire intrarenal venous circulation by simple hand injection of contrast medium. Another cause of renal artery thrombosis is retrograde propagation of aortic thrombus (Fig. 16–17).

Iatrogenic causes of renal artery occlusion are inadvertent migration of embolization coils placed in the contralateral renal artery and guide wire or catheter-induced dissection or plaque dislodgment in severely diseased and stenotic renal arteries.[32]

## HYPERTENSION

Renovascular disease is responsible for hypertension in between 5 and 10% of patients.

The two major causes are atherosclerosis and FMD. Untreated, both diseases progress to renal artery occlusion. Other causes (about 5%) are renal artery stenosis due to neurofibromatosis or pheochromocytoma, fibrous bands, arteritis, emboli, thrombosis, aneurysms, vascular malformations and fistulae, radiation, cysts, neoplasms, and perirenal hematomas.[33, 34]

### Atherosclerosis

Atherosclerosis is a manifestation of the normal aging process, and not all renal artery stenoses demonstrated on arteriography are associated with renovascular hypertension. Thus, in one arteriographic study, renal artery disease was found in 45% of normotensive individuals over 60 years of age.[35] On the other hand, the presence of a renal artery stenosis in patients less than 50 years of age is usually associated with hypertension.[16]

Atherosclerosis is the most common cause

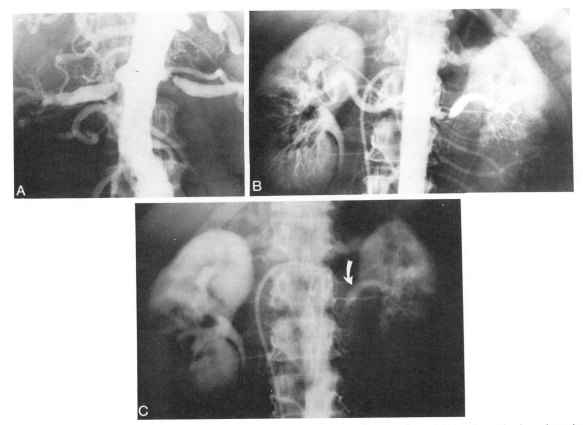

*Figure 16–18.* Atherosclerotic renal artery stenosis. *A,* Abdominal aortogram shows bilateral renal artery stenosis with post-stenotic dilatation. *B,* Early and *C,* late frames from an aortogram in another patient show stenosis of the left renal artery and poor opacification of lower pole branches in the absence of an accessory vessel. Persistent opacification of the left renal artery (*arrow*) after contrast medium has cleared from the aorta and right renal artery indicates the presence of a severe, hemodynamically significant stenosis.

of renovascular hypertension (approximately 60% of patients). The majority of patients are men and are older than 50 years. The stenosis is most commonly located in the proximal renal artery and frequently involves the orifice and is due to a mural aortic plaque (Fig. 16–18). This relationship of the renal artery stenosis to the aortic plaque is often not demonstrated until such a plaque is broken by balloon dilatation.[36]

Thirty-one per cent of patients with renovascular hypertension due to atherosclerosis have bilateral renal artery stenoses.[37] In 93% of patients, the lesion involves the main renal artery, and in the remainder, main renal artery and branch stenoses are present. Isolated branch vessel stenosis due to atherosclerosis is rare. Severe bilateral renal artery stenosis or severe stenosis in the renal artery to a solitary kidney may also be responsible for oliguric renal failure.

## Fibromuscular Dysplasia (FMD)

FMD is the cause of renal artery stenosis in approximately one third of patients with renovascular hypertension. It is observed in all age groups, and the majority of patients are women (ratio of 3:1).[38–41] The patients are younger than those affected by atherosclerosis, and, typically, the lesions occur in the mid- and distal renal artery. Occasionally, the entire renal artery is affected, ie, also the proximal segment. Rarely, the disease may affect only the proximal one third of the renal artery.

The disease is bilateral in two thirds the patients.[38] Unilateral disease occurs more frequently in the right renal artery.[39] In 79% of patients, the lesions involve the main renal artery; in approximately 17%, the branch vessels are also involved; and in about 4%, there are isolated lesions of the branches.[38]

**TABLE 16–3.** Classification of Fibromuscular Dysplasia*

| Type | Incidence (%) | Location | Pathology | Angiography |
|---|---|---|---|---|
| Intimal fibroplasia | 1–2 | Main RA, large branch | Circumferential or eccentric intimal proliferation | Focal stenosis |
| Medial fibroplasia | 60–70 | Mid–distal RA, branches | Multiple fibromuscular ridges causing stenosis and mural thinning leading to aneurysm formation | "String of beads," alternating areas of stenosis and aneurysms |
| Medial hyperplasia | 5–15 | Main RA, branches | Smooth muscle hyperplasia | Long, smooth narrowing |
| Perimedial fibroplasia | 15–25 | Main RA | Fibroplasia of outer media | Irregular stenoses, beading (without aneurysm formation)†; rarely, true aneurysms |
| Medial dissection | ~5 | Main RA, branches | Dissection in outer third of media | False channel, aneurysms |
| Adventitial fibroplasia | <1 | Main RA, large branch | Adventitial and periarterial proliferation | Long, segmental stenosis |

*Includes data from references 32, 39, and 40.
†Beaded segment not wider than unaffected arterial segments.
  RA = renal artery.

FMD is the most common cause of renovascular hypertension in children, and branch vessel disease predominates either as an isolated abnormality or in association with main renal artery disease.[38, 41] In older patients, FMD and atherosclerosis may coexist.

FMD is an arterial disease, and convincing evidence of venous abnormalities in these patients is lacking.[42] Classification and the angiographic appearance of the different types of FMD are listed in Table 16–3 (Figs. 16–12 and 16–19 to 16–22).

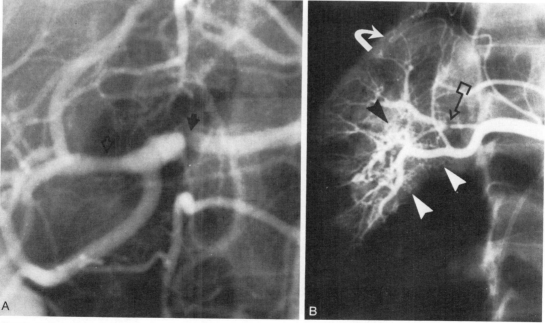

**Figure 16–19.** Intimal fibroplasia. *A*, Closeup of a right renal arteriogram shows a focal ringlike stenosis of the distal renal artery (*arrow*). There is poststenotic dilatation, and another severe focal ringlike stenosis is present at the renal artery bifurcation. Open arrow points to a long, smooth stenosis of a branch vessel. *B*, Focal stenosis (*arrow*) in another patient with severe hypertension. A myriad of intrarenal collaterals is seen (*arrowheads*). In addition, the capsular artery is enlarged and anastomoses with an interlobar branch (*curved arrow*).

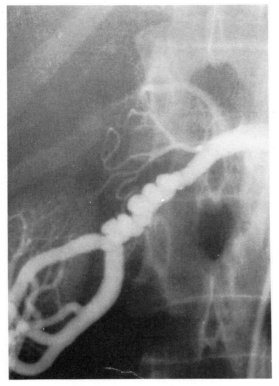

**Figure 16–20.** Medial fibroplasia. Alternating areas of aneurysm formation and narrowing give the "string of beads" appearance. Note that the aneurysmal segments are wider than the normal artery.

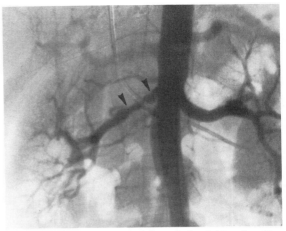

**Figure 16–21.** Perimedial fibroplasia. Subtraction film from an AP abdominal aortogram shows an irregular and narrowed lumen of the right renal artery (*arrowheads*).

## Neurofibromatosis (Fig. 16–23)

The arterial stenoses caused by neurofibromatosis are mainly due to intimal proliferation and occasionally to the presence of neurofibromata.[43] Hypertension due to neurofibromatosis is observed mainly in children. In addition to renal artery abnormalities, abdominal aortic coarctation has also been reported.[44] The vascular changes in-

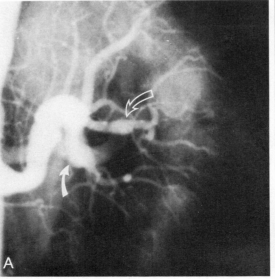

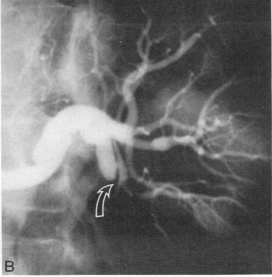

**Figure 16–22.** Spontaneous renal artery dissection in a patient with FMD. *A,* The lumen of the distal renal artery is wider than that of the proximal vessel. In addition there is widening of the lumina of two of its branches (*arrows*). A dissection is seen in one of the branches (*open arrow*). *B,* RPO renal arteriogram shows the dissection in the other branch (*arrow*) in addition to the dissection in the main renal artery. *Note:* Such fusiform arterial dilatation in young patients is highly suggestive of FMD with spontaneous dissection.

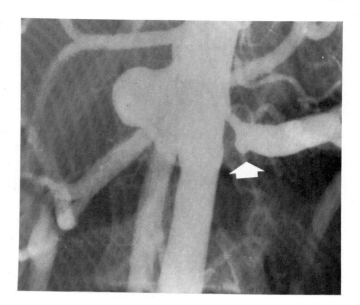

Figure 16–23. Neurofibromatosis. AP abdominal aortogram shows a large aneurysm of the right and a small aneurysm of the left renal artery (*arrow*). In addition, there is a stenosis of the left renal artery orifice. (From Kadir S et al: *In* Athanasoulis CA, et al (Eds): Interventional Radiology. Philadelphia, WB Saunders, 1982.)

clude smooth or nodular-appearing stenosis and saccular aneurysms. Both types may coexist. The stenotic lesions may simulate intimal FMD or congenital renal artery stenosis. Typically, the proximal renal artery or orifice is affected in neurofibromatosis, whereas FMD occurs in the mid- and distal segments and only rarely involves the proximal renal artery.

## Congenital Stenosis (Fig. 16–24)

Congenital bands are a rare cause of renal artery stenosis.[45, 46] These are composed of muscular and fibrous tissue originating from the diaphragmatic crura or psoas muscle and neural tissue from the sympathetic aortic and sympathetic renal ganglia and may affect either side.

On arteriography, the proximal renal artery appears kinked or may demonstrate a circumferential stenosis. Poststenotic dilatation is present in severe stenoses.

## Page Kidney

This refers to renin-angiotensin–mediated hypertension[47] caused by renal compression by a process (hematoma, cyst, tumor) in the perinephric or subcapsular space. The most common etiology is hematoma following blunt trauma (recent or remote). Sonography and CT are usually diagnostic. On arteriography, the intrarenal vessels are stretched and splayed. There is a slow arterial washout and the nephrogram shows distortion of the renal contour and thinning of the parenchyma. The capsular artery is often enlarged and displaced.

## Angiography

The hemodynamic significance of a stenotic lesion is determined by the demonstration of:

1. Elevated renin levels from the renal vein of the affected kidney by a ratio of $\geq 1.5:1$.

2. Collateral vessels in the presence of a renal artery stenosis.

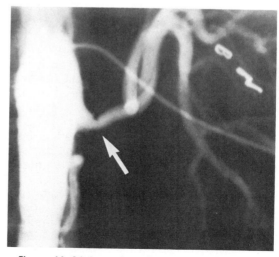

Figure 16–24. Asymptomatic congenital renal artery stenosis. Aortogram performed for evaluation of lower extremity vascular disease shows a stenosis of the proximal left renal artery (*arrow*).

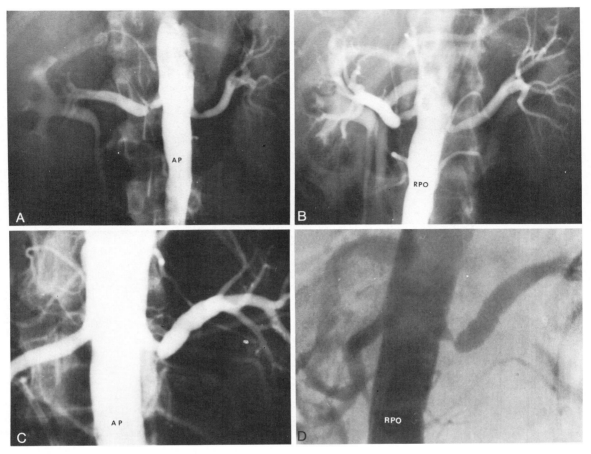

*Figure 16–25.* Importance of multiple projections for the detection of renal artery stenosis. *A* and *B,* The severe right renal artery stenosis is obscured on the aortogram performed in the RPO projection. *C* and *D,* A critical stenosis of the left renal artery is obscured on the AP aortogram, in another patient.

3. Greater than 70% stenosis of the arterial lumen with poststenotic dilatation.

4. Decrease in size of the kidney.

5. Measurement of an intraarterial pressure gradient $\geq$ 40 mm Hg. However, measurement of a pressure gradient is not recommended as a routine procedure. It should be used only when other findings are equivocal.

Intravenous DSA may be used as an outpatient screening procedure in conjunction with venous sampling for renin. Abdominal aortography is an essential part of the workup of patients with suspected renovascular hypertension. Although some reports suggest that an RPO projection is preferable,[48, 49] anatomical considerations and clinical experience indicate that the RPO projection alone is inadequate in close to half the patients with an abnormality of the proximal renal arteries (Fig. 16–25).

An AP abdominal aortogram is performed first. If a lesion is demonstrated, no further arteriography is necessary. If the AP aortogram does not show a lesion and/or the renal artery orifices are obscured, oblique aortograms (first RPO and, if necessary, LPO) are obtained. In children and young adults, selective renal arteriograms should be obtained to evaluate the intrarenal vessels if the main renal arteries are normal on the aortogram.

PITFALLS IN DIAGNOSIS (Figs. 16–25 to 16–27)

1. Obscured stenoses: The severity of a stenosis may not be apparent on either the AP or the oblique projection alone. Thus, oblique arteriograms must be obtained if the lesion is not well defined on the AP study. Similarly, if an oblique arteriogram is obtained first, a stenosis may also be obscured, necessitating an AP study. However, the presence of poststenotic dilatation often provides the clue to the presence of a stenosis.

Intrarenal disease and occasionally mild

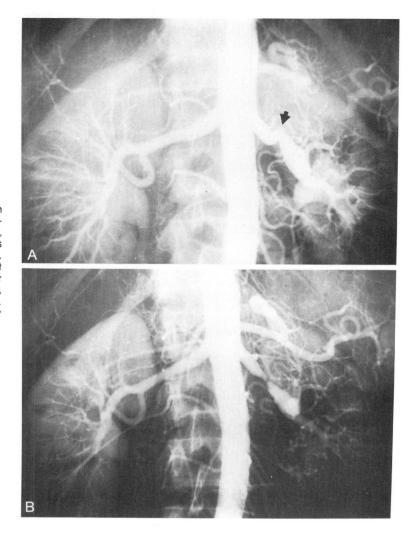

*Figure 16–26.* Effect of respiration on the arteriographic demonstration of a renal artery stenosis. *A,* Aortogram in end expiration shows a kink in the left renal artery (*arrow*). A stenosis is not demonstrated, but the artery distal to the kink is wider than the proximal renal artery. *B,* Aortogram in maximal inspiration. There is a critical left renal artery stenosis with post-stenotic dilation.

stenoses of the main renal artery may not be detected without the aid of selective renal arteriography.

2. Effect of phase of respiration on demonstration of renal artery stenosis: Sometimes a stenosis may only be demonstrated in end expiration or inspiration. If the diameter of the distal renal artery is wider than that of the proximal vessel, poststenotic dilatation beyond a severe stenosis must be suspected.

3. Change in arterial caliber during systole/diastole: During rapid sequence imaging, a change in opacified arterial diameter is observed in relationship to the cardiac cycle. This should not be mistaken for an anatomical abnormality.

4. Technical considerations: The use of straight catheters without tip-occluding devices or a high (above renal) or low catheter position may result in incomplete opacifica-

tion of the renal arteries and may thus simulate a stenosis or lead to obscuration of a lesion because of superimposition of opacified mesenteric vessels. If only selective renal arteriography is performed, an orifice stenosis may be overlooked because of inadequate reflux of contrast medium into the aorta. In addition, catheter-induced renal artery spasm (which occurs frequently in young patients) or intimal dissection may simulate primary renal artery disease. Occasionally, the reflux of contrast medium into the aorta during selective arteriography is in the form of a jet, and thus simulates an orifice stenosis.

5. Subtraction artefacts: When using DSA, subtraction artefacts must be taken into consideration. Different oblique views and craniocaudad or a complex angulation may be necessary to define the anatomy.

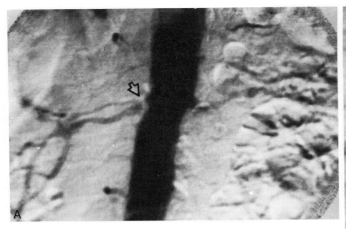
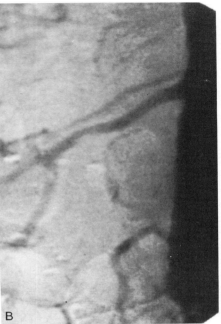

**Figure 16–27.** Subtraction artefact simulating renal artery stenosis. *A*, Intravenous DSA in the AP projection suggests the presence of a proximal stenosis (*arrow*) and early bifurcation of the right renal artery. *B*, Repeat intravenous DSA in the RPO projection with craniocaudad angulation. The orifice of the main renal artery is normal. No early branching is seen but there are two renal arteries originating separately from the aorta.

6. Superimposition of arterial segments: In tortuous or redundant renal arteries, superimposition of segments of the main renal artery and/or its branches may obscure a lesion or simulate disease (eg, aneurysm). The situation is easily clarified by oblique selective arteriography.

7. Renal artery spasm causing a pseudostenosis: This is catheter-induced spasm that is seen on selective arteriography and not on aortography.

8. Standing waves: During selective arteriography, these may occasionally simulate medial fibroplasia. The absence of uneven sacculations (ie, normal arterial diameter) and the regular interval of alternating narrowings permit easy differentiation. Alternatively, an aortogram is obtained for clarification.

## INFLAMMATORY/PARENCHYMAL DISEASES

Although rarely indicated in chronic glomerulo- or pyelonephritis, the angiographic picture in these diseases is quite characteristic.[50, 51] In *chronic glomerulonephritis*, there is marked reduction in renal blood flow, and often there is reflux of contrast medium into the aorta even at an injection rate as low as 1 to 2 ml/sec. The intrarenal vessels, especially the interlobar and arcuate arteries, are severely pruned and tortuous, and interlobular arteries are not visualized. The nephrogram is usually homogeneous, but the corticomedullary junction is indistinct.

In *chronic pyelonephritis*, the intrarenal arteries are also small and are often tortuous in affected areas. Blood flow is diminished, but is normal or only minimally diminished in patients without renal failure.[50] There is pruning of the intrarenal vessels and the nephrogram is inhomogeneous. In addition, stenoses, occlusions, and occasionally aneurysms of the intrarenal vessels are seen. The presence of pyelonephritic scars and segmental or asymmetrical involvement of the kidneys permits differentiation between pyelo- and glomerulonephritis. In xanthogranulomatous pyelonephritis, fine neovascularity may be observed, which cannot be differentiated from that seen in uroepithelial neoplasms.

In *acute tubular necrosis*, the extra- and intrarenal arteries are normal. Although normal blood flow is maintained, there is delayed emptying of the intrarenal vessels. The nephrogram is normal, although diminished cortical perfusion is occasionally observed. The venous opacification is slightly delayed or normal.

## RENAL TRANSPLANT

The right iliac fossa is the usual location for the first renal transplant. In adults, the transplant renal artery is anastomosed end to end with the recipient internal iliac artery. In children and occasionally in adults, the external iliac artery is used and, rarely, the abdominal aorta. The renal vein is anastomosed to the external iliac vein.

Hypertension is observed in approximately 50% of patients undergoing renal transplantation.[52] The most frequent cause is allograft rejection, but hypertension may also be secondary to renal artery stenosis. In either case, the etiology is renal ischemia.

### Complications of Renal Transplant

Complications of renal transplantation (including vascular complications) can conveniently be divided into three groups: pre-, intra-, and postrenal.[53]

**Prerenal.** Renal artery stenosis is observed in approximately 5% of transplants, but according to some reports it can occur in as many as 23%.[54, 55] Renal failure may occur in severe stenoses without occlusion (see Fig. 16–28). Both focal and long stenoses are observed. Most focal stenoses occur at the anastomosis between the donor renal and the recipient iliac arteries. These are usually due to technical factors (operative), clamp or perfusion cannula trauma, or ischemia of the donor vessel. Approximately 75% of such stenoses are due to technical errors and are potentially avoidable.[55] Long segments of stenosis can be due to trauma occurring during allograft harvesting, to operative technique, or as a manifestation of rejection.

**Intrarenal.** In acute rejection there is renal enlargement. Multiple stenoses and occlusion are present, and there is rapid tapering and pruning of the interlobar arteries, and poor cortical perfusion. Arterial opacification is prolonged (normal, < 2 seconds; mildly prolonged, 2 to 4 seconds; moderate, 4 to 7 seconds; severe, > 7 seconds),[56] and the interlobular arteries are not demonstrated. The nephrogram is poor and inhomogeneous, the corticomedullary junction is ill defined, and occasionally arteriovenous shunting is observed. Arteriography can often be used to estimate severity and to predict recovery from rejection.[53]

In chronic rejection, the kidney is small and the number of intrarenal vessels is diminished. Vascular pruning or stenoses and occlusions may also be present. The arterial transit time is either normal or prolonged.

**Postrenal.** Venous thrombosis may involve the renal or iliac vein. Venography is essential for the diagnosis. The arteriographic findings may mimic acute rejection, ie, enlargement of the transplant, prolonged arterial transit time, diminished cortical perfusion, arterial spasm, and absent venous opacification.[53] Arterial occlusions are absent.

### Arteriography (Table 16–4 and Figs. 16–28 to 16–30)

Evaluation of hypertension and differentiation between surgical and medical complications are the main indications for angiography. Although hypertension is observed in about half the patients after renal transplantation, only a small number of them actually require arteriography. Furthermore, a stenosis with at least a 70% reduction in arterial lumen is necessary for the development of renovascular hypertension.

Although intravenous DSA can be used for transplant evaluation, this necessitates a large volume of contrast medium (approximately 25 ml/injection), and overlapping vessels often do not permit an optimal study. Many patients have compromised renal function and cannot tolerate large volumes of contrast medium. In our experience, intraar-

#### TABLE 16–4. Renal Transplant Arteriogram

| | |
|---|---|
| Approach | Contralateral femoral artery for internal iliac anastomosis |
| | Ipsilateral femoral artery for external iliac anastomosis |
| Catheter: | Cobra (end and side holes), cobra in loop configuration, visceral hook, sidewinder |
| | Multipurpose (ipsilateral approach) |
| Position | Recipient iliac artery proximal to anastomosis |
| Guide wire | 1.5 mm LLT J |
| Contrast medium | 76% diatrizoate meglumine sodium* |
| Injection rate/volume | 4–5 ml/sec, total 10–12 ml |
| Films: | 10 |
| Rate | 2 per second for 6 films |
| | 1 per second for 4 films |
| Projections | AP, steep ipsilateral posterior oblique (near lateral) |

*20% concentration for DSA.

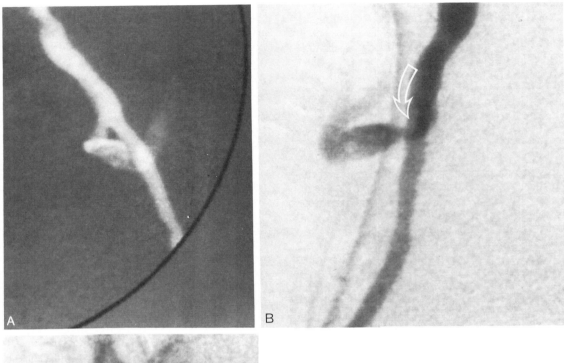

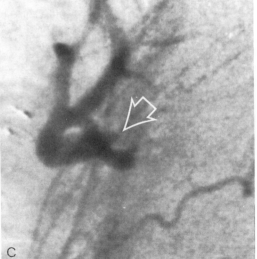

**Figure 16–28.** Oliguric renal failure in a patient with transplant renal artery stenosis. *A,* AP intraarterial DSA of the left common iliac artery. There is no evidence of a stenosis. *B,* Intraarterial DSA in a near lateral projection. The anastomotic stenosis overlies the external iliac artery (*arrow*). *C,* Later frame from the same arteriogram. The contrast medium persists in the transplant renal artery, whereas it has cleared from the external iliac artery. A beaklike stenosis is present (*arrow*).

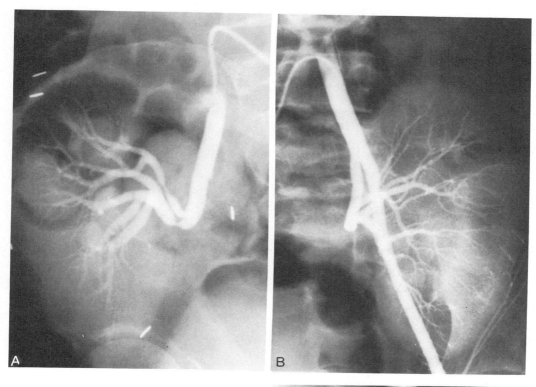

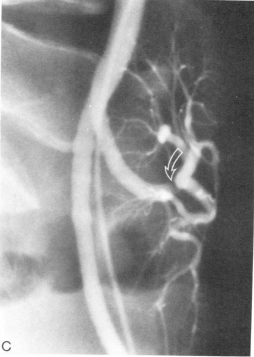

*Figure 16–29.* Transplant renal artery stenosis. *A*, Focal and long stenoses in the transplant renal artery. *B*, and *C*, Severe transplant renal artery stenosis in another patent. The stenosis is seen only on the lateral arteriogram (*arrow*).

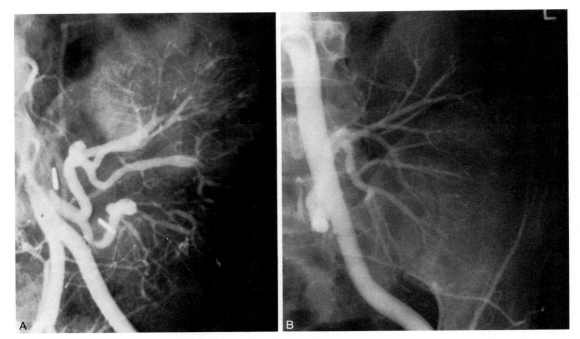

*Figure 16–30. A,* Acute transplant rejection. Left common iliac arteriogram shows multiple stenoses and occlusions of the intrarenal arteries. The transplant renal artery is anastomosed to the common iliac artery. *B,* Chronic transplant rejection. Left common iliac arteriogram shows pruning of the intrarenal branches. (*A,* Courtesy of Dr. CA Athanasoulis.)

terial DSA has provided the optimal method for evaluating renal transplants. Comparison with the donor renal arteriogram also helps in evaluating disease of the intrarenal arteries after transplantation.

From the contralateral femoral artery approach, a cobra catheter (5 Fr, end and side holes) is placed in the common or proximal internal iliac artery on the side of the transplant. Alternatively, a single curve or sidewinder catheter is placed in the recipient common iliac artery. Stiff catheters or excessive manipulation should be avoided in order to prevent arterial trauma in the transplant/recipient vessels. Arteriograms are obtained in both an AP (for evaluation of intrarenal vessels and nephrogram) and a steep ipsilateral posterior oblique projection (for evaluation of the anastomosis).

Venous catheterization for the detection of renal vein thrombosis or venous sampling for renin can be performed from the cubital vein or from the ipsilateral femoral vein, ie, same side as the transplant.

PITFALLS IN DIAGNOSIS

1. Normal AP arteriogram: A stenosis at the anastomosis between the donor renal and the recipient internal iliac arteries is fre-

quently not visualized on the AP arteriogram. A steep oblique (often a near lateral) projection and selective arteriography may be required to demonstrate the anastomosis without overlapping vessels (Fig. 16–29).

2. Vessels overlapping and obscuring the anastomosis: Selective arteriography should be performed with a slower injection rate (3 to 4 ml/sec) to avoid reflux into the external iliac artery. If this is not possible, the arterial washout time should be assessed (Fig. 16–28). Persistent renal artery opacification after contrast medium has cleared from the iliac arteries indicates the presence of a hemodynamically significant stenosis.

3. Hypertension with a normal anastomosis: This is observed in allograft rejection.

4. Occasionally, acute tubular necrosis may be difficult to differentiate from acute rejection. In the former, the intrarenal vasculature is normal but cortical perfusion is diminished.

TRAUMA

Renal parenchymal or vascular injury may occur as a result of blunt or penetrating abdominal trauma or it may be iatrogenic, occurring after interventional radiological procedures (angioplasty, nephrostomy), renal biopsy, or operation. The most common clinical manifestation of renal injury, ie, hematuria (micro- or macroscopic), is observed in more than 90% of patients.[57, 58] Hypertension is a late manifestation of vascular injury.

**Blunt Injury.** Blunt abdominal trauma may result in parenchymal injury, ie, contusion, laceration, rupture (fracture), or vascular injury. Visualization of the kidney on intravenous urography does not exclude vascular injury. The affected kidney fails to visualize only if the vascular pedicle has been severed or arterial thrombosis has occurred. This must be differentiated from congenitally absent or dysplastic kidneys (see section on Miscellaneous Application of Angiography). Vascular pedicle injury occurs as a result of the shear stress from deceleration.[59, 60] This leads to intimal disruption, dissection, and thrombosis of the renal artery. Occasionally, there is traumatic dissection or intimal disruption without thrombosis (Fig. 16–31B).

In renal contusion, the nephrogram appears striated, and cortical hypoperfusion and arteriovenous shunting may be present.[61] Severe blunt trauma may cause parenchymal tears and associated hematoma formation but may also result in injury to larger vessels with formation of aneurysms or arteriovenous fistulae.

**Penetrating Injury.** In one series, penetrating injury to the kidney or renal vessels was observed in 12.6% of patients with abdominal stab wounds.[57] Penetrating injuries may result in subcapsular hematoma (eventually leading to a Page kidney), formation of an aneurysm or arteriovenous fistula, or arterial occlusion.

**Iatrogenic Injury.** Percutaneous renal biopsy, operation (eg, nephrolithotomy), percutaneous transluminal angioplasty, and intravascular drug abuse are also associated with vascular injury. Arteriovenous fistula or aneurysm formation and retroperitoneal hemorrhage (following arterial perforation or aneurysm rupture) may be observed.

**Arteriography.** This is indicated for both assessment of vascular injury and nonoperative treatment of certain lesions.[23] The main indications for arteriographic evaluation are:

1. Blunt or penetrating abdominal or flank trauma with hematuria.
2. Nonvisualization of the kidney on intra-

venous urography in patients with abdominal or flank trauma.
3. Evaluation of hypertension or persistent hematuria following abdominal or flank trauma.
4. Hypotension (due to blood loss), persistent hematuria or hypertension (suspected renal artery occlusion or perirenal hematoma) following operation, percutaneous biopsy, or interventional radiological procedure.

The following arteriographic findings may be observed:

1. Arterial occlusion (Fig. 16–31): This occurs in blunt deceleration and occasionally in iatrogenic injury.[62]
2. Intimal disruption or dissection without arterial occlusion (Fig. 16–31).
3. Arteriovenous fistula (Figs. 16–32 and 16–33): This can occur after blunt or penetrating injury or following diagnostic (biopsy) or therapeutic medical procedures (eg, percutaneous transluminal angioplasty, operation, or nephrostomy). Although most small fistulae close spontaneously, some may persist for long periods.[57]
4. Aneurysms (Figs. 16–32, 16–34, and 16–35): These may occur after blunt or penetrating injury.
5. Arteriocalyceal fistula: This is a rare complication of penetrating renal injury.[63]
6. Renal fracture (Fig. 16–35): This occurs in severe blunt trauma.
7. Perirenal hematoma (Fig. 16–34): On arteriography, this shows the typical configuration also observed in subcapsular hepatic and splenic hematomas, ie, lateral concave margin and compression of the renal parenchyma.[64] The Page kidney is a late manifestation of blunt or penetrating renal injury.
8. Retroperitoneal hematoma (Fig. 16–32).

## TUMORS

### Benign Renal Tumors

Most benign renal tumors are small, rarely gain clinical significance, and are discovered incidentally at autopsy. They become clinically significant if they grow large and cause symptoms. Of the cortical tumors, the *adenoma* is the most common lesion. It occurs more frequently in men, and symptoms include hematuria, pain, and rarely hypertension.[65] At autopsy, an adenoma is found in about 1% of individuals.[66] Four different types are observed: papillary or cystadenoma (38%), tubular (38%), alveolar (3%), and

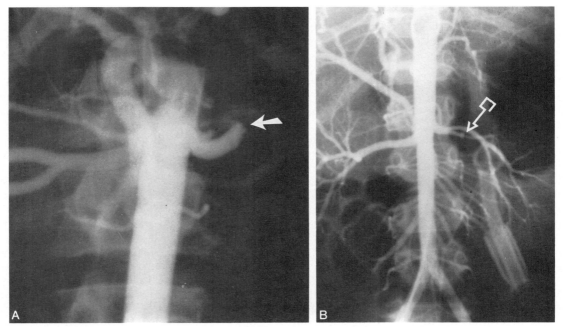

*Figure 16–31.* Renal artery injury following blunt abdominal trauma. *A,* Abdominal aortogram shows occlusion of the left renal artery (*arrow*). *B,* Abdominal aortogram from a child shows intimal disruption without arterial thrombosis (*arrow*). The intrarenal branches distal to the traumatized artery are attenuated.

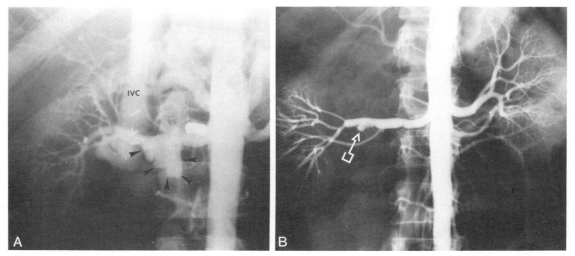

*Figure 16–32.* Traumatic renal artery aneurysm. *A,* From penetrating injury. Abdominal aortogram shows a false aneurysm (*arrowheads*) with renal artery to IVC fistula following a bullet injury. Surgical clips are from a preceding surgical exploration. IVC = inferior vena cava. *B* and *C,* Following percutaneous transluminal angioplasty for FMD. *B,* Early arterial phase from an abdominal aortogram shows a traumatic aneurysm of the right renal artery (*arrow*). The right kidney is displaced laterally and inferiorly by a retroperitoneal hematoma. There is spasm of the segmental arteries (compare with left kidney).

*Illustration continued on opposite page*

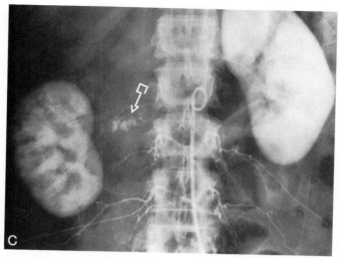

**Figure 16–32** *Continued. C,* Parenchymal phase from the same study shows contrast extravasation (*arrow*). The nephrogram of the right kidney is inhomogeneous. The latter is most likely due to the arterial spasm.

**Figure 16–33.** Arteriovenous fistula following blunt flank trauma. The patient developed hematuria following a fall from a tree. Renal arteriogram shows an arteriovenous fistula and a small traumatic aneurysm (*arrow*). V = renal vein. On repeat arteriography 1 week later, the fistula had closed spontaneously.

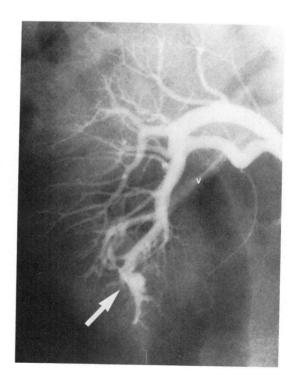

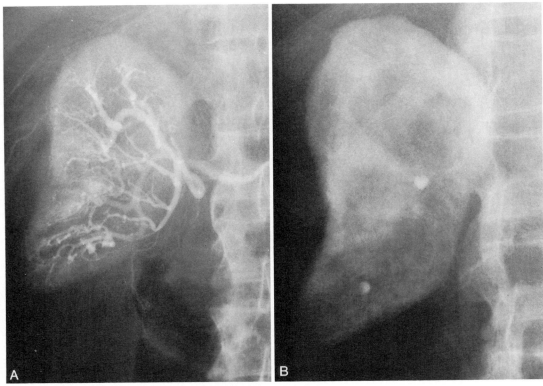

*Figure 16–34.* Perirenal hematoma and false aneurysms following attempted nephrostomy. *A*, Early arterial phase and *B*, parenchymal phase from a right renal arteriogram show compression of the lateral margin of the kidney from the hematoma. On the parenchymal phase, persistent contrast accumulation is seen in two false aneurysms. (Reprinted with permission from Kadir S, Athanasoulis CA: CRC Crit Rev Diag Imaging, 1979, pp 35–78. Copyright CRC Press, Inc.)

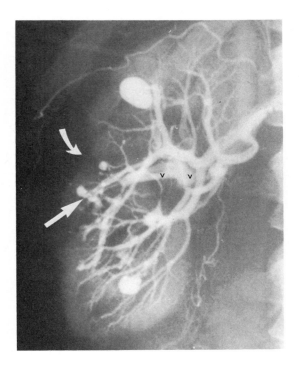

*Figure 16–35.* Blunt renal trauma. Renal arteriogram shows multiple false aneurysms and an arteriovenous fistula (*straight arrow*). The kidney is fractured through its mid-portion (*curved arrow*). v = vein.

mixed types (21%).[65] Histologically, adenoma may be difficult to differentiate from adenocarcinoma. Classicially, tumor size has been used to differentiate between benign and malignant lesions, with tumors less than 3 cm considered benign. However, lesions less than 3 cm have been known to metastasize and demonstrate intravenous growth, indicating that size alone is not sufficient for differentiation.

On arteriography, the papillary type is hypovascular, whereas the others are generally hypervascular.[65] Fine neovascularity is present; the lesion is well circumscribed, with either a homogeneous or a heterogeneous tumor stain; and arteriovenous shunting is infrequent. In contradistinction, malignant tumors are poorly marginated.

The benign *oxyphilic adenoma* (oncocytoma) is a variant of the tubular adenoma. The lesion arises in the proximal renal tubules where the epithelial cells have transformed into oncocytes. It grows exophytically and has a relatively characteristic angiographic picture[67, 68] (Fig. 16–36). The tumor is well circumscribed with a characteristic "spoke wheel" arrangement of the arteries. However, such a pattern is not observed in all lesions.[67] The parenchymal phase is relatively homogeneous, and the wild neovascularity

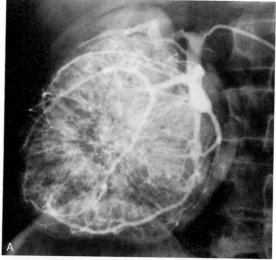

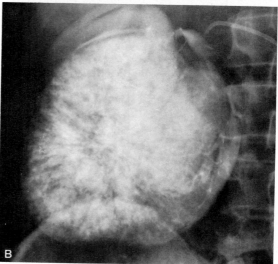

*Figure 16–36.* Renal oncocytoma. *A,* Arterial and *B,* parenchymal phases of a right renal arteriogram show a highly vascular tumor with a spoke-wheel configuration of the tumor vessels. (Courtesy of Dr. SN Weiner. From Weiner SN, Bernstein RG: Radiology, 125:633, 1977. Used with permission.)

observed in malignant lesions is absent. Nevertheless, differentiation from adenocarcinoma is not always possible.[67]

The *renin-secreting adenoma* is a rare cortical tumor found in young individuals.[69] Arteriographic demonstration of this lesion has not always been successful.[70] However, the tumor may be detectable with selective magnification arteriography and pharmacological enhancement. Measurement of high renin levels from segmental renal veins may be the only indicator of its presence.

Of the mesenchymal tumors, the *angiomyolipoma* is of interest, as it is often symptomatic and because of its angiographic similarity to adenocarcinoma. Histologically, it is a hamartoma, comprised of normal tissue (vascular, fatty, and muscular elements), which are present in a disorganized and disproportionate fashion. Vascularity of the lesion depends upon the relative abundance of the different elements.

The angiomyolipoma occurs as an isolated lesion or in association with tuberous sclerosis. The isolated lesion (occasionally two or more tumors are found) occurs predominantly in women (ratio > 4:1) in the third to sixth decades of life.[71] Most solitary tumors are symptomatic, ie, there is a mass, pain (caused by spontaneous hemorrhage into the tumor or infarction), and hematuria. Rarely, spontaneous rupture may occur into the retroperitoneum. Multiple angiomyolipomas, which are seen in patients with tuberous sclerosis, are usually asymptomatic.

On arteriography, the typical features are present in less than half the cases.[71] Most lesions are hypervascular, but if fatty elements predominate, the tumor is hypovascular. The arteries supplying the tumor are enlarged and tortuous (Fig. 16–37). Often there is a single large vessel.[71] Neovascularity and saccular aneurysms are seen. The tumor stain is inhomogeneous because of the presence of fat, and arteriovenous shunting is absent. Angiographic differentiation from adenocarcinoma may be very difficult because all the arteriographic features described above may also be observed in adenocarcinoma.

## Malignant Renal Tumors

### Adenocarcinoma

The adenocarcinoma (hypernephroma, renal cell carcinoma), which arises from the renal tubules, is the most frequent malignant

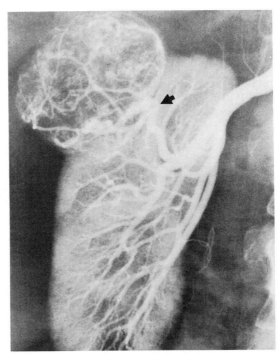

**Figure 16–37.** Angiomyolipoma. Renal arteriogram shows a highly vascular exophytic tumor. A single, enlarged, tortuous artery (*arrow*) supplies the tumor. (Courtesy of Dr. MA Bosniak. From Bosniak MA: Urol Radiol 3:135, 1981.)

tumor, constituting approximately 80% of all renal lesions. It occurs more frequently in men (ratio of 2:1) in the fifth to seventh decades of life, but may be seen in younger individuals (including children). Symptoms are weight loss, anemia, hematuria, flank pain, and a palpable mass. Occasionally, spontaneous retroperitoneal hemorrhage may be the initial presentation. Rarely, the tumor may produce renin and be responsible for hypertension.[72]

Although the majority of tumors are single, bilateral tumors occur in up to 5% of patients in the absence of von Hippel–Lindau disease.[73] The most frequent locations for metastases are the lungs, lymph nodes, and liver. Ten per cent of adenocarcinomas demonstrate calcification on the plain abdominal radiograph.[74] CT is the procedure of choice for establishing the diagnosis and staging:

Stage I: Tumor confined to the kidney.

Stage II: Tumor confined to Gerota's fascia.

Stage III: Extension of tumor into the perinephric fat, renal vein, and IVC, and regional lymph node involvement.

Stage IV: Extension into adjacent organs; distant metastases.

Multiple bilateral renal carcinomas are observed in patients with von Hippel–Lindau disease.[75] In addition, the disease is characterized by angiomatosis retinae, hemangioblastomas, and pheochromocytomas. The renal tumors are often very small and intracystic[76] (Fig. 16–38). Arteriography is essential for the detection of smaller lesions if conservatory surgery is to be performed. Since many of the lesions are small and do not enhance more than the normal renal parenchyma, they escape detection by CT.

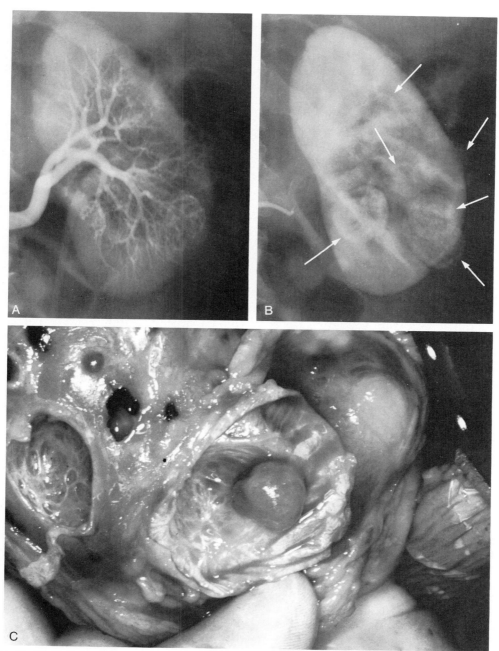

*Figure 16–38.* Multiple renal cell carcinomas in a patient with von Hippel–Lindau disease. *A,* Arterial and *B,* parenchymal phase from a left renal arteriogram shows multiple carcinomas (*arrows*). *C,* Intraoperative photograph shows a small intracystic tumor. (From Kadir S et al: J Urol 126:316, 1981. Used with permission.)

**Angiography.** In renal cell carcinoma, angiography is indicated for the:

1. Evaluation of large tumors (usually Stage II or more).

2. Determination of vascular supply, vascularity, and sources of parasitized blood supply. This helps in planning the operation and estimating intraoperative blood loss.

3. Detection of venous extension.

4. For preoperative devascularization (transcatheter embolization) in hypervascular lesions.

5. Diagnosis of some small tumors (eg, in von Hippel–Lindau disease) and those with equivocal CT findings.

6. Definition of vascular anatomy in patients who are to undergo bench surgery or partial nephrectomy.

7. Differentiation between caval invasion and paracaval lymphadenopathy.

8. Treatment of spontaneous hemorrhage by transcatheter embolization.

The accuracy of angiography for the diagnosis of renal carcinoma has been reported as 97%.[77] Reports that suggest a much lower accuracy must be interpreted with caution. In addition, for a meaningful comparison of angiography with CT,[78] a complete angiographic study with a careful review of the films is absolutely essential.

An abdominal aortogram should be a part of the angiographic evaluation of all large renal masses. This serves primarily to evaluate the sources of blood supply and evaluate the proximal renal artery of the opposite kidney for occlusive disease. Selective arteriography characterizes the tumor, defines vascular supply, and evaluates the need for preoperative embolization. If a tumor is not readily identified on AP renal arteriography, oblique views are essential. Selective arteriography of the opposite kidney is used to exclude a contralateral metastasis or a second primary tumor. In the pre-CT era, hepatic arteriography was performed routinely for the detection of hepatic metastases. Presently, this is no longer necessary because these patients have undergone CT evaluation.

Techniques to enhance angiographic visualization of poorly vascularized neoplasms are high dose angiography (with or without pharmacological enhancement),[79] epinephrine pharmacoangiography, and renal venography. The last can also be used to differentiate between cystic tumors and benign simple cysts. For high dose arteriography, 20 to 30 ml of contrast medium is injected into the renal artery. The flow rate is increased by about 25% if a vasodilator is used.

Demonstration of venous extension of renal carcinoma may have prognostic and surgical implications. Therefore, determination of renal vein patency and, more important, of caval extension of tumor is necessary. Although the renal veins and IVC are easily evaluated by CT, a nonoccluding tumor thrombus may go undetected. The inferior venacavogram, although less sensitive than CT for the assessment of paracaval lymphadenopathy, may be able to differentiate between caval invasion by tumor and adenopathy.

Although angiography may not be required for preoperative assessment of small renal carcinomas, some surgeons may desire preoperative definition of the blood supply to the affected kidney. This can be assessed in a relatively noninvasive fashion by intravenous DSA. If the femoral vein approach is used, the inferior vena cava can also be evaluated.

The typical adenocarcinoma is hypervascular and shows several of the angiographic features listed below, but up to 22% of these tumors are hypovascular[77] (Fig. 16–40). This hypovascularity may be a manifestation of a necrotic tumor, cystic degeneration, or carcinoma arising within a cyst. The last is observed in 3% of patients[80] and must be suspected if hemorrhagic aspiration fluid is obtained.

The angiographic features of renal cell carcinoma are described below. Not all features are seen in every tumor (Figs. 16–38 to 16–44):

1. Enlarged, tortuous, poorly tapering feeding vessels.

2. Coarse neovascularity and formation of small aneurysms.

3. Parasitization of adjacent vessels (lumbar, adrenal, subcostal, inferior and superior mesenteric artery branches).

4. Hypervascular lesions show a dense, inhomogeneous tumor stain, puddling of contrast medium, and occasionally arteriovenous shunting. The tumor margins are poorly defined.

5. Tumor growth into the renal vein and IVC: This is observed in one third of patients.[81] It is more likely to occur in large tumors and in those located on the right side. Caval extension may lead to IVC and hepatic vein obstruction and the Budd-Chiari syndrome.[82]

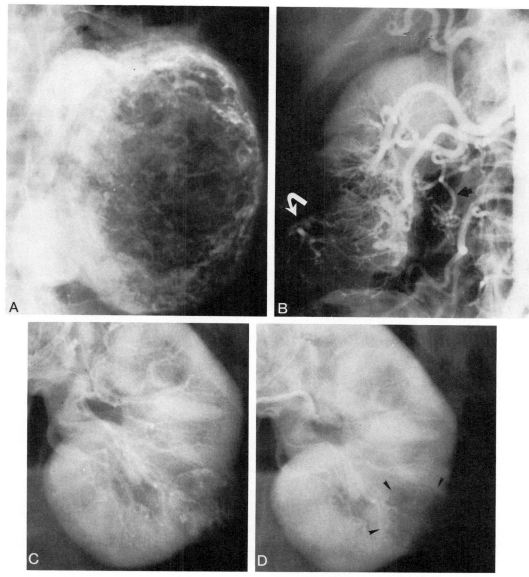

*Figure 16–39.* Renal cell carcinomas. *A,* Parenchymal phase from a left renal arteriogram shows a large, hypervascular carcinoma. *B,* Hypervascular lower pole carcinoma in another patient. The pelvic branch is enlarged (*arrow*) and supplies the tumor. Coarse tumor vessels are seen (*curved arrow*). *C* and *D,* Small, well-marginated renal cell carcinoma in a different patient. *C,* Late arterial phase of left renal arteriogram shows a small tumor. *D,* Repeat arteriogram following intraarterial injection of epinephrine. The tumor is less well seen (*arrowheads*) because of constriction of the abnormal vessels in response to intraarterial epinephrine.

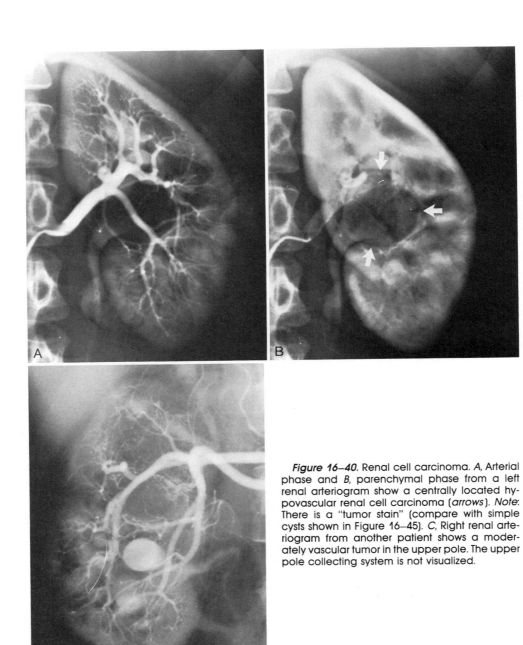

***Figure 16–40.*** Renal cell carcinoma. *A,* Arterial phase and *B,* parenchymal phase from a left renal arteriogram show a centrally located hypovascular renal cell carcinoma (*arrows*). *Note*: There is a "tumor stain" (compare with simple cysts shown in Figure 16–45). *C,* Right renal arteriogram from another patient shows a moderately vascular tumor in the upper pole. The upper pole collecting system is not visualized.

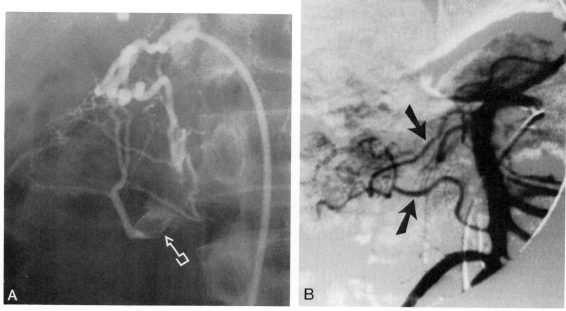

*Figure 16–41.* Parasitization of blood supply in renal cell carcinoma. *A,* Lumbar arteriogram shows tumor vessels and retrograde opacification of the renal artery (*arrow*). (Same patient as in Figure 16–40*C.*) *B,* DSA of the superior mesenteric artery in another patient shows parasitization of superior mesenteric branches (*arrows*) by a right-sided renal cell carcinoma.

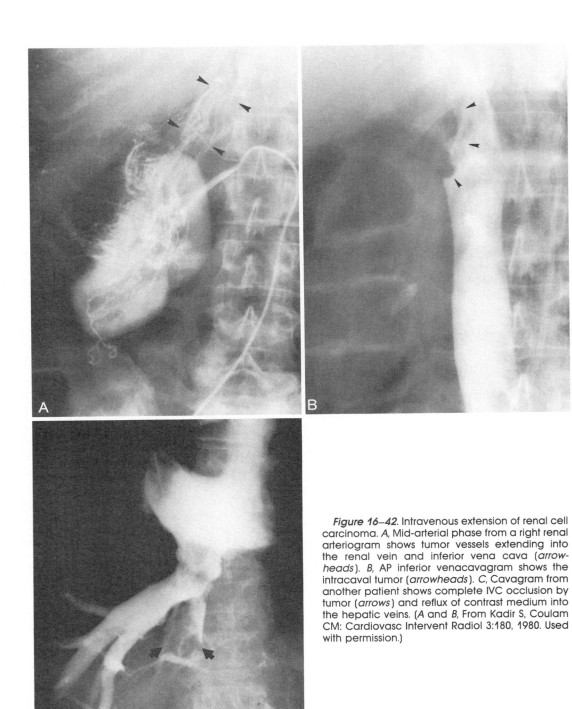

*Figure 16–42.* Intravenous extension of renal cell carcinoma. *A,* Mid-arterial phase from a right renal arteriogram shows tumor vessels extending into the renal vein and inferior vena cava (*arrowheads*). *B,* AP inferior venacavagram shows the intracaval tumor (*arrowheads*). *C,* Cavagram from another patient shows complete IVC occlusion by tumor (*arrows*) and reflux of contrast medium into the hepatic veins. (*A* and *B,* From Kadir S, Coulam CM: Cardiovasc Intervent Radiol 3:180, 1980. Used with permission.)

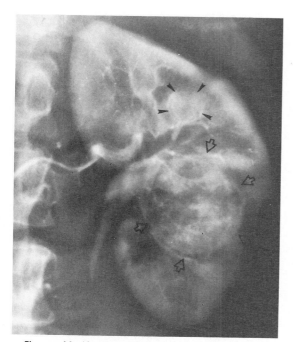

*Figure 16–43.* Minimally vascular renal cell carcinoma in a patient with von Hippel–Lindau disease. Renal arteriogram shows a tumor that is isodense with the normal renal parenchyma (*open arrows*). In addition, there is a small benign cortical rest causing splaying of arterial branches (*arrowheads*).

6. Demonstration of hypervascular metastases in the regional lymph nodes.

7. Demonstration of collateral veins. This is not necessarily an indicator of the presence of venous occlusion but may be a manifestation of the immense hypervascularity of the tumor.

8. Hypovascular tumors show vascular displacement, and a faint or absent tumor stain. Capsular feeding vessels may be seen. High volume pharmacoangiography and renal venography may be necessary for the evaluation of such tumors.

PITFALLS IN DIAGNOSIS

1. Cystic lesion (Figs. 16–44 and 16–45): Cyst versus cystic tumor? Cystic tumors are thick walled and poorly marginated. Benign simple cysts are thin walled. Some cystic carcinomas may be indistinguishable from cysts with inflammatory reaction or infection.

2. CT shows an isodense mass: Tumor versus column of Bertin? Small tumors may enhance to the same degree as the normal renal parenchyma and may therefore remain undetected by CT.

A benign cortical rest (column of Bertin) shows smooth arcuate displacement of normal arterial branches. There is no vascular

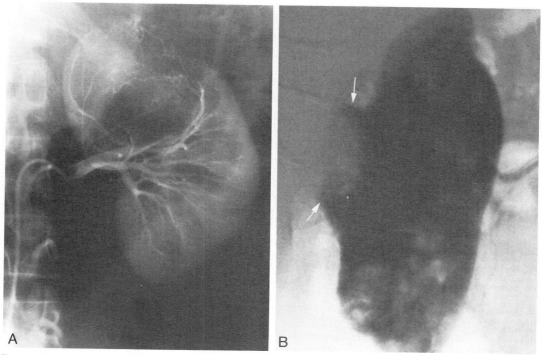

*Figure 16–44.* Hypovascular cystic renal cell carcinomas. *A,* There is minimal coarse neovascularity in the upper pole tumor. Such a lesion can be difficult to distinguish from a cyst with chronic inflammation. *B,* Thick-walled, exophytic cystic tumor in another patient (*arrows*).

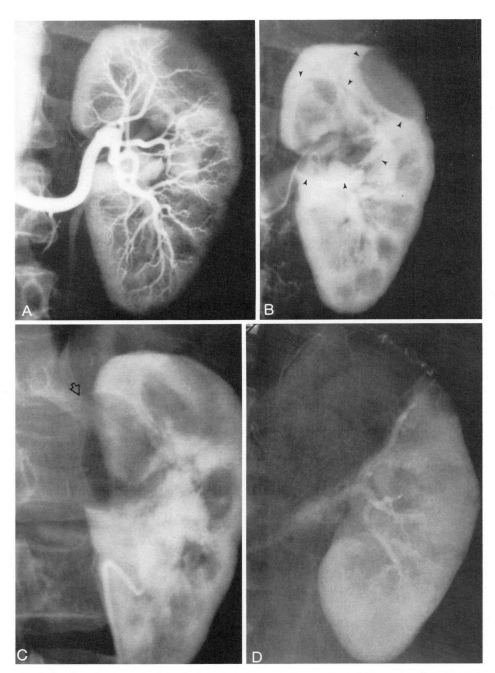

**Figure 16–45.** Benign simple cysts. *A* to *C*, Note the absence of vascular enlargement, neovascularity, or tumor blush and the presence of a sharp interphase with the renal parenchyma (*arrowheads*) and thin wall (*arrow*). D, Benign renal cyst with chronic inflammatory reaction.

enlargement or abnormal vessels and the parenchymal phase is homogeneous (Fig. 16–43). In tumors, there is abnormal vasculature and the parenchymal stain is nonhomogeneous.

The importance of preoperative distinction

lies herein: that in patients with small solitary tumors or suspected bilateral tumors (eg, von Hippel–Lindau disease) a heminephrectomy may be performed.

3. AP arteriogram is normal (Fig. 16–46): Oblique arteriography is absolutely essential

for complete evaluation. The ipsilateral posterior oblique projection usually provides the most information.

4. Inconclusive arteriogram: If the arteriogram is not convincing, renal venography should be performed. Distortion of the venous pattern in the tumor establishes the diagnosis (Fig. 16–46D).

### Mesenchymal Tumors

The sarcomas account for 3% of primary tumors of the kidney, and the fibrosarcoma is the most common type.[83] Renal sarcomas may be hypo- or hypervascular. Hemangiopericytomas are generally hypervascular.

### Uroepithelial Carcinomas

The most common uroepithelial malignancies are the transitional and squamous cell carcinomas, which account for about 12% of all renal malignancies.[84] The angiographic abnormalities observed in these tumors are caused by infiltration of the renal parenchyma. Infiltrative growth is characteristic of

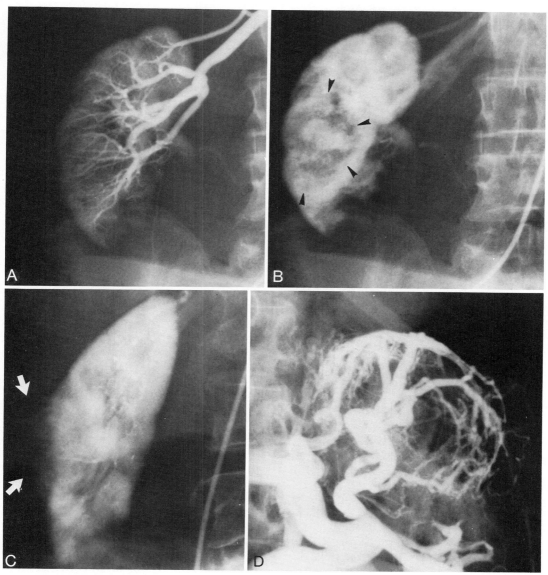

*Figure 16–46.* Exophytic, hypovascular renal cell carcinoma. *A,* Arterial phase shows no abnormality. *B,* On the parenchymal phase, there is some inhomogeneity of the nephrogram (*arrowheads*) with a central hypervascular nodule. The lower margin of the kidney is jagged. This is the typical appearance of the nephrogram when a part of the kidney is supplied by an accessory renal artery. *C,* RPO arteriogram shows the hypovascular neoplasm (*arrows*). *D,* Distorted venous pattern in renal cell carcinoma in another patient.

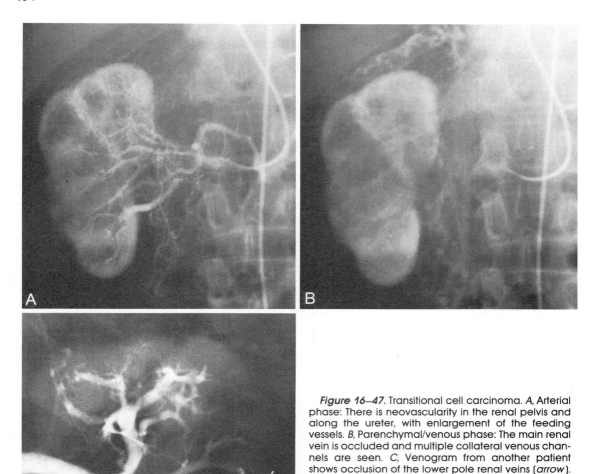

**Figure 16–47.** Transitional cell carcinoma. *A,* Arterial phase: There is neovascularity in the renal pelvis and along the ureter, with enlargement of the feeding vessels. *B,* Parenchymal/venous phase: The main renal vein is occluded and multiple collateral venous channels are seen. *C,* Venogram from another patient shows occlusion of the lower pole renal veins (*arrow*).

the nonpapillary type carcinomas (squamous cell and some transitional cell).

Most uroepithelial carcinomas are hypovascular. In small noninvasive tumors, no angiographic abnormality may be seen. In invasive tumors, there is arterial encasement and occlusion: neovascularity and enlarged pelvic and ureteric arteries are demonstrated in the region of the tumor[85] (Fig. 16–47). Occlusion of the renal vein and/or branches is observed in 41% of cases.[84] Rarely, renal and transitional cell carcinomas may coexist, giving a complex angiographic picture.[86]

On arteriography, uroepithelial tumors cannot always be differentiated from xanthogranulomatous pyelonephritis, which may show similar angiographic features, ie, ve-

nous encasement and occlusion[87] and fine neovascularity.

### Wilms' Tumor

This is the most common intraabdominal malignant neoplasm in children but is rare in adults. Arteriography is rarely indicated for diagnosis but may be required in very large masses and if bilateral tumors (approximately 9%) are suspected.[88] On the other hand, inferior venacavography is indicated for the evaluation of caval involvement since this alters the surgical approach.

On arteriography, the majority of tumors are hypervascular.[89] Enlarged, tortuous vessels, coarse neovascularity, small arterial aneurysms, vascular lakes, and, rarely, arte-

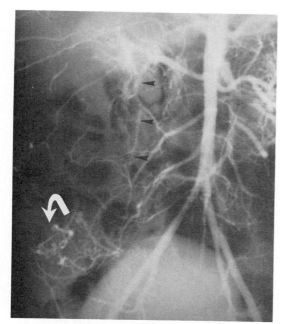

*Figure 16–48.* Large Wilms' tumor. The right kidney is displaced craniad. Normal renal vasculature is present only in the upper portion of the kidney. A branch of the renal artery feeding the tumor is markedly enlarged (*arrowheads*). Large tumor vessels (*curved arrow*) are seen in the lower portion of the lesion, which is partially hypovascular.

riovenous shunting may be seen. In large tumors, the aorta and often the hepatic or splenic arteries are displaced (Fig. 16–48). Parasitization of the vascular supply from adjacent organs also occurs. The abdominal aortogram defines the vascular anatomy satisfactorily if the tumor is large and hypervascular.

### Secondary Tumors of the Kidney

Metastases are the most common malignant tumors of the kidney. They are twice as common as primary tumors.[90] Most metastatic lesions are asymptomatic and without clinical significance and are detected only at autopsy. The most common primary lesions are bronchial, breast, and stomach carcinomas. Arteriography is indicated only if complications develop (eg, hemorrhage) or if operation is contemplated. The arteriographic appearance of metastases usually corresponds to that of the primary lesion.

The kidney may also be involved by retroperitoneal disease, lymphomas, leukemic infiltration, and myeloma. In lymphoma, renal involvement occurs in between 13% (for Hodgkin's disease) and 63% of patients

(for lymphosarcoma with bone marrow involvement).[91] In lymphoma, arteriography may show either a hypovascular or a moderately vascular lesion. Neovascularity (occasionally a palisade-like configuration), vascular displacement, and encasement are seen[92] (Fig. 16–49). This palisade appearance has also been observed in plasmacytoma.[93]

## VENOUS DISEASES

### Renal Vein Thrombosis

In children, common causes of renal vein thrombosis are maternal diabetes, dehydration (diarrheal diseases), and sepsis.[94] Clinical findings include flank mass, uremia, and the nephrotic syndrome. In adults, renal vein thrombosis may be due to glomerulonephritis, diabetic nephropathy, collagen diseases, trauma, amyloidosis, thrombophlebitis, or tumor and manifests with the nephrotic syndrome.[95] It occurs more frequently in males and involves the left side more often.

The diagnosis can often be made by ultra-

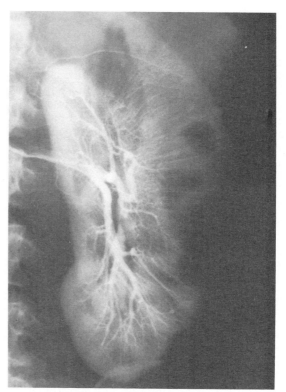

*Figure 16–49.* Lymphoma of the kidney. There is a characteristic palisade configuration of the vessels over the lateral aspect of the kidney.

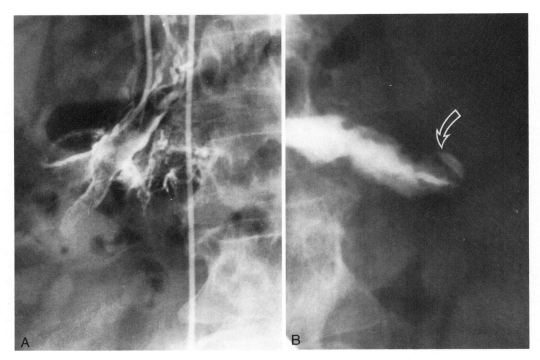

**Figure 16–50.** Renal vein thrombosis. *A,* Manual injection of contrast medium into the right renal vein shows a fresh thrombus outlined by contrast medium. *B,* Manual injection of contrast medium into left renal vein shows an older occusion. The thrombus is adherent to the vein wall. Some of the contrast medium is in the thrombus. Arrow points to a renal vein valve.

sonography or CT. The latter shows an enlarged renal vein.[96] In partial recanalization there is contrast enhancement of the lumen. Angiography is indicated for confirmation of the diagnosis. Renal arteriography is usually not necessary, but when it is performed, the renal artery may appear attenuated and slow antegrade contrast flow is observed. In acute occlusion, the kidney is enlarged and venous opacification is absent.

The diagnostic angiographic procedure is inferior venacavography with or without renal vein catheterization.[95] On cavography, venous inflow from the renal vein(s) is absent. A thrombus may also be identified if it extends into the cava. If a thrombus is not seen in the IVC, or the diagnosis of renal vein thrombosis cannot be established from the inferior venacavogram, a cobra catheter is used to gently probe for the renal vein orifice. Injection of 2 to 3 ml of contrast medium confirms the diagnosis if the main renal vein is thrombosed, and spot films are used for documentation. In our experience, gentle and minimal catheter manipulation with slow injection of no more than 2 to 3 ml of contrast medium has not resulted in clinically evident thromboembolism.

In recent thrombosis with incomplete obstruction, the thrombus is outlined by contrast medium. In complete obstruction, the contrast medium appears as an irregular collection. Washout is slow or absent (Fig. 16–50). In partial recanalization, irregular vascular channels are seen. Extensive collaterals may also be visualized in longstanding obstruction.

If the main renal vein is patent, epinephrine-aided or balloon occlusion (of the renal artery) retrograde renal venography is performed to evaluate the smaller intrarenal branches.

### Varicocele/Gonadal Vein Catheterization

Approximately 10% of males have a testicular varicocele.[97] The etiology of most varicoceles is unclear. Compression of the left renal vein and/or valvar incompetence or absence may play some role in its predisposition. However these do not appear to cause a varicocele. Incompetent or absent valves are found in about half the male population,[98] whereas testicular varicocele occurs only in 10%. In our own experience, supine pressure measurements in the testicular and renal veins and the IVC have rarely revealed a gradient greater than 2 to 3 mm Hg, indicating that superior mesenteric artery (SMA) compression is not an etiological factor. A secondary varicocele may be due to tumor, an aberrant renal artery, or obstruction of the renal vein central to its junction with the testicular vein.[98, 99]

Clinically, the symptoms may include scrotal pain or swelling and infertility due to impaired sperm motility, immature sperm, and oligospermia. A testicular varicocele is found in almost half the infertile males. In an analysis of over 200 patients referred for testicular vein occlusion, we found 78% left-sided, 16% bilateral, and 6% right-sided varicoceles.[100]

**Angiography.** The indications for catheterization of the gonadal veins are:

1. Testicular venography and transcatheter embolization in an attempt to improve sperm quality and fertility or for pain.

2. Localization of maldescended testes.[101]
3. Determination of testicular absence.
4. Venous sampling for hormonally active tumors.

Reflux of contrast medium into the testicular vein may occur during retrograde renal venography. On the other hand, selective catheterization is relatively simple in almost all patients. From the femoral vein approach (preferably the right), a specially designed single curve catheter (Hopkins curve) or a modified cobra C2 catheter (without the tertiary curve) is used for the left gonadal vein. For the right gonadal vein, a sidewinder I catheter is used. From the cubital vein approach, a multipurpose catheter is employed for both gonadal veins.

In individuals with varicoceles, testicular vein valves are either incompetent (in most patients) or only partially competent. In the latter, there is reflux of selectively injected contrast medium into the distal vein, but the catheter or guide wire may not advance past

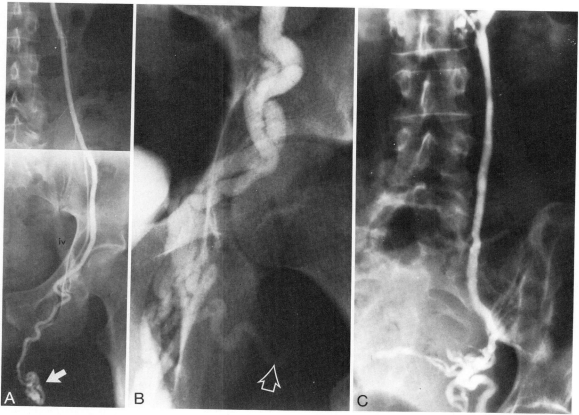

*Figure 16–51.* Gonadal venography. *A,* Left testicular varicocele. Contrast medium injected into the left testicular vein refluxes down io the testicle and opacifies the varicocele (*arrow*). The external iliac vein (iv) is also opacified via communicating channels. *B,* Testicular venogram in another patient shows the external spermatic vein (*arrow*). *C,* Ovarian venogram from the cubital vein approach shows absence of valves.

the valve. With the catheter about 2 to 3 cm from the valve, a straight or 7.5 mm J LLT wire is used to gently probe the orifice during different phases of respiration. With these maneuvers, catheter placement beyond the valve is usually possible. For venography, manual injection of 5 to 10 ml of 60% contrast medium is used and one or two films (single exposures with upper and lower radiographic positioning) are obtained (Fig. 16–51). In most cases, it is not necessary to image the varicocele, ie, the testicle is not exposed to radiation. The diagnosis of a varicocele is based upon the physical examination and is confirmed by the presence of an enlarged testicular vein and incompetent valves.

In patients with varicoceles, venography shows an enlarged testicular vein (4 to 12 mm in diameter), and there is free reflux of contrast medium into the intrascrotal veins (Fig. 16–51). Often two channels of the internal spermatic vein are observed in the pelvis. These may be of equal or different calibers and usually unite at the level of L4 or L5. Collateral venous channels are observed frequently. These usually parallel the testicular vein or drain into the intrarenal or renal capsular veins. Occasionally, collateral venous channels are demonstrated to the inferior epigastric vein via the external spermatic vein or to the internal iliac vein via the ductus deferens vein (Fig. 16–51). The latter collaterals are more likely to be demonstrated on upright venography and play a significant role in the development of recurrent varicoceles after surgical ligation or transcatheter embolization. Rarely, transscrotal collaterals are observed.[98]

In testicular absence, the testicular vein ends blindly. In individuals with a maldescended testis, contrast opacification of the pampiniform plexus helps to locate the gonad (Fig. 16–52).

## "Nutcracker" Phenomenon/Ovarian Vein Syndrome

The former refers to compression of the left renal vein as it passes between the angle formed by the SMA and aorta. Although in most individuals this phenomenon is of questionable clinical significance, in some it may be the cause of symptoms.[102] Acquired causes of left renal vein compression are pancreatic and retroperitoneal neoplasms and lymphadenopathy.[103] In patients with hemodynamically significant compression of the left

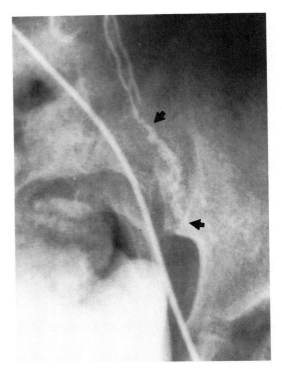

**Figure 16–52.** Undescended testis in a 2 year old boy. Left testicular venogram shows the pampiniform plexus of the abnormally located, hypoplastic testicle (*arrows*).

renal vein, a pressure gradient is measured between the renal vein and the IVC. Normally the pressure difference is less than 2 cm $H_2O$.[102] On the late phase of the aortogram, retrograde flow is observed in the left gonadal vein. In one series, it was observed in 12% of abdominal aortograms.[9] In our own experience with several hundred abdominal aortograms, this phenomenon was observed only a few times, indicating that it is indeed rare (Fig. 16–53).

Ovarian vein dilatation has been incriminated as the cause of distal ureteric obstruction, leading to symptoms of pyelonephritis.[104, 105] A causal relationship between ureteric obstruction and the dilated vein, which occurs most frequently on the right side, is not completely understood, since ovarian vein dilatation is a relatively common occurrence in asymptomatic multiparous women. On aortography, retrograde flow may be observed in patients with this syndrome.

## Renal Vein Varix

Isolated renal vein varices are a rare but angiographically detectable cause of recur-

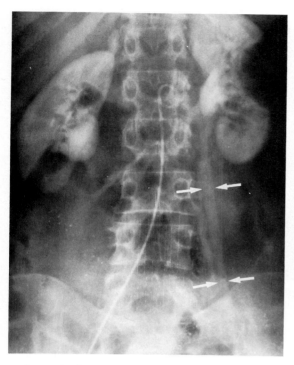

**Figure 16–53.** "Nutcracker" phenomenon. Late film from an abdominal aortogram shows contrast opacification of the left ovarian vein (*arrows*).

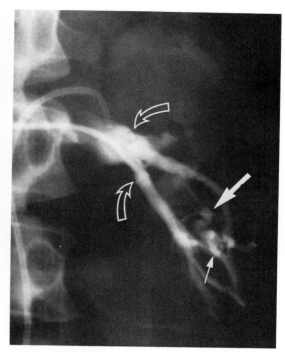

**Figure 16–54.** Left renal venogram shows focal lower pole varices (*arrows*) in a patient with intermittent hematuria. Valves are seen in the main renal vein and proximal branches (*curved arrows*).

rent gross hematuria. In one series, a varix was observed in 2 of 48 patients with gross hematuria evaluated by angiography.[106] In another review of 132 consecutive renal venograms, renal vein varices were found in 8 patients (6%) (Beckmann CF: personal communication). Only one of these patients had experienced hematuria. The arteriogram is usually normal, and retrograde renal venography demonstrates intrarenal varices (Fig. 16–54).

## MISCELLANEOUS APPLICATIONS OF ANGIOGRAPHY

### Renal Agenesis, Dysgenesis, Hypoplasia

Visualization of a single kidney on intravenous urography may be due to unilateral renal agenesis, dysgenesis, hypoplasia (dysplasia), or vascular insult. In renal *agenesis*, there is complete absence of renal tissue and the renal vessels. The adrenal gland is absent in approximately 11% and the other kidney is hypertrophied in 50% of the individuals.[107, 108] Absence of the ureteric orifice and

hemitrigone are considered diagnostic of unilateral renal agenesis.

In renal *dysgenesis*, a nubbin of renal tissue is present. However, this has no resemblance to renal parenchyma. The renal vessels are usually absent, although small vascular channels supplying the tissue nubbin may occasionally be present.[107] In *hypoplasia*, the kidney is very small but resembles the normal organ. The renal vein is hypoplastic and intrarenal veins are disorganized,[109] but the renal artery is usually absent.

In *vascular insult* (longstanding thrombosis or embolic occlusion), the kidney is small, but the intrarenal venous architecture is normal. Intrarenal arteries usually visualize on the late phase of the abdominal aortogram.

Differentiation between agenesis, dysgenesis, dysplasia, and shrunken kidney due to vascular occlusion is possible by venography. In agenesis and dysgenesis, the left renal vein is formed by confluence of the gonadal and adrenal veins, which has a characteristic appearance (Fig. 16–55). There is no vein extending into the renal fossa. On the right side, the renal vein is absent. In the dysplastic kidney, a nonreniform collection of veins is observed.[109] In renal artery occlu-

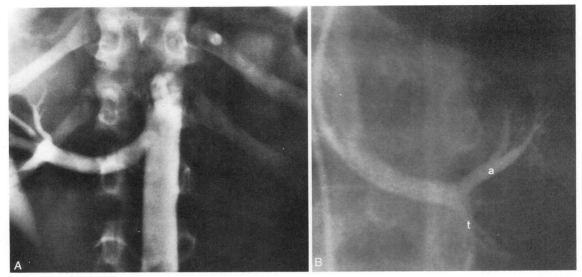

*Figure 16–55.* Congenitally absent left kidney. The patient was evaluated for microscopic hematuria following blunt abdominal trauma. *A,* Abdominal aortogram shows no left renal artery. *B,* Left renal venogram. The left renal vein is formed by the adrenal (a) and testicular (t) veins.

sion, the intrarenal venous architecture is normal. The same is found in end-stage renal parenchymal disease.

## Evaluation of the Kidney Following Revascularization

In most instances, a postoperative arteriogram is obtained only if there is a problem, eg, recurrent hypertension or decreasing renal function. Thus, many abnormalities that are hemodynamically insignificant remain undetected. Postoperative arteriography may be used to exclude nonvascular causes for postoperative problems in some patients,[110] whereas in others this may permit early intervention, eg, surgical or radiological. In our own experience, a standard arteriogram is necessary if the study is performed within 7 to 10 days of the operation. Disturbances in bowel motility and excessive intestinal gas preclude evaluation by intravenous or intraarterial DSA.

In one series of 128 patients studied by arteriography following revascularization for hypertension, several abnormalities were detected; however, no correlation was made with clinical symptoms.[111] The delineation of some of these abnormalities often requires multiple projections, including craniocaudad or other complex angulation of the C or U arm.

The most frequent angiographic abnormalities seen with the use of saphenous vein bypass grafts are diffuse and progressive dilatation and stenosis, each occurring in about one third of the patients.[111] Occasionally, there is aneurysm formation. Other complications following renovascular surgery are (Fig. 16–56):

1. Stenosis of the proximal or distal anastomosis of aorto-renal bypass grafts: In our experience, the distal anastomotic stenosis occurs more frequently.

2. Graft occlusion.

3. Aneurysm formation: This is a complication of saphenous vein grafts. Endarterectomized vessels also appear diffusely dilated but do not result in aneurysm formation.

4. Segmental infarct secondary to occlusion of a branch vessel.

5. Ringlike stenosis at the distal margin of the endarterectomy. A late complication of endarterectomized vessels is a diffuse stenosis.

Fate of the native artery: If the bypassed vessel is not ligated, rapidly progressive narrowing and subsequent occlusion are observed on follow-up arteriograms in patients with normally functioning grafts. If there is an anastomotic stenosis, occlusion of the native artery (if this was not ligated at the time of operation and provided this was not severely stenotic) does not occur (Fig. 16–57).

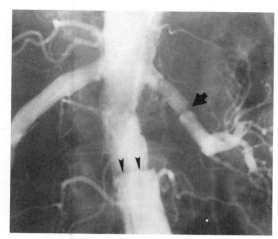

Figure 16–56. Complication of renal artery endarterectomy. Abdominal aortogram shows focal ringlike stenosis of the left renal artery (*arrow*). This is located at the point where the endarterectomy was terminated. The right renal artery shows the normal appearance after endarterectomy. Arrowheads point to distal extent of aortic endarterectomy.

## Evaluation of the Hemodialysis Fistula

Surgically created arteriovenous fistulae provide access for chronic hemodialysis. A commonly used fistula is the Gore-Tex (expanded polytetrafluoroethylene) shunt. Internal fistulae and treated bovine grafts are used less frequently. The fistula is usually created in the nondominant forearm, between the proximal radial artery and the basilic vein. The graft is anastomosed end-to-side to the artery. Either a loop configuration or a straight graft is used. A normally functioning fistula should provide between 250 and 300 ml of continuous blood flow.

Angiography is indicated for evaluation of the fistula if there is diminished blood return or difficulty in cannulation during dialysis, diminished graft pulsation or a mass (pulsatile, nonpulsatile, or expanding), venous stasis of the forearm and hand, or digital ischemia. Since interventional radiological techniques can be used to restore blood flow, ie, balloon dilatation of stenoses or infusion of thrombolytic agents in occluded grafts, angiographic evaluation should not be delayed if graft malfunction is suspected.

The fistula can be evaluated by antegrade brachial artery or direct graft puncture.

**Brachial Artery Puncture.** Antegrade brachial artery puncture is performed with a sheath needle. Either DSA (20% contrast medium) or standard cut film angiography (60% diatrizoate meglumine sodium) is performed. Contrast medium is injected at 5 to 6 ml/sec for a total of 15 ml. Films/images are obtained in the AP projection at 2/sec for 6 films/image and 1/sec for another 4 films/images. The forearm and upper arm are evaluated. If no abnormality is seen, the proximal brachial and axillary veins are also evaluated for stenoses.

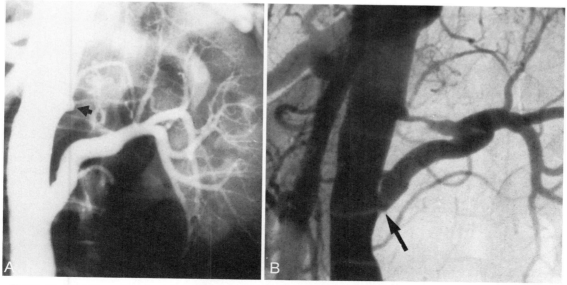

Figure 16–57. A, Normal aorto–left renal artery bypass graft. The native renal artery is occluded (*arrow*). B, Patent native renal artery in another patient with a stenosis of the aortorenal bypass graft (*arrow*).

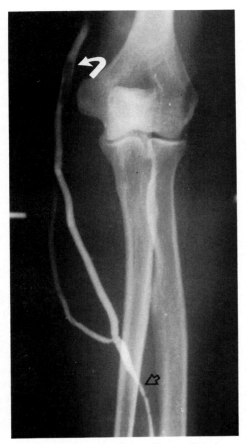

**Figure 16–58.** Complications of hemodialysis access fistula. Angiogram of the venous limb shows a stenosis (*open arrow*) at the venous anastomosis, and a non-occluding thrombus (*curved arrow*) is present in the brachial vein.

**Graft Puncture.** Alternatively, the graft is punctured in a retrograde fashion, close to the arterial anastomosis, using a No. 19 butterfly or a pediatric arterial puncture needle. Two sets of films are obtained. For assessment of the proximal (arterial) anastomosis, a blood pressure cuff is placed over the upper arm and inflated to about 50 mm Hg above the systolic brachial artery pressure. Contrast medium is injected by hand or via pressure injector (5 to 6 ml/sec for a total of 15 ml), and a single film (or 2 to 3 films at 1/sec) is obtained. The brachial cuff is deflated immediately thereafter. Such occlusion permits reflux of contrast medium into the brachial artery and thus allows evaluation of the arterial anastomosis.

The second contrast injection is performed without the brachial pressure cuff in order to evaluate the venous limb. Again, a single film is obtained at the peak of the contrast injection. DSA can be used with either technique and provides superior quality images with minimal patient discomfort.

In an alternative technique, the pressure cuff is released halfway through the contrast injection, which permits assessment of both proximal and distal anastomoses and brachial veins.[112] This technique requires serial filming (3/sec for 6 films and 1/sec for another 4 films).

The following angiographic abnormalities may be observed (Figs. 16–58 and 16–59):

1. Thrombosis: This is the most frequent cause of graft failure and is most often due

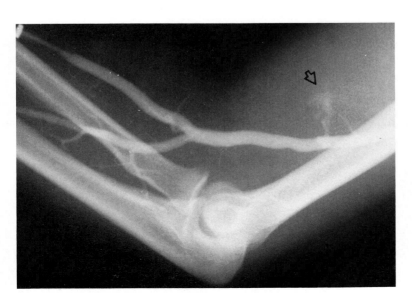

**Figure 16–59.** Complication of hemodialysis. Brachial arteriogram shows a large hematoma probably secondary to rupture of a pseudoaneurysm. A jet of contrast medium is seen extravasating from the brachial artery (*arrow*).

to obstruction at or in the vicinity of the venous anastomosis. Other causes include progressive stenosis due to pseudointimal hyperplasia, venous obstruction, and errors in surgical technique.

2. Stenosis: Accelerated atherosclerosis or pseudointimal hyperplasia occurs secondary to the high flow and turbulence. This occurs most frequently at the venous anastomosis but may also occur in the graft as a result of the repeated cannulations. Occasionally, the stenosis occurs remote from the fistula, ie, in the axillary vein.

3. Aneurysms and pseudoaneurysms: Venous aneurysms occur as a result of the high flow and turbulence. Pseudoaneurysms also occur at the graft puncture sites.

4. Other, less frequent complications include venous hypertension, digital ischemia, and occasionally claudication and high output cardiac failure.[112-114]

PITFALLS IN DIAGNOSIS

Extrinsic compression of the axillary vein may simulate a stenosis or occlusion. This occurs if the angiogram is performed in adduction.

## REFERENCES

1. Graves FT: The arterial anatomy of the congenitally abnormal kidney. Br J Surg 56:533–541, 1969.
2. Spring DB, Salvatierra O Jr, Palubinskas AJ, et al: Results and significance of angiography in potential kidney donors. Radiology 133:45–47, 1979.
3. Merklin RJ, Michels NA: The variant renal and suprarenal blood supply with data on the inferior phrenic, ureteral and gonadal arteries. A statistical analysis based on 185 dissections and review of the literature. J Intern Coll Surg 29:41–76, 1958.
4. Odman P, Ranninger K: The location of the renal arteries. An angiographic and post mortem study. AJR 104:283–288, 1968.
5. Beckmann CF, Abrams HL: Renal venography. Anatomy, technique, applications. Analysis of 132 venograms and a review of the literature. Cardiovasc Intervent Radiol 3:45–70, 1980.
6. Kahn PC: Selective venography of the branches. In Ferris EJ, et al (eds): Venography of the Inferior Vena Cava and Its Branches. Huntington, NY, RE Krieger, 1973, pp 154–224.
7. Beckmann CF, Abrams HL: Circumaortic venous ring: Incidence and significance. AJR 132:561–565, 1979.
8. Ahlberg NE, Bartley O, Chidekel N: Right and left gonadal veins. An anatomical and statistical study. Acta Radiol Diagn 4:593–601, 1966.
9. Ahlberg NE, Bartley O, Chidekel N: Retrograde contrast filling of the left gonadal vein. A roentgenologic and anatomic study. Acta Radiol Diagn 3:385–392, 1965.
10. Hammersen F, Staubesand J: Medulläre Äste des Plexus perivascularis als Fortsetzung der Nieren-

beckenstrombahn beim Menschen. Angioarchitektonische Studien an der Niere. Z Anat Entwicklungsgesch. 122:349–362, 1961.
11. Rosenbusch G, van Douveren WI, Penn WM, et al: Stenosen bei multiplen Nierenarterien und Ausbildung eines reno-renalen Kollateralkreislaufs. Fortschr Roentgenstr 120:164–173, 1974.
12. Abrams HL, Cornell SH: Patterns of collateral flow in renal ischemia. Radiology 84:1001–1012, 1965.
13. Ambos MA, Bosniak MA, Lefleur RS: Blood flow to the kidney via the gonadal-renal capsular artery. Urol Radiol 1:11–16, 1979.
14. Cochran ST, Waisman JI, Pagani JJ, et al: Nephrotoxicity of epinephrine assisted venography. Invest Radiol 17:583–592, 1982.
15. Kadir S: Balloon occlusion technique for renal venography. Fortschr Roentgenstr 131:185–186, 1979.
16. Holley KE, Hunt JC, Brown AL Jr, et al: Renal artery stenosis. A clinical-pathological study in normotensive and hypertensive patients. Am J Med 37:14–22, 1964.
17. Davidson AJ, Talner LB, Downs WM III: A study of the angiographic appearance of the kidney in an aging normotensive population. Radiology 92:975–983, 1969.
18. Tham G, Ekelund L, Herrlin K, et al: Renal artery aneurysms: Natural history and prognosis. Ann Surg 197:348–352, 1983.
19. Abeshouse BS: Aneurysm of the renal artery: Report of two cases and review of the literature. Urol Cutan Rev 55:451–463, 1951.
20. Cummings KB, Lecky JW, Kaufman JJ: Renal artery aneurysms and hypertension. J Urol 109:144–148, 1973.
21. Nuzum JW Jr, Nuzum JW Sr: Polyarteritis nodosa. Statistical review of one hundred seventy five cases from the literature and report of a "typical" case. Arch Intern Med 94:942–955, 1954.
22. Capps JH, Klein RM: Polyarteritis nodosa as a cause of perirenal and retroperitoneal hemorrhage. Radiology 94:143–146, 1970.
23. Kadir S, Marshall FF, White RI, et al: Therapeutic embolization of the kidney with detachable silicone balloons. J Urol 129:11–13, 1983.
24. Buck SW, Joshi SJ, Sunwoo YC, et al: Cholesterol embolization with renal arterial aneurysms. J Nat Med Assn 74:903–907, 1982.
25. Oxman HA, Sheps SG, Harrison EG Jr: An unusual cause of renal arteriovenous fistula—Fibromuscular dysplasia of the renal arteries. Mayo Clin Proc 48:207–210, 1973.
26. Bosniak MA: Radiographic manifestations of massive arteriovenous fistula in renal cell carcinoma. Radiology 85:454–459, 1965.
27. Ekelund L, Göthlin J: Renal hemangiomas: An analysis of 13 cases diagnosed by angiography. AJR 125:788–794, 1975.
28. Rao CN, Blaivas JG: Primary renal artery dissecting aneurysms: a review. J Urol 118:716–719, 1977.
29. Hare WSC, Smith PK: Dissecting aneurysm of the renal artery. Radiology 97:255–263, 1970.
30. Gewertz BL, Stanley JC, Fry WR: Renal artery dissections. Arch Surg 112:409–414, 1977.
31. Dean RH, Lawson JD, Hollifield JW, et al: Revascularization of the poorly functioning kidney. Surgery 85:44–52, 1979.
32. Wirthlin LS, Gross WS, James TP, et al: Renal artery occlusion from migration of stainless steel coils. JAMA 243:2064–2065, 1980.
33. Mena E, Bookstein JJ, Holt JF, et al: Neurofibro-

matosis and renovascular hypertension in children. AJR:118:39–45, 1973.

34. Jensen SR, Novelline RA, Brewster DC, et al: Transient renal artery stenosis produced by a pheochromocytoma. Radiology 144:767–768, 1982.

35. Eyler WR, Clark MD, Garman JE, et al: Angiography of the renal areas including a comparative study of renal artery stenosis in patients with and without hypertension. Radiology 78:879–892, 1962.

36. Kadir S, Russel RP, Kaufman SL, et al: Renal artery angioplasty. Technical considerations and results. Fortschr Roentgenstr 141:378–383, 1984.

37. Bookstein JJ, Maxwell MH, Abrams HL, et al: Cooperative study of radiologic aspects of renovascular hypertension. JAMA 237:1706–1709, 1977.

38. Stanley JC, Fry WJ: Renovascular hypertension secondary to arterial fibroplasia in adults. Arch Surg 110:922–928, 1975.

39. Harrison EG Jr, Hunt JC, Bernatz PE: Morphology of fibromuscular dysplasia of the renal artery in renovascular hypertension. Am J Med 43:97–112, 1967.

40. Harrison EG Jr, McCormack LJ: Pathologic classification of renal arterial disease in renovascular hypertension. Mayo Clin Proc 46:161–167, 1971.

41. Clayman AS, Bookstein JJ: The role of renal arteriography in pediatric hypertension. Radiology 108:107–110, 1973.

42. Ekelund L, Gerlock AJ, Goncharenko V, et al: Renal venographic findings in 29 kidneys with fibromuscular dysplasia of the renal artery. Radiology 125:631–632, 1977.

43. Feyrter F: Über die vasculäre Neurofibromatose, nach Untersuchungen am menschlischen Magen-Darmschlauch. Virchows Arch 317:221–265, 1949.

44. Rosenbusch G, Hoefnagels WHL, Koene RAP, et al: Renovaskuläre Hypertension bei Neurofibromatose. Gleichzeitige Kasuistik multipler abdominaler und zerebraler Gefässveränderungen. Fortschr Roentgenstr 126:218–227, 1977.

45. D'Abreu F, Strickland B: Developmental renal artery stenosis. Lancet 2:517–521, 1962.

46. Silver D, Clements JB: Renovascular hypertension from renal artery compression by congenital bands. Ann Surg 183:161–166, 1976.

47. Spark RF, Berg S: Renal trauma and hypertension. The role of renin. Arch Intern Med 136:1097–1100, 1976.

48. Foster JH, Klatte EC, Burko H: Arteriographic pitfalls in the diagnosis of renovascular hypertension. Arch Surg 99:792–801, 1969.

49. Gerlock AJ, Goncharenko V, Sloan OM: Right posterior oblique: The projection of choice in aortography of hypertensive patients. Radiology 127:45–48, 1978.

50. Mena E, Bookstein JJ, Gikas PW: Angiographic diagnosis of renal parenchymal disease. Chronic glomerulonephritis, chronic pyelonephritis, and arteriolonephrosclerosis. Radiology 108:523–532, 1973.

51. Friedenberg MJ, Eisen S, Kissane J: Renal angiography in pyelonephritis, glomerulonephritis, and arteriolar nephrosclerosis. AJR 95:349–363, 1965.

52. Bachy C, Alexandre GPJ, Van Ypersele de Strihou, C: Hypertension after renal transplantation. Br Med J 2:1287–1289, 1976.

53. Kaude, JV, Hawkins IF Jr: Angiography of renal transplant. Radiol Clin North Am 14:295–308, 1976.

54. Lacombe M: Arterial stenosis complicating renal allotransplantation in man. A study of 38 cases. Ann Surg 181:283–288, 1975.

55. Ricotta JJ, Schaff HV, Williams GM, et al: Renal artery stenosis following transplantation: Etiology, diagnosis and prevention. Surgery 84:595–602, 1978.

56. Hamway S, Novick A, Braun WE, et al: Impaired renal allograft function: a comparative study with angiography and histopathology. J Urol 122:292–297, 1979.

57. Bernath AS, Schutte H, Fernandez RRD, et al: Stab wounds of the kidney: conservative management in flank penetration. J Urol 129:468–470, 1983.

58. Javadpour N, Guinan P, Bush IM: Renal trauma in children. Surg Gynecol Obstet 136:237–240, 1973.

59. Stables DP, Fouche RF, van Niekerk JPDV, et al: Traumatic renal artery occlusion: 21 cases. J Urol 115:229–233, 1976.

60. Collins HA, Jacobs JK: Acute arterial injuries due to blunt trauma. J Bone Joint Surg 43A:193–197, 1961.

61. Lang EK: The role of arteriography in trauma. Radiol Clin North Am 14:353–370, 1976.

62. Andersson I: Renal artery lesions after pyelolithotomy. A potential cause of renovascular hypertension. Acta Radiol Diagn 17:685–695, 1976.

63. Sclafani SJA, Stein K: Arteriographic management of traumatic arteriocalyceal fistula. Urol Radiol 3:177–179, 1981.

64. Kadir S, Athanasoulis CA: Angiographic diagnosis and control of postoperative bleeding. CRC Crit Rev Diag Imag 35–78, 1979.

65. Bruneton JN, Ballanger P, Ballanger R, et al: Renal adenomas. Clin Radiol 30:343–352, 1979.

66. Apitz K: Die Geschwülste und Gewebsmissbildungen der Nierenrinde: Die Adenome. Virchows Arch Path Anat Physiol 311:328–359, 1944.

67. Ambos MA, Bosniak MA, Valensi QJ, et al: Angiographic patterns in oncocytomas. Radiology 129:615–622, 1978.

68. Weiner SN, Bernstein RG: Renal oncocytoma: Angiographic features of 2 cases. Radiology 125:633–635, 1977.

69. Lam ASC, Bedard YC, Buckspan MB, et al: Surgically curable hypertension associated with reninoma. J Urol 128:572–575, 1982.

70. Conn JW, Bookstein JJ, Cohen EL: Renin secreting juxtaglomerular cell adenoma. Radiology 106:543–544, 1973.

71. Bosniak MA: Angiomyolipoma (hamartoma) of the kidney: A preoperative diagnosis is possible in virtually every case. Urol Radiol 3:135–142, 1981.

72. Hollifield JW, Page DL, Smith C, et al: Renin secreting clear cell carcinoma of the kidney. Arch Intern Med 135:859–864, 1975.

73. Beyer D, Fiedler V, Terwort H: Lohnt sich die doppelseitige Durchführung der selectiven Nierenangiographie? Fortschr Roentgenstr 130:278–286, 1979.

74. Daniel WW Jr, Hartman GW, Witten DM, et al: Calcified renal masses: A review of 10 years experience at the Mayo Clinic. Radiology 103:503–508, 1972.

75. Horton WA, Wong V, Eldridge R: von Hippel–Lindau disease: Clinical and pathological manifestations in nine families with 50 affected members. Arch Intern Med 136:769–777, 1976.

76. Kadir S, Kerr WS Jr, Athanasoulis CA: The role of arteriography in the management of renal cell car-

cinoma associated with von Hippel–Lindau disease. J Urol 126:316–319, 1981.

77. Watson RC, Flemming RJ, Evans JA: Arteriography in the diagnosis of renal cell carcinoma: Review of 100 cases. Radiology 91:888–897, 1968.

78. Richie JP, Garnick MB, Seltzer S, et al: Computerized tomography scan for diagnosis and staging of renal cell carcinoma. J Urol 129:1114–1116, 1983.

79. Chuang VP, Fried AM: High dose renal pharmacoangiography in the assessment of hypovascular renal neoplasms. AJR 131:807–811, 1978.

80. Brannan W, Miller W, Crisler M: Coexistence of renal neoplasms and renal cysts. South Med J 55:749–752, 1962.

81. Goncharenko V, Gerlock AJ, Kadir S, et al: Incidence and distribution of venous extension in 70 hypernephromas. AJR 133:263–265, 1979.

82. Kadir S, Coulam CM: Intracaval extension of renal cell carcinoma. Cardiovasc Intervent Radiol 3:180–183, 1980.

83. Lucke B, Schlumberger HG (eds): Tumors of the kidney, renal pelvis and ureter. Cited by Selli C, Stefani P, Carcangiu ML, et al: Cardiovasc Intervent Radiol 5:275–278, 1982.

84. McDonald JR, Priestly JT: Malignant tumors of the kidney: surgical and prognostic significance of tumor thrombosis of the renal vein. Surg Gynecol Obstet 77:295–306, 1943.

85. Apitzsch DE, Meiisel P: Die Angiographie des Nierenbeckenkarzinoms. Fortschr Roentgenstr 124:350–355, 1976.

86. Lundell C, Kadir S, Engel R, et al: Concurrent renal cell and transitional cell carcinoma in a single kidney: A case report. J Urol 127:761–763, 1982.

87. Goldman ML, Gorelkin L, Rude JC III, et al: Epinephrine renal venography in severe inflammatory disease of the kidney. Radiology 127:93–101, 1978.

88. Bond JV: Bilateral Wilms' tumour. Age at diagnosis, associated congenital anomalies and possible pattern of inheritance. Lancet 2:482–484, 1975.

89. Clark RE, Moss AA, DeLormier AA, et al: Arteriography of Wilms' tumor. AJR 113:476–490, 1971.

90. Newsam JE, Tulloch WS: Metastatic tumors in the kidney. Br J Urol 38:1–6, 1966.

91. Richmond J, Sherman RS, Diamond HD, et al: Renal lesions associated with malignant lymphomas. Am J Med 32:184–207, 1962.

92. Jafri SZH, Amendola MA, Brady TM, et al: Angiographic patterns of involvement in renal and perirenal lymphoma. Urol Radiol 6:14–19, 1984.

93. Siemers PT, Coel MN: Solitary renal plasmacytoma with palisading tumor vascularity. Radiology 123:597–598, 1977.

94. Gonzalez R, Schwartz S, Sheldon CA, et al: Bilateral renal vein thrombosis in infancy and childhood. Urol Clin North Am 9:279–283, 1982.

95. Clark RA, Wyatt GM, Colley DP: Renal vein throm-

bosis: An undiagnosed complication of multiple renal abnormalities. Radiology 132:43–50, 1979.

96. Adler J, Greweldinger J, Hallac R, et al: Computed tomographic findings in a case of renal vein thrombosis with nephrotic syndrome. Urol Radiol 3:181–183, 1981.

97. Johnson DE, Pohl DR, Rivera-Correa H: Varicocele: an innocuous condition? South Med J 63:34–36, 1970.

98. Ahlberg NE, Bartley O, Chidekel N, et al: Phlebography in varicocele scroti. Acta Radiol Diagn 4:517–528, 1966.

99. Campbell MF: Varicocele due to anomalous renal vessel: An instance in a 13 year old boy. J Urol 52:502–504, 1944.

100. Kadir S: Unpublished data.

101. Weiss RM, Glickman MG: Venography of the undescended testis. Urol Clin North Am 9:387–395, 1982.

102. Sacks BA, Gomori J, Lerner M, et al: Left renal venous hypertension in association with the nutcracker phenomenon. Cardiovasc Intervent Radiol 4:253–255, 1981.

103. Cope C, Isard HJ: Left renal vein entrapment. A new diagnostic finding in retroperitoneal disease. Radiology 92:867–872, 1969.

104. Smith PD: Ovarian syndrome: Is it a myth? Urology 11:355–364, 1979.

105. Melnick GS, Bramwit DN: Bilateral ovarian vein syndrome. AJR 113:509–517, 1971.

106. Mitty HA, Goldman H: Angiography in unilateral renal bleeding with a negative urogram. AJR 121:508–517, 1974.

107. Ashley DJB, Mostofi FK: Renal agenesis and dysgenesis. J Urol 83:211–230, 1960.

108. Collins DC: Congenital unilateral renal agenesia. Ann Surg 95:715–726, 1932.

109. Athanasoulis CA, Brown B, Baum S: Selective renal venography in differentiation between congenitally absent and small contracted kidney. Radiology 108:301–305, 1973.

110. Cornell SH: Renal angiography after revascularization operations. Radiology 92:880–884, 1969.

111. Ekelund L, Gerlock AJ Jr, Goncharenko V, et al: Angiographic findings following surgical treatment for renovascular hypertension. Radiology 126:345–349, 1978.

112. Glanz S, Bashist B, Gordon DH, et al: Angiography of upper extremity access fistulas for dialysis. Radiology 143:45–52, 1982.

113. Swayne LC, Manstein C, Somers R, et al: Selective digital venous hypertension: A rare complication of hemodialysis arteriovenous fistula. Cardiovasc Intervent Radiol 6:61–62, 1983.

114. Ahearn DJ, Maher JF: Heart failure as a complication of hemodialysis arteriovenous fistula. Ann Intern Med 77:201–204, 1972.

# Angiography of the Spine

Frederick A. Eames, M.D.
Glenn H. Robeson, M.D.

## ANATOMY

### Arterial Anatomy

The major blood supply to the spinal cord is through the anterior spinal artery, which runs the length of the cord in the anterior median sulcus. The sulcocommissural branches penetrate the cord parenchyma and supply the anterior 70 to 80% of the spinal cord, including the corticospinal tracts, via the central arteries (Fig. 17–1).

The posterior spinal arteries are smaller and are usually paired. They may anastomose with each other extensively through an arterial plexus on the posterior aspect of the spinal cord. The posterior spinal arteries supply the posterior 20 to 30% of the spinal cord, including the posterior columns, the outer ends of the posterior horns, and most of the white matter, via peripheral arteries of the cord parenchyma. There are small anastomoses between the anterior and posterior spinal arteries in the pia mater, but parenchymal arteries do not anastomose.[1] The only important collateral pathway between the two systems is the anastomotic loop or "rami cruciantes" around the conus medullaris.

The anterior spinal artery is formed near the vertebral-basilar junction from the union of two spinal rami from the vertebral arteries. The posterior spinal arteries are formed from the posterior spinal rami, which arise from the vertebral arteries or the posterior inferior cerebellar arteries. Inferiorly, both the anterior and the posterior systems are supplied at multiple levels by radicular branches of extraspinal arteries (vertebral, subclavian, posterior intercostal, lumbar, or internal iliac arteries). The radicular arteries accompany their respective nerve roots through the intervertebral foramina. The radicular arteries that continue to supply the spinal cord itself are termed radiculomedullary arteries. The distributions of the anterior and posterior radiculomedullary arteries are generally divided by the plane of the dentate ligament. Each anterior radiculomedullary artery has a characteristic "hairpin loop" configuration, which is a consequence of the differential growth of the spinal cord and the vertebral column. After entering the dural sac, the vessel ascends to a variable degree before dividing into a large branch running caudad in the anterior median sulcus and a much smaller branch running cephalad. These

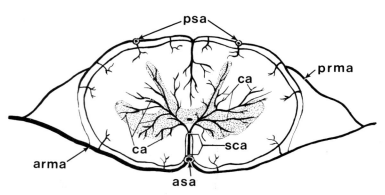

*Figure 17–1.* Arterial blood supply to the spinal cord. There are pial anastomoses between the anterior and posterior spinal arteries, but the parenchymal arteries do not anastomose. arma = anterior radiculomedullary artery, asa = anterior spinal artery, ca = central arteries, prma = posterior radiculomedullary artery, psa = posterior spinal arteries, sca = sulcocommissural arteries.

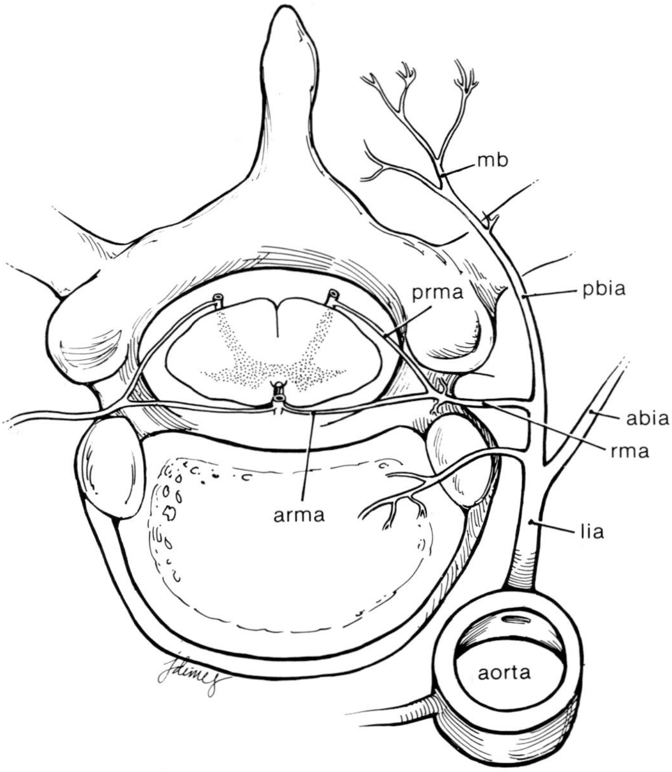

*Figure 17–2.* Segmental (lumbar or intercostal) artery distribution. The posterior branch supplying the spinal cord also supplies the vertebra and paravertebral muscles. abia = anterior branch intercostal artery, arma = anterior radiculomedullary artery, lia = left intercostal artery, mb = muscular branches, pbia = posterior branch of intercostal artery, prma = posterior radiculomedullary artery, rma = radiculomedullary artery.

branches anastomose with others superiorly and inferiorly to form a more or less continuous anterior spinal artery.

In early fetal life there is a uniform metameric vascular pattern consisting of 31 pairs of anterior and posterior radiculomedullary arteries, one pair for each vertebral segment. As development progresses, the great majority of these arteries regress, so that in the adult there are usually six to eight anterior radiculomedullary arteries and 10 to 20 posterior radiculomedullary arteries.[1, 2]

The anatomy of the radicular arteries is shown in Figure 17–2. Each intercostal, subcostal, or lumbar artery has a dorsal branch that supplies the vertebra itself, the dorsal ganglion, the meninges, and the paravertebral and paraspinal musculature as well as the nerve roots and spinal cord. When enlarged, the long dural branches may occasionally be seen on arteriography and have a characteristic spiral configuration.[3] The dural branches are uniformly metameric in distribution.

In contrast to the large number of radiculomedullary arteries supplying the posterior spinal arterial system, anterior radiculomedullary arteries are fewer and more variable.

The typical pattern of distribution is shown in Figure 17–3. The blood supply to the anterior spinal artery is summarized as follows:

1. Two anterior spinal rami off the vertebral arteries.

2. A radiculomedullary artery at C2 or C3, usually a branch of the vertebral artery.

3. A C5 or C6 radiculomedullary artery arising from the deep cervical branch of the costocervical trunk or, less often, from the ascending cervical branch of the thyrocervical trunk. This is a fairly constant large feeder, termed the "artery of cervical enlargement" by Lazorthes (Fig. 17–4).

4. A C8 radiculomedullary artery from the first intercostal branch or another branch of the costocervical trunk. The first and second intercostal arteries usually arise from the superior intercostal branch of the costocervical trunk. On the left side, the second intercostal artery may arise directly from the aorta.

5. A T4 or T5 radiculomedullary artery from a posterior intercostal artery, usually on the left side.

6. A thoracolumbar radiculomedullary artery (the artery of lumbar enlargement, artery of Adamkiewicz, or arteria radiculomedul-

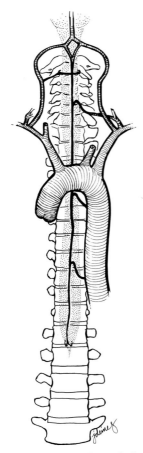

*Figure 17–3.* Anatomy of the anterior spinal arteries. The radiculomedullary arteries have a characteristic hairpin-loop configuration. In this diagram the dominant feeders, the arteries of the cervical and lumbar enlargements, are on the left side at C5–6 and T10–11, respectively.

laris magna). This usually arises on the left side (80%) from a lower thoracic intercostal artery (T9–T12 in 75% of individuals), but can be found as high as T5 or as low as L2. The T12 segmental branch is properly termed a subcostal artery.

7. One or two lower lumbar or lateral sacral radicular arteries may constitute the inferior medullary supply to the cauda equina. The first three lumbar arteries arise directly from the aorta. The fourth lumbar arteries may arise from the aorta or the middle (median) sacral artery. The fifth lumbar arteries may arise from the median sacral or the iliolumbar arteries. The latter, like the lateral sacral arteries, are branches of the posterior trunk of the internal iliac (hypogastric) artery.

Although radicular or segmental arteries

exist at every vertebral level, only a few anterior radiculomedullary arteries continue to supply the anterior spinal artery; and of these, the arteries of the cervical and lumbar enlargements are the dominant feeding vessels.

The implications of this unique pattern of arterial supply to the spinal cord are readily apparent. The lower cervical and thoracolumbar portions of the cord receive a relatively generous blood supply from their respective radiculomedullary arteries. In contrast, the upper thoracic section, which may receive only one small radiculomedullary artery, is considered a watershed area and is more susceptible to ischemic injury. Angiographically, the anterior spinal artery is often discontinuous in this segment. Furthermore, because of individual variation in a given patient, there is potentially a radiculomedullary artery at any vertebral level. Therefore, the angiographer must be aware of the possibility of inadvertent contrast injection into spinal cord vessels during aortography or bronchial or visceral angiography and must recognize possible neurological complications if they occur.

### Anatomical Variations and Normal Radiographic Appearance

The anterior spinal artery in the cervical area is frequently paired (45%),[4] although the paired arteries are totally separate in only 60% of these individuals. Whether paired or single, it can often be visualized in a normal selective vertebral angiogram. In the lateral projection, it marks the ventral border of the spinal cord, and the average separation of the artery from the posterior margin of the C2 vertebral body is 0.3 cm.[5] The posterior spinal arteries are rarely well visualized, but the posterior spinal veins or venous plexus are more frequently apparent in the cervical area.[6, 7]

The anterior spinal artery lies in the anterior medial sulcus. It may be tortuous in the cervical and lumbar enlargements, especially in older individuals. Thus, myelographic demonstration of a tortuous anterior spinal artery is not unusual.

The posterior intercostal arteries arise in symmetrical segmental fashion from the posterior wall of the aorta. Their orifices are approximately 5 to 10 mm apart and are located slightly below each intervertebral disc space. Variations are frequent, and occasion-

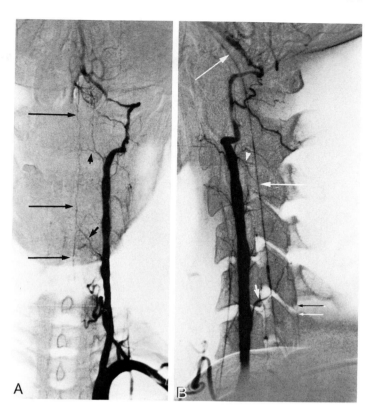

*Figure 17–4.* Patient with occlusive disease of the vertebrobasilar system. Subclavian arteriogram (*A,* AP view; *B,* lateral view) shows the anterior spinal artery (*long arrows*) and the artery of the cervical enlargement (*short arrows*). In this case, it is a branch of the ascending cervical artery accompanying the left C6 spinal nerve. A small radiculomedullary artery is also present at C2–3 (*arrowhead*). The posterior spinal artery is seen faintly (*double arrows in B*).

ally both the left and the right arteries originate from a common trunk or, more often, a single trunk divides into two adjacent ipsilateral intercostal arteries (see also Chapter 8). With advancing age and tortuosity of the thoracic aorta, the location of the orifices of the intercostal arteries comes to lie on the right posterior-lateral aortic wall.

In the cervical area, either the anterior or the posterior radiculomedullary artery is dominant at a given level and only occasionally are both vessels of significant size.[8] Rarely, the anterior and posterior radicular arteries may have separate origins from the dorsal branch of the intercostal artery.

## Venous Anatomy

Venous drainage of the spinal cord is in a pattern similar to the arterial supply, except that the dominant venous channels are posterior.[6, 9] Only the anteromedian portion of the cord drains via radial and sulcal veins to the anterior median spinal veins. The greater part of the cord drains via radial veins to the large coronal venous plexus in the pia, which is posterior and lateral in position. Although not always present, a single large posterior spinal vein may be dominant. Both the anterior and the posterior systems drain by means of medullary or radiculomedullary veins to the epidural (internal vertebral) plexus. As with the arterial supply, the posterior radiculomedullary veins are more numerous than the anterior veins. A dominant "vena radiculomedullaris magna" may be present anteriorly or posteriorly in the thoracolumbar area.[10]

The epidural veins consist of a longitudinal (vertical) system of paired anterior internal vertebral veins and smaller posterior internal vertebral veins that are interconnected by short transverse intraspinal veins enveloping the dural sac (Fig. 17–5).[11, 12] These intraspinal veins also receive the basivertebral veins from the vertebral bodies. The extraspinal longitudinal channels are the paravertebral veins, lateral to the pedicles, and are connected to the epidural veins by suprapedicular and intrapedicular communicating (intervertebral) veins in a coarse plexus around the spinal nerve. The paravertebral channels consist of the vertebral vein in the neck, azygos and hemiazygos veins in the thorax, and ascending lumbar and internal iliac veins. The paravertebral channels com-

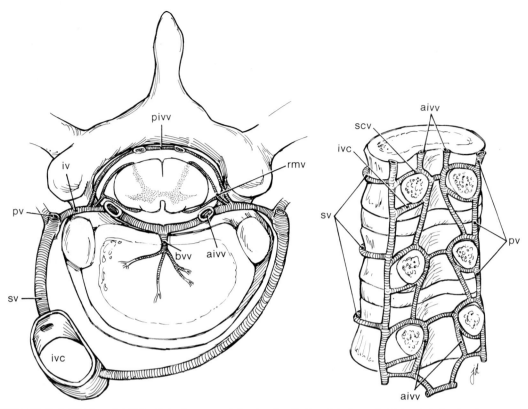

**Figure 17–5.** Anatomy of epidural and paravertebral veins (*left*, axial view; *right*, frontal view). aivv = anterior internal vertebral veins, bvv = basivertebral vein, icv = infrapedicular communicating vein, iv = intervertebral vein, pivv = posterior internal vertebral veins, pv = paravertebral vein, rmv = radiculomedullary vein, scv = suprapedicular communicating vein, sv = segmental vein. The terms "intervertebral" and "communicating" vein are used interchangeably.

municate with the caval system at multiple levels: vertebral with the subclavian veins, azygos/hemiazygos with the superior vena cava, and ascending lumbar with the common iliac veins. In addition, the ascending lumbar veins communicate directly with the inferior vena cava via the segmental lumbar veins.

## ANGIOGRAPHY

Early angiographic studies of the spine and spinal cord described midstream aortography as a means of opacifying all feeding vessels to vascular malformations.[13-15] Subsequently, it was shown that selective arteriography not only produced superior opacification of the spinal cord vasculature but was also associated with a lower morbidity. Earlier fears of spinal cord injury were based more on the effects of inadvertent contrast injection into the spinal artery during aortography or bron-

chial, intercostal, or subclavian arteriography than on the experience with selective spinal arteriography.

Before proceeding to spinal arteriography, other diagnostic procedures (eg, myelography, radioisotope studies,[16, 17] and computed tomography[18] should be considered. Digital subtraction angiography (DSA) also provides a relatively safe and accurate means for diagnosis.[19-21] The possibility of spinal cord injury as a potential complication of spinal angiography should be discussed with the patient.

Premedication of the patient is not essential. Intravenous diazepam (Valium) or fentanyl may be used during the procedure to insure patient comfort and cooperation without masking any signs if neurological complications do develop. Since a large volume of contrast medium may be used, patient hydration is essential.

Although standard angiography can be used, magnification studies may provide some advantage.[22, 23] A strip of marking numbers is placed on the patient's back to help in identifying vertebral segments in the thoracic region. The femoral artery route is used for selective catheterization, and a catheter-introduced sheath is inserted to facilitate catheter manipulation.

In pediatric patients, an aortogram is performed initially, and it may be the only examination necessary.[24] For the aortogram, the LPO view is used, since this projects the aorta off the spine. In addition, film subtraction is essential. In adults, midstream aortography is no longer used, since it does not provide satisfactory information and may be associated with a higher morbidity than that occurring with selective studies.[25-27] In the elderly patient, selective studies occasionally may not be possible because of severe atherosclerosis of the aorta. For selective spinal arteriography, iothalamate meglumine (Conray-60) is the least neurotoxic contrast agent.

In the cervical region, bilateral subclavian arteriograms may provide sufficient information. If the cord vessels are not well visualized, selective vertebral, costocervical, or thyrocervical arteriography may be necessary. For catheterization of these vessels, a catheter with a simple curve, such as an H1 configuration, is used (Fig. 17–6A). This catheter configuration can also be used for intercostal and lumbar arteriography. Occasionally, the catheter configuration may be modified to prevent recoil and dislodgment during contrast injection (Fig. 17–6B). For lower intercostal and lumbar arteries with a caudad directed course, a reverse curve such as the Simmons 1 or 2 catheter is used (Fig. 17–6C).

For intercostal and lumbar arteriography, 3 to 5 ml of contrast medium is injected by hand (the filming sequence is shown in

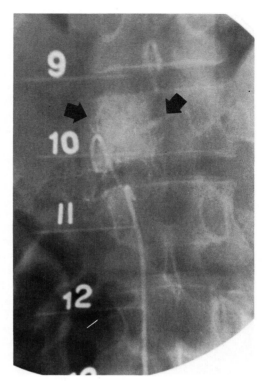

**Figure 17–7.** Selective injection of right subcostal (12th intercostal) artery shows normal muscular branches and staining of the ipsilateral hemivertebra (*arrows*).

Chapter 8, Table 8–7). For vascular malformations, the duration of filming is increased to 10 to 15 seconds to facilitate visualization of the venous drainage.

Since the posterior branch of the intercostal or lumbar artery also supplies the vertebra and adjacent muscles, a selective arteriogram shows the fine vascularity and parenchymal staining of bone and muscle. Under normal circumstances, the stain of the vertebral body is confined to the ipsilateral hemivertebra (Fig. 17–7).[28] If contrast medium is injected into the anterior branch, this parenchymal stain is not seen, necessitating catheter repositioning.

## Complications

Contrast injection into the intercostal and lumbar arteries is associated with a burning or irritating sensation in the back (in the corresponding dermatome). Therefore, the catheter should be withdrawn from the vessel orifice immediately after each selective injection. Contrast injection at the midthoracic level should be performed with particu-

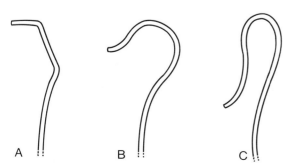

**Figure 17–6.** Catheters used in selective spinal angiography. *A*, H1 catheter; *B*, modified cerebral catheter; *C*, Simmons 2 catheter.

lar caution because the cord in this region is especially susceptible to ischemic and toxic damage.

Symptoms of spinal cord irritation may occur during arteriography. These may be in the form of minor paresthesias of the lower limbs or painful paroxysmal spasms of the trunk and lower extremities. The latter may occur at regular intervals (4 to 6 seconds apart) and have also been called "medullary epilepsy."[27] This is more frequently associated with aortography than with selective arteriography and occurs more often in patients with arteriovenous malformations.[25] In the latter patients during aortography, there may be flooding of the cord with contrast medium via multiple radiculomedullary arteries, and in patients with impaired venous drainage, there is prolonged contact of the contrast medium with the cord parenchyma. Medullary epilepsy can be treated by intraarterial injection of 5 mg of diazepam (diluted with 5% dextrose) if the catheter remains in the selective position when the spasms occur.

Spinal cord injury resulting in permanent neurological deficit (eg, paraplegia or quadriplegia) has generally been attributed to direct neurotoxicity of contrast medium. Previous reports indicated that in the majority of cases such injury occurred following inadvertent contrast injection into spinal arteries during aortography or bronchial arteriography rather than during selective spinal arteriography.[29-35] Use of contrast agents other than iothalamate methylglucamine has also been implicated.

The incidence of permanent cord damage following spinal arteriography is estimated to be between 0.2 and 1.0%. In a series of over 300 cases, there was only one incident of permanent cord injury, which was attributed to multiple contrast injections in the cervical area bilaterally and/or possibly to an allergic type reaction.[27, 36]

Symptoms of cord irritation may occur despite a meticulously performed study. If these are in the form of severe paresthesias or involuntary motor activity, the procedure should be terminated. Since the onset of myelopathy can be delayed by several hours, avoidance of additional contrast injection at this stage may be crucial in preventing irreversible damage. In addition, some authors recommend that multiple bilateral selective contrast injections of cervical cord vessels not be performed during one session.[22]

Although there are no data to prove their efficacy, intravenous steroids have been used when signs of cord injury develop during or after arteriography. In addition, the systemic blood pressure should be maintained at normal or minimally elevated levels. Cerebrospinal fluid lavage has also been used, but its effectiveness remains uncertain.[37]

## SPINAL ARTERIOVENOUS MALFORMATIONS

Spinal arteriovenous malformations (AVMs) are uncommon, making up approximately 5% of all spinal tumors,[38] but these lesions constitute the principal indication for selective spinal angiography. Although other diagnostic methods may be useful for screening or postsurgical follow-up, only selective spinal angiography provides the detailed vascular anatomy that is required for complete evaluation.

Vascular malformations of the central nervous system have been broadly grouped as (1) capillary telangiectasias, (2) cavernous angiomas, and (3) arteriovenous and venous malformations.[39] All of the important vascular lesions of the spinal cord fall into the third category. These have acquired various names, including arteriovenous aneurysms, cirsoid aneurysms, venous angiomas, racemose angiomas, and spinal varices.[38] Most authors, although recognizing significant differences in morphology among the various lesions, tend to group all of these into the general category of AVMs. Those lesions with a predilection for the thoracolumbar cord, previously classified as venous malformations, are now generally considered to be AVMs that have a small arteriovenous nidus but are drained by enlarged, tortuous intradural veins. The syndrome of Foix-Alajouanine, formerly described as a subacute necrotic myelitis or spinal thrombophlebitis, is now understood to represent the chronic sequelae of a spinal AVM.[40]

AVMs may present in all age groups. The majority of patients are in the fourth through sixth decades and have symptoms of progressive myelopathy. Overall there is a male predominance of approximately three to one. A minority of patients present with acute neurological deficits (especially motor impairment) or subarachnoid hemorrhage. Acute deficit or subarachnoid hemorrhage is more common in children.[24] In adults, subarachnoid hemorrhage is unusual (less than

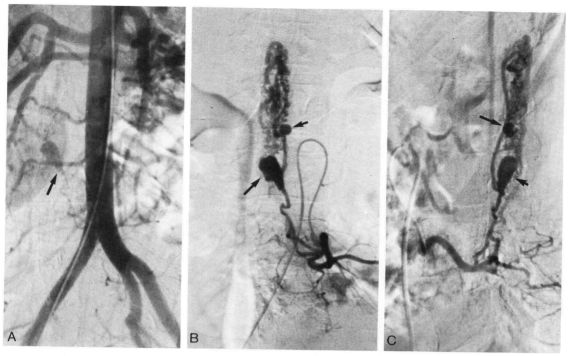

*Figure 17–8.* A 27 year old woman with Klippel-Trenaunay-Weber syndrome and myelographic findings suggesting arachnoiditis in the lumbar area. *A*, Abdominal aortogram demonstrates an intraspinal aneurysm (*arrow*). Selective AP (*B*) and lateral (*C*) arteriogram shows an arteriovenous malformation supplied by a branch of the left fourth lumbar artery. Two aneurysms are present (*arrows*). The malformation extends from L4 to the mid-L1 level and is predominantly posterior in location.

30% of cases) and almost always indicates the presence of an associated aneurysm[41] (Fig. 17–8).

Myelography usually precedes angiography and demonstrates typical serpiginous intradural filling defects in 50 to 70% of cases (Fig. 17–9). Myelography may be omitted only if there are clinical and radiological signs (vertebral scalloping or pedicle erosion) of a large intraspinal mass that is suspected to be vascular and may make lumbar puncture hazardous.

Spinal vascular malformations are occasionally associated with cutaneous or other angiomatous lesions. These include port-wine stains, multiple hereditary telangiectasias (Weber-Rendu-Osler disease), vertebral hemangiomas (Cobb's syndrome), and cutaneous angioma of an extremity with hypertrophy of the limb (Klippel-Trenaunay-Weber syndrome). The dermatomal location of a cutaneous angioma may be related to the site of an intraspinal AVM at the corresponding segmental level.

The anatomical location and configuration of AVMs are variable. Lesions are predominantly retromedullary and are most commonly located in the thoracic or thoracolumbar area. The "malformation" consists of large arterialized veins draining a relatively small nidus,[42] and the blood supply to this nidus is usually from the posterior radiculomedullary arteries or from dural vessels. The arterialized veins commonly appear as a "single coiled vessel"[40] (Fig. 17–10).

Recent studies have shown that in most cases the dilated coronal veins drain a nidus that is extradural, often a dural AV fistula near the intervertebral foramen.[43-45] The AV fistula is convincingly demonstrated only by angiotomography.[44]

There is congestion of the coronal venous plexus with absence of normal medullary veins.[44, 46] Ischemia due to the venous congestion has been held responsible for the gradual progression of symptoms. The dilated veins may be prominent at some distance from the actual fistula and can occasionally extend the entire length of the thoracolumbar spine. Flow through these veins may be quite slow, and complete opacification on angiography may take 40 to 60 seconds.

Intramedullary lesions are more often true

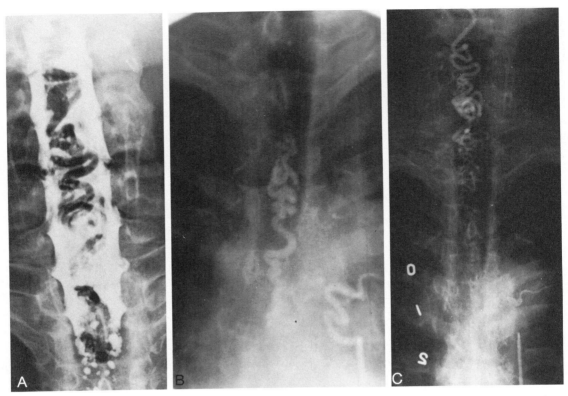

*Figure 17–9.* A 58 year old man with an 8 month history of spastic paraparesis. *A,* Pantopaque myelogram shows typical intradural serpiginous filling defects in the lower cervical area. Spinal angiography (*B,* 1 second; *C,* 6 seconds) demonstrates a large arteriovenous malformation supplied from the left sixth intercostal artery. Surgical exploration revealed at least three other feeding pedicles. The major portion of the intradural vessels were enlarged "arterialized" veins in the coronal plexus.

AVMs that are supplied by multiple radiculomedullary arteries, including the artery of Adamkiewicz. These are usually high flow lesions that are more commonly located in the cervical cord, especially in children (DiChiro's "juvenile" type III lesion) (Fig. 17–10).[40] Clinical symptoms may be due to a "steal" phenomenon or to actual cord compression by the angiomatous mass.

Another type of malformation described by DiChiro is the "glomus" (type II) lesion.[40] On arteriography, this appears as a small tuft or plexus of vessels, usually supplied by a single artery and without prominent draining veins (Fig. 17–11). AVMs that are entirely epidural occur less frequently and may have a completely different clinical presentation, eg, as cervical radiculopathy.[47, 48]

### Arteriography

Arteriographic evaluation should include demonstration of the extent of the AVM, its relationship to the cord and conus medul-

laris, and its arterial supply, including all possible feeding pedicles and venous drainage. It is also important to demonstrate the blood supply to the cord, including the artery of Adamkiewicz and other radiculomedullary arteries near the malformation. The arterial supply to the AVM cannot be assumed to be separate from the blood supply to the cord unless the latter is clearly demonstrated.[49] Such information is important for planning therapy, whether surgical or embolization or both. Thus, a complete study requires injection of all segmental arteries in the vicinity of the AVM.

Lateral arteriograms are important for demonstrating the relationship of the AVM to the spinal cord, for distinguishing anterior from posterior vascular blood supply, and for evaluating venous drainage and length of the sulcocommissural arteries if the AVM is supplied by the anterior spinal artery. Even with biplane arteriography, it is often difficult to predict with certainty whether an AVM is intra- or extramedullary in location.[50]

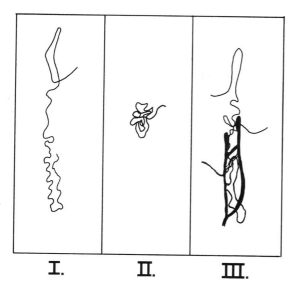

**Figure 17–10.** Representation of three types of arteriovenous malformations. I, single coiled vessel; II, glomus; III, juvenile. (After DiChiro G, et al: Prog Neurol Surg 4:329, 1971.)

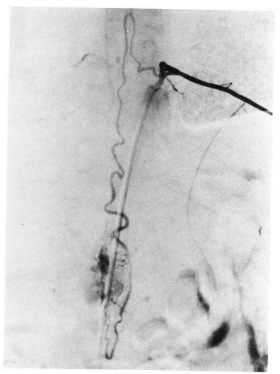

**Figure 17–11.** Small arteriovenous malformation of the "glomus" type is supplied by the anterior spinal artery.

Although angiotomography and myeloangiography have been recommended for demonstration of such relationships,[24] these techniques are not widely practiced.

In the adult patient, aortography is of little use and should not be performed for "orientation." Instead, selective spinal arteriography is performed. However, in children and young adults, aortography is often diagnostic because of the presence of multiple large feeding vessels to AVMs of the high flow type. Aortography can also be helpful when an AVM is supplied by a pedicle from an unusual or unexpected location (see Fig. 17–8).

## TUMORS

Most intramedullary tumors do not have a specific angiographic appearance, and arteriography does not play a significant role in their diagnosis or management. The common lesions, ie, ependymomas and astrocytomas, are hypovascular and only show displacement of the spinal arteries. Occasionally, there is a faint tumor stain and, less frequently, arteriovenous shunting is present.

### Hemangioblastoma

Hemangioblastomas (angioblastomas, angioreticulomas) are benign neoplasms of endothelial origin. They constitute approximately 2% of spinal cord tumors, and most of them occur sporadically.[51] Multiple tumors are associated with von Hippel–Lindau's disease and may be located in the cerebellum and spinal cord.

Approximately 75% of hemangioblastomas are intramedullary and are usually located in the posterior half of the cord.[27, 52, 53] Twenty per cent are radicular in origin, arising from either a root of the cauda equina or a root along the dural sac. Five per cent are intradural-extramedullary.

Arteriography is the most sensitive and specific method for evaluation of suspected hemangioblastomas. Nodules less than 3 mm in size can be detected, often before they become symptomatic. In such patients, intraarterial DSA can now be used as a safe and reliable means of tumor localization.[19, 20]

Since most hemangioblastomas are intramedullary, the cord appears expanded on myelography, and large draining veins can be outlined (Fig. 17–12).[51, 53, 54] Selective spinal arteriography demonstrates a densely staining tumor nodule, often persisting for 15 to 20 seconds. Arterial supply is usually from

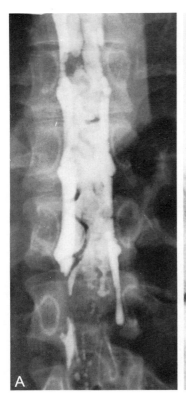
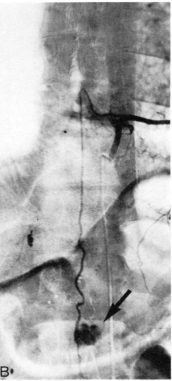

*Figure 17–12.* Intramedullary hemangioblastoma. *A,* Myelogram demonstrates expansion of the conus medullaris and enlarged intradural vessels. *B,* Spinal arteriogram shows a densely staining tumor nodule supplied by the enlarged anterior spinal artery (*arrow*).

the anterior spinal artery, and unlike an AVM, a coil of vessels and arteriovenous shunting are usually absent in a hemangioblastoma, despite the presence of large draining veins.[55] Such veins may appear late (after 12 seconds), whereas the veins in an AVM are seen early (within 6 seconds).[53] The tumor stain is much smaller than the shadow of the expanded cord. The latter is due to an associated syrinx.

## Miscellaneous Tumors

Other intraspinal and vertebral lesions that have been studied by spinal angiography include neurinoma, meningioma, metastases, bone tumors (aneurysmal bone cyst, giant cell tumor, cartilaginous tumors, hemangioma, osteoid osteoma), and tuberculous spondylitis.[3, 53, 56-58]

Arteriography is indicated in some cases to determine the extent and vascularity of lesions. Preoperative localization of the artery of Adamkiewicz may be important if a difficult surgical resection is anticipated. In addition, complete arteriographic evaluation is required for lesions that are to be treated by embolotherapy.

## MISCELLANEOUS INDICATIONS FOR SPINAL ARTERIOGRAPHY

Preoperative spinal angiography may be indicated in some patients prior to surgery for scoliosis or resection of thoracic aortic aneurysms.[59-62] Identification and preservation of the artery of Adamkiewicz or other important radiculomedullary arteries may prevent ischemic injury to the cord.

Arteriography has occasionally been performed in patients with spinal trauma but has seldom contributed significantly to patient management.[26, 63-65] The anterior spinal artery may remain unaffected even in severe cord injury and quadriplegia. The intrinsic vessels of the cord parenchyma are not visualized and have not been evaluated in such cases.

Arteriography is rarely indicated in occlusive diseases of the spinal arteries, since this is an infrequent clinical diagnosis, and effective therapy is not available.[26, 66]

## EPIDURAL VENOGRAPHY

Since the availability of CT, epidural venography is rarely performed. It is occasionally

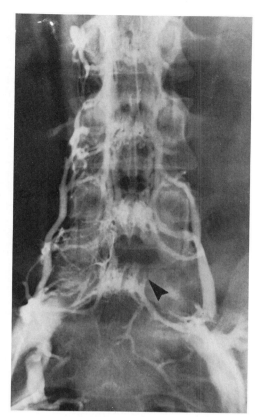

*Figure 17– 13.* Epidural venogram. There is obstruction of the left anterior internal vertebral vein (*arrowhead*) at L4–5 and non-filling of the left intervertebral (communicating) veins at the same level. Left L4–5 disc herniation confirmed at surgery. (Courtesy of Dr. Fredie P. Gargano, Palmetto General Hospital, Hialeah, Florida.)

useful for the diagnosis of certain intraspinal abnormalities and it has been used primarily for the diagnosis of herniated lumbar discs when myelography is negative.[11, 12] Epidural venography of the cervical and thoracic canal has limited clinical applicability.[67, 68] Occasionally, other lesions (eg, an epidural vascular malformation) have been diagnosed by venography.[69]

The lumbar epidural plexus is studied by catheterization of ascending lumbar or lateral sacral veins via the femoral approach. Twenty-five ml of contrast medium is injected at 5 ml/sec into the ipsilateral side during a Valsalva maneuver. This usually opacifies the entire epidural plexus, since these veins do not have valves. Films are obtained at 3 per second for 6 films and 1 per second for an additional 3 films.

Disc herniation is recognized by compression of the epidural veins, most importantly,

compression or occlusion of the anterior internal vertebral vein at a given level, when veins above and below that segment are well filled (Fig. 17–13).

*Frederick A. Eames, M.D.:* Assistant Professor of Radiology, Albany Medical College; Assistant Attending Radiologist, Albany Medical Center Hospital, Albany, New York.

*Glenn H. Robeson, M.D.:* Professor and Chairman, Radiology Department, Albany Medical College; Radiologist-in-Chief, Albany Medical Center Hospital, Albany, New York.

## REFERENCES

1. Tveten L: Spinal cord vascularity. III. The spinal cord arteries in man. Acta Radiol (Diagn) 17(Fasc 3):257–273, 1976.
2. Tveten L: Spinal cord vascularity. I. Extraspinal sources of spinal cord arteries in man. Acta Radiol (Diagn) 17(Fasc 1):1–16, 1976.
3. Herdt JR, Shimkin PM, Ommaya AK, et al: Angiography of vascular intraspinal tumors. AJR 115:165–170, 1972.
4. Kawamura J, Matsubayashi K, Fukuyama H, et al: Paired anterior spinal arteries in a case of locked-in syndrome. Neuroradiology 22:107–110, 1981.
5. Schechter MM, Zingesser LH: The spinal arteries. Acta Radiol (Diagn) 5:1124–1131, 1966.
6. Fried LC, Doppman JL, DiChiro G: Venous phase in spinal cord angiography. Acta Radiol (Diagn) 11:393–401, 1971.
7. Gabrielsen TO, Seeger JF: Vertebral angiography in the diagnosis of intraspinal masses in the upper cervical region. Neuroradiology 5:7–12, 1973.
8. Chakravorty BG: Arterial supply of the cervical spinal cord (with special reference to the radicular arteries). Anat Rec 170:311–330, 1971.
9. Launay M, Chiras J, Bories J: Angiography of the spinal cord: Venous phase. J Neuroradiol 6:287–315, 1979.
10. Gillian LA: Veins of the spinal cord. Neurology 20:860–867, 1970.
11. Drasin GF, Daffner RH, Sexton RF, et al: Epidural venography: Diagnosis of herniated lumbar intervertebral disc and other diseases of the epidural space. AJR 126:1010–1016, 1976.
12. Gargano FP, Meyer JD, Sheldon JJ: Transfemoral ascending lumbar catheterization of the epidural veins in lumbar disc disease. Radiology 111:329–336, 1974.
13. Baker HL, Love JG, Layton DD: Angiographic and surgical aspects of spinal cord vascular anomalies. Radiology 88:1078–1085, 1967.
14. Doppman JL, DiChiro G: Subtraction angiography of spinal cord vascular malformation. J Neurosurg 23:440–443, 1965.
15. Houdart R, Djindjian R, Hurth M: Vascular malformations of the spinal cord. J Neurosurg 24:583–594, 1966.
16. DiChiro G, Jones AE, Johnston GS, et al: Radioisotope angiography of the spinal cord. J Nuc Med 13:567–569, 1972.
17. Obayashi T, Furuse M, Nakama M: Radionuclide angiography of vascular lesions of the spinal cord. Arch Neurol 37:572–574, 1980.

18. DiChiro G, Doppman JL, Wener L: Computed tomography of spinal cord arteriovenous malformations. Radiology 123:351–354, 1977.

19. DiChiro G, Rieth KG, Oldfield EH, et al: Digital subtraction angiography and dynamic computed tomography in the evaluation of arteriovenous malformations and hemangioblastomas of the spinal cord. J Comp Asst Tom 6:655–670, 1982.

20. Yeates, A, Drayer B, Heinz ER, et al: Intra-arterial digital subtraction angiography of the spinal cord. Radiology 155:387–390, 1985.

21. Doppman JL, Krudy AG, Miller DL, et al: Intraarterial digital subtraction of spinal arteriovenous malformations. AJNR 4:1081–1085, 1983.

22. Djindjian R: Vascular malformations. In Shapiro R (ed): Myelography, 4th Ed. Chicago, Year Book Medical Publishers, 1984, pp. 318–344.

23. Shiozawa Z, Tanaka Y, Makino N, et al: Spinal cord angiography using 4× magnification. Radiology 127:181–184, 1978.

24. Riche MC, Modenesi-Freitas J, Djindjian M, et al: Arteriovenous malformations of the spinal cord in children. Neuroradiology 22:171–180, 1982.

25. DiChiro G, Doppman J, Ommaya AK: Selective arteriography of arteriovenous aneurysms of the spinal cord. Radiology 88:1065–1077, 1967.

26. DiChiro G, Wener L: Angiography of the spinal cord. A review of contemporary techniques and applications. J Neurosurg 39:1–29, 1973.

27. Djindjian R: Angiography of the Spinal Cord. Baltimore, University Park Press, 1970.

28. DiChiro G: Recent successes and failures in radiographic and radioisotopic angiography of the spinal cord. Br J Radiol 45:553–560, 1972.

29. DiChiro G: Unintentional spinal cord arteriography: A warning. Radiology 112:231–233, 1974.

30. Ederli A, Sassaroli S, Spaccarelli G: Vertebral angiography as a cause of necrosis of the spinal cord. Br J Radiol 35:261–264, 1962.

31. Feigelson HH, Ravin HA: Transverse myelitis following selective bronchial arteriography. Radiology 85:663–665, 1965.

32. Kardjiev V, Symeonov A, Chankov I: Etiology, pathogenesis, and prevention of spinal cord lesions in selective angiography of the bronchial and intercostal arteries. Radiology 112:81–83, 1974.

33. Killen DA, Foster JH: Spinal cord injury as a complication of contrast angiography. Surgery 59:969–981, 1966.

34. Mosely IF, Tress BM: Extravasation of contrast medium during spinal angiography: A cause of paraplegia. Neuroradiology 13:55–57, 1977.

35. Ramirez-Lassepas M, McClelland RR, Snyder BD, et al: Cervical myelopathy complicating cerebral angiography. Neurology 27:834–837, 1977.

36. Djindjian R: Arteriography of the spinal cord. AJR 107:461–478, 1969.

37. Mishkin MM, Baum S, DiChiro G: Emergency treatment of angiography-induced paraplegia and tetraplegia (letter). N Engl J Med 288:1184–1185, 1973.

38. Yasargil MG: Intradural spinal arteriovenous malformations. In Vinkin PJ and Bruyn GW (eds): Handbook of Clinical Neurology, Vol 20. Amsterdam, North Holland Publishing Co, 1976, pp. 481–523.

39. Rubinstein LJ: Tumors of the central nervous system. Fascicle 6 of Atlas of Tumor Pathology, Washington, DC, Armed Forces Institute of Pathology, 1972.

40. DiChiro G, Doppman JL, Ommaya AK: Radiology of spinal cord arteriovenous malformations. Progr Neurol Surg 4:329–354, 1971.

41. Herdt JR, DiChiro G, Doppman JL: Combined arterial and arteriovenous aneurysms of the spinal cord. Radiology 99:589–593, 1971.

42. Doppman JL: The nidus concept of spinal cord arteriovenous malformations: A surgical recommendation based upon angiographic observations. Br J Radiol 44:758–763, 1971.

43. Kendall BE, Logue V: Spinal epidural angiomatous malformations draining into intrathecal veins. Neuroradiology 13:181–189, 1977.

44. Merland JJ, Riche MM, Chiras J: Intraspinal extramedullary arteriovenous fistulae draining into the medullary veins. J Neuroradiol 7:271–320, 1980.

45. Oldfield EH, DiChiro G, Quindlen EA, et al: Successful treatment of a group of spinal cord arteriovenous malformations by interruption of dural fistula. J Neurosurg 59:1019–1030, 1983.

46. Aminoff MJ, Bernard RO, Logue V: The pathology of spinal vascular malformations. J Neurol Sci 23:255–263, 1974.

47. Bradac GB, Simon RS, Schramm J: Case report: Cervical epidural AVM. Neuroradiology 14:97–100, 1977.

48. Brooks BS, El Gammal T, Beveridge WD: Erosion of vertebral pedicles by unusual vascular causes: Report of three cases. Neuroradiology 23:102–112, 1982.

49. Doppman JL, DiChiro G, Oldfield EH: Origin of spinal arteriovenous malformation and normal cord vasculature from a common segmental artery: Angiographic and therapeutic considerations. Radiology 154:687–689, 1985.

50. Kasdon DL, Wolpert SM, Stein BM: Surgical and angiographic localization of spinal arteriovenous malformations. Surg Neurol 5:279–283, 1976.

51. Browne TR, Adams RD, Robeson GH: Hemangioblastoma of the spinal cord. Arch Neurol 33:435–441, 1976.

52. Djindjian R, Dublin A, Djindjian M: Angiography of the spinal cord. In Youmans JR (ed): Neurological Surgery, Vol 1. Philadelphia, WB Saunders, 1982, pp. 551–616.

53. Djindjian R, Merland JJ, Djindjian M, et al: Angiography of the Spinal Column and Spinal Cord Tumors. New York, Georg Thieme Verlag, 1981.

54. Huk W, Klinger M: The diagnosis of cervical spinal angioblastomas. Neuroradiology 5:174–177, 1973.

55. DiChiro G, Doppman JL: Differential angiographic features of hemangioblastomas and arteriovenous malformations of the spinal cord. Radiology 93:25–30, 1969.

56. Esparza J, Castro S, Portillo JM, et al: Vertebral hemangiomas: Spinal angiography and preoperative embolization. Surg Neurol 10:171–173, 1978.

57. Kamano S, Fukushima T: Angiographic demonstration of vertebral osteoid osteoma. Surg Neurol 6:167–168, 1976.

58. Karasawa J, Kikuchi H, Takahashi N, et al: Selective spinal angiography for spinal tumor (abst). Neuroradiology 22:53, 1981.

59. Doppman JL, DiChiro G, Morton DL: Arteriographic

identification of spinal cord blood supply prior to aortic surgery. JAMA 204:174–175, 1968.

60. Doppman JL, DiChiro G, Ommaya AK: Selective Arteriography of the Spinal Cord. St Louis, Warren H Green, 1969.
61. Hilal SK, Keim HA: Selective spinal angiography in adolescent scoliosis. Radiology 102:349–359, 1972.
62. Fereshetian A, Kadir S, Kaufman S, et al: Preoperative localization of the anterior spinal artery using digital subtraction arteriography. Presented at the 71st Scientific Assembly of the RSNA, Chicago, 1985.
63. Bussat P, Rossier AB, Djindjian R, et al: Spinal cord angiography in dorsolumbar vertebral fractures with neurological involvement. Radiology 109:617–620, 1973.
64. Theron J, Derlon JM, de Preux J: Angiography of the spinal cord after vertebral trauma. Neuroradiology 15:201–212, 1978.
65. Wener L, DiChiro G, Gargour GW: Angiography of cervical cord injuries. Radiology 112:597–604, 1974.
66. DiChiro G: Angiography of obstructive vascular disease of the spinal cord. Radiology 100:607–614, 1971.
67. Miyasaka K, Takei H, Ito T, et al: Catheter cervical vertebral venography. Neuroradiology 16:413–415, 1978.
68. Theron J, Djindjian R: Cervico-vertebral phlebography using catheterization. Radiology 108:325–331, 1973.
69. Saibil EA, Rowed DW, Gertzbein SD: Epidural vascular malformation demonstrated by epidural venography. AJR 132:987–988, 1979.

# ENDOCRINE SYSTEM

## FOUR

## Angiography of the Parathyroid and Adrenal Glands

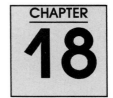

**18**

### ANATOMY

#### Parathyroid Glands

The parathyroid glands are approximately $6 \times 4 \times 2$ mm in size and usually four in number, ie, two on each side of the neck. Additional parathyroid glands are reported in 9% of individuals and are often located in the lower neck and mediastinum.[1] The superior glands have a relatively constant position, ie, posterior to the mid-portion of the thyroid gland. The inferior parathyroid glands, which are subject to greater variation, are located close to the lower poles of the thyroid gland. The left glands (superior and inferior) show more variability of position than the right.

The most frequent source of arterial blood supply to the parathyroid glands is the inferior thyroid artery. In 80% of individuals, a single parathyroid artery supplies each gland.[1] Although multiple arteries to one gland are not uncommon, a single artery rarely supplies two glands. The artery (or arteries) to the superior glands is derived from the inferior thyroid artery in 77% of individuals, from the superior thyroid artery in 15%, and from anastomotic branches of both vessels in the remainder.[1]

The artery to the inferior glands originates from the inferior thyroid artery in 90% of persons.[1] In the remainder, it originates from the superior thyroid artery or from anastomotic vessels between the two thyroid arteries. Rarely, it may arise directly from the subclavian artery, or the gland may be supplied by branches of the internal mammary artery.[2, 3] In individuals with agenesis of the inferior thyroid artery (approximately 9% of persons), the inferior glands are supplied by the thyroidea ima or the superior thyroid artery.[1]

Venous drainage from the parathyroid glands is primarily via the thyroidal veins. The thyroid venous plexus is a system of diffusely communicating veins that drain into the systemic veins via three paired venous trunks (Fig. 18–1). Of these, the inferior thyroid veins are the largest and are the primary drainage pathway for the parathyroid glands.

The *superior thyroid veins* drain the upper portion of the thyroid venous plexus. They are relatively constant in size and location and drain into the internal jugular veins above the level of the vocal cords.[4] The *middle thyroid veins* are the smallest thyroidal veins. Their number, size, and drainage pattern vary greatly. They emanate from the lateral aspect of the thyroid venous plexus and also drain the upper and mid-portions. The middle thyroid veins join the internal jugular veins below the superior thyroid veins. Rarely, they drain into the subclavian or innominate veins.

The *inferior thyroid vein* may be single or paired. It is the largest thyroidal vein that drains the lower portion of the plexus. Veins from both sides may unite to form a single trunk before entering the left brachiocephalic vein, or they may drain separately. The inferior thyroid vein enters the upper wall of

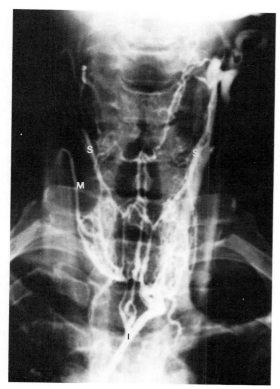

**Figure 18–1.** Retrograde inferior thyroid venogram demonstrating normal venous anatomy of the thyroid venous plexus. I = inferior, M = middle, S = superior thyroid vein. (Courtesy of Dr. J. Doppman.)

the left brachiocephalic vein close to the junction of the latter with the right brachiocephalic vein. If there are two veins, the right vein also enters the left brachiocephalic vein or the right brachiocephalic vein close to its junction with the left. Anomalous drainage into the thymic, azygos, and other mediastinal veins has also been observed.[4] The thyroid venous plexus is devoid of valves. However, a valve with a varying degree of competence is often found in the inferior thyroid vein close to its junction with the brachiocephalic vein.

## Adrenal Glands

At birth the adrenal glands are large (almost one third the size of the kidneys). Involution of the cortex occurs during early infancy, and in the adult the adrenal glands are approximately 1/30 the size of the kidneys, measuring about 5 × 3 × 1 cm.[5] The adrenal cortex, which constitutes 9/10 of the total adrenal weight, envelops the medulla completely.

The right adrenal gland is pyramidal (tri-

angular) in shape, lies anterior and superior to the upper pole of the kidney, and often overlaps its medial border. It is posterolateral to the inferior vena cava. The shape of the left gland is more variable. Most frequently, it is semilunar or leaflike or occasionally triangular[6] and is located along the medial aspect of the upper pole of the kidney. Because it overlaps the kidney, the left gland is often difficult to demonstrate on aortography.

Each adrenal gland is supplied by three groups of arteries (Figs. 18–2 and 18–3):

1. Multiple, slender *superior adrenal arteries* (up to 30)[7] from the posterior division of the inferior phrenic artery: Variations in the origin of the inferior phrenic artery are described in Chapter 10.

2. *Middle adrenal artery* from the aorta immediately above the renal artery: It is usually a single vessel that divides into multiple branches. The middle adrenal artery may also originate from the renal, inferior phrenic, or celiac arteries or from a different level off the aorta.[7]

3. *Inferior adrenal artery* from the proximal renal artery: Several smaller branches may

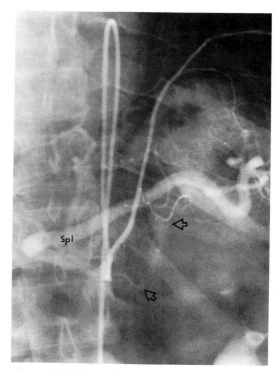

**Figure 18–2.** Normal left inferior phrenic arteriogram showing the superior adrenal arteries (*arrows*). Spl = splenic artery.

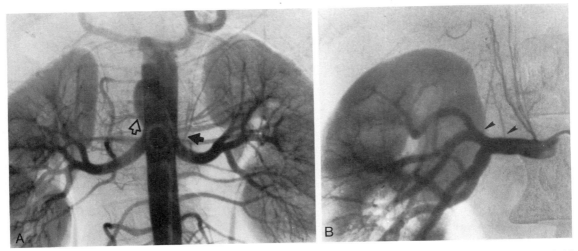

***Figure 18–3.*** Normal adrenal arterial anatomy. *A,* Subtraction film from abdominal aortogram shows the right middle (*open arrow*) and left inferior (*closed arrow*) adrenal arteries. *B,* Subtraction film from a right renal arteriogram shows the inferior adrenal arteries. Arrowheads point to accessory branches arising from the distal renal artery.

arise separately. In the presence of multiple renal arteries, the inferior adrenal artery arises from the uppermost renal artery. This is the major arterial source to the adrenal gland.

Venous drainage from the adrenal glands is via a superficial and a central venous system (Figs. 18–4 and 18–5; see also Figs. 18–11 and 18–15). The superficial system drains the outer cortex via multiple capsular veins, which, in turn, drain into renal capsular, lumbar, phrenic, and hepatic veins. The central venous system drains the inner cortex and medulla.

On the right, three segmental veins unite to form a short (5 to 10 mm) central vein that enters the posterior lateral aspect of the inferior vena cava approximately 2 to 4 cm

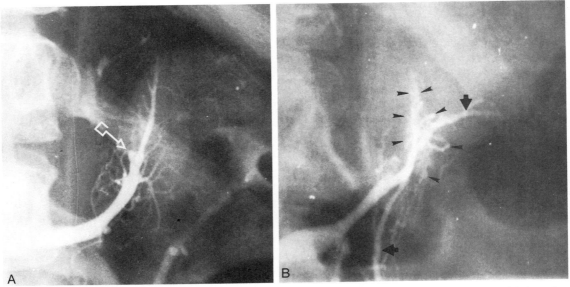

***Figure 18–4.*** Normal retrograde left adrenal venograms in two different patients. In *A,* the arrow points to valve in distal inferior phrenic vein, which prevented reflux of contrast medium into this vessel. In *B,* the arrows point to renal capsular and retroperitoneal veins. The arrowheads point to the normal intraadrenal veins.

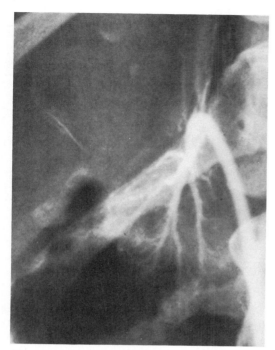

*Figure 18–5.* Normal retrograde right adrenal venogram.

above the right renal vein. However, variant venous anatomy is not uncommon and includes:[8]

1. Two or more adrenal veins entering the inferior vena cava separately.

2. Bifurcation of the main adrenal vein, with each branch entering the cava separately.

3. Drainage of the main adrenal vein or a branch via the hepatic, phrenic, or renal vein.

4. Accessory adrenal veins that drain via the renal vein: This occurs relatively frequently.

On the left side there is a longer single adrenal vein that enters the superior aspect of the renal vein, opposite the gonadal vein. It is joined by the inferior phrenic vein, which lies medially and has a valve approximately 1 cm from its junction with the adrenal vein. Rarely, both veins enter the renal vein separately. The left adrenal vein communicates with lumbar, renal capsular, and other retroperitoneal veins.

## ANGIOGRAPHY OF THE PARATHYROID GLANDS

The main indication for angiography of the parathyroid glands is the localization of a hyperplastic gland or adenoma in patients with persistent or recurrent hypercalcemia following parathyroid surgery. Other indications for preoperative localization are (1) patients who have undergone previous thyroid surgery, since neck reexploration can be difficult, and (2) patients who present diagnostic problems. Preangiographic evaluation should exclude other causes of hypercalcemia, eg, malignancy (primary or metastatic), myeloma, vitamin D intoxication, milk alkali syndrome, and sarcoidosis.

Some authors recommend arteriography as the initial procedure in order to help identify venous drainage, since the normal venous pathways may have been altered by operative ligation.[9] Identification of draining veins on the venous phase of the arteriogram facilitates selective catheterization for venous sampling.[10]

### Arteriography (Table 18–1)

The femoral approach is preferred, since both sides can be catheterized from a single arterial puncture. In patients with a tortuous aorta or redundant brachiocephalic or subclavian arteries, the axillary artery approach is used.

From the femoral approach, either commercially available, preformed 5 to 7 Fr catheters (headhunter, JB-1) are used or a 4.9 or 5 Fr polyethylene catheter is steamed into a headhunter or 45° multipurpose catheter shape. Alternatively, a steerable catheter system (USCI) or coaxial torque wire–guided system can be used for selective catheterization.[10-12]

The arterial study should evaluate both sides and should include:

1. A subclavian arteriogram to define anatomy: This aids in localization of the thyrocervical trunk and identification of its branches to avoid inadvertent injection into the spinal artery if the latter arises as a branch of this trunk.

2. A thyrocervical arteriogram: This is preferred over an inferior thyroid arteriogram because in the latter a parathyroid artery arising either proximally or separately from the thyrocervical trunk (supplying low cervical or mediastinal glands) may be overlooked.

3. An internal mammary arteriogram for detection of mediastinal glands.

4. A superior thyroid arteriogram: This study may not be necessary if the gland has been localized by the previous arteriograms.

**TABLE 18–1.** Parathyroid Angiography

| Vessel | Contrast Injection* | | Filming | | | Remarks |
|--------|---------------------|---|---------|---|---|---------|
| | Rate (ml/sec) | Volume (ml) | Films per Second | Total | Projection | |
| Subclavian artery | 8 | 24 | 2 1 | 4 6 | AP, oblique | Film subtraction |
| Thyrocervical trunk | 3–4 (or hand injection) | 8 | 1 | 8 | AP, 20–30° oblique | Film subtraction |
| Superior thyroid artery | 2–3 (or hand injection) | 6–8 | 1 | 8 | AP, 20–30° oblique | Film subtraction |
| Inferior thyroid artery | 2–3 (or hand injection) | 8–10 | 1 | 8 | AP, 20–30° oblique | Film subtraction |
| Internal mammary artery | 2–3 | 8 | 1 | 8 | AP, oblique | Film subtraction |
| Inferior or superior thyroid venography | 3–4 | 15 | 1 | 6 | AP | Performed during Valsalva maneuver |

*60% Diatrizoate meglumine sodium or iothalamate meglumine.

5. In patients with absent or small inferior thyroid arteries, a search should be made for the thyroidea ima artery off the aortic arch or brachiocephalic artery.[13]

Subclavian arteriography is rarely sufficient for demonstration of smaller lesions, and most patients require selective arteriography. Wedge injections into neck vessels must be avoided. If this occurs, the catheter must be pulled back to permit antegrade flow immediately upon completion of the injection. Both AP and oblique views with film subtraction are essential. Standard cut film arteriography or intraarterial DSA (using 20% concentration of contrast medium) is used. Although iothalamate is recommended by some, we use diatrizoate meglumine sodium as the contrast agent and have not experienced any complications.[10]

## Venous Sampling and Venography

Nonselective venous sampling from large veins (brachiocephalic, jugular) may yield enough information to lateralize a source of excessive hormone production in 56% of cases.[11] However, because of the potential pitfalls (due to anomalous venous drainage and dilution), this is not recommended unless selective catheterization is not possible. Blood samples should be obtained from both the inferior and the superior thyroid veins and, if possible, from the middle thyroid veins. Following each sample, 2 to 3 ml of contrast is injected, and the catheter position is documented on film. Blood samples (10

ml) are obtained by gentle suction or by allowing the blood to drip from the catheter. The samples are put in red top (nonheparinized) tubes and placed on ice until they reach the processing laboratory.

Because of the small size of the thyroid veins, blood withdrawal may not be possible. In such cases the patient is asked to perform a Valsalva maneuver, which often allows gradual withdrawal of blood samples. Alternatively, we have used a coaxial system: A 2.5 or 3 Fr catheter is inserted through the angiographic catheter. The tip is advanced past that of the larger angiographic catheter, which is withdrawn slightly. Venous samples are obtained by allowing the blood to drip from the catheter or by gentle suction. Catheterization of smaller veins is also facilitated by using a catheter with a well-tapered tip. After completion of the sampling, a thyroid venogram is performed by injecting contrast medium into the inferior or superior thyroid vein during a Valsalva maneuver. Occasionally, an adenoma may be demonstrated by retrograde venography.[14]

## DISEASES OF THE PARATHYROID GLANDS

### Hyperparathyroidism

Primary hyperparathyroidism may be caused by an adenoma or hyperplasia and occasionally by carcinoma[15]:

Adenoma (87% of cases):
  Single (80%)
  Multiple (7%)

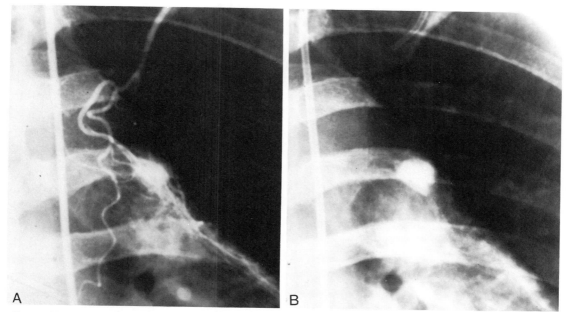

*Figure 18–6.* Mediastinal parathyroid adenoma. Early (*A*) and late (*B*) phases from a left internal mammary arteriogram in the left posterior oblique projection shows a densely staining adenoma. (Courtesy of Dr. CA Athanasoulis.)

Hyperplasia (10% of cases):
  Chief Cell (~ 5%)
  Clear Cell (~ 5%)
Carcinoma (3% of cases)

The symptoms include hypercalcemia, hypophosphatemia, elevated serum parathyroid hormone levels, increased urinary calcium and phosphate loss, nephrolithiasis, and osteopenia (the last in about 25% of patients).

Ninety-five per cent of patients with primary hyperparathyroidism are cured after the first surgical exploration.[16] In patients with recurrent or persistent symptoms, the most frequent location of the surgically missed hyperfunctioning gland is the posterior-superior mediastinum.[17]

An ectopic supernumerary gland may also be a source for excessive hormone production in about 1% of patients.[18] The most frequent location for such glands is the anterior mediastinum, within the thymus, but they can occur anywhere from the mediastinum to the upper neck.

Although most mediastinal glands drain into the inferior thyroid vein, some may drain directly into the brachiocephalic vein, whereas others may drain into the azygos, thymic, or other mediastinal veins.[10, 19] The thymic veins drain into the left brachiocephalic vein but anastomoses between thymic and inferior thyroid veins are common, which makes venous sampling inaccurate.[20] Thus, it is not possible to differentiate between a cervical or mediastinal adenoma on the basis of venous sampling alone.[19]

## Angiography

The normal parathyroid glands cannot be recognized on arteriography. Enlarged glands assume an oval or round configuration, and glands as small as 0.5 cm in diameter can be detected by arteriography.[20] Angiographic signs of the presence of an adenoma are (Fig. 18–6):

1. Enlargement of the parathyroid artery or other branch(es) supplying the involved gland.

2. Round or oval-shaped tumor stain: This is the most reliable sign.

3. Inferior displacement of the caudal loop of the inferior thyroid artery: This sign is unreliable, as a large adenoma may be present without any displacement.

The overall success rates for angiographic localization are approximately 70% for arteriography and 90% for venous sampling.[17] The associated risks, which are few in experienced and cautious hands, include damage to the spinal cord by inadvertent injection into the spinal branch of the costocervical trunk. Occasionally, this vessel arises from the thyrocervical trunk.[21]

PITFALLS IN DIAGNOSIS

1. Dense stain simulating adenoma: This may be due to muscle opacification on thyrocervical arteriography or to intense parenchymal staining of the thyroid gland. A selective arteriogram of the inferior thyroid artery and an oblique projection help in differentiation.

2. AP view only: The thyroid stain may be superimposed and can thus obscure a parathyroid lesion.

3. False-positive stain: This may be due to a lymph node or a thyroid adenoma.[22]

4. An intrathyroid parathyroid adenoma may be obscured by the normal thyroid stain. In this situation, venous sampling is used for lateralization.[23]

# ANGIOGRAPHY OF THE ADRENAL GLANDS

## Arteriography

Adrenal arteriography is indicated for:

1. Evaluation of large masses, both hormone producing and endocrine inactive (all suspected carcinomas and large benign tumors).

2. Pheochromocytoma.

3. Retroperitoneal hemorrhage from a suspected adrenal tumor.

Arteriography is not indicated for the evaluation of patients with benign aldosterone-producing tumors. In most patients these can be detected by computed tomography (CT) and their location confirmed by adrenal venous sampling and venography.

For most adrenal lesions necessitating arteriography, an aortogram should be performed first. This defines the vascular anatomy for selective catheterization (if this becomes necessary) and frequently localizes the lesion.

## Aortography

The AP aortogram is performed in the standard fashion with the tip of the pigtail catheter positioned at T11 (see Chapter 10, Table 10–1). This permits opacification of the celiac artery, which often gives off the inferior phrenic arteries. Cut films are necessary, as they provide better detail than digital subtraction angiography (DSA). Film subtrac-

tion should be used routinely, even in patients in whom an abnormality has been demonstrated, so that additional lesions do not remain undetected.[24]

Unless obscured by more densely opacified organs (ie, kidney, stomach, or liver), the adrenal glands are frequently visualized during the middle and late phases of an abdominal aortogram. Figure 18–7 shows the appearance of the normal adrenal glands on aortography. Initially, the normal adrenal cortex, which measures between 1 and 2 mm, is densely opacified. Later films show medullary opacification, but veins are usually not discernible.

Aortography during a Valsalva maneuver or after epinephrine injection has also been used to enhance visualization of the adrenal glands.[25] However, this is not a reliable method unless larger vascular masses are suspected. Selective adrenal arteriography is necessary in patients with tumors that are not demonstrated by aortography.

## Selective Catheterization (Table 18–2)

Selective catheterization often visualizes only the portion of the adrenal gland supplied by that particular artery, and the search for the different adrenal arteries (unless enlarged) can be tedious and time consuming. Either a cobra or a sidewinder I catheter is used. Inferior phrenic arteriography is associated with chest and shoulder pain, which may simulate angina. Since these vessels are usually very small, the catheter must be withdrawn immediately after the injection is completed if stasis of contrast medium is observed on the test injection.

**Superior Adrenal Arteries.** The inferior phrenic artery may be a branch of the celiac or renal artery or it may arise from the aorta. If it is a branch of the celiac artery, an epinephrine-enhanced celiac arteriogram may be performed in patients in whom selective arteriography is not possible; 10 to 15 μg of epinephrine is injected into the celiac artery followed by injection of 30 ml of contrast medium at a rate of 5 ml/sec. Films are obtained at 1 per second for a total of 12 films.

**Middle Adrenal Arteries.** A cobra or sidewinder catheter is used to search the lateral wall of the suprarenal aorta. When enlarged, the middle adrenal artery is readily opacified on the abdominal aortogram.

**Inferior Adrenal Arteries.** These can be

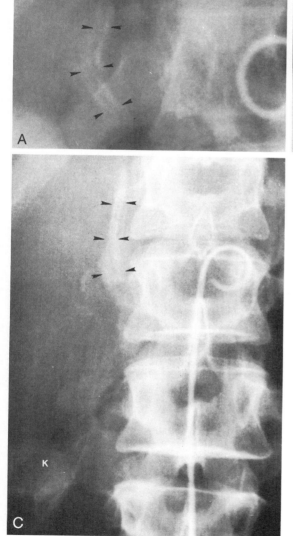

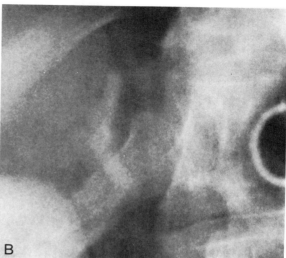

*Figure 18–7.* Appearance of the normal adrenal gland on aortography. *A,* Early parenchymal phase shows dense opacification of the adrenal cortex (*arrowheads*). *B,* Late parenchymal phase shows predominantly medullary opacification. *C,* Mid-parenchymal phase from an abdominal aortogram in another patient with ptotic right kidney. Note that the adrenal gland (*arrowheads*) maintains it normal location. K = kidney.

TABLE 18–2. Selective Adrenal Arteriography

| Artery | Catheter | Contrast Injection* | | Films Rate/Total |
| | | Rate (ml/sec) | Volume (ml) | |
|---|---|---|---|---|
| Superior adrenal† | Cobra, cobra in loop, sidewinder | 2–3 | 6–8 | 1 per sec/8 |
| Middle adrenal | Cobra, Mikaelsson, sidewinder | 1–2 | 4–6 | 1 per sec/8 |
| Inferior adrenal† | Cobra in loop, side-winder | 1–2 | 4–6 | 1 per sec/8 |

*60% Diatrizoate meglumine sodium. For intraarterial DSA, a 20% concentration is used.
†Alternatively, epinephrine-aided celiac or renal arteriography.

catheterized by using the sidewinder or cobra catheter in the loop configuration. If selective catheterization is not possible, an epineph-rine-enhanced renal arteriogram may be performed; 10 μg of epinephrine is injected into the renal artery followed by injection of 8 to 10 ml of contrast medium at a rate of 4 ml/sec. Films are obtained at 1 per second for a total of 10 films.

## Venous Sampling and Venography

Venous sampling should always precede venography. Thus, if contrast extravasation should occur during venography, this will not compromise patient evaluation. On the other hand, contrast extravasation in the adrenal gland should not occur if the venogram is performed carefully. Prior to sampling, a gentle test injection may be used to confirm catheter position. With increasing experience of the vascular radiologist, a test injection may not be necessary. Subsequent to obtaining each venous sample, catheter position must be documented on spot films, using 1 to 2 ml of contrast medium. A 5 to 7 Fr catheter without side holes and a short, well-tapered catheter tip is used.

Catheterization of the right adrenal vein is accomplished by a sidewinder, Mikaelsson, or double renal catheter. In some cases we have also used a cobra catheter. The left adrenal vein can be catheterized with a cobra catheter in the loop configuration or a sidewinder II catheter. For selective catheter placement past the inferior phrenic vein, a 3 Fr catheter is inserted coaxially into the central adrenal vein (Fig. 18–8).

Blood samples are obtained by gentle suction or by allowing the blood to drip out. This may be aided by a Valsalva maneuver. Venous cortisol levels must also be deter-

mined, in addition to the other hormones, in order to confirm the accuracy of the samples. In patients with unilateral adrenal atrophy (in the presence of a contralateral adenoma), blood withdrawal may not be possible from the adrenal vein of the atrophic gland. In such cases, venous samples are obtained from the inferior vena cava adjacent to the adrenal vein orifice. For each sample (for cortisol or catecholamines), 10 ml of blood is obtained. The samples are put in a green top (heparinized) tube and are placed in ice immediately.

Venography is performed by manual injection of contrast medium. Usually 2 to 5 ml is injected in 1 to 2 seconds, and spot films are

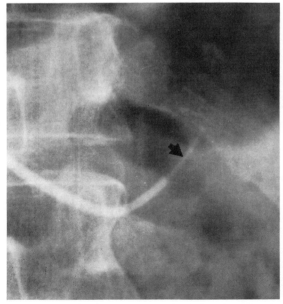

*Figure 18–8.* Coaxial system for left adrenal vein catheterization. Arrow points to the 3 Fr coaxial Teflon catheter that was introduced through a cobra catheter.

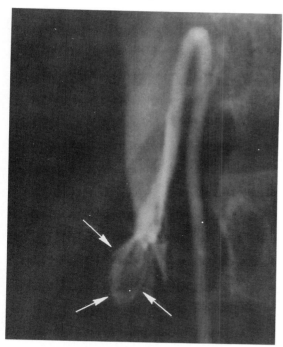

*Figure 18–9.* Pitfall in adrenal venography: adrenal pseudotumor. Retrograde right adrenal venogram. Position of the catheter tip in a branch vessel causes segmental overinjection which simulates a small tumor (*arrows*). (From Kadir S, et al: Cardiovasc Intervent Radiol 4:99–104, 1981. Used with permission.)

obtained at 3 per second for a total of 8 exposures. Prior to the actual venogram, test injections of contrast medium under fluoroscopy are used to assess the rate of contrast injection required to opacify the gland fully without overinjecting. This practice has helped us to avoid contrast ablation of the adrenal glands. Occasionally, rupture of a peripheral (extraadrenal) venule may occur as a result of the increased intravenous pressure. However, this is without clinical consequences.

PITFALLS IN VENOUS SAMPLING AND VENOGRAPHY

1. Improper catheter position during left adrenal vein catheterization, ie, the catheter tip may be in the inferior phrenic vein: This occurs occasionally with the cobra catheter in the loop configuration. To avoid this, a coaxial system is used (Fig. 18–8).

2. Pseudo-tumor blush: A wedged contrast injection into the adrenal vein may result in segmental parenchymal staining and may thus simulate a small adenoma (Fig. 18–9).

3. Hepatic versus adrenal vein: Several small hepatic venules drain directly into the inferior vena cava in the vicinity of the right adrenal vein. One of these may be entered, and on contrast injection (fluoroscopically) the hepatic parenchymogram may simulate the adrenal gland. In such cases, the spot film obtained after venous sampling verifies the position of the catheter (Fig. 18–10). The hepatic parenchymogram has a coarse, granular, geometric appearance, and occasionally other hepatic veins are opacified. In contrast, the adrenal vein injection often opacifies several retroperitoneal and renal capsular veins (Fig. 18–11).

## Complications of Adrenal Angiography

Careful adrenal vein catheterization and venography are rarely associated with clinically significant complications. The overall complication rates are as follows:[26]

*Patients without pheochromocytoma (9%):* Permanent adrenal dysfunction occurred in 1%, whereas 8% had transient symptoms as a result of contrast extravasation, ie, flank pain, bleeding, thrombosis, hematoma, or adrenal necrosis.

*Patients with pheochromocytoma (23%):* A hypertensive episode was the most common complication. The incidence of such complications is much lower in patients who have been pretreated with alpha-adrenergic block-

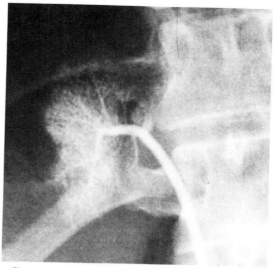

*Figure 18–10.* Hepatic venogram (injection into a small hepatic vein), which can simulate the right adrenal gland on fluoroscopy.

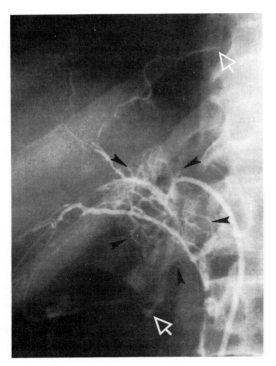

*Figure 18–11.* Right adrenal venogram in a patient with adrenal hyperplasia causing hyperaldosteronism. The gland is enlarged (*arrowheads*), and there is opacification of multiple collaterals, some of which drain into the inferior vena cava via retroperitoneal veins (*open arrows*).

ers. Death following arteriography or venography occurs very rarely.

**Complications Associated with Adrenal Vein Catheterization**

1. Adrenal vein thrombosis: Occlusion of the adrenal vein by the catheter tip may lead to thrombosis. Thus, prolonged catheterization must be avoided.

2. Adrenal infarction: This is a recognized complication of improperly performed adrenal venography. Patients with Cushing's disease or syndrome and less frequently those with hyperaldosteronism appear to have excessive vascular fragility. Thus, even a careful contrast injection into the adrenal vein may result in contrast extravasation. This is often associated with clinical remission of the disease.

3. Extraadrenal hemorrhage: Increase in intravascular pressure in the small retroperitoneal veins during retrograde adrenal venography has occasionally resulted in clinically inconsequential extraadrenal hemorrhage (see Fig. 18–15).

**Complications Associated with Arterial Studies.** Complications of arteriography are

most common in patients with unsuspected pheochromocytoma. A hypertensive episode necessitating intravenous phentolamine (Regitine, Ciba Pharmaceuticals) is the most common complication. In patients who have been premedicated with alpha-adrenergic blockers, a severe contrast-induced hypertensive episode is unlikely. Another complication is the rupture of small retroperitoneal arteries during adrenal arteriography. This is associated with transient flank pain.

## DISEASES OF THE ADRENAL GLANDS

The adrenal gland may be affected by diseases that may or may not be hormonally active. Excessive hormone production by a tumor may not be associated with a clinically manifested syndrome because of synthesis of less potent precursors.[27] Hormonally inactive adenomas of the adrenal cortex are a relatively frequent finding at autopsy. In contrast, hormone-producing tumors are relatively uncommon.

In children, adrenal tumors are almost always malignant and hormone producing. In adults, the majority of carcinomas are also hormone producing. In most cases, more than one hormone is produced, giving rise to a mixed clinical picture. Glucocorticosteroid and androgen production is most common, leading to Cushing's syndrome and virilization. Thus, a single clinical syndrome occurs infrequently, although one clinical picture may predominate.[27-29] Adrenal carcinomas may be locally invasive, and distant metastases, which frequently involve the liver and lungs, may also be hormonally active.[29, 30] Benign tumors and hyperplasia are more likely to be responsible for a single, clear-cut syndrome.[30]

Hormones produced by the different parts of the adrenal gland are:

Cortex:
  Zona glomerulosa—aldosterone.
  Zona fasciculata—cortisol.
  Zona reticularis—progesterone, androgens, and estrogens.
Medulla:
  Epinephrine and norepinephrine.

### Diseases of the Adrenal Cortex

#### Cushing's Syndrome

Cushing's disease refers to bilateral adrenocortical hyperplasia due to excessive ACTH production as a result of a hypothalamic abnormality or is occasionally due to a pituitary tumor, usually a basophilic or chromophobe adenoma. Excessive secretion of ACTH stimulates the adrenal cortex, leading to hyperplasia and the production of excessive amounts of cortisol. Cushing's syndrome is caused by a primary adrenal abnormality in about 20% of patients. Ectopic production of ACTH or substances with ACTH-like activity by nonpituitary, nonadrenal tumors that may stimulate the adrenal cortex is responsible for the syndrome in about 8% of cases. Tumors responsible for ectopic ACTH production are bronchogenic, hepatic, prostatic, ovarian, and breast carcinoma and bronchial adenoma and carcinoid.

**Clinical Aspects.** The clinical features are characteristic and include central obesity, hypertension, purpura, striae, diabetes or impaired glucose tolerance, and osteoporosis. Plasma cortisol levels are elevated, and there is excessive excretion of urinary 17-hydroxycorticosteroids. The diagnosis is easily established by clinical and laboratory methods. The dexamethasone suppression test is used to differentiate between adrenal and pituitary pathology. In the latter, adrenal function is suppressed by administration of dexamethasone (2 mg every 6 hours for 2 days). In addition, an adrenal tumor may be distinguished from hyperplasia by the metyrapone test. In this test, patients with hyperplasia respond with excretion of excessive amounts of 17-hydroxycorticosteroids.

**Pathology.** In the adult, the most common etiology of Cushing's syndrome is bilateral adrenal cortical hyperplasia (70 to 80%).[28, 31] In approximately 10% of cases the syndrome is due to an adenoma, and in another 10% it is due to a carcinoma. Women are affected more frequently than men (ratio of 4:1). In about 8% of patients, adrenal hyperplasia is secondary to ectopic ACTH production.[31] In children, the most frequent cause of Cushing's syndrome is a carcinoma (66%), followed by hyperplasia (about 19%) and adenoma (about 15%).[27, 32]

**Radiology.** Tumors and enlarged hyperplastic adrenal glands are easily diagnosed by CT because of the presence of excessive retroperitoneal fat. However, in one third of the patients with adrenal hyperplasia, the glands are of normal size and weight.[31] Similarly, in patients with micronodular hyperplasia, the glands appear normal on CT, although hypersecretion is documented by venous sampling. Another potential pitfall in CT diagnosis is the presence of a nonfunc-

tioning adenoma in a hyperplastic adrenal gland.[33] Iodocholesterol scanning, although not very reliable, can be used for lateralization of an adrenal tumor.

### Hyperaldosteronism (Conn's Syndrome)

**Clinical Aspects and Pathology.** Diastolic hypertension, hypokalemia in the absence of antidiuretic medication, hyperaldosteronemia, and suppressed plasma renin activity are characteristic features. Hyperaldosteronism occurs more frequently in women than in men (ratio of 2:1). Primary hyperaldosteronism is responsible for hypertension in 2% of patients.[34] Adenoma is responsible for the disease in 89% of patients.[35] In 70% of patients the adenoma is solitary, in 13.5% there are multiple adenomas (often bilateral), and in 5.5% microadenomatosis is present.

The adenomas responsible for hyperaldosteronism are smaller than those seen in Cushing's syndrome. They are usually between 0.5 and 2 cm in size and are frequently on the left side. Bilateral adrenal hyperplasia is responsible for hyperaldosteronism in 11% of patients, but in some series it is reported in as many as 27% of patients.[36, 37] Hyperplasia may be diffuse or nodular. Adrenal carcinoma causing hyperaldosteronism is very rare.[38]

**Radiology.** Differentiation between adenoma and hyperplasia is essential because the treatment of choice for the former is surgical removal, whereas the latter is managed by medical therapy. Bilateral adenomatosis is treated by subtotal (90%) adrenalectomy. Localization of an adenoma by CT is possible in only two thirds of patients because of the small size of the tumors.[33] Hyperactive adrenal glands may also appear normal on CT. With venous sampling and adrenal venography, the diagnosis can be established in 100% of patients. In experienced hands, venography may detect even small adenomas (< 8 mm) in 76% of patients, whereas venous sampling localizes the abnormal side in 91% of patients.[39]

Aldosterone-producing adenomas are usually hypervascular. Some adenomas may be hypovascular and may thus escape arteriographic detection,[40] making arteriography an unreliable method for localization. In hyperplasia, both glands are usually enlarged but can also be of normal size. In the presence of an adenoma, the contralateral gland is atrophic. Venous sampling may be very difficult or impossible in such cases. Errors due to episodic aldosterone production can be eliminated by sampling during ACTH infusion.[39]

### Virilization and Feminization Syndromes (Adreno-Genital Syndromes)

These may be caused by an adrenal abnormality (hyperplasia, adenoma, carcinoma), an ovarian or testicular tumor, or an ACTH- or gonadotropin-producing tumor (pineal, hypothalamic, choriocarcinoma).[41-43]

In the *congenital type,* which affects females more frequently than males, an enzyme defect is responsible for impaired cortisol and aldosterone synthesis, which leads to increased ACTH secretion as a result of the negative feedback. ACTH stimulation leads to adrenal cortical hyperplasia, which results in excessive production of androgens.

There are several different types of enzyme defects. Most frequently, the defect is due to a deficiency of 21-hydroxylase and less frequently of 11-beta-hydroxylase. Clinically, these deficiencies result in virilization of the female fetus and pseudohermaphroditism with development of a urogenital sinus, clitoral hypertrophy, and ambiguous external genitalia. In the older child, there is isosexual precocious puberty in the male and masculinization in the female.

The *acquired type,* which is also more common in females, is due to a tumor, frequently a carcinoma. Clinically, this is manifested by virilization and is associated with Cushing's syndrome.[30] Tumors causing feminization are very rare.[30, 38] Evaluation of the virilization syndrome in females must include sampling of both the adrenal and the ovarian venous effluent for hormonally active substances in order to localize the source.[44]

### Angiography of Adrenal Cortical Diseases

The indications for adrenal angiography are:

**Arteriography.** This is indicated for the evaluation of large tumors and in suspected carcinoma. In the latter, cavography may be needed to evaluate involvement of the inferior vena cava.

**Venous Sampling and Venography.** Adrenal venous sampling and venography are used to differentiate between bilateral nodular hyperplasia and adenomas, in patients with suspected ectopic ACTH production (to exclude an adrenal source) and in patients in whom CT demonstrates normal or minimally enlarged glands.

Venous sampling from the inferior petrosal sinuses may be required for the exclusion of a pituitary/hypothalamic source. In addition, ovarian vein sampling is used for differentiation between adrenal and hormone-producing ovarian tumors.

Arteriography or venography cannot determine whether the tumor is hormonally active. Although differentiation between malignant tumors with extraadrenal extension and benign tumors is often possible, a localized malignant lesion cannot be distinguished from a benign tumor. It may, however, be possible on occasion to differentiate between cortical and medullary lesions by arteriography (Fig. 18–12). In the latter, a normal adrenal cortex is demonstrated, whereas in an autonomous cortical adenoma, the uninvolved cortex and the opposite gland are atrophic. Because of the absence of any characteristic distinguishing features in le-

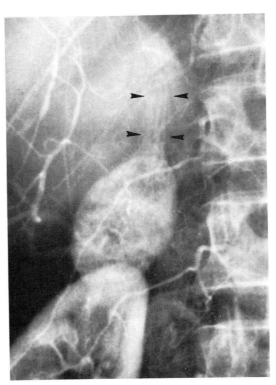

*Figure 18–12.* Parenchymal phase of abdominal aortogram shows a homogeneously staining, exophytically growing pheochromocytoma. The adrenal cortex above the tumor shows a normal, undistorted configuration (*arrowheads*).

sions giving rise to the various syndromes, these lesions are discussed together.

**Hyperplasia** (Figs. 18–13 and 18–14). Arteriography or venography may not show any abnormality if the adrenal gland is normal in size. The enlarged gland often assumes a rounded configuration. Enlargement and splaying of the arteries and minimal hypervascularity may be present. On venography, the adrenal veins are splayed and often dilated. Focal accumulations of contrast medium may be seen on arteriography or retrograde venography.[45, 46] These represent micronodular hyperplasia or microadenomas. Differentiation between these two entities may not be possible even by histological examination.[30] In micronodular hyperplasia, some of the nodules can become quite large (up to 1 cm in size).

**Adenoma** (Figs. 18–15 and 18–16). The adenomas in hyperaldosteronism are small (< 2 cm) and often are only a few millimeters in size. Adenomas associated with Cushing's syndrome are usually larger.

On arteriography, most adenomas are vascular and have neovasculature and a tumor

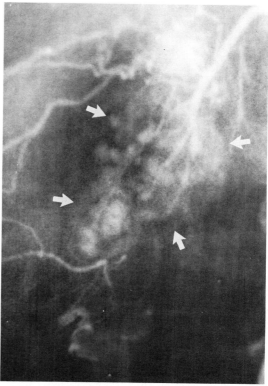

**Figure 18–14.** Nodular hyperplasia. Right adrenal venogram shows an enlarged gland (arrows) and opacification of multiple nodules.

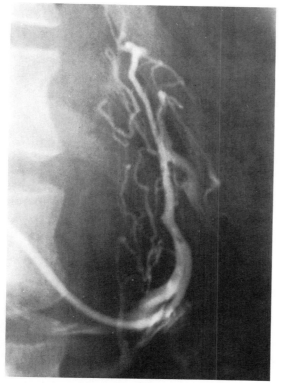

**Figure 18–13.** Diffuse enlargement of the left adrenal gland due to hyperplasia in a patient with hyperaldosteronism. Note that the intraadrenal veins are dilated.

blush. Occasionally, they can be hypovascular.[47] Venous drainage in the form of circumferential veins at the tumor periphery is occasionally demonstrated. In autonomous adenomas, the contralateral gland is atrophic.

On venography, the following findings may be observed:

1. Discretely displaced (occasionally circumferential) adrenal vein branches: These are often seen only in an oblique projection.

2. A more forceful contrast injection may opacify irregularly coursing tumor veins, and a tumor stain may be demonstrated.

3. Pooling of contrast medium in dilated vascular spaces, small adenomas, or hyperplastic nodules.

4. An enlarged central vein with high flow of effluent: For this reason, reflux of contrast medium may not be sufficient to opacify the intraadrenal branches.

Venography does not permit differentiation between medullary and cortical tumors. In addition, smaller adenomas (< 5 mm) may not be demonstrated. Both AP and oblique

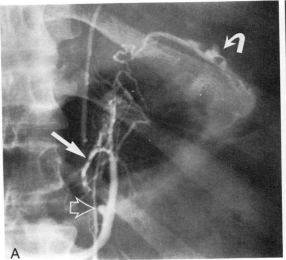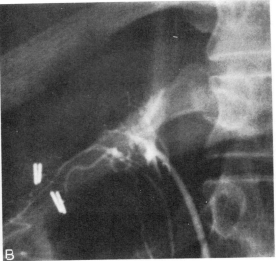

**Figure 18–15.** Aldosterone-producing autonomous adenoma (aldosteronoma). *A*, Left adrenal venogram shows an enlarged and bowed adrenal vein branch (*arrow*). Contrast extravasation is observed from an extraadrenal retroperitoneal branch (*curved arrow*). Open arrow points to the inferior phrenic vein valve. *B*, Right adrenal venogram from the same patient shows an atrophic gland.

venograms may be necessary for establishing the diagnosis.

**Carcinoma** (Fig. 18–17). Malignant adrenal tumors are usually larger than benign lesions, and nonfunctioning tumors are usually the largest. The adrenal arteries are enlarged, there is neovascularity and occasionally parasitization, and arteriovenous shunting and multiple draining veins may be demonstrated. The tumor blush may show areas of hypovascularity resulting from tumor necrosis or hemorrhage. The tumor may extend into and occlude the inferior vena cava and may occasionally extend into the right atrium. This is best demonstrated by inferior and superior venacavography.

PITFALLS IN DIAGNOSIS

1. Adrenal versus renal tumor: Occasionally, adrenal tumors derive a portion of their blood supply from intrarenal branches.[48] If there is uncertainty about tumor origin, selective and oblique arteriography can make differentiation possible. In addition, on retrograde renal venography, communication of the tumor veins with the intrarenal veins confirms a renal origin.

2. Adrenal versus retroperitoneal tumor: In the absence of a well-defined cleavage plane, it may not be possible to localize the origin of the tumor by CT.[49, 50] Differentiation may be possible by selective arteriography.

## Diseases of the Adrenal Medulla

### Pheochromocytoma

Pheochromocytoma is a rare tumor of the chromaffin tissue that is responsible for hypertension in approximately 0.1% of cases. Its incidence at autopsy is 0.13%.[51] Pheochromocytoma may occur sporadically as solitary or multiple tumors (94%) or in association with familial syndromes (6%), ie, multiple endocrine neoplasia (MEN) syndromes, types II and III (see Chapter 15, Table 15–11), von Hippel–Lindau disease, neurofibromatosis, and familial pheochromocytosis.[51]

**Clinical Aspects.** In one autopsy series, the diagnosis was established ante mortem in only 24% of cases, and 9% of the tumors were clinically silent.[51] Symptoms are due to excessive catecholamine secretion and include hypertension, which may be episodic or sustained, headaches, excessive sweating, palpitations, chest and abdominal pain, anxiety, and nausea and vomiting. Rarely, the initial presentation may be a hypertensive crisis induced by massive catecholamine release as a result of tumor necrosis[52] or a massive retroperitoneal hemorrhage.

Sustained hypertension occurs more frequently in children. The diagnosis is established by the measurement of excessive uri-

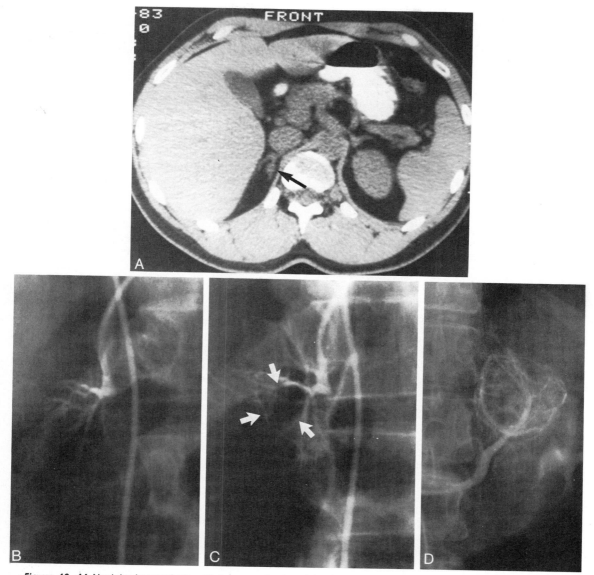

**Figure 18–16.** Nodular hyperplasia with large cortical nodule. *A,* CT scan shows enlargement of both glands and a cortical nodule on the right (*arrow*). *B,* Adrenal venogram in the AP projection shows glandular enlargement but a nodule is not demonstrated. *C,* Venogram in the left posterior oblique projection shows a nonstaining nodule with circumferential displacement of intraadrenal veins (*arrows*). *D,* Left adrenal venogram from another patient shows a large cortical adenoma. (*D,* From Kadir S: AJR 134:31, 1980. Used with permission.)

nary catecholamines, metanephrines, and vanillylmandelic acid (VMA). However, in 21% of patients excessive VMA is not excreted and 25% have normal catecholamine excretions.[53]

Hypertension may also be due to coexisting renal parenchymal or renal artery disease.[54, 55] The latter may be functional (vasoconstrictive response to catecholamines), anatomical and related to the pheochromo-cytoma (fibrosis, intimal proliferation, tumor encasement, or postoperative), or due to a coexisting, unrelated renal artery stenosis (eg, fibromuscular disease).

**Pathology.** Ninety-eight per cent of pheochromocytomas are subdiaphragmatic in location.[56] The adrenal gland is the most common location, but the tumor may arise anywhere from the chromaffin tissue along the sympathetic chain. In the adult, approx-

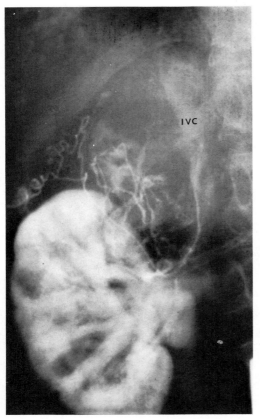

**Figure 18–17.** Large adrenal carcinoma. Right renal arteriogram shows a partially hypovascular tumor. Neovasculature, tumor stain in a portion of the lesion, and arteriovenous shunting with opacification of the inferior vena cava (IVC) are seen.

imately 90% of pheochromocytomas arise in the adrenal glands. Ten per cent are extraadrenal, 10% are bilateral, and about 14% are malignant.[56] Although some reports indicate a higher incidence of extraadrenal and malignant pheochromocytomas,[48] others suggest a much lower incidence of malignancy.[55] The incidence of extraadrenal tumors in children is 31%, and frequently these tumors arise adjacent to the adrenal gland or in the renal hilus.[48, 57] Other common extraadrenal locations are the base of the urinary bladder and the organ of Zuckerkandl, located at the origin of the inferior mesenteric artery.

The incidence of multiple tumors is 32% in children,[57] approximately 10% in adult patients without familial syndromes, and 60 to 70% in patients with a familial syndrome. In patients with a MEN syndrome, a spectrum of adrenal medullary changes may be encountered.[58] These most likely represent the different phases of development of pheochromocytoma. Initially, diffuse medullary hyperplasia may be present. Subsequently, there is nodular hyperplasia, which is followed by the development of larger nodules representing pheochromocytomas.

Whereas adrenal tumors produce both epinephrine and norepinephrine, extraadrenal tumors are primarily norepinephrine producing. The diagnosis of malignancy can be established only by demonstration of metastases or local tumor invasion. The most frequent sites for metastases are bone, lymph nodes, liver, and lung.[56] Metastases may also be hormonally active.

**Radiology.** Intraarterial injection of contrast medium may stimulate catecholamine release and induce a hypertensive crisis. In fact, such a maneuver was used as a "provocative test" for the detection of pheochromocytomas.[59] To avoid this complication, all patients with suspected pheochromocytoma must be premedicated with alpha-adrenergic blockers (phenoxybenzamine). In addition, blood pressure must be monitored carefully during the study. Phentolamine should be on hand to treat a hypertensive episode. Because of the availability of better and safer tests, the use of arteriography as a provocative test should be abandoned.

In the patients evaluated by us, intravenous injection of contrast medium for CT or urography has not resulted in clinically detectable symptoms attributable to excessive catecholamine release.

The overall accuracy of CT for the localization of pheochromocytomas is 91%.[33] In adults, adrenal and large extraadrenal lesions are easily detected. In children, extraadrenal tumors often remain undetected, owing to the paucity of retroperitoneal fat.[24]

**Angiography.** Arteriography is indicated for tumor localization and not as a diagnostic test. Abdominal aortography is performed first with a pigtail catheter placed at T12. If this fails to demonstrate a lesion, selective arteriography of the adrenal and renal arteries is performed. Ninety per cent of pheochromocytomas can be localized by aortography alone and the remainder by selective arteriography.[48] Film subtraction should be used routinely to facilitate detection of lesions obscured by bone.[24, 60]

Venous sampling for catecholamines and adrenal venography are used in patients with a nondiagnostic arteriogram, recurrent disease, metastases, or persistent symptoms postoperatively. Figure 18–18 shows the sites

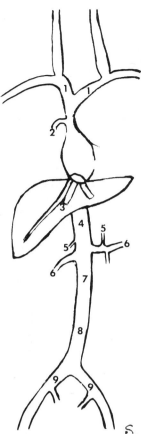

**Figure 18–18.** Schema showing sites for venous sampling for localization of endocrine-active pheochromocytomas/paragangliomas. 1 = brachiocephalic vein; 2 = azygos vein; 3 = hepatic vein; 4 = suprarenal inferior vena cava; 5 = adrenal veins; 6 = renal veins; 7 = infrarenal IVC; 8 = IVC above junction of iliac veins; 9 = common iliac veins. (From Kadir S, Robinette C: J Urol 126:789–793, 1981. Used with permission.)

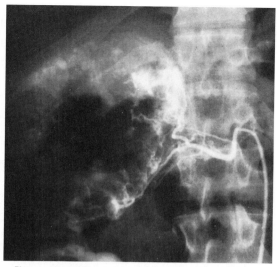

**Figure 18–19.** Pheochromocytoma. Right middle adrenal arteriogram shows a large tumor with central hypovascularity due to hemorrhage.

of venous sampling. Adrenal venography should be performed after the venous sample has been obtained, since contrast injection or excessive catheter manipulation may stimulate catecholamine release from the adrenal gland. In the majority of patients, the tumors are 2 cm or larger and a normal venogram serves to exclude the adrenal gland as the location of the tumor.

Arteriographic findings are (Figs. 18–19 to 18–23; see also Fig. 18–12):

1. Pheochromocytomas are usually hypervascular, but some tumors may be extremely hypovascular or may demonstrate a faintly vascular rim (halo) with central hypo- or avascularity. The latter sign is suggestive of a centrally necrotic tumor.[61]

2. The arteries supplying the tumor are usually (but not always) enlarged.

3. Neovascularity may be seen and may have a spoke wheel configuration.

4. An intense tumor blush may be noted. This is homogeneous in small tumors and inhomogeneous in large tumors (due to the presence of necrosis or hemorrhage).

5. Arteriovenous shunting is observed occasionally.

6. A portion of the arterial supply may be derived from the intrarenal (perforating) branches and the pheochromocytoma may thus simulate a renal mass (Fig. 18–20).

7. Intravenous growth of the tumor may be demonstrated.[46]

Extraadrenal pheochromocytomas arising adjacent to a normal adrenal gland cannot be distinguished from adrenal lesions, except by adrenal venography. Similarly, it is not possible to differentiate between benign and malignant tumors unless there is evidence of metastases or local invasion. Metastases are often hypervascular and hormone producing (Fig. 18–22).[48]

PITFALLS IN DIAGNOSIS

1. Extremely hypovascular tumors: Such lesions may not be detected by selective arteriography and the use of film subtraction. Arteries supplying these tumors may not be enlarged. Such tumors, if hormonally active, can be localized by venous assay or venography.[62]

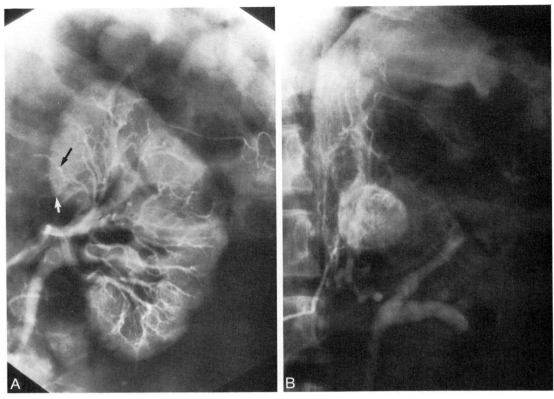

*Figure 18–20.* Adrenal pheochromocytoma deriving a portion of its blood supply from intrarenal branches of the renal artery. *A,* Left renal arteriogram shows arterial supply to the pheochromocytoma from perforating branches of the renal artery (*arrows*). *B,* Middle adrenal arteriogram shows a hypervascular tumor. (From Kadir S, Robinette C: J Urol 126:789–793, 1981. Used with permission.)

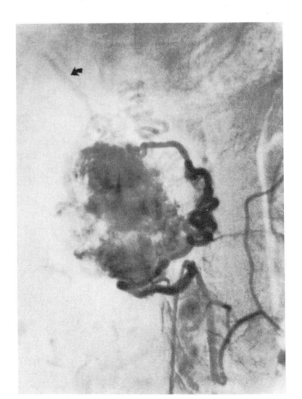

*Figure 18–21.* Pheochromocytoma arising from the organ of Zuckerkandl. Subtraction film from an inferior mesenteric arteriogram shows a hypervascular tumor with arteriovenous shunting (*arrow*). (From Kadir S, et al: Cardiovasc Intervent Radiol 4:99–104, 1981. Used with permission.)

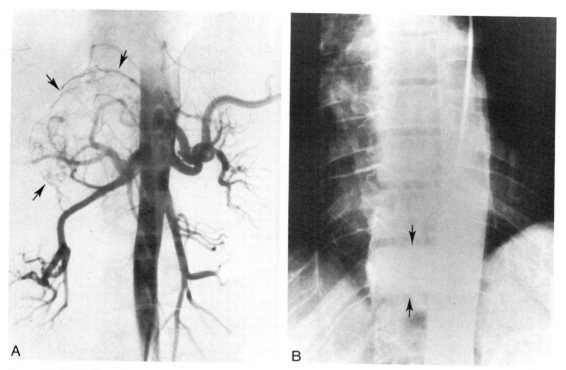

**Figure 18–22.** Malignant pheochromocytoma. *A,* Subtraction film from an abdominal aortogram shows a large, vascular, paraaortic, extraadrenal pheochromocytoma (*arrows*) in a 38 year old woman. *B,* The symptoms recurred several months after operation, and a thoracic aortogram performed for evaluation of elevated catecholamines derived from the azygos vein showed a hypervascular metastasis at T11 (*arrows*). (From Kadir S, Robinette C: J Urol 126:789–793, 1981. Used with permission.)

**Figure 18–23.** Venographic appearance of an adrenal pheochromocytoma. Only a portion of the tumor (*arrowheads*) is opacified on the retrograde venogram. K = kidney. Same patient as in Figure 18–12.

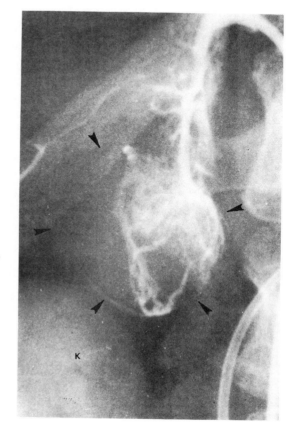

2. Missed extraadrenal tumors: In children and in patients with a familial syndrome, multiple lesions must be suspected. In such patients, film subtraction is an invaluable aid[24] (Fig. 18–24).

3. Elevated catecholamines in venous effluent from a normal adrenal gland as demonstrated by CT and venography: This may be due to catecholamine release as a result of catheter manipulation or contrast injection, or the patient may have adrenal medullary hyperplasia.[63]

4. Renal artery stenosis: This may be due to the pheochromocytoma or an unrelated coexisting abnormality.[54, 64]

## Neuroblastoma, Ganglioneuroblastoma, and Ganglioneuroma

Neuroblastoma is the second most common malignant tumor of childhood. Approximately half the tumors originate in the adrenal medulla, but the lesion may arise anywhere along the sympathetic chain. Approximately 50% of neuroblastomas have calcification and 69% have metastases at the time of diagnosis.[65] Rarely, the tumor may be hormonally active or familial. Caval involvement, which occurs with a high frequency, is an indicator of unresectability.[66]

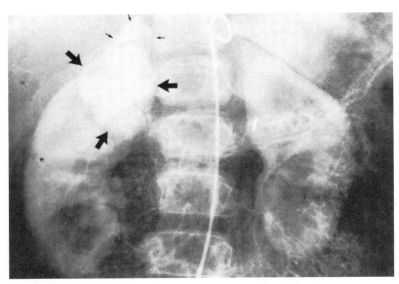

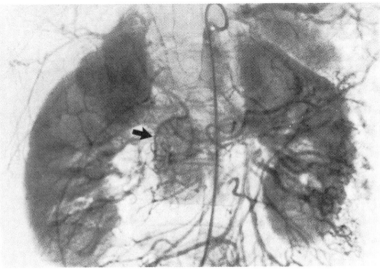

*Figure 18–24.* Importance of film subtraction for the detection of extraadrenal pheochromocytomas. *A,* Abdominal aortogram in a 13 year old girl shows multiple adrenal (*small arrows*) and paraadrenal (*large arrows*) pheochromocytomas. No other lesions are identified. *B,* Subtraction film from the same aortogram reveals another paraaortic tumor (*arrow*) that is not demonstrated on the unsubtracted film. (From Kadir S, et al: Cardiovasc Intervent Radiol 4:99–104, 1981. Used with permission.)

The ganglioneuroblastoma is a transitional tumor (transition of cellular maturity from neuroblastoma to ganglioneuroma) that contains cellular elements of both the highly malignant neuroblastoma and the benign ganglioneuroma.

The ganglioneuroma is a rare benign tumor. It is often discovered incidentally, occurs most frequently in young females, and may represent the end stage of maturation of a neuroblastoma.[67] Although 60% of patients are younger than 20 years, the age at which the tumor is diagnosed is generally greater than that of patients with neuroblastoma.[68] A ganglioneuroma may be located anywhere along the sympathetic chain and occurs in the adrenal gland in approximately 20% of patients. The most common location is the mediastinum (43%), where it may present as a paraspinal mass.[68] Rarely, the tumor may produce catecholamines.[69]

**Angiography** (Figs. 18–25 and 18–26). Arteriography is rarely indicated for preoperative evaluation. On the other hand, assessment of caval involvement is important, as it determines resectability (encasement and occlusion versus compression).

On arteriography, neuroblastomas may be (1) hypervascular with demonstration of neovascularity, (2) hypovascular, or (3) both hyper- and hypovascular. Arteriovenous shunt-

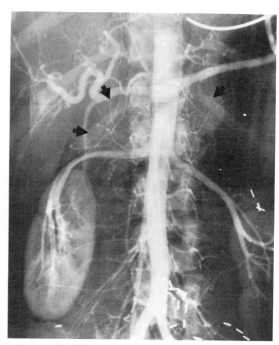

**Figure 18–26.** Large ganglioneuroma. Abdominal aortogram shows displacement and malrotation of the right kidney and inferior displacement of the left kidney. The right renal artery is narrowed slightly. A few tumor vessels are seen in the suprarenal (*arrows*) and pararenal areas.

ing may be demonstrated by some tumors. Ganglioneuromas are often very large. They can also be hypervascular and may demonstrate neovascularity and areas of hypovascularity.[70] In our own experience and that of some others,[68] these tumors can also be completely hypovascular but may cause considerable distortion of the vascular anatomy by displacement.

## MISCELLANEOUS DISEASES OF THE ADRENAL GLANDS AND THE PARAGANGLIA

**Adenoma.** Nonfunctioning adrenal adenomas are found in 3% of patients at autopsy and are more common in the hypertensive and diabetic population.[71] This incidence increases four-fold in patients with a malignant tumor. Differentiation between a benign adenoma and a metastatic deposit is not possible by arteriography.[72]

**Adrenal Hyperplasia.** Hyperplasia of the adrenal gland not associated with a clinically manifested hormone-induced syndrome has also been observed in patients with a

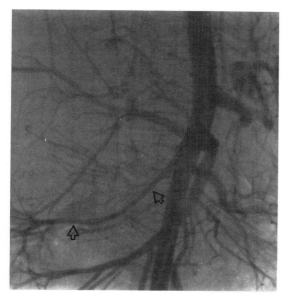

**Figure 18–25.** Large neuroblastoma arising from the right adrenal gland. The aorta is displaced to the left, and the right renal artery is stretched and displaced inferiorly (*arrows*). Tumor vascularity is present in the suprarenal area.

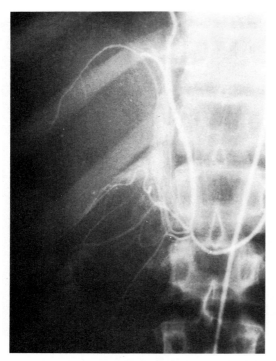

*Figure 18–27.* Adrenal hyperplasia in a patient with chronic renal failure. Right inferior phrenic arteriogram shows an enlarged, hyperemic adrenal gland. The gland has maintained its normal configuration.

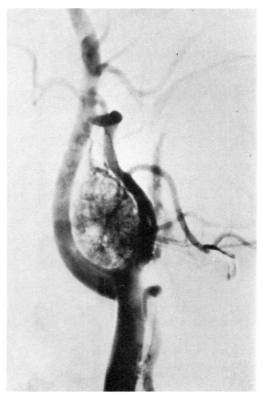

*Figure 18–28.* Cervical paraganglioma (carotid body tumor). Subtraction film from a common carotid arteriogram shows a widened bifurcation and a hypervascular tumor. The tumor was hormonally inactive.

malignancy[73] or other chronic illnesses (eg, chronic renal failure) (Fig. 18–27). The causal relationship remains undetermined, but it may be due to chronic stress. Such hyperplasia may also be diffuse or nodular.[46]

**Metastases.** Hematogenous metastases to the adrenal gland are observed in 27% of all tumors.[74] The most frequent primary cancers are breast, lung, and renal carcinomas, gastrointestinal malignancies, and melanoma. Most metastases are located in the adrenal medulla.[75]

Arteriography is not indicated for the evaluation of hormonally inactive metastases. However, if it is performed, the metastases frequently show the same vascularity as the primary tumor, including neo- and hypervascularity and arteriovenous shunting.[45]

**Myelolipoma.** This is a benign tumor, consisting of fat and hematopoietic cells, that is usually discovered at autopsy. The tumor may become quite large and give rise to symptoms. The high fat content results in a characteristic CT and ultrasound appearance. On arteriography, these tumors are usually hypovascular.[76]

**Paragangliomas of the Head and Neck.** The paraganglia cells are of neuroectodermal origin and belong to the APUD (amine precursor uptake and decarboxylation) system. They also store catecholamines and differ from the adrenal medulla only in that they are nonchromaffin. The most prominent paraganglionic tissue is located in carotid, aortic, and ciliary bodies and the glomus jugulotympanicum. Tumors arising from these paraganglia had previously been called chemodectomas or glomus tumors. Histologically, they are similar to pheochromocytomas but are usually nonfunctioning and unilateral. Bilateral and hormonally functioning tumors are seen in association with familial syndromes and other endocrine and nonendocrine tumors.[77-80] Tumors of the carotid bodies are bilateral in about 3% and malignant in 6.4% of patients.[78]

On arteriography, most paragangliomas are hypervascular (Figs. 18–28 and 18–29). There is neovascularity and an intense tumor blush. Carotid body tumors often cause a

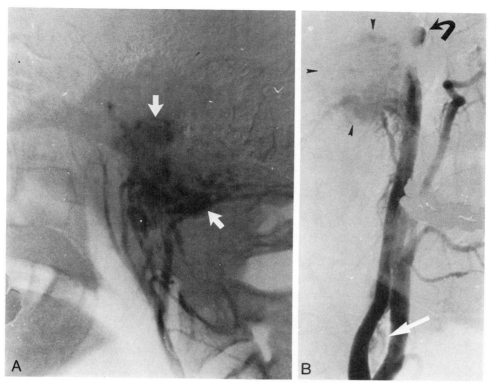

**Figure 18–29.** Hormonally functional cervical paragangliomas in a patient with the triad of gastric leiomyoma, pulmonary chondroma, and extraadrenal paragangliomas. *A,* Subtraction film from an external carotid arteriogram shows a hypervascular tumor arising from the glomus jugulotympanicum. (*arrows*). *B,* Subtraction film from the opposite common carotid arteriogram shows another vascular tumor arising from the glomus jugulotympanicum (*arrowheads*). Curved arrow points to the internal carotid artery. Another small tumor is seen arising from the carotid body (*arrow*).

widening of the angle of the common carotid bifurcation. Since the paragangliomas that do not occur sporadically are often multiple and may occur anywhere in the paraganglionic tissue (glomus jugulotympanicum to the base of the urinary bladder), an arteriographic search must include selective carotid arteriography, arch and abdominal aortography, and pelvic arteriography. Functioning tumors not detected by arteriography may be localized by venous sampling for catecholamines.

**Stressed Adrenal Glands.** In patients in acute stress (gastrointestinal bleeding, shock, severe trauma, complicated postoperative course), the adrenal gland is intensely hypervascular on arteriography[81] and may occasionally simulate contrast extravasation (see Chapter 14, Fig. 14–42). Frank contrast extravasation can also occur. This must be differentiated from overinjection into an adrenal artery that is inadvertently catheterized. In addition, rupture of fragile retroperitoneal and periadrenal branches and

contrast extravasation can occur during carefully performed arteriography in patients with Cushing's syndrome and hyperaldosteronism.

## REFERENCES

1. Flament JB, Delattre JF, Pluot M: Arterial blood supply to the parathyroid glands: Implications for thyroid surgery. Anat Clin 3:279–287, 1982.
2. Jander HP, Diethelm AG, Russinovich NAE: The parathyroid artery. AJR 135:821–828, 1980.
3. Doppman JL: Parathyroid localization. Arteriography and venous sampling. Radiol Clin North Am 14:163–188, 1976.
4. Shimkin PM, Doppman JL, Pearson KD, et al: Anatomic considerations in parathyroid venous sampling. AJR 118:654–662, 1973.
5. Warwick R, Williams PL: Gray's Anatomy, 35th Brit. Ed. Philadelphia, WB Saunders Company, 1973, pp. 1377–1382.
6. Lindvall N, Slezak P: Arteriography of the adrenals. Radiology 92:999–1005, 1969.
7. Merklin RJ, Michels NA: The variant renal and suprarenal blood supply with data on the inferior phrenic, ureteral and gonadal arteries. A statistical

analysis based on 185 dissections and review of the literature. J Int Coll Surg 29:41–76, 1958.

8. El-Sherief MA: Adrenal vein catheterization. Anatomic considerations. Acta Radiol Diagn 23:345–360, 1982.

9. Doppman JL: The localization and treatment of parathyroid adenomas by angiographic techniques. Ann Radiol 23:253–258, 1980.

10. Doppman JL, Hammond WG: The anatomic basis of parathyroid venous sampling. Radiology 95:603–610, 1970.

11. Powell D, Shimkin PM, Doppman JL, et al: Primary hyperparathyroidism. Preoperative tumor localization and differentiation between adenoma and hyperplasia. N Engl J Med 286:1169–1175, 1972.

12. Eisenberg H, Palotta J, Sherwood LM: Selective arteriography, venography and venous hormone assay in diagnosis and localization of parathyroid lesions. Am J Med 56:810–820, 1974.

13. Krudy AG, Doppman JL, Brennan MF: The significance of the thyroidea ima artery in arteriographic localization of parathyroid adenomas. Radiology 136:51–55, 1980.

14. Shimkin PM, Doppman JL, Powell D, et al: Demonstration of parathyroid adenomas by retrograde thyroid venography. Radiology 103:63–67, 1972.

15. Cope O, Nardi GL, Castleman B: Carcinoma of the parathyroid glands: 4 cases among 148 patients with hyperparathyroidism. Ann Surg 138:661–671, 1953.

16. Satava RM, Beahrs OH, Scholz DA: Success rate of cervical exploration for hyperparathyroidism. Arch Surg 110:625–628, 1975.

17. Wang C-A: Parathyroid re-exploration. A clinical and pathological study of 112 cases. Ann Surg 186:140–145, 1977.

18. Russel CF, Grant CS, van Heerden JA: Hyperfunctioning supernumerary parathyroid glands. An occasional cause of hyperparathyroidism. Mayo Clin Proc 57:121–124, 1982.

19. Doppman JL, Mallette LE, Marx SJ, et al: The localization of abnormal mediastinal parathyroid glands. Radiology, 115:31–36, 1975.

20. Krudy AG, Doppman JL, Brennan MF, et al: The detection of mediastinal parathyroid glands by computed tomography, selective arteriography and venous sampling. Radiology 140:739–744, 1981.

21. Gold RP: An anatomic consideration in angiography of the neck: replacement of part of the costocervical trunk to the inferior thyroid artery. Cardiovasc Intervent Radiol 4:105–107, 1981.

22. Efsen F, Bruun E, Lockwood K, et al: Arteriographic exposition of the parathyroids. Br J Surg 62:96–99, 1975.

23. Spiegel AM, Marx SJ, Doppman JL, et al: Intrathyroidal parathyroid adenoma or hyperplasia. An occasionally overlooked cause of surgical failure in primary hyperparathyroidism. JAMA 234:1029–1033, 1975.

24. Kadir S, Robertson D, Coulam CM: Pitfalls in the diagnosis of extraadrenal pheochromocytoma. Cardiovasc Intervent Radiol 4:99–104, 1981.

25. Ludin H: Angiographische Nebennierendarstellung. Fortschr Roentgenstr 99:654–666, 1963.

26. Lecky JW, Wolfman NT, Modic CW: Current concepts of adrenal angiography. Radiol Clin North Am 14:309–352, 1976.

27. Lipsett MB, Hertz R, Ross GT: Clinical and pathophysiological aspects of adrenocortical carcinoma. Am J Med 35:374–383, 1963.

28. Heger N, Taubert M, Ruile K, et al: Nebennierenrinden-karzinome. Med Welt 25:1531–1536, 1968.

29. Case Records of the Massachusetts General Hospital: Case 40-1976. N Engl J Med 295:774–782, 1976.

30. Richter HJ: Zur pathologischen Anatomie der Nebennierentumoren. Radiologe 20:149–157, 1980.

31. Falke THH, Te Strake L, van Seters AP: CT of the adrenal glands: Adenoma or hyperplasia? Scientific exhibit. Radiological Society of North America, 1984.

32. Gilbert MG, Cleveland WW: Cushing's syndrome in infancy. Pediatrics 46:217–229, 1970.

33. Dunnick NR, Korobkin M: Computed tomography of the adrenal gland in hypertension. Urol Radiol 3:245–248, 1982.

34. Streeten DHP, Tomycz N, Anderson GH Jr: Reliability of screening methods for the diagnosis of primary aldosteronism. Am J Med 67:403–413, 1979.

35. Brown JJ, Davies DL, Fraser R, et al: Plasma electrolytes, renin, and aldosterone in the diagnosis of primary hyperaldosteronism with a note on plasma corticosterone concentration. Lancet 2:55–59, 1968.

36. Horton R, Finck E: Diagnosis and localization in primary aldosteronism. Ann Intern Med 76:885–890, 1972.

37. Vetter H, Brecht G, Fischer M, et al: Lateralization procedures in primary aldosteronism. Klin Wochenschr 58:1135–1141, 1980.

38. Foye LV Jr, Feichtmeir TV: Adrenal cortical carcinoma producing a solely mineralocorticoid effect. Am J Med 19:966–975, 1955.

39. Weinberger MH, Grimm CE, Hollifield JW, et al: Primary aldosteronism. Diagnosis, localization, and treatment. Ann Intern Med 90:386–395, 1979.

40. Colapinto RF, Steed BL: Arteriography of adrenal tumors. Radiology 100:343–350, 1971.

41. Besser GM, Witt M: Hirsutes. Br J Med 2:264–266, 1971.

42. Jones KL: Feminization, virilization, and precocious sexual development that results from neoplastic processes. Ann NY Acad Sci 230:195–203, 1974.

43. Gyepes MT, Lindstrom R, Merten D, et al: Hormonally active adenomas and carcinomas in children. Ann Radiol 20:123–131, 1976.

44. Kirschner MA, Jacobs JB: Combined ovarian and adrenal vein catheterization to determine the site(s) of androgen overproduction in hirsute women. J Clin Endocrinol 33:199–209, 1971.

45. Hoevels J, Eklund L: Angiographic findings in adrenal masses. Acta Radiol Diagn 20:337–352, 1979.

46. Costello P, Clouse ME, Kane RA, et al: Problems in the diagnosis of adrenal tumors. Radiology 125:335–341, 1977.

47. Kahn PC, Kelleher MD, Egdahl RH, et al: Adrenal arteriography and venography in primary aldosteronism. Radiology 101:71–78, 1971.

48. Kadir S, Robinette C: Accuracy of angiography in the localization of pheochromocytoma. J Urol 126:789–793, 1981.

49. Kuribayashi S, Harrington DP, Petersen LM: Massive nonfunctioning adrenal cortical adenoma: complementary roles of computed tomography and angiography in the diagnosis. Cardiovasc Intervent Radiol 5:271–274, 1982.

50. Kadir S: Fetus in fetu. Angiographic CBT and ultrasound findings. Fortschr Roentgenstr 134:449–452, 1981.

51. St John Sutton MG, Sheps SG, Lie JT: Prevalence of clinically unsuspected pheochromocytoma. Review of 50 year autopsy series. Mayo Clin Proc 56:354–360, 1981.

52. Jacobs LM, Williams LF, Hinrichs HR: Hemorrhage into a pheochromocytoma. JAMA 239:1156, 1978.

53. Sheps SG, Tyce GM, Flock EV, et al: Current expe-

rience in the diagnosis of pheochromocytoma. Circulation 34:473–483, 1966.

54. Naidich TP, Sprayregen S, Goldman AG, et al: Renal artery alterations associated with pheochromocytoma. Angiology 23:488–499, 1972.

55. Sutton D: The radiological diagnosis of adrenal tumors. Br J Radiol 48:237–258, 1975.

56. James RE, Baker HL Jr, Scanlon PW: The roentgenologic aspects of metastatic pheochromocytoma. AJR 115:783–793, 1972.

57. Stackpole RH, Melicow MM, Uson AC: Pheochromocytoma in children. Report of 9 cases and review of the first 100 published cases with follow-up studies. J Pediatr 63:315–330, 1963.

58. Carney JA, Sizemore GW, Tyce GM: Bilateral adrenal medullary hyperplasia in multiple endocrine neoplasia, Type 2. The precursor of bilateral pheochromocytoma. Mayo Clin Proc 50:3–10, 1975.

59. Meaney TF, Buonocore E: Selective arteriography as a localizing and provocative test in the diagnosis of pheochromocytoma. Radiology 87:309–314, 1966.

60. Reuter SR, Talner LB, Atkin T: The importance of subtraction in the angiographic evaluation of extraadrenal pheochromocytomas. AJR 117:128–131, 1973.

61. Velasquez, G, Nath PH, Zollikofer C, et al: The "ring sign" of necrotic pheochromocytoma. Radiology 131:69–71, 1979.

62. Baltaxe HA, Levin DC, Imperato JL: The angiographic demonstration of partially infarcted pheochromocytomas of the adrenal gland. AJR 119:793–795, 1973.

63. Bauman A: Unilateral adrenal catecholamine excess. Pheochromocytoma or possible sporadic medullary hyperplasia. Arch Intern Med 142:377–378, 1982.

64. Liedmerer KM, Kissane JM: Persistent hypertension after resection of a pheochromocytoma. Am J Med 73:97–104, 1982.

65. Kincaid OW, Hodgson JR, Dockerty MB: Neuroblastoma: A roentgenologic and pathologic study. AJR 78:420–436, 1957.

66. Allen JE, Morse TS, Frye TR, et al: Venacavagrams in infants and children. Ann Surg 160:568–574, 1964.

67. Aterman K, Schueller EF: Maturation of neuroblastoma to ganglioneuroma. Am J Dis Child 120:217–222, 1970.

68. Bunn ND Jr, King AB: Cervical ganglioneuroma: a case report and review of the literature. Guthrie Clin Bull 30:5–14, 1961.

69. Hamilton JP, Koop CE: Ganglioneuromas in children. Surg Gynecol Obstet 121:803–812, 1965.

70. Dunnick NR, Castellino RA: Arteriographic manifestations of ganglioneuromas. Radiology 115:323–328, 1975.

71. Commons RR, Callaway CP: Adenomas of the adrenal cortex. Arch Intern Med 81:37–41, 1948.

72. Ambos MA, Bosniak MA, Lefleur RS, et al: Adrenal adenoma associated with renal cell carcinoma. AJR 136:81–84, 1981.

73. Parker TG, Sommers SC: Adrenal cortical hyperplasia accompanying cancer. Arch Surg 72:495–499, 1956.

74. Abrams HL, Spiro R, Goldstein N: Metastases in carcinoma. Analysis of 1000 autopsied cases. Cancer 3:74–85, 1950.

75. Burke EM: Tumors of the adrenals. Am J Cancer 20:338–351, 1934.

76. Behan M, Martin EC, Muecke EC, et al: Myelolipoma of the adrenal: Two cases with ultrasound and CT findings. AJR 129:993–996, 1977.

77. Chedid A, Jao W: Hereditary tumors of the carotid bodies and chronic obstructive pulmonary disease. Cancer 33:1635–1641, 1974.

78. Staats EF, Brown RL, Smith RR: Carotid body tumors, benign and malignant. Laryngoscope 76:907–916, 1966.

79. Carney JA, Sheps SG, Go VLW, et al: The triad of gastric leiomyosarcoma, functioning extraadrenal paraganglioma and pulmonary chondroma. N Engl J Med 296:1517–1518, 1977.

80. Karasov RS, Sheps SG, Carney JA, et al: Paragangliomatosis with numerous catecholamine-producing tumors. Mayo Clin Proc 57:590–595, 1982.

81. Lunderquist A, Voegeli E: Angiographic findings in the adrenals during stress. AJR 119:560–563, 1973.

# VENOUS SYSTEM

## FIVE

## Venography

### ANATOMY

#### Upper Extremities and Superior Vena Cava (Fig. 19–1)

The main venous drainage pathway in the upper extremities is the superficial venous system. In contrast to those of the lower extremities, the deep veins of the upper extremities are small. They are paired, intercommunicate with each other, and accompany the arteries.

The main superficial arm veins are the:

1. Cephalic vein: This begins in the distal forearm, over the radial aspect, from the dorsal venous network of the hand. It continues over the anterior-lateral aspect of the forearm and upper arm and joins the axillary vein just below the clavicle. It receives tributaries from the deep veins of the forearm and communicates with the basilic vein via the medial cubital vein.

2. Basilic vein: This begins over the ulnar aspect of the distal forearm. Immediately below the elbow, it courses over to the anterior surface, ascends along the medial border of the upper arm, and continues as the axillary vein. Its tributaries include the brachial veins.

3. Median vein of the forearm: This vein is located over the anterior aspect of the forearm and drains the palmar venous plexus. It joins the basilic or medial cubital vein.

The axillary vein continues as the subclavian vein past the lateral border of the first rib. At the medial border of the anterior scalene muscle, it is joined by the internal

jugular vein to form the brachiocephalic vein. The external jugular vein also joins the subclavian vein. The lymphatic ducts empty into the venous system at the junction of the internal jugular and subclavian veins. Valves are present in the arm, axillary, and subclavian veins. The brachiocephalic veins have no valves. The main tributaries of the brachiocephalic veins are the vertebral, internal mammary, superior intercostal, first posterior intercostal, and inferior thyroid veins.

Both brachiocephalic veins unite at the level of the first costosternal junction to form the superior vena cava (SVC). The SVC is approximately 2 cm wide and 7 cm long and does not have any valves. The azygos vein drains into the SVC proximal to its entry into the right atrium.

#### Azygos/Hemiazygos System (Fig. 19–2)

The azygos vein originates in the abdomen at the level of the right renal vein (lumbar azygos vein), or it may be a continuation of the ascending lumbar vein. It ascends anterior to the vertebral bodies, to the right of the midline. At T4, it courses anteriorly to join the SVC. The azygos vein carries blood from the posterior intercostal, right superior intercostal, mediastinal, esophageal, pericardial, and bronchial veins. Valves are present in the azygos vein, and occasionally a prominent valve is located at its junction with the SVC.

The hemiazygos vein also begins at the level of the renal vein and ascends anterior to the vertebral bodies, to the left of the

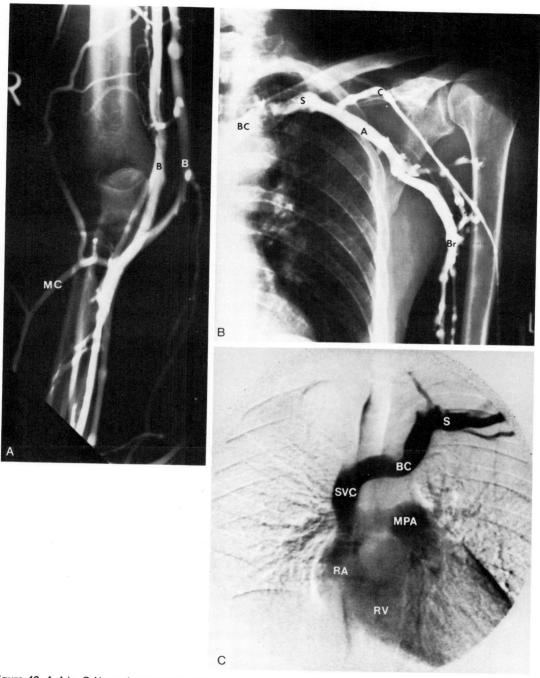

***Figure 19–1.*** *A* to *C*, Normal upper extremity venograms. The basilic vein is duplicated. A = axillary, B = basilic, BC = brachiocephalic, Br = brachial, C = cephalic, MC = median cubital, MPA = main pulmonary artery, RA = right atrium, RV = right ventricle, S = subclavian vein, SVC = superior vena cava.

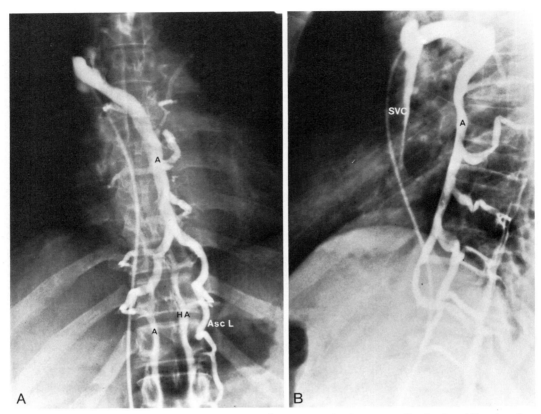

**Figure 19–2.** Normal AP and lateral azygos venogram. A = azygos, Asc L = ascending lumbar, HA = hemiazygos veins; SVC = superior vena cava.

midline, lying parallel to the azygos vein. At T8, it crosses over to the right to join the latter vein. Occasionally, both veins converge to a midline position. It carries blood from the lower left posterior intercostal, subcostal, and ascending lumbar veins and communicates with the left renal vein.

The accessory hemiazygos vein lies anterior to the upper thoracic vertebrae, to the left of the midline. It drains the upper (fourth to eighth) posterior intercostal veins and in some cases the bronchial vein. It may communicate with the hemiazygos vein inferiorly and the superior intercostal vein superiorly.

### Lower Extremities, Pelvis, and Inferior Vena Cava (Figs. 19–3 to 19–5)

The lower extremities are also drained by a deep and a superficial venous system. Unlike drainage in the upper extremities, the majority of the venous return is via the deep system. Communications between the deep and the superficial veins are present in the form of perforating veins, which are located at the ankle, lower leg, and distal thigh. Under normal circumstances, valves in these perforating veins permit unidirectional blood flow from the superficial to the deep system.

### Superficial Venous System

1. Greater saphenous vein: This is the longest vein in the body. It originates from the medial marginal vein of the foot and continues along the anterior-medial aspect of the tibia and along the medial aspect of the thigh, terminating in the common femoral vein below the inguinal ligament. It is often duplicated below the knee and communicates with the deep veins at several levels.

2. Lesser saphenous vein: This vessel originates from the lateral marginal vein of the foot, behind the lateral malleolus, and ascends over the posterior aspect of the calf, passing between the two heads of the gastrocnemius muscle. Above the knee joint, it joins the popliteal, greater saphenous, or deep calf veins.

3. Accessory saphenous vein: This is an inconstant vessel that is located over the posterior-medial aspect of the thigh. Distally,

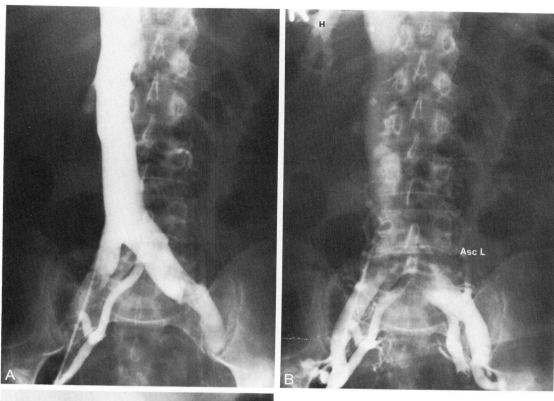

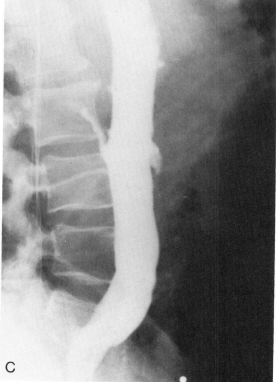

*Figure 19–3.* Normal inferior vena cavagram. *A,* Early phase. *B,* Later film shows reflux of contrast medium into pelvic and hepatic (H) veins. *C,* Lateral film shows the normal relationship of the inferior vena cava to the spine. Asc L = ascending lumbar vein.

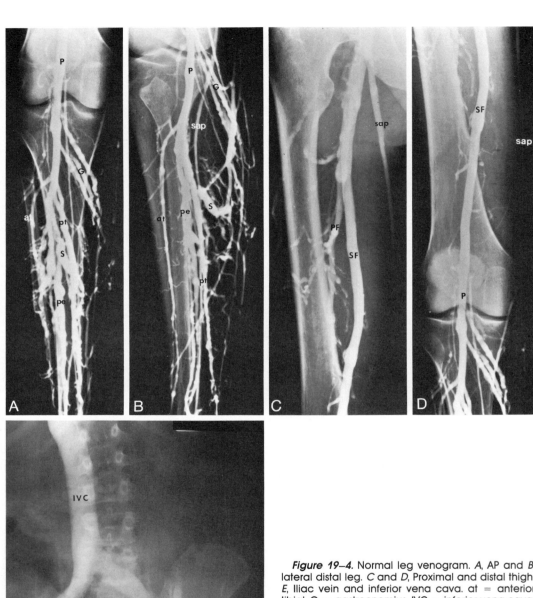

**Figure 19–4.** Normal leg venogram. *A*, AP and *B*, lateral distal leg. *C* and *D*, Proximal and distal thigh. *E*, Iliac vein and inferior vena cava. at = anterior tibial, G = gastrocnemius, IVC = inferior vena cava, P = popliteal, pe = peroneal, PF = profunda femoris, pt = posterior tibial, S = soleal, sap = saphenous, SF = superficial femoral veins.

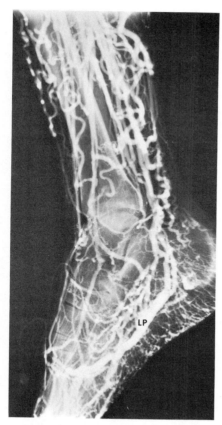

*Figure 19–5.* Venous anatomy of the foot. Numerous incompetent perforating veins are present in the lower leg, along with opacification of varicosities. LP = lateral plantar vein.

it communicates with the lesser saphenous vein and usually terminates in the greater saphenous vein.

**Deep Venous System.** The deep veins in the lower leg are paired and accompany the arteries. The medial and lateral plantar veins unite to form the deep plantar arch and continue behind the medial malleolus as the posterior tibial veins. The popliteal vein is formed by the junction of the tibial and peroneal veins at the lower border of the popliteus muscle, below the knee joint space. The veins from the soleus muscle, which are often bulbous, join the posterior tibial or peroneal veins. The veins from the gastrocnemius muscle drain into the popliteal vein. In the mid-thigh, the latter continues as the superficial femoral vein after passing through the adductor canal. The superficial femoral and popliteal veins are duplicated or bifid in approximately 25% of individuals.

The deep femoral vein enters the superficial femoral vein posteriorly, 4 to 10 cm below the inguinal ligament, to form the common femoral vein. The latter is joined by the saphenous vein, which enters it anteriorly. Above the inguinal ligament, the common femoral vein continues as the external iliac vein. The latter is joined by the internal iliac vein at the level of the sacroiliac joint and forms the common iliac vein. Tributaries of the internal iliac vein correspond to the branches of the internal iliac artery. The iliolumbar vein joins the common iliac veins directly and is often entered during femoral vein catheterization.

The common iliac veins unite at L5 to form the inferior vena cava (IVC). The IVC lies to the right of the abdominal aorta and anterior to the lumbar vertebrae. The main tributaries are the renal, lumbar, right gonadal, right adrenal, inferior phrenic, and hepatic veins. A rudimentary valve is present proximal to the junction of the IVC with the right atrium.

### Variant Anatomy

**Anomalies of the SVC** (see Fig. 19–7). Persistence of the left anterior cardinal vein gives rise to the left SVC. Rarely, this is present as an isolated asymptomatic anomaly (eg, in association with situs inversus) but is more commonly associated with cardiac anomalies.[1, 2] In one series, a left SVC was observed in 3% of patients with congenital heart disease.[2] The left SVC usually drains into the right atrium via the coronary sinus and occasionally into the left atrium. Duplication of the SVC is almost always associated with congenital heart disease and occasionally is associated with anomalous pulmonary venous return.[1, 3]

**Anomalies of the IVC** (Figs. 19–6 and 19–7). In one autopsy study, duplication of the IVC was found in 2.2% of individuals.[4] The left renal and adrenal veins drain into the left IVC, which then crosses over to the right to unite with the right IVC at L1–L2. This anomaly is of clinical significance in patients with recurrent thrombolic disease. A left IVC occurs in 0.2% of individuals.[4] It also crosses over to the right side at the level of the renal veins.

Absence of the IVC (interruption of the hepatic segment) is observed in 0.6% of patients with congenital heart disease and is more common in those with cyanotic heart

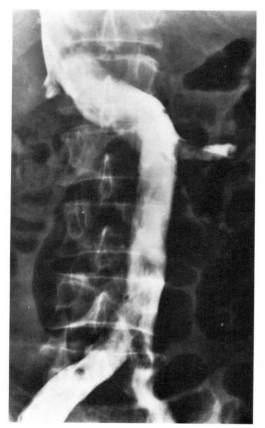

*Figure 19–6.* Left-sided inferior vena cava.

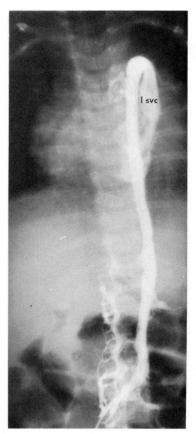

*Figure 19–7.* Absence of the inferior vena cava with hemiazygos continuation and drainage into a left superior vena cava (l svc) in a patient with an ostium primum defect.

disease.[5] Venous drainage to the heart occurs via the azygos or hemiazygos system. The latter often drains into a left SVC and is more frequently associated with congenital anomalies.[5, 6] The hepatic veins are normally formed and drain into the right atrium. Although by itself, azygos continuation of the IVC is not symptomatic and may occur in the absence of other congenital anomalies, it is frequently observed in patients with congenital heart disease, especially those with discordant cardiac-visceral situs.[7]

## PHYSIOLOGY OF VENOUS BLOOD FLOW

The capacity of the venous bed is larger than that of the arteries and contains up to two thirds of the circulating blood. The main venous reservoir is located in the lower extremities.

Propagation of venous blood in the lower extremities occurs mainly with the aid of the calf muscle pump.[8] In the deep venous system, muscular contraction facilitates flow of blood towards the heart. Retrograde blood flow into the distal leg and into the superficial venous system is prevented by the presence of valves. In addition, the presence of a tight deep fascia in the calf contributes towards the effectiveness of the muscular pump. Venous contractions also assist in the propagation of blood.

## ANGIOGRAPHY

Both standard film venography and digital subtraction angiography (DSA) can be used for the assessment of the venous system. The latter is particularly applicable to patients with compromised cardiac and renal function and in children. In general, a 20% concentration of contrast medium is used for DSA. The rate and volume of power-injected contrast medium are similar to that used for conventional venography. For hand injections utilizing the digital technique (usually for smaller veins), the volume of contrast injected can be decreased by approximately 25 to 33%.

Figure 19–8 shows the setup used for manual contrast injection. The venipuncture needle is connected to heparinized flushing solution (D5W) over a three-way stopcock and extension tubing. Upon completion of the contrast injection, 50 to 100 ml of heparinized flushing solution (D5W) is rapidly injected (or infused) into the veins in order to "flush out" the contrast medium and thus minimize contact with the venous intima to prevent contrast-induced thrombophlebitis.

Tables 19–1 and 19–2 list the approach, injection rates and volume, and filming (using a rapid film changer) for the different procedures. In patients on therapeutic doses of heparin, contrast venography of the extremities or a venacavogram via the cubital vein approach can be performed safely without discontinuing the heparin.

## Upper Extremities

A 19 gauge butterfly or angiocath is used for venipuncture. If the entire upper extremity is to be evaluated, a distal forearm vein is chosen. For evaluation of the axillary or more central venous structures, the cubital or proximal forearm veins are used.

With the arm in neutral position (palm facing up), a tight tourniquet is placed (or a blood pressure cuff is inflated) several centimeters proximal to the venipuncture. Twenty-five ml of contrast medium (60%) is delivered by rapid hand injection. Immediately thereafter, while continuing to inject another 5 ml of contrast medium with one hand, the tourniquet is released with the other hand and filming is begun.

In cooperative patients and especially those in cardiac or renal failure and in children, DSA provides an excellent alternative method for venography. The injection technique is the same as that just described. The absence of pain, because of the injection of diluted contrast medium, is particularly helpful in children.

## Superior Vena Cava

The SVC can be evaluated by simultaneous bilateral cubital vein injections or catheter angiography. In the former, a 18 gauge or larger angiocath is inserted in the median cubital vein of each arm. If access to the upper extremity veins is not available, the external jugular vein may be used for contrast injection, or the femoral vein is used for catheterization of the SVC.

With the extremities in neutral position, 25 ml of contrast medium is injected simultaneously through each angiocath, using the tourniquet technique described previously.

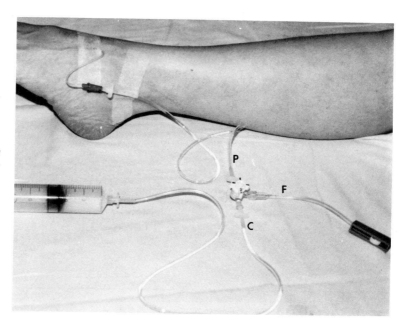

*Figure 19–8.* Set-up for extremity venography. C = to contrast syringe, F = to heparinized flush, P = to patient.

**TABLE 19–1.** Venography of the Upper Extremities, SVC, and Azygos Vein

| Venography | Approach (Venipuncture) | Catheter | Contrast Rate (ml/sec) | Volume (ml) | Conc. (%) | Filming Rate (per sec) | Total No. | DSA* | Comments |
|---|---|---|---|---|---|---|---|---|---|
| Arm | Distal forearm, hand | — | Manual | 30 | 60 | 1 | 8 | Yes | Tourniquet technique |
| Axillary, subclavian | Cubital | — | Manual | 30 | 60 | 1 | 8 | Yes | Tourniquet technique |
| SVC | Bilateral cubital | — | Manual | 50† | 60 | 1 | 8 | Yes | Tourniquet technique |
|  | Cubital/ femoral | Pigtail | 15 | 30 | 76 | 2 1 | 6 2 | Yes | Biplane for mediastinal tumor evaluation |
| Azygos | Cubital | Multipurpose | 5 | 12 | 76 | 1 | 6 | Yes | Biplane for mediastinal tumor evaluation |
|  | Femoral | Cobra, visceral hook | 5 | 12 | 76 | 1 | 6 | Yes | Biplane for mediastinal tumor evaluation |

*With 20% concentration contrast medium.
†25 ml per arm.

Filming is begun as the tourniquets are released.

For the catheter technique via the cubital or femoral vein, a 5 or 6 Fr pigtail catheter is placed at the junction of the brachiocephalic veins. DSA can be used in conjunction with either technique (catheter or cubital/jugular vein injection).

### Azygos Vein

The main indications for azygos venography are the assessment of resectability of mediastinal carcinoma (bronchogenic and esophageal) and venous sampling for hormone-producing tumors.[9, 10] The azygos vein can be catheterized from the femoral or cubital vein approach. From the femoral vein approach, a cobra or visceral hook catheter is used. From the cubital vein approach, a multipurpose catheter is used.

### Inferior Vena Cava

The IVC can be evaluated from the femoral or cubital vein approach. The latter approach

**TABLE 19–2.** Venography of the IVC and Pelvic Veins

| Venography | Approach (Venipuncture) | Catheter | Contrast Rate (ml/sec) | Volume (ml) | Conc. (%) | Filming Rate (per sec) | Total No. | DSA* | Comments |
|---|---|---|---|---|---|---|---|---|---|
| Pelvis | Bilateral femoral | Sheath Multiple hole straight | 20† | 40† | 76 | 2 1 | 8 2 | Yes | During Valsalva |
| External/ common iliac | Femoral ipsilateral | Sheath Multiple hole straight | 10 | 20 | 76 | 2 1 | 8 2 | Yes | |
|  | Femoral contralateral | Multiple hole straight‡ cobra | 10 | 20 | 76 | 2 1 | 8 2 | Yes | |
|  | Cubital | Multipurpose | 10 | 20 | 76 | 2 1 | 8 2 | Yes | |
| Internal iliac | Femoral | Cobra with side holes | 6–8 | 12–15 | 76 | 2 1 | 8 2 | Yes | During Valsalva |
| IVC | Femoral | Pigtail | 20 | 40 | 76 | 4 | 8 | Yes | Mid-respiration |
|  | Cubital | Pigtail | | | | 1 | 4 | | |

*With 20% concentration contrast medium.
†10 per sec for 20 ml total per side injected simultaneously.
‡With aid of tip deflector.

should not be used if thrombosis is suspected. From the femoral vein approach, a 60 cm long 5 or 6 Fr pigtail catheter is placed at the confluence of the common iliac veins. From the arm approach, either a 100 cm long pigtail or an end hole–occluded multipurpose catheter is used. The latter is inserted through a sheath.

For evaluation of thrombotic disease, an AP inferior venacavogram is usually sufficient. If retroperitoneal disease, tumor, or caval compression due to the presence of ascites is being evaluated, a biplane study is necessary.

Images are obtained either by standard cut film angiography or by DSA. For the latter, 20% contrast medium is used, and the injection sites and rates are the same as those for cut film angiography.

## Pelvis

For evaluation of the pelvic veins, both femoral veins are punctured. A short Teflon sheath (from the Amplatz needle) or a short catheter is inserted on each side. Both catheters are connected to the injector over a metal "Y" connector and high pressure tubing. Contrast medium is injected during a Valsalva maneuver to facilitate reflux of contrast into the internal iliac veins.

For unilateral iliac venography, the ipsilateral femoral vein is catheterized, and a short sheath or catheter is inserted. In the absence of thrombus, either the contralateral femoral vein approach (cobra catheter with end and side holes or multiple hole straight or pigtail catheter with the aid of a tip deflector) or the cubital vein approach (100 cm multipurpose catheter) may be used.

The internal iliac veins can be catheterized from the contralateral approach and occasionally from the ipsilateral side (cobra catheter with side holes) or the cubital vein approach (multipurpose catheter).

## Lower Extremities

**Venipuncture.** The most suitable site for venipuncture is over the instep. A 19 gauge butterfly is used, and the needle tip is directed towards the toes. An angiocath can also be used, especially if large veins are present. We prefer the butterfly, since it permits an easier and relatively less painful venipuncture (compared with the sheath cannula). Local skin anesthesia with lidocaine (Xylocaine) is avoided in order not to obscure the vein.

Direction of the needle tip towards the toes facilitates filling of the foot veins, which are widely anastomosing, and thus insures maximal mixing of contrast medium with blood, resulting in optimal opacification of the deep veins of the calf. An atraumatic puncture is important. If the position is not satisfactory, it is advisable to tape the needle in place and use another needle for a subsequent attempt. This prevents extravasation of contrast medium from unsuccessful puncture sites.

Upward direction of the needle often fills the superficial venous system preferentially and is useful for the evaluation of the saphenous veins prior to bypass surgery.

Aids for successful venipuncture:

1. Patients with edema of the extremity: Prior to venography, elevation of the extremity for several hours or wrapping it with an elastic bandage is often helpful. At the time of venography, the edema fluid can be dispersed by local digital compression or by inflating a blood pressure cuff over the instep for a few minutes.

2. Poorly visible veins: Useful procedures are application of warm compresses and dependent position of the extremity (have the patient sit up with legs dangling down). Rarely, a cutdown may be necessary.

**Tourniquets.** Tourniquets (usually two) should be used if venography is performed in the supine or shallow upright ($< 30°$) position. A tight tourniquet is placed above the ankle. This obstructs the superficial veins and facilitates passage of contrast medium into the deep venous system, thereby improving venous filling and diminishing opacification of the superficial veins. However, the tourniquet is often responsible for incomplete or absent filling of the anterior tibial veins.[11] A second tourniquet is placed immediately above the knee. This delays emptying of the superficial veins and thus indirectly enhances deep venous filling. If the semi-upright position ($> 45°$) is used with the needle tip pointing towards the toes, tourniquets are not necessary.

**Contrast Medium.** We routinely use 60% contrast medium for venography. This provides superior opacification of the venous system in comparison with 40 or 45% contrast medium and, with appropriate precautions, contrast-induced complications can be reduced significantly.

The use of 60% contrast medium is usually associated with burning and cramplike foot and calf pain, which is often severe in patients with venous obstruction. The pain can be reduced by adding Xylocaine (2mg/ml contrast medium) or by using low osmolarity agents.[12, 13] A total of 70 to 80 ml of contrast medium is used per extremity, and it is injected within 1½ to 2 minutes.

There are several techniques for contrast injection: hand injection, slow power injection, or drip infusion by gravity. We prefer the controlled rapid manual injection.

**Venous Manometry.** Venous pressure measurements have been used to assess abnormalities of the perforating veins (valve incompetence) and malfunction of the calf muscle pump. The normal venous pressure in the upright individual is about 90 mm Hg. It falls to below 50 mm Hg during calf muscle exercise. In the presence of incompetent perforating veins, such a fall in pressure is not observed.

## Venography Techniques

There are several methods for leg venography. The popularity of each method is subject to the type of equipment available and the individual preference of the vascular radiologist. When performed properly, they all provide satisfactory results.[14–17]

Venography may be performed in the supine or semi-upright position, with 100 or 105 mm spot film, 14 × 17 inch film, or long film changers or with the aid of DSA. The supine or semi-upright technique may be used with or without fluoroscopy, using spot films and/or 14 × 17 inch film. Long film changers are used in conjunction with the supine technique. Fluoroscopy and spot films can be used to evaluate areas not adequately defined on the large film. A single extremity should be evaluated at one time.

The advantage of fluoroscopy is that it permits assessment of the pattern of blood flow and filling of incompetent perforating veins and allows the reevaluation of poorly opacified segments.

During contrast injection, the site of venous puncture must be kept under constant observation. If this area begins to swell or if the patient complains of excessive foot pain or a burning sensation or both, the injection is terminated immediately, as these could be due to contrast extravasation. The venous puncture site must be inspected carefully before proceeding with the study. A frequent pitfall is that blood return is observed upon suction and the operator is misled into believing that the needle position is satisfactory, not realizing that blood return will also

be observed if the needle tip is partially extravascular. This complication is less likely to occur with the use of the angiocath.[18] Contrast medium may also extravasate from the site of a previous failed venipuncture. Thus, if there is any doubt with respect to needle position, a radiograph is obtained or fluoroscopy is used to assess the situation.

The puncture site may not be easy to evaluate visually in severely edematous extremities, and in this case one may have to use an angiocath, or the procedure may have to be performed under fluoroscopic monitoring.

### Ascending Venography

**Semi-Upright Non–Weight Bearing Venography** (Fig. 19–9). After successful venipuncture, the patient is brought into a semi-erect position (45 to 60°). A wooden box (4 to 6 inches high) is placed under the other extremity to permit a non–weight bearing position of the leg being examined. This prevents calf muscle contraction and results in better opacification of the deep veins. A continuous injection of contrast medium is important. Tourniquets may be used to enhance deep venous opacification for the shallow upright position.

If fluoroscopy is used, ascent of the contrast medium is monitored and either large spot or 14 × 17 inch overhead films are obtained. Filming is begun after approximately 35 to 40 ml of contrast medium has been injected (if fluoroscopy is not used) or when the contrast column has reached the

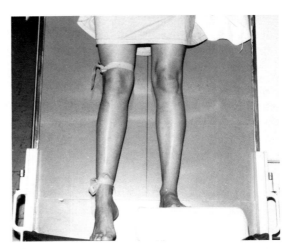

*Figure 19–9.* Patient positioning for non–weight-bearing ascending leg venography. The tourniquets shown in the illustration are not used if the patient can be brought into a semi-upright position (>45°).

proximal popliteal vein. The following films are obtained in sequence:

1. Calf: three films—AP, internal, and external rotation (lateral).

2. Distal thigh and knee: one film—AP.

3. Pelvis/proximal thigh: one film—AP (patient horizontal).

The first four films are obtained in the semi-upright position. As the patient is brought back into the supine position for the last film, manual compression is applied to the femoral vein at the groin, and the patient is asked to perform a Valsalva maneuver. Once the patient is in the supine position, femoral compression is released, the extremity is elevated, normal respiration is resumed, and the last film is exposed. In addition to elevation of the extremity, gentle manual calf compression (not massage, as this could dislodge thrombi) may be applied to facilitate emptying of the deep veins. All of these maneuvers are used to enhance pelvic and distal caval opacification.

**Supine Leg Venography.** This technique is used if a tilt table is not available for venography, the patient cannot tolerate an upright position, or a long leg changer is to be used. A tourniquet is applied above the ankle and another above the knee. After 35 to 40 ml of contrast medium has been injected, the lower tourniquet is released and the three films of the calf (AP, obliques) are obtained. Subsequently, the upper tourniquet is released prior to obtaining films of the upper leg and pelvis. The contrast volume and filming are the same as for the semi-upright technique.

The injection of contrast medium should be continuous to prevent dilution and streaming artefacts. Caval, thigh, and pelvic vein opacification can be enhanced by leg elevation, calf compression, and the Valsalva maneuver. The last is particularly helpful for opacification of the deep femoral and internal iliac vein branches.

### Descending Leg Venography

This is used mainly to evaluate valve competency in patients with varicose veins and for preoperative evaluation prior to valve surgery.[19, 20] After femoral vein puncture, a short catheter or sheath is inserted in the femoral vein, and the patient is brought into the upright or semi-upright position. A slow bolus of 20 to 25 ml of contrast medium (60%) is injected and observed fluoroscopically, and spot or overhead films are obtained. A variant of this technique utilizes the Valsalva maneuver with the patient in the horizontal position.[21]

Retrograde flow of contrast medium into the femoral and saphenous veins depends upon the competence of the femoral vein valves. If these are competent, contrast medium does not reflux beyond the proximal thigh. In the presence of incompetent valves, contrast medium opacifies the distal thigh and calf veins. In the upright position, some contrast medium may get past competent valves, thus limiting the usefulness of the technique.[21]

### Intraosseous Venography

The main indications for intraosseous venography are the evaluation of the deep venous system (1) in patients without access for percutaneous venography (eg, the presence of skin disease or ulcerations) and (2) following inadequate visualization of the deep system by standard venography.

The procedure is very painful and hence requires very heavy premedication or general anesthesia. A sternal puncture trocar is inserted into the bone marrow at the appropriate site and 40 to 50 ml of 60% contrast medium is injected. Films are obtained at 1 per second for a total of 8 to 10 films. Details for this technique are described in references 22 and 23.

Some of the sites for contrast injection and areas evaluated thereby are listed below[22–24] (Fig. 19–10):

Ribs: Azygos and hemiazygos system.

Iliac crest: Gluteal and common iliac veins, IVC.

Pubic bones: Obturator plexus, internal iliac vein.

Greater trochanter: Iliac veins, IVC.

Proximal tibia: Femoral veins.

Calcaneus/malleoli: Deep veins of the calf.

### Varicography

Contrast medium can be injected directly into a varicose vein for the demonstration of incompetent perforating veins.[24a] The varicose veins are most pronounced when the extremity is in a dependent position. Thus, the venous puncture (of a varicose vein) is performed with the patient sitting or standing. A 19 gauge butterfly or an angiocath is used. The study is performed on a tilting table in order to facilitate examination in the semi-upright, horizontal, and Trendelenburg (head-down) positions. The contrast medium

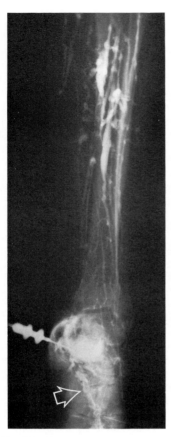

*Figure 19–10.* Intraosseous venogram with injection into the calcaneus. A thrombus is present in the lateral plantar vein (*arrow*).

injection is observed fluoroscopically and spot films are used for documentation. The commonly used ionic contrast agents are thrombogenic, and prolonged contact with the intimal surface due to the slow washout from the varicose veins predisposes to thrombosis. Therefore, diluted contrast medium (45% concentration) or the low osmolality contrast media should be used for varicography.

## The Normal Venogram (see Figs. 19–1 to 19–4)

The normal veins are homogeneously opacified (see later section on Pitfalls and Artefacts). The walls of the normal veins are smooth and parallel, and abrupt caliber changes are absent. At the valves, there is a slight widening of the diameter of the veins. The normal soleal veins have a bulbous appearance.

## The Abnormal Venogram

The shape of a thrombus varies with its age and size. A fresh thrombus appears as a constant defect in the contrast-opacified lumen of a vein. The shape and location are constant on two or more films. In older thrombi that have undergone retraction, the shape may appear different in another projection. Smaller thrombi are often lobulated and eccentric. The different stages in the thrombotic process are as follows:

1. Acute thrombosis: The fresh thrombus has a smooth surface and is outlined by a thin layer of contrast medium. As it becomes older and adherent to the vein wall, the thrombus is no longer outlined completely by contrast medium.

2. Clot retraction: This occurs in about 2 weeks. A thicker column of contrast medium can now get by the thrombus, and the surface is irregular or undulating. Such a thrombus is usually adherent to a section of the vein wall.

3. Recanalization: After several weeks to months, one or more irregular smaller channels may be present, but the valves are no longer seen.

Thrombi that are adherent to the vein wall are less likely to embolize than are non-adherent thrombi or those with a "tail." A thrombus that has broken off and embolized may have a "square cut" appearance.[23]

On venography, the following features may be demonstrated (Figs. 19–11 to 19–15; see also Fig. 19–51):

1. Thrombus cast fills the entire vein: A thin outline of contrast medium surrounds the thrombus. Failure of contrast medium to get past the occlusion may leave the more proximal veins unopacified.

2. Complete occlusion: Contrast medium does not get past the thrombus. This may be due to elevated perivenous pressure, which does not permit contrast opacification of the obstructed veins, or to adherence of the thrombus to the vein wall. The superficial veins are well opacified unless these too are thrombosed.

3. A thrombus "tail" or meniscus proximal to the occluded vein.

4. Enlarged collateral veins bypassing the obstructed segment.

5. The retracted thrombus is eccentric, lobulated, and adherent.

6. Irregular streaky appearance of the recanalized vein: Valves are usually not recognizable. Occasionally, the vein may appear normal after recanalization.[23]

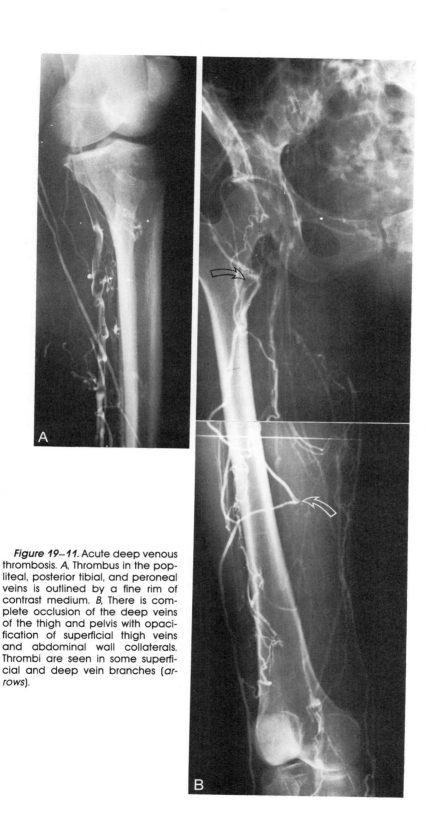

***Figure 19–11.*** Acute deep venous thrombosis. *A,* Thrombus in the popliteal, posterior tibial, and peroneal veins is outlined by a fine rim of contrast medium. *B,* There is complete occlusion of the deep veins of the thigh and pelvis with opacification of superficial thigh veins and abdominal wall collaterals. Thrombi are seen in some superficial and deep vein branches (*arrows*).

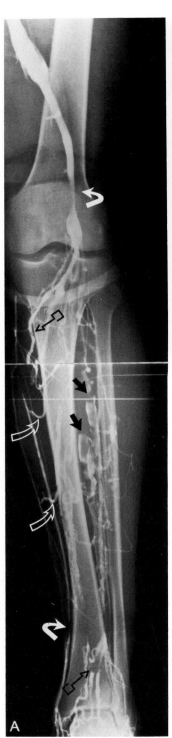

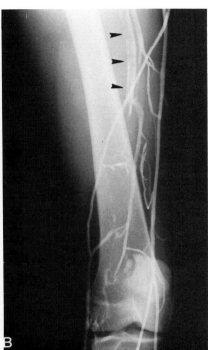

**Figure 19–12.** *A,* Slightly older thrombus than that shown in Fig. 19–11A. There is a thicker rim of contrast medium around the thrombus and it is adherent to the vein wall. Segments of the veins (*black arrows*) remain unopacified. Curved arrows point to compression artefacts caused by the tourniquets. Perforating veins are demonstrated (*open arrows*). Several air bubbles are also seen (*hooked arrows*). *B,* Retracted thrombus in the superficial femoral vein (*arrowheads*).

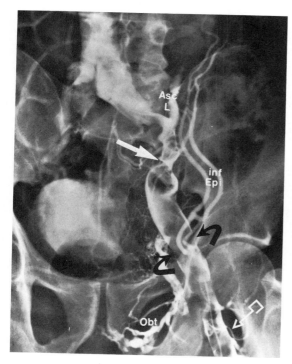

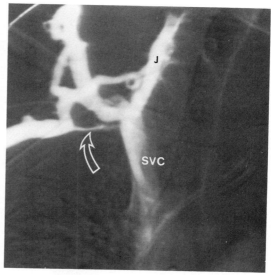

**Figure 19–14.** Subclavian venogram using DSA shows thrombosis (*arrow*) of the subclavian vein following central venous catheter placement and chemotherapy infusion. Enlarged bypassing collaterals to the jugular vein (J) are present. SVC = superior vena cava.

**Figure 19–13.** Common femoral venogram shows encasement of the common iliac vein by prostatic carcinoma (*white arrow*). A partially adherent thrombus (*curved arrows*) is present in the external iliac and common femoral veins. An older retracted thrombus is present in the distal common femoral vein (*hooked arrow*). Enlarged venous collaterals are opacified. Asc L = ascending lumbar, inf Epi = inferior epigastric, Obt = obturator veins.

## Pitfalls and Artefacts (Figs. 19–16 to 19–19; see also Fig. 19–12)

The two most frequent errors that decrease the accuracy of contrast venography of the extremities are attempting to interpret an incomplete or poorly performed examination (Fig. 19–16) and failure to recognize artefacts. Some of the pitfalls in the interpretation of leg venograms are:

1. Absent or poor filling of deep veins (occlusion versus artefact): Poor filling of deep calf veins can be due to technical factors (inappropriate needle position, supine technique without tourniquet, calf muscle contraction due to pain or weight bearing, inadequate volume of contrast medium) or venous thrombosis. For the latter, the veins adjacent to the nonopacifying segments should be evaluated for the presence of thrombi. In normal veins, the walls are smooth and the contrast column often terminates at a valve. In thrombosis, the walls

are often irregular and a "tail" of the thrombus may be outlined by the contrast. If a tourniquet is used, the anterior tibial veins are often not opacified, as these can be easily obstructed by the tourniquet.

2. Preferential filling of the superficial veins: This is most frequently due to a poor technique (upward-directed needle, supine technique without tourniquet), but also occurs in extensive deep venous thrombosis (DVT) (see Fig. 19–11B).

3. Pseudo-thrombus: Segments of a vein may remain unopacified on one or more films, suggesting the presence of a thrombus. This is due to absent or incomplete contrast opacification. A thrombus is usually outlined by contrast medium. Smaller pseudo-thrombi are frequently observed in valve cusps. Enhancement of venous filling with the Valsalva maneuver should be used to clarify the situation.

4. Streaming artefacts: These are caused by inflow of unopacified blood from tributaries or layering of contrast medium and may simulate a thrombus. Poor mixing of contrast medium with blood gives rise to streaking, which may simulate a recanalized vein.[23] Such artefacts are often due to inadequate contrast volume or an intermittent injection technique (injection interrupted when the tourniquet is unfastened or the extremity is turned for oblique films). This is avoided by

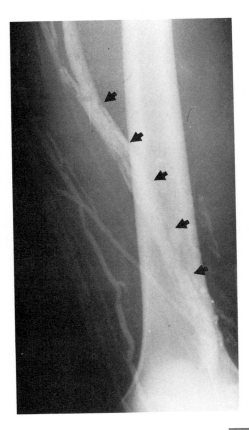

**Figure 19–15.** Typical appearance of a recanalized vein (*arrows*). Multiple neochannels are present and the valves have been destroyed.

**Figure 19–16.** Pitfall of interpreting an incomplete and improperly performed study. *A,* There is incomplete filling of the deep femoral vein. The superficial femoral vein is not opacified and no thrombi are seen. *B,* Repeat venogram shows an abrupt occlusion of the superficial femoral vein by a thrombus, which is faintly outlined by contrast medium.

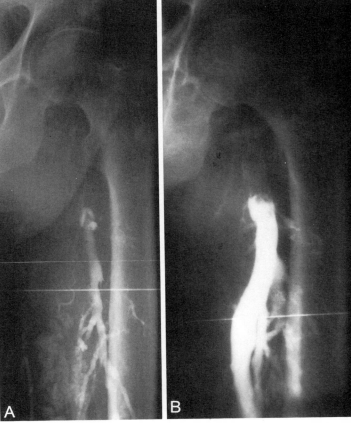

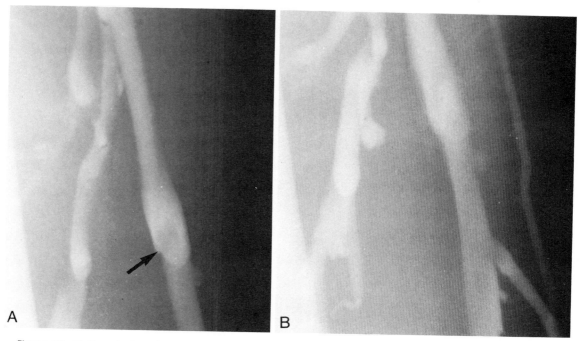

*Figure 19–17.* Pseudo-thrombus due to unopacified blood. *A*, A well-defined defect is seen in a valve cusp (*arrow*). *B*, Spot film obtained at the time of reevaluation shows better filling of the tributaries, and the defect is no longer present. *Note*: The valve cusps are a frequent location for initial thrombus formation. Therefore, differentiation between artefact and thrombus is important.

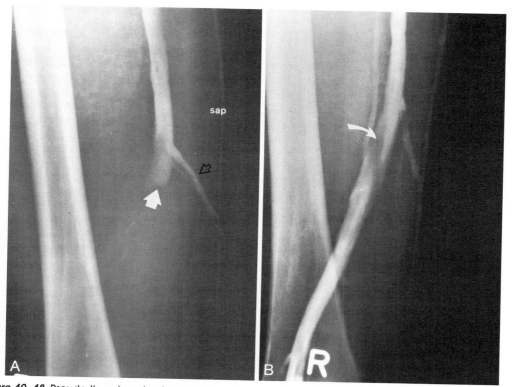

*Figure 19–18.* Pseudo-thrombus due to nonmixing of unopacified blood. *A*, There is an abrupt termination of the contrast column in the superficial femoral vein (*arrow*). The contrast medium appears less dense below the junction of the perforating vein (*open arrow*). *B*, Later film shows a flow defect (*curved arrow*) with opacification of the popliteal vein. sap = saphenous vein.

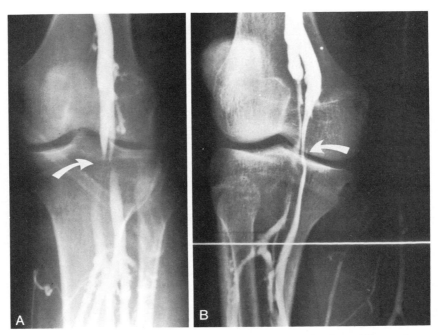

*Figure 19–19.* Compression artefacts in the popliteal vein. *A,* Due to contraction of the gastrocnemius muscle (*arrow*). *B,* Due to a ruptured Baker's cyst (*arrow*). *Note:* The popiteal vein is duplicated in both these patients.

operating the syringe with one hand while the other is used to unfasten the tourniquet or turn the extremity. In addition, for the pelvic veins and IVC, the Valsalva maneuver can be used.

5. Compression artefacts: These are caused by tight tourniquets (anterior tibial veins) or hyperextension and affect the femoral, popliteal, and muscular veins. Frequent compression artefacts are seen in the proximal left common iliac vein at the point where it crosses the aorta, and popliteal vein compression is seen between the heads of the gastrocnemius muscle (see Fig. 19–19). Baker's cysts (ruptured or nonruptured) may also compress the popliteal vein.

6. Inadvertent injection of air: These artefacts may simulate thrombi. However, in most instances, they are easily recognized, as they are round in configuration and do not have a constant location (see Fig. 19–12).

7. In the calf, projection of the deep veins over bone or partial overlapping with another vein can often simulate a thrombus.

## Local Complications of Extremity Venography

**Needle Dislodgment.** This is most frequently due to faulty fixation of the needle or venipuncture close to the ankle or toes. In the latter situation, the needle is dislodged by inadvertent or pain-induced motion of the foot or toes.

**Pain.** By itself, pain is not a complication. It is associated with the use of ionic hyperosmolar contrast agents or is due to the toxicity of the sodium salt.[25] It is most intense in patients with DVT. Pain during contrast injection may also indicate extravasation. Delayed pain often indicates post-venography thrombophlebitis.

Pain can be decreased by diluting the contrast medium to 45%, by adding Xylocaine (2 to 4 mg/ml of contrast medium),[13, 26] or using sodium-free contrast medium.[23] In children and other sensitive individuals, 20% contrast medium can be used in conjunction with DSA. With the use of nonionic and low osmolarity contrast agents, this side effect is observed less frequently.[12, 27]

**Thrombophlebitis and Embolism.** Delayed pain may be indicative of thrombophlebitis. Although this complication has not been observed in some series, other studies report an incidence of up to 29%.[12, 26–28] In our experience, thrombophlebitis occurs very infrequently (< 1 to 2%) and has rarely been of clinical significance. The volume of contrast medium used in some of the studies reporting this complication was significantly higher (125 ml) than is our practice.[14, 26] In addition, contact time of contrast medium with the vein may have been longer because of the upright technique.

Post-venography thrombophlebitis can be avoided or its incidence can be reduced significantly by using nonionic or low osmolarity agents,[12, 27] early ambulation,[23] leg elevation, and vigorous flushing with heparinized solution. In addition, supine venography may be associated with fewer such complications.[29]

Symptoms of post-venography DVT (pain, swelling, tenderness, temperature elevation) are absent in as many as 20% of patients, and 50% may not have pain.[27] Symptoms may occur as early as 2 hours after venography, with a peak incidence at about 24 hours. Most of the studies reporting post-venography thrombophlebitis were done with [125]I-fibrinogen. The limitations of such studies are discussed in the section on Nonangiographic Methods for Evaluation.

Pulmonary embolization is a rare complication of leg venography. It is more likely to occur during femoral vein catheterization, in which a thrombus is dislodged during guide wire or catheter insertion. Fat embolization may occur after intraosseous venography.

**Contrast Extravasation.** Extravasation can occur from the site of venipuncture or from the site of an attempted venipuncture. In one series, contrast extravasation was observed in 78% of patients in whom a metal cannula was used for venipuncture versus only 4.5% in whom a plastic cannula was utilized.[18] In our experience and that of others, clinically significant contrast extravasation occurs very infrequently.[23]

A small extravasation (< 10 ml) in the foot or hand is usually insignificant clinically in patients without DVT or compromised arterial circulation. In patients with compromised circulation, a small extravasation may lead to severe cellulitis, ulceration, skin necrosis, and rarely gangrene. Contrast extravasation at the groin is rare with the current techniques.

Histologically, contrast extravasation is characterized by edema and a severe inflammatory response, which is maximal at 24 hours.[30] The reaction begins to subside after 72 hours, leading to scarring. Contrast extravasation can be avoided by:

1. Careful monitoring of the venipuncture site during contrast injection.

2. Avoiding multiple venipunctures or excessive needle manipulation to achieve intravascular position. It is best to leave the needle in place if the venipuncture has failed.

If contrast extravasation should occur, the following are usually effective:

1. Immediate local massage in order to dissipate the contrast medium.

2. Leg elevation.

3. Application of warm compresses over the site of extravasation to promote vasodilation in an attempt to improve peripheral perfusion.

In addition, the following measures have been recommended by some authors:

1. Injection of physiological saline:[23] However, histological studies show that this in itself elicits an inflammatory response, and, on the other hand, dilution of the contrast medium does not alter the histological tissue response.[30]

2. Injection of hyaluronidase:[18] However, histological studies indicate that tissue response is adversely modified by use of this agent.[30]

## NONANGIOGRAPHIC METHODS FOR EVALUATION

Several noninvasive or less invasive (than angiography) procedures have been utilized to establish the diagnosis of venous disease, primarily venous thrombosis of the extremities.[31–34] Although some of these can be used as a substitute for contrast studies in certain cases, most are useful primarily as screening procedures.[28] When used in combination, they do provide a high degree of accuracy. The results from such studies are likely to be more accurate than results from poorly performed contrast venography.

**Radionuclide Venography.** This can be used in conjunction with lung scanning and permits evaluation of patency of the major veins of the leg and pelvis and of the IVC. It can also be used to evaluate patency of the upper extremity veins and the SVC. To perform this study, [99m]technetium-labeled microspheres are injected into a foot or peripheral arm vein to obtain a venogram.

Although the accuracy for detecting thrombi in the main venous channels is between 80 and 90%, there are several limitations to the study, ie, inability to detect thrombi in smaller branches and inability to detect nonocclusive thrombi in major veins. Another potential source of error is the presence of a bifid or duplicated superficial femoral vein with occlusion of one limb. Radionuclide venography in combination with radionuclide plethysmography using tagged erythrocytes may improve the sensitivity of this technique.[35]

**Fibrinogen Scanning.** [125]I-fibrinogen may also be used for the detection of venous thrombosis. The overall accuracy is reported to be about 90% for thrombi in the calf veins.[36] Accuracy is much lower for thrombi in the thigh and pelvic veins. Major limitations are false-positive scans due to cellulitis or other inflammatory processes, recent surgery, or trauma close to the site of suspected venous thrombosis.[37] In 10 to 20% of patients with positive scans, thrombi are not demonstrated on venography.[36] Furthermore, fibrinogen is not incorporated into a mature thrombus, and the scans cannot be used to determine extent of disease.

**Impedance Plethysmography.** This study measures the changes in the electrical resistance (impedance) caused by changes in blood volume of the leg. An accuracy rate of 97% has been reported for the detection of venous thrombi in the popliteal and proximal veins.[38] In the same study, the accuracy rate for the calf veins, where most thrombi originate, was only 22%. In another study, the impedance plethysmogram was normal in 83% of symptomatic and in over 90% of asymptomatic calf vein thrombi.[39]

Other limitations of this study are its inability to distinguish old from fresh thrombotic occlusion or thrombotic from nonthrombotic occlusion. In addition, false-negative test results may occur in patients with nonoccluding thrombi and in the presence of occlusion with collaterals. False-positive results are obtained in patients with congestive heart failure and severe occlusive peripheral arterial disease.[38]

**Ultrasound Imaging.** The popliteal and femoral/external iliac veins are readily accessible to imaging by ultrasound. Preliminary studies indicate that this method is accurate in identifying venous thrombosis or obstruction in over 95% of cases (Fakhri A, Sanders R: Personal communication). Venous obstruction proximal to the area being imaged is identified by incompressibility and nondistensibility of the vein during a Valsalva maneuver.

## DISEASES AFFECTING THE UPPER EXTREMITY VEINS

### Thrombosis

The incidence of DVT of the upper extremities is very low in comparison with that of the lower extremities and accounts for less than 2% of all deep venous thromboses.[40] Thrombosis may be idiopathic or may occur in association with systemic disease (Trousseau's phenomenon or migratory thrombophlebitis, polycythemia vera, congestive heart failure, vasculitis, rapid dehydration), following trauma or exertion, or as a result of a more central obstruction (cervical rib, central venous catheter, tumor- or radiation-induced stenosis).[40–45]

The most frequent symptom is nonpitting edema. In women, this may lead to unilateral breast enlargement on the involved side. Other symptoms are pain, weakness, paresthesias, and dependent cyanosis. On physical examination, a strand (thrombosed vein) may be palpable. In over half the patients, the occlusion involves the axillary vein.[41] Upper extremity DVT may also be a source for pulmonary emboli.[42, 45, 46] Spontaneous thrombosis without known predisposing factors, as part of a paraneoplastic syndrome, may occur several months before the tumor is manifested.[42] Tumors associated with Trousseau's phenomenon include bronchial, pancreatic, and gastric carcinoma.

### Axillary/Subclavian Vein Obstruction Due to the Thoracic Outlet Syndrome

A detailed discussion of the thoracic outlet syndrome is found in Chapter 9.

### Trauma

Trauma may be extrinsic, eg, from a clavicular fracture or shoulder or elbow dislocation, or iatrogenic, eg, due to an operation or from central venous or hyperalimentation catheters, transvenous cardiac pacing leads, or infusion of drugs that may damage the venous intima and predispose to thrombosis (chemotherapeutic agents and some antibiotics). In infants and small children, the central venous catheter may obstruct the subclavian vein and cause thrombosis.

Effort thrombosis (Paget–von Schroetter syndrome) is a form of post-traumatic thrombosis of the axillary vein. It is usually observed in younger individuals following strenuous exercise or occupational activity.[45] The etiology is a compression of the axillary vein by the subclavius muscle and/or costocoracoid ligament during forced abduction.[40]

## Tumors

Primary or metastatic neoplasms may obstruct the axillary or subclavian veins, leading to severe stenosis without thrombosis or complete obstruction with thrombosis. Stenosis may be due to compression by lymphadenopathy or primary neoplasm (eg, neurofibromatosis) or venous encasement and/or invasion by the tumor (eg, apical lung carcinoma). Postoperative or radiation-induced fibrosis may also lead to stenosis or occlusion.

### Angiography

Venography is indicated for evaluation of the site and extent of obstruction. If thrombolytic therapy is instituted, a follow-up venogram may become necessary to evaluate the degree of thrombolysis. Venography may also be indicated for assessment of vein patency in certain patients prior to placement of a hyperalimentation catheter and for differentiation between venous and lymphatic

obstruction in patients with arm swelling following mastectomy.

The angiographic findings are shown in Figures 19–20 to 19–22. In acute obstruction by thrombus, an intraluminal defect is seen, and only a few deep and superficial veins may be opacified. In chronic obstruction, multiple collaterals are seen. Radiation- or tumor-induced stenosis appears as a focal area of narrowing in the region of the radiation portal or tumor. Insidious onset or chronic obstruction facilitates the formation of extensive collaterals. Recanalization of upper extremity veins occurs less frequently than that of the lower extremity veins. This may be due to the presence of a vast collateral network in this region. Obstruction of the axillary or subclavian veins is bypassed by the supra- and subscapularis, circumflex humeral, transverse cervical, and long thoracic veins.[41]

PITFALLS IN DIAGNOSIS (Fig. 19–23)

1. Pseudo-obstruction of the axillary vein in hyperabduction: In certain individuals normal anatomical structures may cause extrinsic compression of the axillary vein in hyperabduction. These include the pectoralis minor muscle and the humeral head.[47]

2. Pseudo-obstruction of the brachial or axillary vein in adduction: In obese individ-

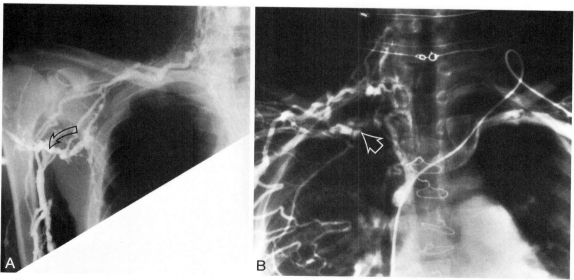

*Figure 19–20.* A, Axillary and subclavian vein thrombosis responsible for pulmonary embolus. Arrow points to the distal end of the thrombus. Enlarged bypassing collaterals are present. B, Another patient with right subclavian and brachiocephalic vein thrombosis due to a previous right subclavian transvenous cardiac pacer. Arrow points to the distal end of the thrombus. Extensive collaterals are present. A left-sided transvenous pacemaker has been implanted.

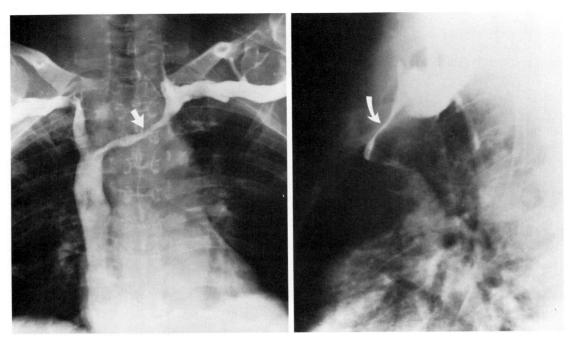

*Figure 19–21.* Tumor encasement. AP (*left*) and lateral (*right*) superior venacavagrams using the bilateral cubital vein technique show encasement of the left brachiocephalic vein by adenocarcinoma of the lung (*arrow*).

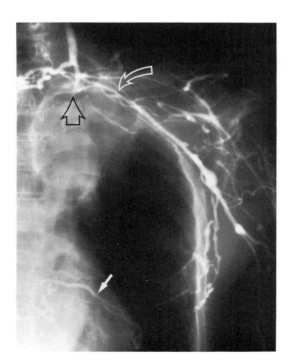

*Figure 19–22.* Tumor encasement and occlusion. Left arm venogram shows encasement of the subclavian vein (*curved arrow*) and occlusion of the brachiocephalic vein (*straight open arrow*) by carcinoma of the lung. Enlarged intercostal veins serve as collaterals (*solid arrow*).

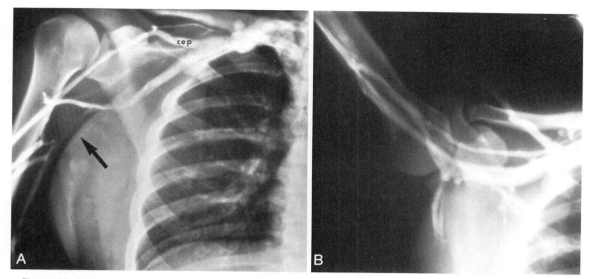

*Figure 19–23.* Spurious occlusion of the axillary vein in an obese female patient. *A,* The axillary vein is not opacified on the venogram in the neutral position (*arrow*). *B,* Repeat study in abduction shows a normal axillary vein. cep = cephalic vein.

uals (especially women), spurious occlusion of the brachial or axillary vein may be observed.

## Venous Ectasia

Fusiform or saccular dilation of the internal or external jugular vein has been reported in children and adults.[48, 49] Clinically, this may present as a pulsatile neck mass that typically enlarges during a Valsalva maneuver. Histological examination of some specimens has shown absence of elastic tissue.[49] The disorder is usually an isolated benign abnormality that does not require any therapy. Venous ectasia of the mediastinal veins has also been reported.[50] Diagnosis is established by contrast venography via the femoral approach using a multiple hole catheter (Fig. 19–24).

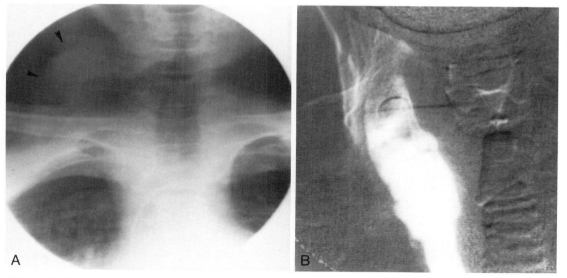

*Figure 19–24.* Jugular venous ectasia presenting as a pulsatile neck mass. *A,* A soft tissue neck mass is seen (*arrowheads*). *B,* Jugular venogram from the femoral approach using DSA shows a dilated vein.

## DISEASES AFFECTING THE SVC AND THE AZYGOS/HEMIAZYGOS SYSTEM

### Thrombosis/SVC Syndrome

In 80 to 90% of patients, obstruction of the SVC is due to a malignant process. The most frequent etiology is carcinoma of the lung (over 50% of cases), followed by lymphoma and other primary and metastatic tumors of the mediastinum.[51, 52]

In the past, tuberculosis and ascending aortic aneurysms were the most common benign causes.[53] More recently, iatrogenic SVC obstruction due to central venous and hyperalimentation catheters and transvenous pacer electrodes appears to be among the more common causes. Other benign causes include substernal goiter, constrictive pericarditis, histoplasmosis, sarcoidosis, and other forms of mediastinitis.[44, 54, 55] Ascending aortic–SVC fistula due to rupture of an aneurysm can be responsible for a dynamic SVC syndrome without obstruction.[53]

With the more frequent use of both short- and long-term indwelling venous catheters, an increasing number of thrombotic complications are to be expected. A thrombus sleeve around indwelling catheters can be detected in up to 90% of patients,[56] and venous thrombosis is reported in 23% of patients.[57] Thrombosis is usually associated with some other predisposing factors (eg, sepsis, multiple catheter exchanges) but may also occur in apparently uncomplicated cases.[58]

Symptoms usually develop insidiously and manifest as swelling of the face, neck, and upper extremities, venous congestion with dilated collateral veins, dyspnea, and cyanosis. Acute onset of symptoms is characteristic of acute SVC thrombosis.

### Trauma

Injury to the SVC may occur in blunt and penetrating chest trauma or may be iatrogenic following placement of central venous catheters.[59] In severe chest trauma, angiography is usually performed to detect arterial injuries and, rarely, for venous injuries. SVC obstruction may occur from a mediastinal hematoma.

### Tumor

Primary tumors of the major veins of the mediastinum are rare. The most frequent causes of SVC obstruction are bronchial carcinoma, lymphoma, and metastases.[53] Invasion and occlusion of the SVC give rise to the SVC syndrome. Venography of the azygos vein (to demonstrate encasement) has been used to assess resectability of mediastinal lesions. Rarely, tumor growth into the SVC has been observed.[60]

### Angiography

Neoplastic involvement of the SVC or azygos vein should be evaluated by a biplane study for the purpose of staging. Other forms of SVC thrombosis or occlusion can be evaluated by an AP study. DSA is an excellent method for the evaluation of patency and the demonstration of collaterals.

The angiographic findings in neoplastic involvement of the SVC and azygos vein are (Figs. 19–25 and 19–26):

1. Smooth, serrated, or undulating narrowing due to encasement and/or compression.

2. Occlusion, with or without demonstration of a proximal thrombus.

3. Demonstration of dilated collaterals, the extent of which depends upon the severity and duration of obstruction.

In non-neoplastic SVC obstruction, the angiographic picture varies with the etiology of the occlusion (Figs. 19–27 to 19–30; see also Chapter 7, Fig. 7–18). In fibrotic processes (eg, radiation, histoplasmosis), the SVC lumen is either severely distorted or obliterated and numerous dilated collaterals are seen. In SVC obstruction following placement of indwelling catheters, a thrombus is usually seen. The thrombus may extend into the right atrium, and pulmonary emboli may be demonstrated.

In complete obstruction of the SVC, blood return to the heart is via the IVC. The main venous collaterals to the IVC are via the azygos, lateral thoracic, and internal mammary veins and the vertebral plexus.[61]

## DISEASES AFFECTING THE IVC

### Obstruction

**Intrinsic Obstruction/Thrombosis.** The most frequent cause of IVC obstruction is a malignancy. Non-neoplastic obstruction of the IVC may be due to multiple causes. It is frequently idiopathic or occurs as a thrombus

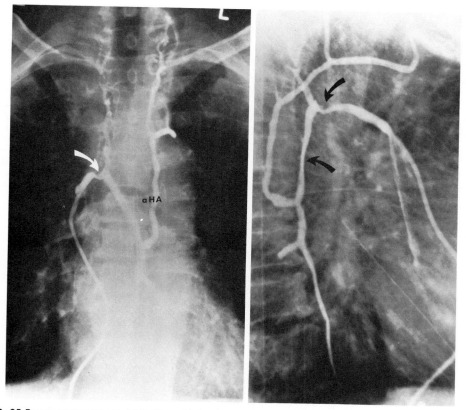

**Figure 19-25.** Tumor encasement. AP (*left*) and lateral (*right*) azygos venograms show encasement of the azygos vein by carcinoma of the esophagus (*arrows*). aHA = accessory hemiazygos vein.

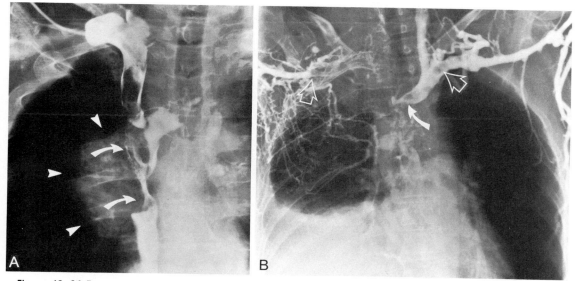

**Figure 19-26.** Tumor encasement and occlusion. *A*, Encasement of the superior vena cava (*curved arrows*) by oat cell carcinoma (*arrowheads*). A thrombus is present in the right brachiocephalic vein. *B*, Superior venacavogram via bilateral cubital vein injection demonstrates occlusion of the superior vena cava and right brachiocephalic vein by metastatic breast carcinoma. Thrombi are present in both brachiocephalic veins (*open arrows*). The left brachiocephalic vein is also encased by tumor (*curved arrow*).

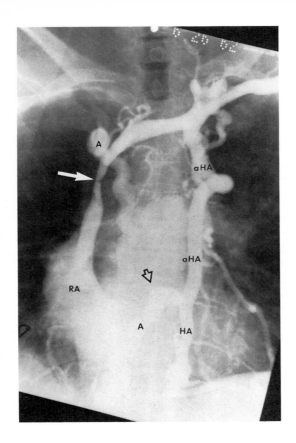

*Figure 19–27.* SVC stenosis and obstruction of the azygos vein due to tuberculosis. Superior venacavogram shows a severe stenosis of the superior vena cava (*arrow*). The azygos vein is dilated and occluded distal to the confluence with the hemiazygos vein (*open arrow*). There is reversal of blood flow in the azygos and hemiazygos system, which now carries blood to the IVC. A = azygos, αHA = accessory hemiazygos, HA = hemiazygos veins; RA = right atrium.

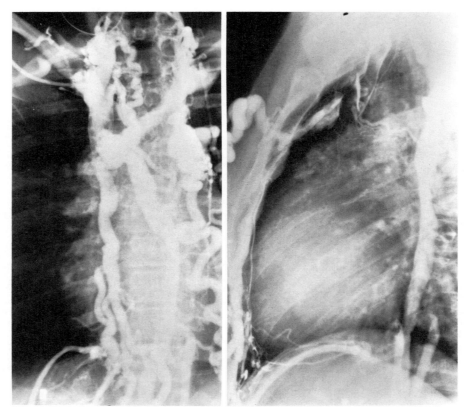

*Figure 19–28.* Superior vena caval occlusion due to fibrosing mediastinitis following histoplasmosis. AP (*left*) and lateral (*right*) right brachiocephalic venograms demonstrate occlusion of the superior vena cava. Extensive intra- and extrathoracic collaterals are present. (Courtesy of Dr. CA Athanasoulis.)

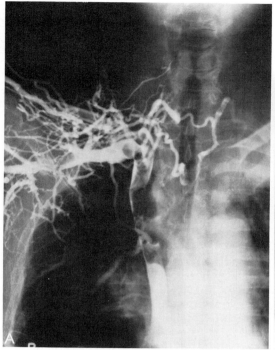 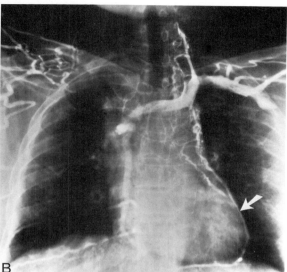

*Figure 19–29. A*, Acute thrombosis of the superior vena cava, right brachiocephalic, and axillary veins. *B*, Thrombosis of the arm veins and superior vena cava in a patient with leukemia. Bilateral cubital vein injection demonstrates occlusion of the right axillary, subclavian, and brachiocephalic veins. The superior vena cava below the azygos vein is also occluded. Arrow points to the left pericardiophrenic vein.

in the femoroiliac system extends proximally. Other causes are systemic or generalized disorders (eg, coagulopathy, Budd-Chiari syndrome, infection, sepsis, congestive heart

*Figure 19–30.* Bilateral brachiocephalic vein and superior vena caval thrombosis following central line placement in a newborn. Blood return to the inferior vena cava is via the azygos (A) and the accessory hemiazygos (aHA) veins.

failure), postoperative (eg, phlebitis, ligation, plication, clip, umbrella), severe exertion, trauma, and congenital membranes.[62–64]

A caval thrombus represents a potential source for life-threatening pulmonary embolus. Following caval ligation, the proximal cava is usually free of thrombus, whereas the cava below the ligation contains thrombi in 50% of cases.[62] Similarly, thrombi may also form distal to intraluminal caval occlusion devices (Fig. 19–31).

Recurrent pulmonary emboli may occur after caval ligation. These may originate from the retroperitoneal veins (eg, ascending lumbar and renal veins) or more distally. In the latter situation, enlarged bypassing collaterals (gonadal and lumbar veins or a left IVC) may serve as a pathway for the emboli.[62, 64]

**Extrinsic Compression/Constriction.** Extrinsic compression or displacement of the IVC may occur at any level. The mid-IVC (L2–L3) is most frequently involved. In the adult, the most common cause is retroperitoneal lymphadenopathy. In children, renal and adrenal tumors are the most frequent causes. Other lesions or conditions that indent, displace, or obstruct the cava in the adult are hepatic masses or hepatomegaly, large adrenal and renal tumors, pancreatic

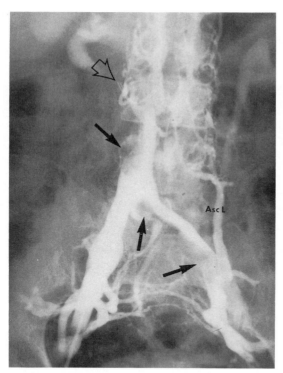

*Figure 19–31.* Inferior vena caval thrombus (*straight arrow*) below a Mobinuddin caval umbrella (*open arrow*). The lower arrows point to thrombus in the left common iliac vein. Asc L = ascending lumbar vein.

tumors, tortuous aorta and aortic aneurysms, retroperitoneal hematoma, and retroperitoneal neoplasms.

In patients with massive ascites, the cava is constricted at and above the hepatic segment. Removal of the ascitic fluid results in relief of the obstruction.[65] Retroperitoneal fibrosis and tumor-induced desmoplastic reaction (eg, metastatic carcinoid) may also constrict or occlude the IVC either focally or diffusely.[66]

**Functional     Obstruction/Pseudo-obstruction** (Fig. 19–32). Functional caval obstruction can be caused by the pregnant uterus or a Valsalva maneuver.[67–69] In children, IVC obstruction occurs relatively frequently in association with straining or crying, resulting in opacification of the paravertebral plexus.

Pseudo-obstruction of the IVC may be observed in large abdominal masses if the venacavagram is performed in the supine position. This is frequently observed in children, in whom the mass compresses the IVC against the spine in the supine position. If the venacavagram is repeated with the patient in the lateral decubitus position, the weight of the mass no longer compresses the IVC and, if patent, the lumen is demonstrated.[70]

## Trauma

Injury to the IVC is associated with a high mortality.[71, 71a] Survival is determined by the location and type of injury, among other factors. The most frequent injuries are due to penetrating trauma (bullet and knife injuries) and are associated with a mortality rate of 21 and 50%, respectively.[71, 71a] Blunt injuries, although less frequent, carry a significantly higher mortality (85%) because of associated injuries of the parenchymal organs and other blood vessels. The most frequently associated parenchymal injury is to the liver. Vascular injuries involve the portal vein and hepatic artery. Such patients are rarely studied by angiography because of their hemodynamic instability and severity of injury, which necessitates immediate surgical exploration. Trauma of lesser severity may result in a retroperitoneal hematoma with caval displacement. Occasionally, a pelvic hematoma may dissect upward and masquerade as a retroperitoneal hematoma.

Penetrating injuries to the cava may result in the formation of an arterio-caval fistula. Such fistulae have also been reported after lumbar disc operations.[72] Other iatrogenic causes for retroperitoneal hematoma are translumbar aortography, percutaneous nephrostomy, caval filters, and occasionally percutaneous biopsy.

## Tumor

Primary tumors of the IVC are rare. Leiomyoma, leiomyosarcoma, and endothelioma have been reported.[62, 64] Neoplasms are by far the most common cause of IVC obstruction. In one series, renal carcinoma was responsible for obstruction in 31% of patients and pancreatic carcinoma in 9%.[63] Obstruction may also be due to intracaval extension of tumor, encasement/invasion, regional lymph node metastases, lymphomas, and sarcomas. Intracaval growth is observed most frequently in renal carcinoma and occasionally in adrenal carcinoma and other tumors (eg, uterine leiomyomatosis).[73–75]

## Miscellaneous

**Collateral Circulation in IVC Occlusion.** (Fig. 19–33; see also Figs. 19–38 and 19–39).

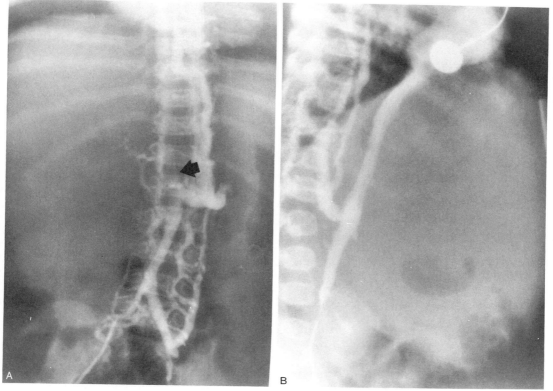

**Figure 19–32.** Pseudo-obstruction of the inferior vena cava in a 4 month old child with hepatoblastoma. *A,* Supine inferior venacavagram shows obstruction of the inferior vena cava at T12 (*arrow*). *B,* Left lateral decubitus cavagram shows a normal inferior vena cava. (From Kadir S, O'Neal JA: Cardiovasc Intervent Radiol 5:25–29, 1982. Used with permission.)

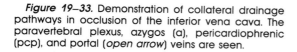

**Figure 19–33.** Demonstration of collateral drainage pathways in occlusion of the inferior vena cava. The paravertebral plexus, azygos (a), pericardiophrenic (pcp), and portal (*open arrow*) veins are seen.

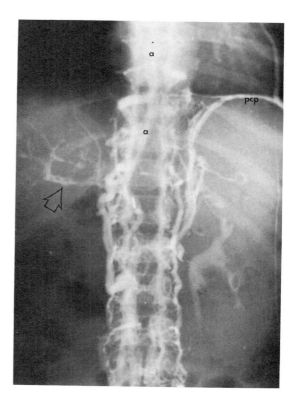

In the event of occlusion of the IVC, numerous deep and superficial collaterals are available for venous return to the right heart. A detailed description of these collaterals can be found in references 62, 76, and 77. Some of the main channels are listed below:

*Upper IVC (hepatic segment):* Occlusion may be congenital (membrane, congenital absence) or due to a tumor or thrombus. Venous drainage from the lower IVC is primarily via the paravertebral plexus, ascending lumbar–azygos/hemiazygos system, and superficial abdominal wall venous communications.

*Mid and lower IVC:* The most frequent cause of obstruction of the mid IVC is tumor. Frequent causes of lower IVC obstruction are thrombosis and tumor. Venous drainage is similar to that seen in obstruction of the upper IVC but with two additional pathways: (1) the portal system, which serves as a collateral via the superior hemorrhoidal → inferior mesenteric → portal → hepatic vein route, and (2) via the left gonadal and ureteric → left renal → ascending lumbar → hemiazygos vein route.

The superficial veins play a major role as collaterals in obstruction of the lower IVC. The superficial veins may connect directly to tributaries of the SVC (superficial epigastric → lateral thoracic → axillary veins; inferior epigastric → internal mammary veins) or via the portal system (paraumbilical veins → recanalized umbilical → portal vein).

**Foreign Bodies.** The most frequent intracaval foreign bodies are short guide wires or catheters that are inadvertently advanced into the IVC during catheterization of the femoral vein. An inferior venacavogram is indicated in such patients to exclude thrombus around the foreign body and caval perforation prior to percutaneous retrieval.[78]

### Angiography

Cavography is indicated to evaluate the extent of occlusion (due to thrombosis or neoplasm). In patients with benign disease (eg, Budd-Chiari syndrome), patency of the IVC must be determined before a meso- or portacaval shunt can be performed. In patients with neoplasm, demonstration of caval invasion or occlusion may determine resectability and prognosis.[79]

Angiographic findings (Figs. 19–34 to 19–41; see also Fig. 19–49):

1. Displacement: Anterior or lateral displacement is observed in the presence of masses or hematoma. Displacement is usu-ally smooth, but may be associated with nodular impressions if it is caused by enlarged lymph nodes or a nodular tumor. IVC displacement alone is a poor indicator for the presence of retroperitoneal lymphadenopathy. Sensitivity for detecting anteriorly located lymph nodes is very low.

2. Indentation: This is most frequently caused by enlarged lymph nodes and is located in the mid-portion of the cava. It is smooth and may be posterior and/or lateral. Occasionally, indentation is caused by a nodular tumor.

3. Narrowing/encasement: Smooth tubular narrowing of the lower IVC is seen in patients with retroperitoneal fibrosis. Focal constriction in the absence of a shelflike mural abnormality is seen in other fibrotic processes (eg, metastatic carcinoid). Smooth narrowing of the upper IVC is also seen in hepatomegaly, massive ascites, and retroperitoneal lymphoma. In most cases, tumor invasion or encasement is associated with an abrupt narrowing of the lumen, which may demonstrate a shelflike transition. Serrations of the lumen or tumor nodules may be seen projecting into the lumen (see Chapter 13, Fig. 13–3, and Chapter 16, Fig. 16–42).

4. Thrombus/occlusion: Thrombosis may partially or completely occlude the IVC lumen. Nonoccluding thrombi appear as intraluminal defects and are most frequently infrarenal. IVC occlusion may also be due to intraluminal growth of tumor and is difficult to differentiate from thrombus on a venacavogram. In the majority of patients, tumor extends towards the right atrium, but occasionally growth may be centrifugal. The IVC below the segment obstructed by tumor may contain a thrombus. Differentiation between intracaval tumor and thrombus is usually possible by arteriography, which demonstrates tumor vascularity extending into the cava.

There are few descriptions of the angiographic findings in IVC trauma because most patients with severe abdominal trauma who are not in hemodynamic shock are studied by arteriography only. Intimal tears, similar to those seen in arterial injury,[80] and arteriovenous fistulae have been observed (Fig. 19–41) (see also Chapter 16, Fig. 16–32A).

Pitfalls in Diagnosis (Figs. 19–42 to 19–44)

1. Posterior indentation due to osteophytes may simulate lymphadenopathy. Lateral caval indentation has also been observed in massive enlargement of the renal pelvis.[81]

*Text continued on page 573*

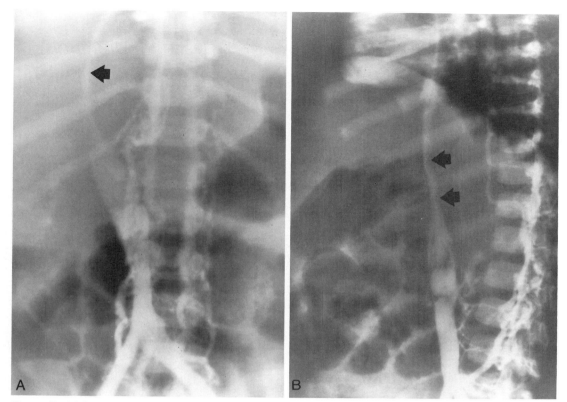

*Figure 19–34.* Displacement and encasement of the upper inferior vena cava in a 2 year old child with non-Hodgkin's lymphoma. *A,* AP cavogram shows narrowing and lateral displacement (*arrow*) of the hepatic segment of the inferior vena cava. *B,* Lateral cavagram also shows encasement and anterior displacement (*arrows*). (From Kadir S, O'Neal JA: Cardiovasc Intervent Radiol 5:25–29, 1982. Used with permission.)

*Figure 19–35.* Indentation and displacement of the inferior vena cava. *A,* Posterior indentation and anterior displacement of the inferior vena cava by enlarged lymph nodes in a patient with lymphoma (*arrows*). A small mural thrombus is also present (*open arrow*). *B,* Displacement and compression (*arrows*) of the infrarenal inferior vena cava by a large, nodular Wilms' tumor in a 4 year old child. (From Kadir S, O'Neal JA: Cardiovasc Intervent Radiol 5:25–29, 1982. Used with permission.)

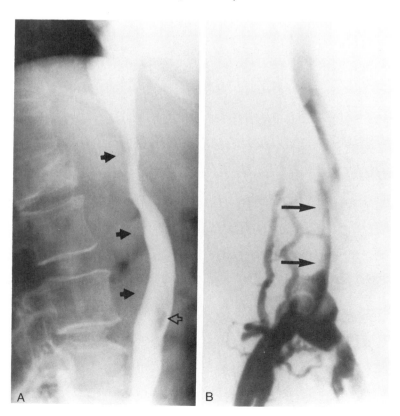

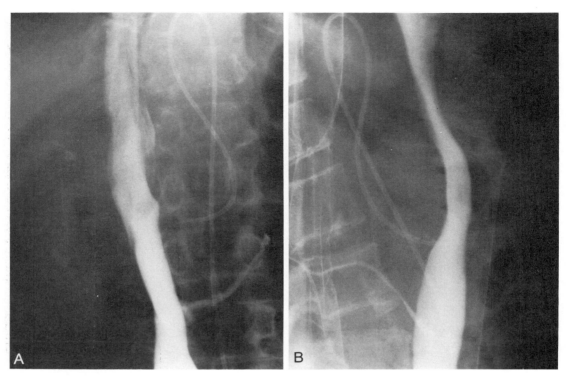

*Figure 19–36.* Inferior vena caval displacement by retrocaval lymphadenopathy from renal carcinoma. Significance of lateral projection. *A*, AP inferior venacavogram shows minimal lateral displacement at the level of the renal veins. Inflow of unopacified blood from the renal veins is seen. *B*, The lateral projection shows marked anterior displacement of the inferior vena cava.

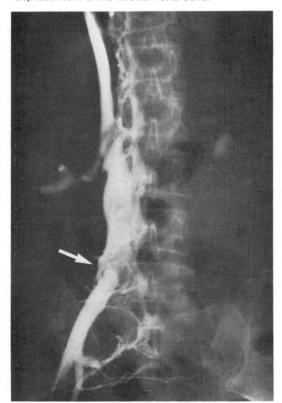

*Figure 19–37.* Constriction of the distal inferior vena cava and iliac veins (*arrow*) by carcinoid-induced fibrosis.

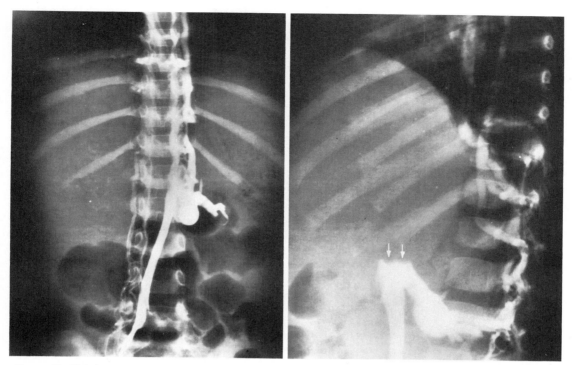

*Figure 19–38.* Inferior vena caval occlusion by tumor. AP (*left*) and lateral (*right*) inferior venacavograms show abrupt occlusion with opacification of collaterals. On the lateral study, intracaval tumor is seen (*arrows*).

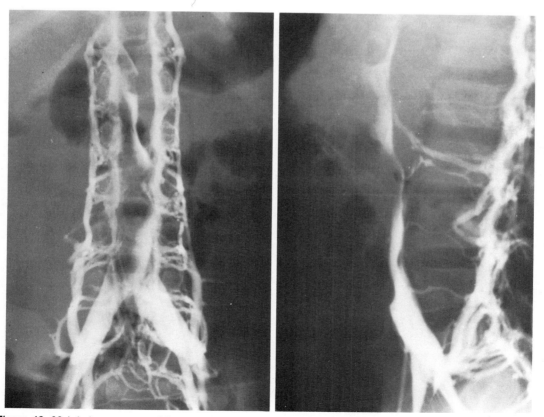

*Figure 19–39.* Inferior vena caval thrombus. AP (*left*) and lateral (*right*) inferior venacavograms show a partially occluding caval thrombus with opacification of the paravertebral plexus.

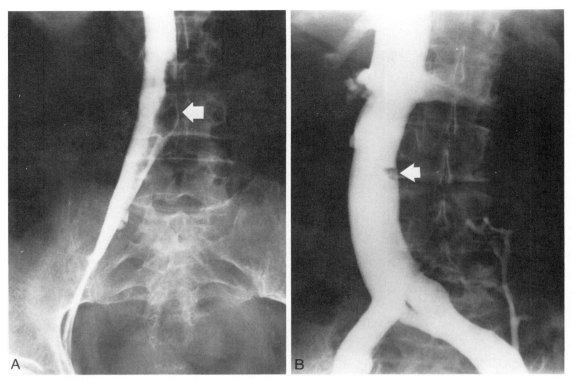

*Figure 19–40.* Nonoccluding thrombus. *A,* Right iliac venogram shows a nonoccluding thrombus extending into the distal cava from the left iliac vein (*arrow*). *B,* There is a small mural thrombus (*arrow*). This defect is sharply marginated and should not be mistaken for inflow from a retroaortic left renal vein. Note the bowing of the inferior vena cava due to the scoliosis.

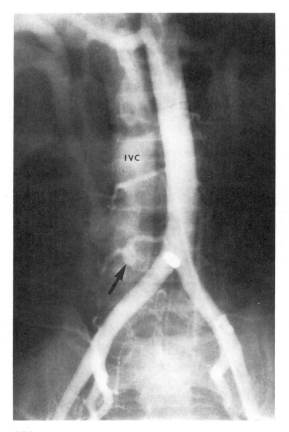

*Figure 19–41.* Traumatic arteriocaval fistula. Aortogram shows an aneurysm of a right lumbar artery (*arrow*) and opacification of the inferior vena cava (IVC).

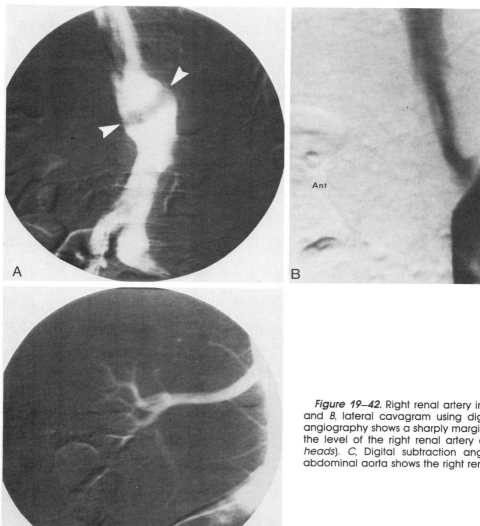

**Figure 19–42.** Right renal artery impression. *A,* AP and *B,* lateral cavagram using digital subtraction angiography shows a sharply marginated defect at the level of the right renal artery crossing (*arrowheads*). *C,* Digital subtraction angiogram of the abdominal aorta shows the right renal artery.

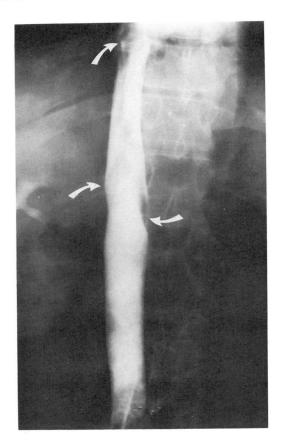

Figure 19–43. Artefacts from inflow of unopacified blood from the renal and hepatic veins (*arrows*). Characteristically, the appearance of inflow artefacts varies on different films from the same cavagram.

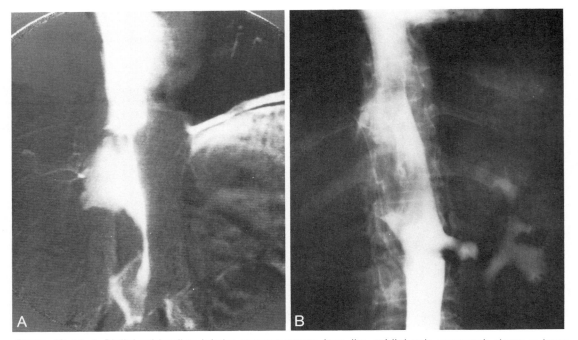

Figure 19–44. *A*, Digital subtraction inferior venacavagram from the cubital vein approach shows a large intraluminal tumor. The infrarenal cava appears occluded. *B*, Repeat study from the femoral approach shows that the cava below the tumor is patent.

2. Posterior indentation by the right renal artery is sharply marginated and may also be demonstrated on the AP projection.[82]

3. Scoliosis of the spine may simulate anterior-lateral displacement of the IVC.

4. Flow artefacts: Inflow of unopacified blood from the tributaries of the IVC may simulate a mural abnormality. In our experience, such defects are due to a slow contrast injection rate (< 20 ml/second), distal injection site (external iliac, often unilateral), and slow filming sequence (< 3 films/second). Common locations for such artefacts are the renal veins, especially the retroaortic branches. Such flow artefacts are not constant, unlike the mural thrombus seen in Figure 19–40B.

5. In patients with retroperitoneal tumors, the CT scan may suggest caval invasion or occlusion, and angiography is indicated to evaluate patency and venous extension of tumor. Contrast injection in the upper IVC from the cubital vein approach is frequently not sufficient, as reflux of contrast medium into the infrarenal IVC may not occur, suggesting complete caval occlusion. If the venacavagram is performed from the femoral approach, the true extent of disease is demonstrated (Fig. 19–44).

## DISEASES AFFECTING THE LOWER EXTREMITY AND PELVIC VEINS

### Thrombosis

Autopsy studies on hospitalized patients indicate that the incidence of deep venous thrombosis (DVT) in this group is between 34 and 53% and the incidence of pulmonary thromboembolism is about 15%.[83, 84] Using [125]I-fibrinogen, a 30% incidence of DVT was detected in postoperative patients.[85] Conditions that predispose to DVT are obesity, previous DVT or pulmonary emboli, varicose veins, underlying malignancy, oral contraceptives, prolonged immobilization, postoperative or post-partum period, and old age.[86, 87] Spontaneous venous thrombosis has also been reported in patients with thromboangiitis obliterans, lupus erythematosus and ulcerative colitis.[88, 89]

**Location of DVT.** In most patients, thrombosis begins in the calf veins and may extend proximally into the popliteal/femoral veins or distally into the foot.[85] Thrombosis may also develop simultaneously at multiple noncontiguous locations. If untreated, propagation of DVT may occur in as many as two thirds of patients. Propagation of thrombosis and pulmonary thromboembolism are also observed in patients on heparin therapy and oral anticoagulants.[86, 90]

DVT may also begin in the foot veins, or these vessels may be the only location of DVT[91, 92] (see Fig. 19–10). In one series, thrombi were detected in the foot veins in 56% of venograms positive for DVT.[91] In 10%, the thrombus was confined to the foot veins, being most frequently located in the lateral plantar vein.

The frequency and location of DVT are shown in Table 19–3. DVT involves the calf (91%), the thigh (55%), and the veins proximal to the inguinal ligament (25%).[93] The process is bilateral in 35 to 44% of individuals, and involvement is symmetrical in 58% of these extremities.[84, 93]

**Symptoms.** The most frequent symptoms of DVT are swelling in 89% and pain in 69% of patients.[90] In addition, there may be temperature elevation and cyanosis and the superficial veins are distended. In superficial venous thrombosis, a tender, indurated cord is usually present with focal inflammatory reaction. Superficial venous thrombosis is more commonly seen in patients with varicose veins and occasionally in patients with an occult malignancy or thromboangiitis obliterans.[94]

Whereas the symptoms and physical signs suggesting the diagnosis of DVT can be misleading in two thirds of patients, 50% of thromboses may be silent clinically.[85, 87, 93] Although less invasive or noninvasive studies may be used to screen patients with a high degree of accuracy, leg venography remains the single most reliable test for the

**TABLE 19–3. Frequency and Location of DVT in the Lower Extremity**

| Location | Frequency (%)* | | |
|---|---|---|---|
| | *Ref. 91* | *Ref. 93* | *Ref. 90* |
| Foot veins only | 10 | | |
| Foot and other veins | 56 | | |
| Calf and distal veins | | 42 | 46 |
| Popliteal vein | | | 11 |
| Thigh and distal veins | | 29 | |
| Thigh veins only | | 5 | 24 |
| Profunda femoris vein | | 9 | |
| Pelvic† and distal veins | | 22 | 19 |
| Pelvic† veins only | | 3 | |

*Of lower extremity venograms positive for DVT.
†Iliac and common femoral veins with extension into lower IVC.

diagnosis of DVT. Venography provides a very high degree of accuracy for the detection of DVT (about 97%), and a therapeutic decision can safely be based upon results of venography, since a negative leg venogram excludes the presence of clinically significant DVT.[95]

Clinically, a ruptured Baker's (popliteal) cyst, cellulitis, lipedema, or gas gangrene may simulate DVT.[96, 97] The venogram is usually normal, but popliteal vein compression or displacement may be seen in unruptured popliteal cysts (see Fig. 19–19). On the other hand, DVT and ruptured popliteal cyst may coexist.[98]

**Sequelae of DVT.** Spontaneous thrombolysis also occurs in the venous system, and in one study this was suggested in 35% of patients.[85] Lysis occurred within 72 hours, and all thrombi were smaller than 5 cm. In the majority of patients with DVT, the valves are damaged permanently, predisposing to chronic venous insufficiency. The process of recanalization begins within 1 week, and up to 75% of the cross-sectional area is recanalized in 2 to 3 months.[99]

PULMONARY EMBOLI. Pulmonary emboli may originate from any site of DVT, including the foot veins. Although there does not appear to be any predilection for a particular site, over 50% of the pulmonary emboli originate from the calf and about 25% originate from the thigh veins.[90] This reflects the relative frequency of DVT in these locations and not the propensity for thromboembolism. Emboli originating from the more proximal veins are more likely to be lethal because of their large size, whereas those from the smaller distal veins may remain clinically silent.

The incidence of pulmonary emboli in patients with DVT is between 9 and 15%[83, 85, 90] and is 30% in postoperative patients.[87] As many as 45% of the emboli (especially those from the smaller calf veins) may be clinically silent.[100] In up to 66% of patients with documented pulmonary emboli, the proximal extension of the thrombus is into the popliteal vein.[100] However, the actual embolus may have arisen from a more proximal location.

PHLEGMASIA CERULEA DOLENS. This condition occurs in extensive DVT of the iliofemoral veins and their branches, leading to a severely edematous, cyanotic extremity that may progress to gangrene. There is trapping of blood distal to the obstruction, which may lead to hemodynamic instability and impairment of arterial circulation to the leg.

POST-PHLEBITIC SYNDROME. Destruction of the valves in the calf and perforating veins leads to failure of the calf muscle pump and chronic venous insufficiency. Venous return is established via collaterals and the superficial veins, giving rise to secondary varicosities. Rupture of small venules and capillaries leads to subcutaneous bleeding and is responsible for the characteristic skin pigmentation around the ankles, which is observed in almost 25% of patients. Other clinical manifestations are swelling, pain, skin induration, varicosities, and skin ulceration.

**Angiography.** Venography is indicated to confirm the presence of venous thrombosis and to determine its extent. Determination of extent (proximal extension) is crucial for assessing the type of therapy required. Although venous thrombosis is bilateral in over one third of patients, simultaneous bilateral venography is not recommended, especially in ambulant patients. A single leg venogram should be performed first, and if no thrombus is identified, the other leg may be studied if bilateral disease is suspected. Since the therapy for bilateral DVT is essentially the same as for single leg DVT, if a thrombus is demonstrated in one leg, it is not necessary to subject the other extremity to venography.

The venographic findings in acute DVT have been described earlier and are shown in Figures 19–11 to 19–16 and Figure 19–45. In chronic DVT (post-phlebitic syndrome), the following may be observed (Figs. 19–46 and 19–47):

1. Persistent occlusion of the deep veins with opacification of multiple collaterals. Occasionally, there is persistent occlusion of a segment of a deep vein and opacification of one or more markedly dilated, tortuous bypassing collaterals.

2. Recanalization: A single channel or multiple irregular channels are present.

3. Incompetent perforating veins and opacification of varicosities.

4. Vein valves are either partially or totally destroyed.

## Varicose Veins

Varicose veins are defined as tortuous, dilated, redundant veins that are deficient in competent valves. Primary varicose veins may be due to multiple causes (eg, genetic predisposition, obesity, pregnancy). The varicosities involve the saphenous system primarily, and the deep veins are normal.

Secondary varicose veins are most fre-

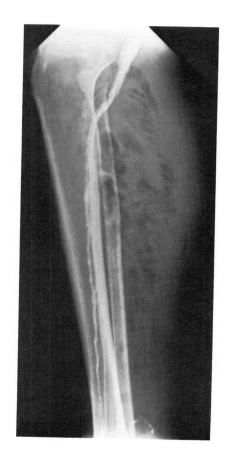

*Figure 19–45.* Gas gangrene and deep venous thrombosis in a middle-aged diabetic male patient. Lateral film from the leg venogram shows gas in the soft tissues. The posterior tibial and peroneal veins and muscular branches are occluded.

quently a part of the post-phlebitic syndrome. Other causes include chronic alcoholism, arteriovenous malformations, and congenital venous abnormalities (eg, Klippel-Trenaunay-Weber syndrome). The deep veins are abnormal, with incompetent or absent valves.

Pelvic varicosities may be responsible for the pelvic congestion syndrome in premenopausal women.[101, 102] The varicosities may involve the external and internal genitalia and are demonstrated by retrograde ovarian venography or by direct varicography of vulval varicose veins.[101] Vulval varicose veins are observed in 1% of patients with leg varicose veins[101] and may also be seen in association with pelvic masses. Pelvic (and vulval) varices are also observed in patients with thrombosis of the common femoral and iliac veins and IVC (Figs. 19–47 and 19–49).

**Venography.** For the demonstration of primary varices, venography is performed in the supine position. Tourniquets are not used, and the needle tip is pointed towards the ankle. Alternatively, the varicosities can be punctured directly (varicography), or descending venography is used with the aid of the Valsalva maneuver. For the evaluation of secondary varices and demonstration of the level of incompetent perforating veins, routine supine or upright venography can be used.

Venographic findings (Figs. 19–48 and 19–49; see also Fig. 19–5):

1. In primary varicose veins, varicosities of the superficial system and a normal deep venous system are demonstrated. During ascending venography, the communicating veins may opacify in the normal fashion (from superficial to deep system).

2. In secondary varicose veins, the varicosities opacify via incompetent perforating veins. Typically, these are dilated, tortuous, valveless channels that narrow as they pass through the fascia and enter into a dilated saccular varix.[103] Most incompetent perforating veins are located over the medial aspect of the leg. In the presence of paired perforating veins, the upper channel is usually larger.[103]

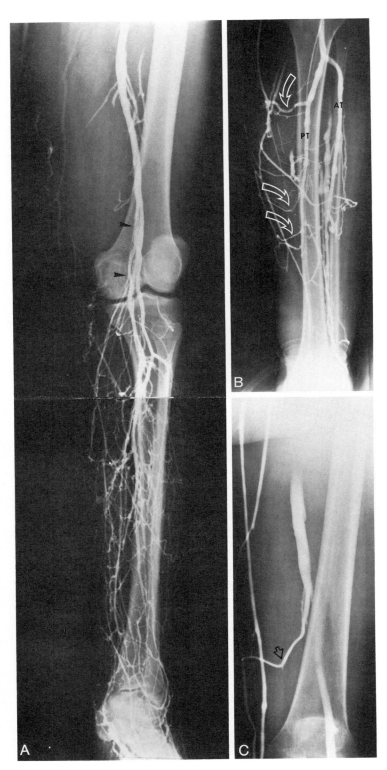

**Figure 19–46.** Post-phlebitic changes. *A,* The deep veins of the lower calf are attenuated and there is opacification of numerous nonvaricose superficial veins. The popliteal vein is duplicated and one of the limbs shows recanalization (*arrowheads*). *B* and *C,* Venogram from another patient. *B,* Valveless, incompetent perforating veins are seen (*arrows*) and there is filling of the superficial veins from the deep veins. There is also edema of the leg. *C,* In the thigh, which was uninvolved by deep venous thrombosis, there is normal flow from superficial to deep veins via a perforating vein (*arrow*). AT = anterior tibial, PT = posterior tibial veins.

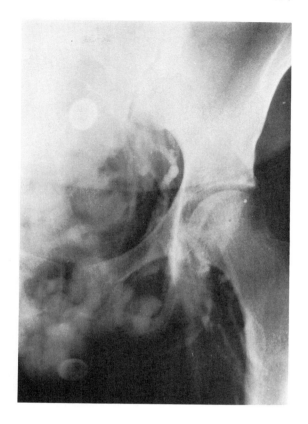

**Figure 19–47.** Pelvic varices in a patient with chronic occlusion of the iliofemoral veins.

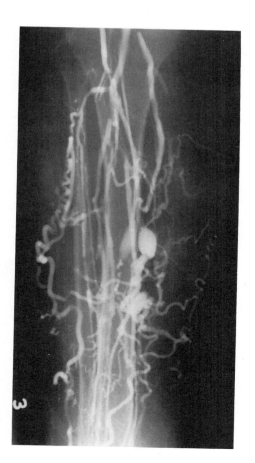

**Figure 19–48.** Leg venogram showing varicose veins.

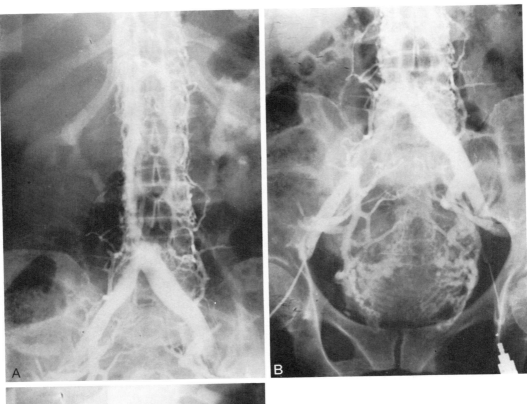

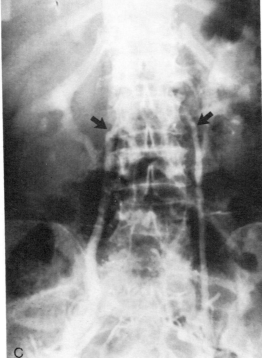

*Figure 19–49.* Pelvic varices in a patient with nephrotic syndrome and inferior vena caval obstruction. *A,* Early film from a pelvic venogram shows caval obstruction with opacification of paravertebral collaterals. *B,* Later film shows dilated uterine, ovarian, and bladder veins. *C,* On a later film, the ovarian veins are opacified (*arrows*) and serve as a collateral pathway.

## MISCELLANEOUS INDICATIONS FOR VENOGRAPHY

### Venography of the Corpora Cavernosa

The corpora cavernosa of the penis can be visualized by direct puncture (19 gauge needle) and injection of diluted contrast medium (30 to 45%). Corpus cavernosography is indicated for the evaluation of Peyronie's disease, priapism, trauma, and impotence. The technique is described in references 104 and 105.

### Congenital Abnormalities

Congenital abnormalities of the veins of the lower extremity are seen in patients with the Klippel-Trenaunay-Weber syndrome. A detailed discussion of this abnormality can be found in Chapter 10. A single extremity is usually affected. Dilated, bulbous-appearing, anomalous veins are present, and valves and occasionally the deep venous system are absent. Angiomatous or plexiform lesions have also been observed.[106]

### Iliac Compression Syndrome

In some individuals, there is obstruction of the left (and occasionally of the right) common iliac vein caused by the crossing of the right iliac artery or distal aorta and predisposes to thrombosis of the iliac vein(s). In susceptible individuals, this chronic compression leads to fibrous constriction of the vein.[107] This syndrome is usually observed in young persons (< 30 years of age) and most frequently involves the left leg. It occurs after operation or other conditions that require bed rest.

On venography, the vein appears flattened as a result of extrinsic compression (Fig. 19–50). In severe obstruction or occlusion, there is opacification of pelvic collaterals and drainage via the contralateral iliac system.

### Trauma

In leg trauma, the veins may be injured directly or DVT may occur as a consequence of the immobilization. Venography is vastly underutilized for the assessment of venous injury.[108] Recognition of injury to the major

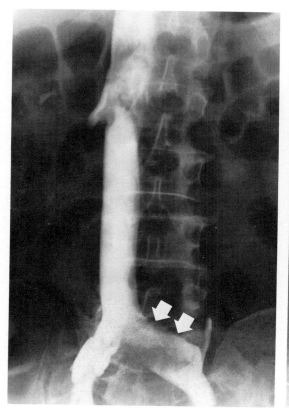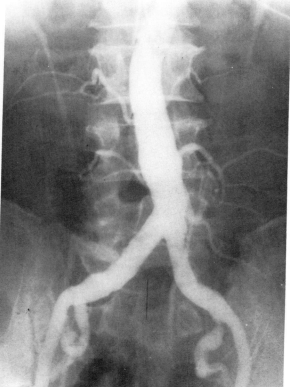

**Figure 19–50.** Extrinsic compression of iliac vein. Inferior vena cavagram (*left*) shows compression of the left common iliac vein (*arrows*) by the distal aorta and proximal iliac arteries (*right*).

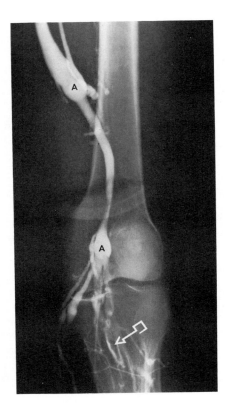

*Figure 19–51.* Idiopathic venous aneurysms (A). The patient was evaluated for calf deep venous thrombosis. A partially retracted thrombus is present in the popliteal vein (*arrow*). Same patient as in Figure 19–12.

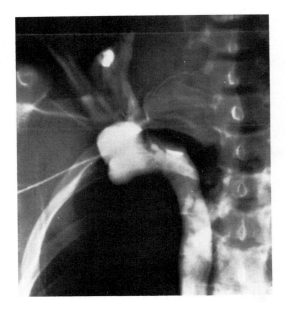

*Figure 19–52.* Aneurysm of the subclavian vein in a patient with Ehlers-Danlos syndrome. Same patient as in Figure 8–55, Chapter 8.

veins is important, as operative repair based upon these findings may avoid late sequelae of impairment of venous circulation. Chronic venous insufficiency as a late sequela of immobilization-induced DVT is observed in 40% of young patients with lower leg fractures.[109]

## Venous Aneurysms

Dilatation of the femoral or popliteal vein segments is seen occasionally in the absence of a venous dysplasia syndrome (Fig. 19–51). Isolated venous aneurysms may also develop as a complication of intravenous drug abuse.[110] Thrombus formation in venous aneurysms can be the source of pulmonary emboli.[111] Venous aneurysms are also seen in patients with the Ehlers-Danlos syndrome (Fig. 19–52).

## REFERENCES

1. de Leval MR, Ritter DG, McGoon DC, et al: Anomalous systemic venous connection. Surgical considerations. Mayo Clin Proc 50:599–610, 1975.
2. Campbell M, Deuchar DC: The left sided superior vena cava. Br Heart J 16:423–439, 1954.
3. Gensini GG, Caldini P, Casaccio F, et al: Persistent left superior vena cava. Am J Cardiol 4:677–685, 1959.
4. Reis RH, Esenther G: Variations in the pattern of renal vessels and their relation to the type of posterior vena cava in man. Am J Anat 104:295–318, 1959.
5. Anderson RC, Adams P Jr, Burke B: Anomalous inferior vena cava with azygous continuation (infrahepatic interruption of the inferior vena cava). Report of 15 new cases. J. Pediatr 59:370–383, 1961.
6. Haswell DM, Berrigan TJ Jr: Anomalous inferior vena cava with accessory hemiazygos continuation. Radiology 119:51–54, 1976.
7. Elliot LP, Jue KL, Amplatz K: A roentgen classification of cardiac malpositions. Invest Radiol 1:17–28, 1966.
8. Almen T, Nylander G: Serial phlebography of the normal lower leg during muscular contraction and relaxation. Acta Radiol Diagn 57:264–272, 1962.
9. Benfield JR, Bonney H, Crummy AB, et al: Azygograms and pulmonary arteriograms in bronchogenic carcinoma. Arch Surg 99:406–409, 1969.
10. Kadir S, Robinette C: Accuracy of angiography in the localization of pheochromocytoma. J Urol 126:789–793, 1981.
11. Greitz T: Phlebography of the normal leg. Acta Radiol 44:1–20, 1955.
12. Thomas ML, Briggs GM, Kuan BB: Contrast agent induced thrombophlebitis following leg phlebography: Meglumine ioxaglate versus meglumine iothalamate. Radiology 147:399–400, 1983.
13. Silverbach S: The use of Xylocaine to diminish leg cramps in venography. Radiology 133:788–789, 1979.
14. Rabinov K, Paulin S: Roentgen diagnosis of venous thrombosis in the leg. Arch Surg 104:134–144, 1972.
15. Thomas ML: Phlebography. Arch Surg 104:145–151, 1972.
16. DeWeese JA, Rogoff SM: Functional ascending phlebography of the lower extremity by serial long film technique. Evaluation of anatomic and functional detail in 62 extremities. AJR 81:841–854, 1959.
17. Tisnado J, Tsai FY, Beachley MC: An alternate technique for lower extremity venography. Radiology 133:787–788, 1979.
18. Göthlin J: The comparative frequency of extravasal injection at phlebography with steel and plastic cannula. Clin Radiol 23:183–184, 1972.
19. Kistner RL: Surgical repair of the incompetent femoral vein valve. Arch Surg 110:1336–1342, 1975.
20. Queral LA, Whitehouse WM, Flinn WR, et al: Surgical correction of chronic deep venous insufficiency by valvular transposition. Surgery 87:688–695, 1980.
21. Gullmo A: The phlebographic Trendelenburg test. Br J Radiol 36:812–821, 1963.
22. Thomas ML, Fletcher EWL: The techniques of pelvic phlebography. Clin Radiol 18:399–402, 1967.
23. Thomas ML: Phlebography of the Lower Limb. Edinburgh, Churchill Livingstone, 1982.
24. Schneider R: Die ossale Venographie. Unter besonderer Berücksichtigung der Tumordiagnostik. Dtsch Med Wochenschr 92:487–488, 1967.
24a. Thomas ML, Bowles JN: Incompetent perforating veins: Comparison of varicography and ascending phlebography. Radiology 154:619–623, 1985.
25. Sommer FG, Laglia A, Goldberg RT: Pain accompanying leg venography: A comparison of sodium and methylglucamine diatrizoates. Radiology 133:790–791, 1979.
26. Bettmann MA, Paulin S: Leg phlebography: The incidence, nature and modification of undesirable side effects. Radiology 122:101–104, 1977.
27. Walters HL, Clemenson J, Browse NL, et al: 125-I-fibrinogen uptake following phlebography of the leg. Comparison of ionic and nonionic contrast media. Radiology 135:619–621, 1980.
28. O'Donnell TF, Abbott WM, Athanasoulis CA, et al: Diagnosis of deep venous thrombosis in the outpatient by venography. Surg Gynecol Obstet 150:69–74, 1980.
29. Coel MN, Dodge W: Complication rate with supine phlebography. AJR 131:821–822, 1978.
30. McAlister WH, Palmer K: The histologic effects of four commonly used media for excretory urography and an attempt to modify the responses. Radiology 99:511–516, 1971.
31. Wheeler HB, Anderson FA Jr: Impedance phlebography: the diagnosis of venous thrombosis by occlusive impedance plethysmography. In Bernstein EF (ed): Noninvasive Diagnostic Techniques in Vascular Disease. St. Louis, The CV Mosby Company, 1982, pp 482–496.
32. Strandness DE Jr, Sumner DS: Ultrasonic velocity detector in the diagnosis of thrombophlebitis. Arch Surg 104:180–183, 1972.
33. Kakkar VV: Fibrinogen uptake for detection of deep venous thrombosis. A review of current practice. Semin Nucl Med 7:229–244, 1977.
34. Henkin RE, Yao JST, Quinn JL III, et al: Radionuclide venography (RNV) in lower extremity venous disease. J Nucl Med 15:171–175, 1976.
35. Singer I, Royal HD, Uren RF, et al: Radionuclide

plethysmography and Tc-99m red blood cell venography in venous thrombosis: comparison with
contrast venography. Radiology 150:213–217, 1984.

36. Hull RD, Hirsh J: 125-I-fibrinogen leg scanning. In
Bernstein EF (ed): Noninvasive Diagnostic Tech-
niques in Vascular Disease. St. Louis, The CV
Mosby Company, 1982, pp. 497–501.

37. Harris WH, Salzman EW, Athanasoulis C, et al:
Comparison of 125-I-fibrinogen count scanning
with phlebography for detection of venous thrombi
after elective hip surgery. N Engl J Med
292:665–667, 1975.

38. Benedict KT Jr, Wheeler HB, Patwardhan NA:
Impedance plethysmography: Correlation with
contrast venography. Radiology 125:695–699, 1977.

39. Hull RD, Hirsh J: Comparative value of tests for
the diagnosis of venous thrombosis. In Bernstein
EF (ed): Noninvasive Diagnostic Techniques in Vascular Disease. St. Louis, The CV Mosby Company,
1982, pp 522–538.

40. Coon WW, Willis PW III: Thrombosis of the axillary
and subclavian veins. Arch Surg 94:657–663, 1967.

41. Tilney NL, Griffiths HJG, Edwards EA: Natural
history of major venous thrombosis of the upper
extremity. Arch Surg 101:792–796, 1970.

42. Thomas ML, Andress MR: Axillary phlebography.
AJR 113:713–721, 1971.

43. Prescott SM, Tikoff G: Deep venous thrombosis of
the upper extremity: a reappraisal. Circulation
59:350–355, 1979.

44. van Deventer GM, Snyder N III, Patterson M: The
superior vena cava syndrome. A complication of
the LeVeen shunt. JAMA 242:1655–1656, 1979.

45. Adams JT, McEvoy RK, DeWeese JA: Primary deep
venous thrombosis of upper extremity. Arch Surg
91:29–42, 1965.

46. Swinton NW, Edgett JW Jr, Hall RJ: Primary subclavian–axillary vein thrombosis. Circulation
38:737–745, 1968.

47. Hewitt RL: Acute axillary vein obstruction by the
pectoralis minor muscle. N Engl J Med 279:595,
1968.

48. Gordon DH, Rose JS, Kottmeier P, et al: Jugular
venous ectasia in children. A report of 3 cases and
review of the literature. Radiology 118:147–149,
1976.

49. Pataro VF, Crosbie JC, Conde RM: Jugular phle-
bectasias. J Cardiovasc Surg 2:3–8, 1961.

50. Okay NH, Bryk D, Kroop IG, et al: Phlebectasia of
the jugular and mediastinal veins. Radiology
95:629–630, 1970.

51. Tierstein AS: Editorial. Diagnostic procedures in
patients with superior vena cava syndrome. JAMA
245:956, 1981.

52. Lockrich JJ, Goodman R: Superior vena cava syndrome. Clinical management. JAMA 231:58–61,
1975.

53. Hussey HH, Katz S, Yater WM: The superior vena
caval syndrome. Report of thirty-five cases. Am
Heart J 31:1–26, 1946.

54. Lesavoy MA, Norberg HP, Kaplan EL: Substernal
goiter with superior vena caval obstruction. Surgery 77:325–329, 1975.

55. Ochs H, Brecht Th, Brecht G, et al: Idiopathische
Thrombose der oberen Hohlvene. Dtsch Med
Wochenschr 101:1193–1196, 1976.

56. Ahmad N, Payne RF: Thrombosis after central
venous cannulation. Med J Aust 1:217–220, 1976.

57. Foley WJ, Elliott JP Jr, Smith RF, et al: Central

venous thrombosis and embolism associated with
peritoneovenous shunts. Arch Surg 119:713–720,
1984.

58. Calhoun TR, Wright RM Jr, Cimo PL, et al: Use of
cardiopulmonary bypass for thrombectomy in acute
superior vena cava syndrome. Tex Heart Inst J
10:347–350, 1983.

59. Kappes S, Towne J, Adams M, et al: Perforation of
the superior vena cava. A complication of subclavian dialysis. JAMA 249:2232–2233, 1983.

60. Perez D, Brown L: Follicular carcinoma of the
thyroid appearing as an intraluminal superior vena
cava tumor. Arch Surg 119:323–326, 1984.

61. Okay NH, Bryk D: Collateral pathways in occlusion
of the superior vena cava and its tributaries. Radiology 92:1493–1498, 1969.

62. Ferris EJ, Hipona FA, Kahn PC, et al: Venography
of the Inferior Vena Cava and Its Branches. Huntington, NY, RE Krieger Publishing Company,
1973.

63. Siqueira-Filho AG, Kottke BA, Miller WE: Primary
inferior vena cava thrombosis. Report of nine cases.
Arch Intern Med 136:799–802, 1976.

64. Missal ME, Robinson JA, Tatum RW: Inferior vena
cava obstruction. Clinical manifestations, diagnostic methods, and related problems. Ann Intern Med
62:133–161, 1965.

65. Ranninger, K, Switz DM: Local obstruction of the
inferior vena cava by massive ascites. AJR
93:935–939, 1965.

66. Neistadt A, Jones T, Rob C: Vascular system involvement by idiopathic retroperitoneal fibrosis.
Surgery 59:950–954, 1966.

67. Doppman J, Rubinson RM, Rockoff SD, et al:
Mechanism of obstruction of the infradiaphrag-
matic portion of the inferior vena cava in the
presence of increased intraabdominal pressure. Invest Radiol 1:37–53, 1966.

68. Samuel E: The inferior vena cavogram in pregnancy. Proc Roy Soc Med 57:702–704, 1964.

69. Sos TA, Baltaxe HA: Spurious complete obstruction
of the inferior vena cava in an adult as a result of
the Valsalva maneuver. Radiology 119:280, 1976.

70. Kadir S, O'Neal JA: Pseudoobstruction of the inferior vena cava in pediatric abdominal masses. J
Cardiovasc Intervent Radiol 5:25–29, 1982.

71. Kudsk KA, Bongard F, Lim RC Jr: Determinants of
survival after vena caval injury. Analysis of a 14
year experience. Arch Surg 119:1009–1012, 1984.

71a. Ochsner JL, Crawford ES, DeBakey ME: Injuries
of the vena cava caused by external trauma. Surgery 49:397–402, 1961.

72. Brewster DC, May ARL, Darling RC, et al: Variable
manifestations of vascular injury during lumbar
disc surgery. Arch Surg 114:1026–1030, 1979.

73. Kadir S, Coulam CM: Intracaval extension of renal
cell carcinoma. Cardiovasc Intervent Radiol
3:180–183, 1980.

74. Ferris EJ, Bosniak MA, O'Connor JF: An angiographic sign demonstrating extension of renal carcinoma into the renal vein and vena cava. AJR
102:384–391, 1968.

75. Iverson LIG, Lee J, Drew D, et al: Intravenous
leiomyomatosis with cardiac extension. Tex Heart
Inst J 10:275–278, 1983.

76. Albrechtsson U: The portal vein as a collateral in
inferior vena cava obstruction. J Cardiovasc Radiol
2:107–110, 1979.

77. Gorenstein AI, Gordon RL, Shifrin E, et al: Collat-

eral pathways in inferior vena caval obstruction in children, including the cavo-portal route. Pediatr Radiol 10:225–228, 1981.

78. Kadir S, Athanasoulis CA: Percutaneous retrieval of intravascular foreign bodies. *In* Athanasoulis CA et al (eds): Interventional Radiology. Philadelphia, WB Saunders Company, 1982, pp 379–390.

79. Allen JE, Morse TS, Frye TR, et al: Vena cavagrams in infants and children. Ann Surg 160:568–574, 1964.

80. Sclafani SJA, Gordon DH, Mitchell S: Laceration of the inferior vena cava on angiographic demonstration. Cardiovasc Intervent Radiol 6:164–166, 1983.

81. Lien HH, Kolbenstvedt A: Nonmalignant venographic abnormalities of the inferior vena cava. Radiology 122:105–110, 1977.

82. Helander CG, Lindbom A: Venography of the inferior vena cava. Acta Radiol 52:257–268, 1959.

83. Hunter WC, Sneeden VD, Robertson TD, et al: Thrombosis of the deep veins of the leg. Its clinical significance as exemplified in 351 autopsies. Arch Intern Med 68:1–17, 1941.

84. McLachlin J, Paterson JC: Some basic observations on venous thrombosis and pulmonary embolism. Surg Gynecol Obstet 93:1–8, 1951.

85. Kakkar VV, Howe CT, Flanc C, et al: Natural history of postoperative deep vein thrombosis. Lancet 2:230–232, 1969.

86. Dale WA, Lewis MR: Heparin control of venous thromboembolism. Arch Surg 101:744–755, 1970.

87. Kakkar VV, Howe CT, Nicolaides AN, et al: Deep vein thrombosis of the leg. Is there a "high risk" group? Am J Surg 120:527–530, 1970.

88. Angles-cano E, Clauvel JP, Sultan Y: Letter. JAMA 241:2785–2786, 1979.

89. Iyer SK, Handler LJ, Johnston JS: Thrombophlebitis migrans in association with ulcerative colitis. J Nat Med Assn 73:987–989, 1981.

90. Menzoian JO, Sequiera JC, Doyle JE, et al: The therapeutic and clinical course of deep vein thrombosis. Am J Surg 146:581–585, 1983.

91. Thomas ML, O'Dwyer JA: A phlebographic study of the incidence and significance of venous thrombosis in the foot. AJR 130:751–754, 1978.

92. Danecke K: Der Plantarschmerz als Früehsymptom einer beginnender Thrombose der unteren extremitaet. Munch Medizin Wochenschr 76:1912–1913, 1929.

93. Browse NL, Thomas ML: Source of nonlethal pulmonary emboli. Lancet 1:258–259, 1974.

94. Young JR: Thrombophlebitis and chronic venous insufficiency. Geriatrics 28:63–69, 1973.

95. Hull R, Hirsh J, Sackett DL, et al: Clinical validity of a negative venogram in patients with clinically suspected venous thrombosis. Circulation 64:622–625, 1981.

96. Stallworth JM, Hennigar GR, Jonsson HT, et al: The chronically swollen painful extremity. JAMA 228:1656–1659, 1974.

97. Kilcoyne RF, Imray TJ, Stewart ET: Ruptured Baker's cyst simulating acute thrombophlebitis. JAMA 240:1517–1518, 1978.

98. Gordon GV, Edell S, Brogadir SP, et al: Baker's cyst and true thrombophlebitis. Report of two cases and review of the literature. Arch Intern Med 139:40–42, 1979.

99. Flanc C: An experimental study of the recanalization of arterial and venous thrombi. Br J Surg 55:519–524, 1968.

100. Moreno-Cabral R, Kistner RL, Nordyke RA: Importance of calf vein thrombophlebitis. Surgery 80:735–742, 1976.

101. Craig O, Hobbs JT: Vulval phlebography in the pelvic congestion syndrome. Clin Radiol 25:517–525, 1974.

102. Chidekel N: Female pelvic veins demonstrated by selective renal phlebography with particular reference to pelvic varicosities. Acta Radiol 7:193–211, 1968.

103. Mellmann J, Wuppermann Th, von Schweder WJ: Zur Morphometrie primärer Varizen. Fortschr Roentgenstr 126:205–209, 1977.

104. Ney C, Miller HL, Friedenberg RM: Various applications of corpus cavernosography. Radiology 119:69–73, 1976.

105. Velcek D, Evans JA: Cavernosography. Radiology 144:781–785, 1982.

106. Thomas ML, Andress MR: Angiography in venous dysplasias of the limbs. AJR 113:722–731, 1971.

107. Cockett FB, Thomas ML: The iliac compression syndrome. Br J Surg 52:816–821, 1965.

108. Rich NM, Hobson RW II, Collins GJ Jr, et al: The effect of acute popliteal venous interruption. Ann Surg 183:365–368, 1976.

109. Willen J, Bergqvist D, Hallbook T: Venous insufficiency as a late complication after tibial fracture. Acta Orthop Scand 53:149–153, 1982.

110. Johnson JE, Lucas CE, Ledgerwood AM, et al: Infected venous pseudoaneurysm. A complication of drug addiction. Arch Surg 119:1097–1098, 1984.

111. Dahl JR, Freed TA, Burke MF: Popliteal vein aneurysm with recurrent pulmonary thromboemboli. JAMA 236:2531–2532, 1976.

# Pulmonary Angiography

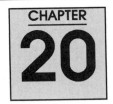

## ANATOMY

The main pulmonary artery arises from the right ventricle, lying anterior to the ascending aorta. It is approximately 5 cm long and 3 cm wide and lies within the pericardium (Fig. 20–1). It courses to the left of the aorta and bifurcates into the left and right pulmonary arteries in the concavity of the aortic arch.

The left pulmonary artery is shorter than the right (Fig. 20–2). At the hilus, it gives off three to five branches to the upper lobe, which may arise independently or as one or two small trunks. It then continues as the interlobar artery in the major fissure and divides into segmental branches for the lower lobe segments.

The right pulmonary artery passes behind the ascending aorta, superior vena cava, and right upper lobe pulmonary vein (Figs. 20–1 and 20–2). It lies anterior to the esophagus and the right upper lobe bronchus. At the hilus, it divides into a smaller upper lobe artery (superior branch) and a larger interlobar artery supplying the lower and middle lobes. The upper lobe artery divides into four branches. The middle lobe artery, which arises close to and occasionally together with the upper lobe artery, subdivides into a lateral and a medial branch. Occasionally, both branches arise independently from the interlobar artery. The lower lobe artery divides into segmental arteries for each lower lobe segment. The branching pattern of the pulmonary arteries corresponds to that of the bronchi.

The pulmonary veins (Fig. 20–3) drain into the left atrium. On the left side, the three segmental upper lobe veins form the superior pulmonary vein. The two main lower lobe veins form the left inferior pulmonary vein. On the right side, the middle lobe vein joins the upper lobe veins to form the right superior pulmonary vein.

## Congenital Anomalies

Most congenital anomalies of the pulmonary vessels are observed in association with congenital cardiac diseases and will not be discussed here.

**Hypoplasia.** Hypoplasia of the right pulmonary artery is seen in the hypogenetic lung syndrome. Other abnormalities associated with this syndrome are hypoplasia of the right lung with systemic arterial supply and partial or totally anomalous venous drainage from the right lung into systemic veins, usually to the IVC. A portion of the venous return may be to the left atrium, and communicating vessels may be present between the normal and the abnormal veins.[1, 2] The anomalously draining vein is frequently seen on the chest radiograph and is also called the "scimitar syndrome"[2] (Fig. 20–4).

On the chest radiograph, the right hemithorax is smaller than the left, and there is a shift of the mediastinal structures to the right side. In addition, reticular-appearing densities (enlarged bronchial and transpleural collaterals) and rib notching are seen.[3] The right hilus appears small, owing to the absence of the right pulmonary artery. Systemic arterial supply to the affected lung is derived from the thoracic (bronchial, intercostal, transpleural) or abdominal (celiac artery, transdiaphragmatic) aorta.[2, 3]

**Agenesis.** In agenesis of the lung, the ipsilateral pulmonary artery is absent and the affected hemithorax is small. The normal opposite lung occupies the entire thoracic cavity and the mediastinal structures are shifted to the affected side (Fig. 20–5).

**Anomalous Origin of the Pulmonary Arteries.** In the absence of congenital heart

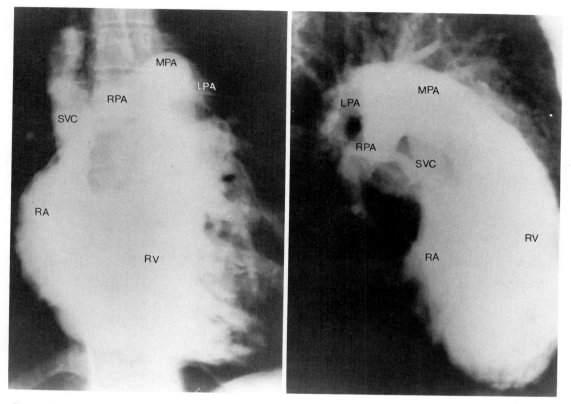

*Figure 20–1.* AP and lateral right ventriculogram showing normal proximal pulmonary artery anatomy. LPA = left pulmonary artery; MPA = main pulmonary artery; RA = right atrium; RPA = right pulmonary artery; RV = right ventricle; SVC = superior vena cava.

disease, an anomalous origin of a pulmonary artery has been reported from the ascending aorta (right pulmonary artery with a left aortic arch; left pulmonary artery with a right aortic arch), left pulmonary artery from the right (pulmonary sling), and rarely from the abdominal aorta or its branches.[4–6] The pulmonary sling is responsible for obstruction of the distal trachea, the right bronchus, or both structures.[7]

## ANGIOGRAPHY

All patients undergoing pulmonary arteriography must have continuous cardiac monitoring, since catheter manipulation in the heart can cause life-threatening conduction defects and arrhythmias. Lidocaine for intravenous injection and a defibrillator must be at hand.

**Pressure Monitoring.** IVC, SVC, and right atrial pressures should be recorded prior to catheter manipulation in the right heart.

Right ventricular pressure may be recorded either before advancing the catheter into the pulmonary artery or upon completion of the contrast study. Pulmonary artery pressure must be measured before contrast medium is injected (see next section). The catheter should be connected to a pressure transducer for continuous pressure monitoring during catheter manipulation through the heart. This aids in identifying catheter position and is particularly helpful in differentiating between the right ventricle and the coronary sinus.

**EKG Monitoring.** Continuous EKG monitoring is mandatory during pulmonary arteriography and in particular during catheter manipulation through the right heart. Premature ventricular contractions occur frequently, but if a "run" of five or more such beats is observed, the catheter must immediately be withdrawn into the right atrium. Catheter manipulation is resumed after the baseline rhythm is restored.

Ventricular tachycardia usually breaks

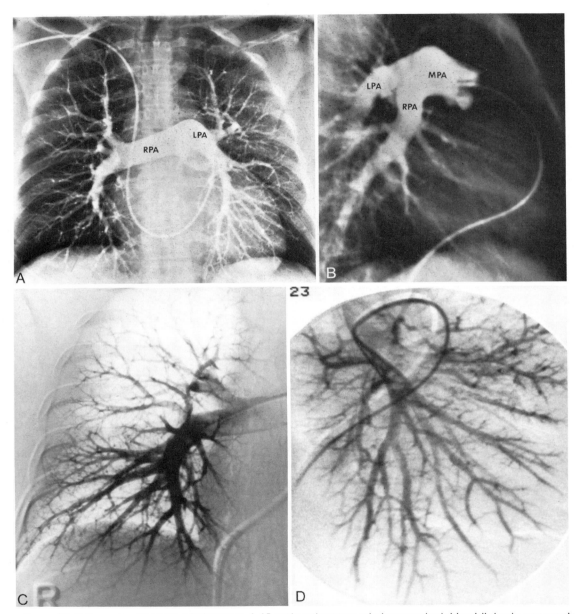

*Figure 20–2.* Normal pulmonary arteriograms. *A,* AP main pulmonary arteriogram via right cubital vein approach. *B,* Lateral main pulmonary arteriogram. *C,* Subtraction film from a normal right pulmonary arteriogram. *D,* Normal left posterior oblique pulmonary arteriogram using intraarterial DSA. For abbreviations see legend for Figure 20–1.

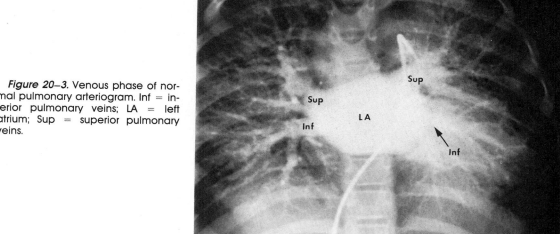

*Figure 20–3.* Venous phase of normal pulmonary arteriogram. Inf = inferior pulmonary veins; LA = left atrium; Sup = superior pulmonary veins.

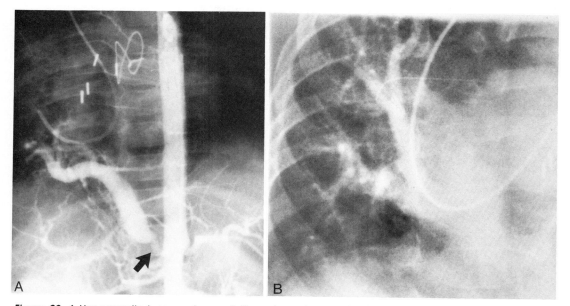

*Figure 20–4.* Hypogenetic lung syndrome. *A,* Thoracic aortogram shows a large, anomalous vessel originating from the abdominal aorta and supplying the right lower lobe. A stenosis is present at the orifice of this vessel (*arrow*). Venous catheter is in the anomalous pulmonary vein. *B,* Venous phase of pulmonary arteriogram shows anomalous venous drainage to the right atrial–inferior vena caval junction. (Courtesy of Dr. Jean Kan.)

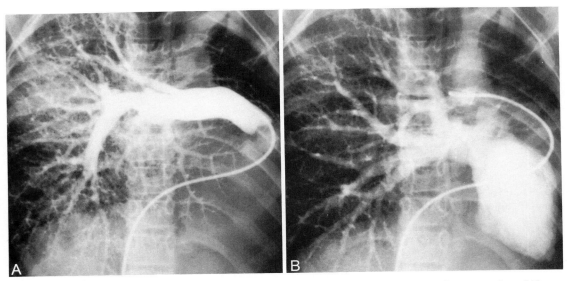

*Figure 20–5.* Agenesis of left lung. *A,* AP pulmonary arteriogram shows absence of left pulmonary artery. *B,* Venous phase shows normal return. Note position of mediastinal structures in the left hemithorax. In addition, the right lung also occupies the left hemithorax.

spontaneously. In patients with excessive ventricular irritability or ventricular tachycardia associated with a decrease in pressure, an intravenous bolus of lidocaine (100 mg) should be injected. Ventricular flutter or fibrillation requires defibrillation.

## Indications, Contraindications, and Precautions

Thromboembolic disease is by far the most common indication for pulmonary arteriography in the adult patient. Other indications include evaluation and treatment of pulmonary arteriovenous malformations and aneurysms and occasionally the evaluation of mediastinal neoplasms.

Pulmonary arteriography is contraindicated in patients with severe pulmonary hypertension (systolic pulmonary artery pressure >100 mg Hg). It should not be considered safe in patients with end-diastolic right ventricular pressure above 20 mm Hg[8] and systolic pulmonary artery pressure over 80 mm Hg. Contrast injection into the right heart chambers or the pulmonary arteries in such patients may lead to acute right heart failure and death. In such patients, balloon occlusion arteriography can be performed safely using 5 to 7 ml of contrast medium per injection, or nonionic contrast agents are used since these do not elevate the pulmonary artery pressure as significantly.[9]

The presence of a left bundle branch block is also a contraindication for catheter manipulation through the heart. Catheter-induced right bundle branch block may occur, leading to complete heart block. In such patients, the indications for pulmonary arteriography must be reevaluated, and intravenous digital subtraction angiography (DSA) must be given consideration. If selective arteriography is considered necessary, a transvenous pacemaker must be inserted before catheterization.

## Arteriographic Techniques

Pulmonary arteriography can be performed from the femoral or the cubital/basilic vein. From the femoral approach, both pigtail and balloon catheters can be used. From the arm approach, the NIH type or balloon catheters are used.

### Femoral Approach for Pulmonary Arteriography

The femoral approach is contraindicated if iliofemoral venous thrombosis is suspected. After venous access is obtained and the sheath from the Amplatz needle or a short 6 Fr vessel dilator is inserted into the femoral vein, 5 to 10 ml of contrast medium is injected, and the bolus is followed through the IVC to assess patency. If no thrombus is seen, the angiographic catheter is inserted.

If an abnormality is detected, a venogram or venacavagram is obtained to document the extent of disease, and the arm approach is used for pulmonary arteriography. In one study, thrombi were detected in the IVC in 14% of patients undergoing pulmonary arteriography.[10] These occurred more frequently in patients with positive pulmonary arteriograms.

### Pigtail Catheter Method

TIP DEFLECTING WIRE TECHNIQUE (Fig. 20–6). A 7 or 7.1 Fr, 100 cm long polyethylene pigtail catheter is advanced to the right atrium. A 100 cm long tip deflecting wire is inserted, and the catheter tip is deflected 90° towards the tricuspid valve. While the deflection is maintained and the wire is held in place, the catheter is advanced into the right ventricle. Once it is in the right ventricle, the deflection is released and the catheter straightens out, bringing the tip into the right ventricular outflow tract. The wire is then advanced to the catheter tip in order to stiffen the catheter, without applying deflection. While holding the wire in place, the catheter is rotated in a counterclockwise direction and advanced into the pulmonary artery.

STIFF GUIDE WIRE TECHNIQUE (Fig. 20–7). The stiff end of a heavy duty guide wire is bent 180° (see Chapter 2, Fig. 2–27). With the pigtail catheter in the right atrium and the pigtail facing the tricuspid valve, the bent stiff end of the guide wire is inserted up to the pigtail. This usually provides a 60 to 70° deflection to the catheter. The wire *must not* straighten out the pigtail or exit from the catheter (end or side holes). While holding the wire in place, the catheter is advanced into the right ventricle. Once in the ventricle, the stiff end is removed, and the soft end of the wire is inserted up to the pigtail to stiffen the catheter. Again, the wire is held in place and the catheter rotated counterclockwise and advanced into the pulmonary artery.

### Grollman Type Pigtail Catheter Method.

A 6.7 Fr Grollman catheter is inserted into the right atrium via the femoral approach.[11] If the right atrium is not enlarged, the catheter can be advanced into the right ventricle (Fig. 20–8). As it enters the right ventricle, a counterclockwise rotation brings the pigtail into the outflow tract, and the catheter is further advanced into the pulmonary artery.

If the right atrium is enlarged, the short limb on the standard Grollman catheter may not negotiate the tricuspid valve. In this case, the bent stiff end of the guide wire or a tip deflecting wire is used to facilitate catheter entry into the right ventricle (see previous section on Pigtail Catheter Method). Alternatively, a Grollman catheter with a longer limb (Hopkins curve) is used.

RIGHT ATRIAL LOOP TECHNIQUE. This is used in individuals with dilated right heart chambers, in whom it is often difficult to negotiate the tricuspid valve and direct the Grollman catheter into the pulmonary artery. The right atrial loop technique is illustrated in Figure 20–9.

### Balloon Catheter Method.

A 7 Fr sheath is placed in the femoral or arm vein. A 7 Fr angiographic balloon catheter (end hole occluded, multiple side holes) is advanced into the right atrium. The balloon is inflated and can usually be advanced through the right ventricle into the pulmonary artery. Again, a rotatory motion may be required to direct the balloon catheter into the pulmonary artery. The catheter has little stiffness and cannot be torqued satisfactorily. It often advances into the right ventricular apex and cannot be brought into the outflow tract or the pulmonary artery. In this case, a loop is formed in the right atrium using the same technique as for the Grollman catheter. As the catheter tip enters the ventricle, the balloon comes to lie in the right ventricular outflow tract. At this point, if the catheter does not advance into the pulmonary artery, a guide wire is inserted up to the catheter tip. This often provides the stiffness required to torque and advance the catheter.

### Arm Approach for Pulmonary Angiography

A balloon or closed end NIH type catheter may be used through a sheath placed percutaneously in the cubital or basilic vein.

### Balloon Catheter Method.

Although a medial (cubital or basilic) vein is preferred, the cephalic vein can be used, provided it is large. A 7 Fr angiographic balloon catheter is used. The balloon is inflated in the right atrium and can usually be advanced into the pulmonary artery without much difficulty.

### NIH Type Catheter Method.

A closed end, multiple side hole catheter is used. The catheter is brought into the right atrium, and the tip is anchored against the lateral right atrial wall for 10 to 15 seconds to form a loop. The catheter is rotated 180° and withdrawn slightly so that the tip enters the right ventricle. Once this happens, the catheter can

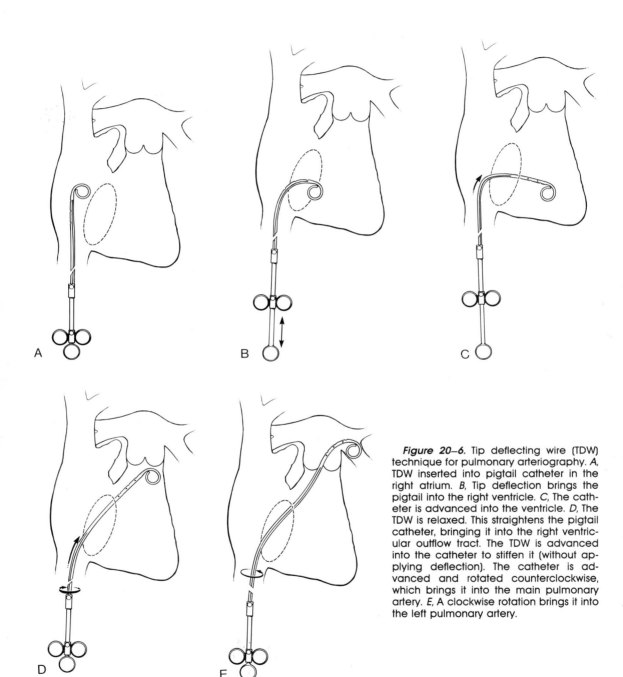

*Figure 20–6.* Tip deflecting wire (TDW) technique for pulmonary arteriography. *A,* TDW inserted into pigtail catheter in the right atrium. *B,* Tip deflection brings the pigtail into the right ventricle. *C,* The catheter is advanced into the ventricle. *D,* The TDW is relaxed. This straightens the pigtail catheter, bringing it into the right ventricular outflow tract. The TDW is advanced into the catheter to stiffen it (without applying deflection). The catheter is advanced and rotated counterclockwise, which brings it into the main pulmonary artery. *E,* A clockwise rotation brings it into the left pulmonary artery.

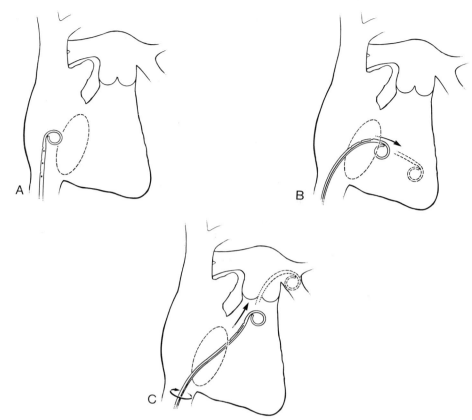

**Figure 20–7.** Stiff guide wire technique for pulmonary arteriography. *A,* Pigtail catheter in right atrium. *B,* As the bent stiff end of a heavy duty guide wire is advanced, the catheter tip is deflected through the tricuspid valve and the pigtail is advanced over the wire into the right ventricle. *C,* The soft end of the wire is inserted to stiffen the catheter, which is rotated counterclockwise and advanced into the pulmonary artery.

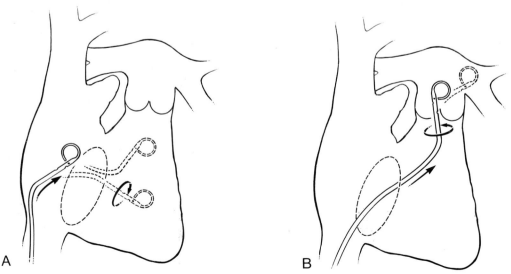

**Figure 20–8.** Grollman catheter method. *A,* Catheter is advanced into the right ventricle and rotated counterclockwise to bring the pigtail into the outflow tract. *B,* Once in the pulmonary artery, it is rotated clockwise to bring the pigtail into the left pulmonary artery.

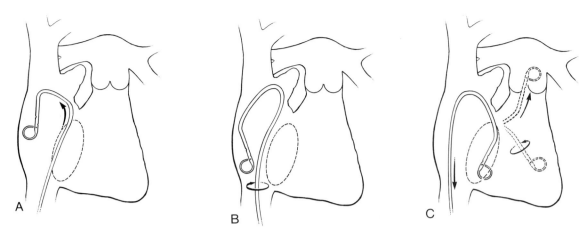

**Figure 20–9.** Right atrial loop technique. *A,* The Grollman catheter is brought against the lateral wall of the right atrium and a loop is formed. *B,* The catheter is rotated to bring the pigtail towards the tricuspid valve. *C,* As the catheter is withdrawn at the groin, the pigtail enters the ventricle. The catheter is rotated counterclockwise and advanced into the pulmonary artery.

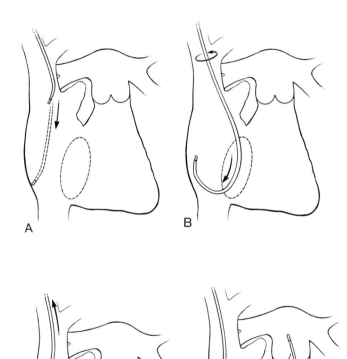

**Figure 20–10.** NIH type catheter method. *A,* The catheter is advanced into the right atrium. *B,* A loop is formed against the atrial wall. *C,* The catheter is rotated to bring the tip towards the tricuspid valve and is withdrawn slightly. *D,* Once the tip is in the ventricle, the catheter is advanced into the pulmonary artery.

be advanced into the pulmonary artery (Fig. 20–10).

## Balloon Occlusion Pulmonary Arteriography

This method may be used as a bedside procedure to confirm the diagnosis of embolism or in the angiographic suite in patients with severe pulmonary hypertension. Contrast injection into the balloon-occluded pulmonary artery is associated with coughing. This can be prevented by adding 2 mg of lidocaine per ml of contrast medium.

**Bedside Method.** This is not a substitute for standard pulmonary arteriography and should be used only in severely ill patients who cannot be moved for arteriography.[12] It provides a nonselective, random pulmonary arteriogram that may not be accurate, ie, the arteriogram may be normal but emboli may be present in other branches.

A pulmonary wedge balloon catheter (end hole only) is flow directed into the pulmonary artery. The catheter is attached to a pressure monitor, and the balloon is test inflated prior to angiography to determine the volume of air or $CO_2$ needed to occlude the branch. Occlusion is confirmed by observation of a dampened pressure wave form. For arteriography, the balloon is reinflated with the predetermined volume of air or $CO_2$; 3 to 5 ml of contrast medium (60% with 2 mg of lidocaine added per ml of contrast) is injected over 2 to 3 seconds; and a portable 14 × 17 inch radiograph is obtained. The balloon is deflated immediately thereafter.

**Fluoroscopic Guided Method.** This is used in patients with severe pulmonary hypertension, in whom standard arteriography is contraindicated. Another indication for this method is an equivocal cut film arteriogram.[13] The absence of flow artefacts and superior pulmonary artery opacification permit accurate detection of smaller thrombi. The radionuclide ventilation/perfusion scan is used as a guide to the area of suspected disease. The small volume of contrast medium used with this method does not precipitate acute right heart failure. When used as the only method, it has the disadvantage of being more time consuming, and selective catheterization of a desired branch may be difficult.

A 7 Fr pulmonary wedge balloon catheter is inserted into the pulmonary artery from the groin or the arm approach. The balloon is slowly inflated with $CO_2$ or diluted contrast medium. As this is accomplished, the balloon begins to bounce back and forth. When occlusion is complete, balloon motion ceases completely. Overinflation must be avoided, as this can rupture the balloon and may result in injury to the pulmonary artery. Contrast medium (usually 5 to 10 ml, 60%) is injected slowly over 3 to 5 seconds until the entire vessel is opacified, and 3 to 4 films (105 mm spot or 14 × 14 inch cut films) are obtained in maximal inspiration at 1 film per second. The balloon is deflated immediately thereafter.

## Digital Subtraction Angiography

DSA can be used if the larger pulmonary artery branches (up to third order) are to be evaluated. This can be combined with selective catheterization or performed via a right atrial–SVC injection. For the latter, undiluted contrast medium is used (76%, approximately 20 ml per second, 30 ml total). Images are obtained at 2 to 3 per second for a total of 12 images and subsequently at 1 per second for an additional 5 images. In the former, about 30% contrast medium is necessary, and the injection and imaging rates are similar to those for cut film arteriography.

There are several disadvantages and limitations of pulmonary DSA with the currently available systems:

1. Comparatively poorer resolution (compared with cut film arteriography) of smaller branches if contrast medium is injected in the right atrium.

2. Applicability limited to cooperative and not very sick patients who can hold respiration for the duration of the imaging.

3. Pressure measurements cannot be obtained with the nonselective (right atrial–SVC contrast injection).

## Wedge Pulmonary Arteriogram

This technique is used for evaluating the pulmonary veins (ie, patency and drainage pattern). An end hole catheter is wedged into a pulmonary artery branch and 7 to 10 ml of contrast medium (60%) is hand injected over 2 to 3 seconds. Films (14 × 17 inch or 105 mm spot films) are obtained at 2 per second for a total of 10 films (Fig. 20–11).

## Selective Catheterization

**Left Pulmonary Artery.** The balloon and pigtail catheters usually advance into the left pulmonary artery. Occasionally, the Grollman catheter advances into the right pulmonary artery. To enter the left pulmonary

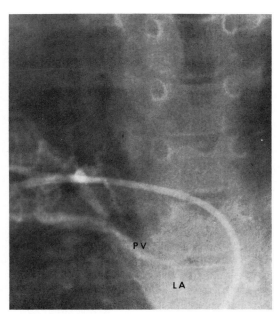

*Figure 20–11.* Wedge pulmonary arteriography. Late phase from a wedge pulmonary arteriogram shows normal pulmonary venous return. LA = left atrium; PV = pulmonary vein.

artery, the catheter is withdrawn into the main pulmonary artery. It is rotated so that the pigtail faces the left side and then advanced into the left pulmonary artery. If this is not successful, the stiff end of a guide wire is inserted to straighten out the distal bend, and both catheter and wire are advanced into the left pulmonary artery as a unit.

**Right Pulmonary Artery**

PIGTAIL CATHETER (Fig. 20–12). The tip deflecting wire is inserted and the catheter is withdrawn into the main pulmonary artery. Deflection is applied and the catheter and wire are rotated to deflect to the right. The wire is held in place as the catheter is advanced into the right pulmonary artery. If the catheter keeps reentering the left pulmonary artery, the tip lies in the left pulmonary artery and must therefore be withdrawn further to bring it into the main pulmonary artery.

GROLLMAN CATHETER. The catheter is withdrawn into the main pulmonary artery. It is rotated to point the pigtail to the right and advanced into the right pulmonary artery. If this is unsuccessful, the distal bend is accentuated by a tip deflecting wire or the bent stiff end of a heavy duty guide wire.

BALLOON CATHETER. The side to be catheterized is elevated by about 45 to 50°. The balloon catheter is withdrawn into the main pulmonary artery, and the balloon is inflated and advanced into the desired branch.

## Technical Problems During Catheterization

1. The catheter tip points in the direction of the right ventricle but will not advance and buckles in the right atrium: This occurs when the catheter tip has entered the coronary sinus. On AP fluoroscopy, it may not be possible to differentiate between catheter position in the coronary sinus or the right ventricle. If continuous pressure monitoring is used, right atrial pressure is measured, indicating that the catheter tip is in the coronary sinus (coronary sinus pressure is the same as the right atrial pressure). Alternatively, injection of 3 to 5 ml of contrast medium confirms the location (Fig. 20–13).

2. The catheter is in the right ventricular outflow tract but does not enter the pulmonary artery in the absence of pulmonary valve stenosis: The systolic-diastolic motion of the catheter tip is observed, and the catheter is advanced in synchronization with systole as the tip moves towards the pulmonary artery and the pulmonary valve is open.

**Catheterization of Segmental Branches.** This is required for balloon occlusion arteriography or for localization of pulmonary arteriovenous malformations for embolotherapy. The pulmonary artery is catheterized with a pigtail, Grollman, or balloon catheter. This is exchanged for a selective catheter over a heavy duty exchange guide wire. The different catheter shapes for selective catheterization are shown in Figure 20–14. These shapes can be steamed onto 6 to 9 Fr polyethylene catheters. In addition, the high torque multipurpose catheters are very useful for selective catheterization of the branches.

## Filming and Contrast Injection

For the evaluation of pulmonary emboli, AP and ipsilateral anterior (and occasionally the ipsilateral posterior) oblique projections are used. For the evaluation of pulmonary arteriovenous malformations, AP, lateral, and oblique arteriograms are obtained. The latter are necessary to define the arterial supply for selective catheterization and therapeutic embolization.

The injection and filming rates for pulmonary arteriography are shown in Table 20–1.

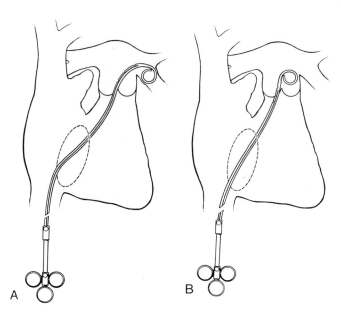

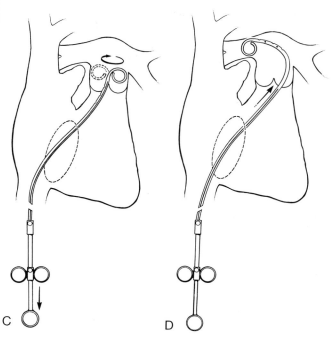

*Figure 20–12.* Selective catheterization of right pulmonary artery. *A,* Tip deflecting wire is inserted into the pigtail catheter, which is then withdrawn into the main pulmonary artery (*B*). *C,* Tip deflection is applied; the catheter is rotated to point towards the right. *D,* The catheter is advanced while holding the wire in place.

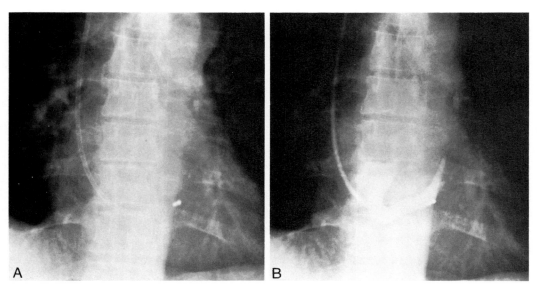

**Figure 20–13.** Catheter in coronary sinus. *A,* Without contrast medium or pressure monitoring, it is impossible to determine catheter position in the AP projection, ie, right ventricle versus coronary sinus. *B,* Contrast injection shows that catheter tip is in the coronary sinus.

Main pulmonary artery injections are avoided, since the diagnostic quality of such studies is inferior to that of selective left and right pulmonary arteriograms. Balloon occlusion or magnification AP or oblique arteriograms should be obtained to assess areas inadequately defined on the standard arteriogram. When using angiographic balloon catheters for arteriography, the balloon should be deflated or only partially inflated during contrast injection. All films are obtained in maximal inspiration.

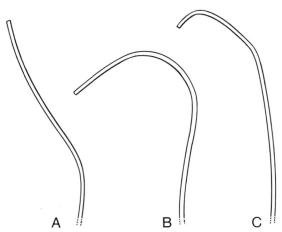

**Figure 20–14.** Catheter shapes for catheterization of segmental branches. *A,* Upper lobes; *B,* lower lobes; *C,* middle lobe and lingula.

**TABLE 20–1.** Pulmonary Arteriography

| | |
|---|---|
| Study | Left/right pulmonary arteriogram |
| Catheter: | 7 Fr pigtail, 6.7 Fr Grollman, 7 Fr angiographic balloon catheter |
| Position | Left or right pulmonary artery |
| Guide wire | Tip deflecting wire, bent stiff end of heavy duty guide wire |
| Contrast medium | 76% diatrizoate meglumine sodium |
| Injection rate/volume | 20–25 ml/sec, total 40–50 ml |
| Films: | 12 |
| Filming rate | 3 per second for 9 films 1 per second for 3 films |
| Projections | AP, obliques, magnification arteriography |
| Optional techniques | DSA, balloon occlusion arteriography |

### Catheter Removal

Upon completion of the arteriogram, pulmonary artery, ventricular, and atrial pressures should be recorded if this was not done prior to arteriography. The pigtail and Grollman catheters must be removed under fluoroscopic observation. The pigtail must be observed closely, especially if the catheter does not come out smoothly. In this case, the pigtail may have hooked a papillary mus-

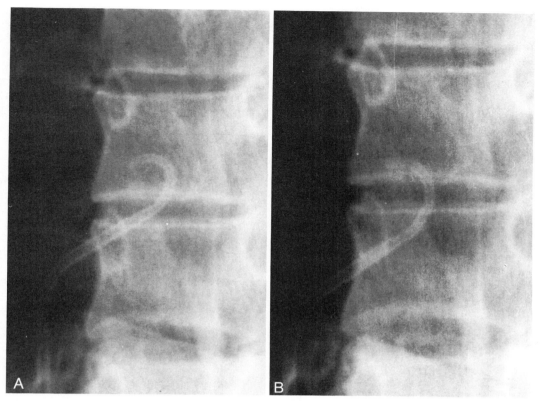

*Figure 20–15.* Hooked pigtail. *A,* Pigtail prior to removal from right ventricle. *B,* As the catheter is withdrawn, the pigtail opens because it has hooked onto a valve leaflet or chordae.

cle, chordae tendineae, or a tricuspid valve leaflet (Fig. 20–15). The catheter is readvanced into the right ventricle and rotated in an attempt to disengage it. If this is unsuccessful, a J LLT guide wire is inserted to straighten the pigtail and facilitate removal. Balloon catheters can be removed without fluoroscopy (with the balloon deflated).

## Complications

The majority of serious complications (with the exception of contrast-related problems) have been associated with the use of nonpigtail and nonballoon catheters. In one large series, major complications were observed in 3.2% of patients undergoing pulmonary arteriography.[8] Cardiac perforation and endomyocardial injury due to contrast jet constituted 46% of all major complications and occurred only with the use of stiffer nonpigtail catheters. Death occurred in 0.2% of patients, all of whom had pulmonary hypertension with an end-diastolic right ventricular pressure ≥ 20 mm Hg.[8] This complication is due to the sudden increase in pulmonary artery pressure following injection of hyperosmolar contrast agents.[9] Acute pulmonary edema can also occur after pulmonary arteriography in patients with poor cardiac function.

Catheter manipulation in the heart is frequently associated with premature contractions. Occasionally, ventricular tachycardia, flutter, fibrillation, or right bundle branch block may occur. Serious arrhythmias or cardiac arrest occurs in about 1% of patients.[8]

**Catheter-Related Complications.** Inappropriate flushing has been responsible for iatrogenic pulmonary thromboemboli. Such emboli are also observed in patients with indwelling pressure monitoring pulmonary artery catheters. Injury may occur to the papillary muscle or tricuspid valve apparatus if the pigtail is not removed carefully (Fig. 20–15). The only serious complication (other than contrast reactions) that we have observed during pulmonary arteriography is attributable to this type of injury.

With proper patient selection and careful

technique, pulmonary arteriography is a safe procedure with extremely few serious complications.

## THROMBOEMBOLIC DISEASE

Pulmonary emboli are diagnosed in about 1% of all hospitalized patients, and nonfatal emboli occur four times as frequently as fatal emboli.[14, 15] Pulmonary emboli are the cause of death in 6.9% of adult patients coming to autopsy.[16] The overall incidence of pulmonary emboli at autopsy is reported to be between 12 and 30%, but a careful search may detect the disease (old or recent) in 64% of cases.[16-18] In patients with clinically suspected or diagnosed deep venous thrombosis (DVT), the incidence of pulmonary emboli is between 9 and 56%, depending upon the type of diagnostic studies used for their detection.[18-20] Conversely, only 10 to 33% of patients with fatal pulmonary emboli have symptoms of DVT,[14, 18] and an ante-mortem diagnosis of pulmonary embolism is made in fewer than one third of patients.[14, 16-18] However, at autopsy 60% of adult patients with pulmonary emboli have DVT, most frequently in the leg veins (47%).[16]

In over half the patients, pulmonary embolization occurs to the lower lobes, in 25% the upper lobes are affected, in 65% the emboli are multiple, and in 42% the process is bilateral.[21] Pulmonary emboli (also massive emboli) may lyse spontaneously and disappear completely,[22] they may be organized and incorporated into the arterial wall as a plaque, or they may recanalize in a fashion similar to that seen in DVT.

The restoration of pulmonary blood flow depends upon the extent of embolization and the presence or absence of underlying cardiovascular disease. Complete recovery is more likely in the absence of underlying cardiovascular problems.[21]

Contrary to the general teaching that pulmonary infarction occurs in about 10% of pulmonary emboli, infarction may be observed in over half the cases.[16, 23] It is more likely to develop if the occlusion involves a segmental or distal branch and in the presence of cardiopulmonary disease with obstruction of the pulmonary venous outflow.[24, 25] The presence of precapillary arterial collaterals between the bronchial and pulmonary circulations and a hypertrophied bronchial circulation contribute significantly towards preventing infarction.[24]

Animal experiments show that partial resolution of nonmassive pulmonary emboli occurs within 24 hours.[26] This is explained by partial thrombolysis and fragmentation with resulting relocation of the fragments. Clinically, restoration of blood flow to the affected lung segment begins within 1 week and complete resolution can occur in 3 to 4 weeks.[21, 22, 27]

### Clinical Aspects

Pulmonary embolism may be difficult to diagnose clinically. The disease is self-limited in patients with nonmassive emboli and in the absence of underlying cardiopulmonary abnormalities. However, the importance of establishing the diagnosis and initiating early treatment is emphasized by the fact that, if left untreated, pulmonary embolization has a mortality of up to 26% as a result of recurrent embolization; with treatment, the mortality is reduced to below 8%.[28, 29]

Pulmonary emboli are fatal if more than 60% of the pulmonary arterial bed is obstructed.[30] Although the most frequent sources of pulmonary emboli are the lower extremity veins, emboli may also originate from the upper extremity veins,[16, 31] mural thrombi in the right heart chambers,[18] the renal veins, and occasionally from metastasizing tumors. Mural intracardiac thrombi occur in 4.5% of patients and are observed more frequently in patients with cardiac disease.[16] Microemboli (occlusion of vessels smaller than 1 mm in diameter) predominate in almost half the patients.[18, 32]

The peak incidence of pulmonary emboli is in patients 70 years and older.[18] The most frequent symptoms are: dyspnea (81%), pleuritic chest pain (72%), apprehension (59%), cough (54%), and hemoptysis (34%).[33] The last is usually in the form of streaking and, less frequently, frank expectoration of blood.[15, 33] Factors or diseases predisposing to pulmonary embolization are prolonged immobilization (due to trauma, operation, or chronic illness), cardiovascular diseases (eg, congestive heart failure), severe trauma, operation, polycythemia, malignancy, pregnancy, oral contraceptive intake, obesity, and a history of previous DVT or pulmonary emboli.

**EKG Changes.** These are observed in 83% of patients but are mostly nonspecific.[33] They include QRS, ST, and T wave changes, arrhythmias, and right bundle branch blocks. The only EKG findings specific for acute, significant pulmonary emboli (in the absence of underlying cardiopulmonary disease) are P-pulmonale, $S_1$ $Q_3$ $T_3$ pattern, and T wave inversion over the right precordial leads.[15]

**Arterial Blood Gases.** A wide range of arterial $pO_2$ values are found, corresponding to the severity of embolization and the presence of underlying cardiopulmonary disease. A fall in arterial $pO_2$ can be observed in obstruction of as little as 13% of the pulmonary arterial bed.[34] In patients without cardiopulmonary disease, the arterial $pO_2$ may be as low as 40 mm Hg or higher than 90 mm Hg. However, the likelihood of pulmonary emboli in patients with a $pO_2$ greater than 90 mm Hg is less than 5%.[34] This wide range of values makes arterial $pO_2$ a less valuable diagnostic aid.

**Chest Radiograph.** An abnormality is observed in 93% of patients with pulmonary emboli.[35] Most frequently, this is an area of consolidation, an elevated hemidiaphragm, atelectasis, or pleural effusion on the affected side. In the absence of cardiopulmonary disease, the presence of consolidation and elevation of the hemidiaphragm are valuable diagnostic signs and are each observed in 41% of patients.[33]

**Ventilation/Perfusion Scans.** A normal study virtually excludes the presence of clinically significant pulmonary emboli.[35, 36] Similarly, a clinically significant pulmonary embolus can be excluded if the V/Q scan is of low probability in the presence of a normal chest radiograph.[35] The accuracy of an abnormal scan varies according to the presence or absence of an abnormality on the plain chest radiograph and whether the defects are matched or mismatched. Under controlled experimental conditions and in the absence of radiographically visible pulmonary parenchymal abnormalities, perfusion scans are highly sensitive for the detection of emboli with a volume as small as 0.1 to 0.2 ml.[37] However, such "ideal" conditions are rarely encountered in the clinical setting.

Table 20–2 shows the incidence of pulmonary emboli in the different types of ventilation/perfusion abnormalities. In general, a ventilation/perfusion mismatch (segmental or larger) indicates a high likelihood of pulmonary emboli, but a match cannot exclude an embolus.[38] Matched V/Q defects occur early in pulmonary embolism as a result of transient reflux bronchoconstriction.[39, 40] In the clinical setting, the incidence of pulmonary emboli in the presence of perfusion defects alone is 71% if one or more segmental or larger defects are present and less than 27% if one or more subsegmental defects are present.[38] Occasionally, nonsegmental and diffuse abnormalities may be seen in association with pulmonary emboli.[35] In the presence of matched V/Q defects and consolidation of the chest radiograph, pulmonary emboli were found in 3 of 10 patients in one report.[41]

**Hemodynamic Changes.** Elevation of the pulmonary artery pressure corresponds to the severity of the embolic occlusion.[34, 42] Hemodynamic changes are usually observed in patients with obstruction of at least 25% of the pulmonary arterial bed. The mean

**TABLE 20–2.** V/Q Scans and Incidence of Pulmonary Emboli*

| Type of Abnormality on V/Q Scan | Incidence of Pulmonary Emboli by Arteriography | Overall Incidence† |
|---|---|---|
| Matched V/Q defect, > segmental, single or multiple | 23% | 46% |
| Matched V/Q defect, < segmental, single or multiple | 13% | 13% |
| V/Q mismatch, > segmental, single or multiple | 86% | 91% |
| V/Q mismatch, < segmental, single or multiple | 27% | 40% |
| Indeterminate | 17% | 58% |

*Adapted from Hull RD, et al: Ann Intern Med 98:891–899, 1983.
†Overall incidence of thromboembolic disease based upon positive pulmonary arteriography and leg venography.

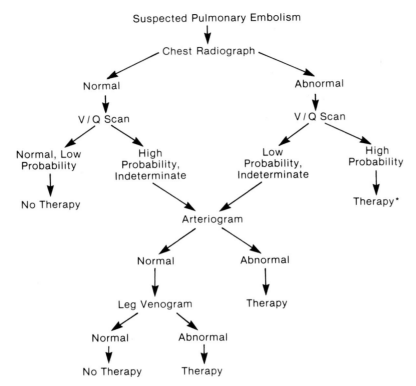

**Figure 20–16.** Sequence of studies for suspected pulmonary embolism. (*Arteriography may be necessary for documentation prior to thrombolytic therapy.)

pulmonary artery pressure is elevated but does not exceed 40 mm Hg even in the presence of massive embolization.[34] A mean pulmonary artery pressure above 40 mm Hg is obtained in patients with chronic recurrent emboli or pulmonary hypertension due to another cause. The cardiac index remains normal or is mildly increased in the presence of hypoxemia ($PO_2 < 60$ mm Hg).[34]

Changes in the right atrial pressure are a less reliable indicator of the severity of pulmonary embolization. Elevation of mean right atrial pressure in the presence of large emboli occurs in about 50% of patients.[34] However, up to 40% of the pulmonary arterial bed can be obstructed without increasing the right atrial pressure. Mean right atrial pressure changes occur in response to changes in the mean pulmonary artery pressure, usually if the latter exceeds 30 mm Hg.[34] Thus, in patients without underlying cardiopulmonary disease, elevation of right atrial pressure is an indicator of the severity of the pulmonary embolic occlusion.

**Sequence of Radiological Studies.** A chest radiograph should be the first study to exclude diseases that may produce similar symptomatology (eg, pneumonia, pneumo-

thorax, congestive heart failure). This should be followed by a V/Q scan. A normal chest radiograph with a normal or low probability scan virtually excludes the diagnosis of pulmonary emboli. A normal chest radiograph with a high probability scan is associated with a 50% incidence of pulmonary emboli.[35] A high probability scan with two or more major abnormalities on the chest radiograph (see earlier discussion) is virtually diagnostic of pulmonary emboli and does not require pulmonary arteriography unless this is indicated for documentation of emboli prior to thrombolytic therapy.

A positive or indeterminate scan should be followed by pulmonary arteriography. If the pulmonary arteriogram is normal, leg venography should be performed to detect DVT. A flow chart for the sequence of studies is shown in Figure 20–16. Since the treatment for DVT and pulmonary emboli is essentially the same, some authors recommend that leg venography, which is less invasive, be performed first and, if positive, pulmonary arteriography is not required.[38] Since about 30% of patients with pulmonary emboli have negative venograms[38] and ultimately may require pulmonary arteriography, we believe

# Zestril

## NOTES

LEFT OR RIGHT PULM ART

40-50d        20-25d / sec        36d

    3 / sec      ×      3 secs

    1 / sec      ×      3 secs

    AP

± Anterior Oblique

---

Rt Atrial Injection DSA.

Undiluted Contrast

30ds @ 20ds / sec

2 or 3 / sec              11 secs.

---

Left or Rt Pulmonary DSA        30%

18d        4 ds at 20ds / sec

3 / sec    for 6 secs

that the latter should be performed first. Serious complications are few, and the mortality associated with pulmonary arteriography can be virtually eliminated by careful patient selection.

## Arteriography

Arteriography must not be used as a screening procedure. However, it should be performed within 24 hours of the acute embolic episode. There are sufficient clinical, autopsy, and experimental data to support the fact that in almost half the patients the emboli affect the smaller vessels (microemboli) and that fragmentation, partial lysis, and relocation of larger (< segmental) emboli occur after 24 hours.[18, 21, 26, 37] Thus, a standard nonmagnification pulmonary arteriogram obtained more than 24 hours after the acute episode can be falsely normal. Therefore, if arteriography is delayed by 24 hours or more and main left or right pulmonary arteriograms are negative, an effort should be made to evaluate the smaller branches (1 to 2 mm diameter) by magnification arteriography. In view of this, the accuracy of arteriography would be enhanced, and it would be more cost efficient to perform arteriography within 24 hours of the episode.

In most cases, and especially if the arteriogram is performed within 24 to 48 hours of the acute episode, left and right pulmonary arteriograms are sufficient for the detection of pulmonary emboli. Oblique arteriograms are necessary if there is overlapping of vessels and if an embolus is not seen on the AP arteriogram. Although the ipsilateral anterior oblique projection (LAO for the left pulmonary arteriogram) is more helpful in most cases, occasionally the ipsilateral posterior oblique projection provides more information (see Fig. 20–17).[43]

Patients with clinically suspected pulmonary emboli, suspicious V/Q scan defects, and positive leg venograms may have normal pulmonary arteriograms (contrast injection into the left or right pulmonary arteries). In such patients, segmental arteriography using magnification techniques is more accurate in detecting the smaller emboli that are likely to be responsible for these defects and are not resolved by standard pulmonary arteriography. The V/Q scan should be used to guide the arteriographic evaluation of the area of suspected abnormality. A normal segmental magnification pulmonary arteriogram thus performed can effectively exclude a clinically significant pulmonary embolus.[44]

Arteriographic findings are as follows (Figs. 20–17 to 20–23; see also Fig. 20–32 and Chapter 7, Fig. 7–6): The two most reliably diagnostic arteriographic abnormalities are an intraluminal defect and an abrupt termination of a branch.

An intraluminal defect is the most frequent arteriographic abnormality and was observed in 94% of pulmonary arteriograms in one series.[38] Other arteriographic abnormalities that are less specific and thus less reliable than an intraluminal defect or an abrupt termination are:

1. Parenchymal hypovascularity (oligemia), which is often wedge shaped, especially when viewed in the lateral or oblique projections.

2. Absence of a draining vein from the affected segment(s).

3. Demonstration of tortuous arterial collaterals, especially in infarcts.

4. Hypervascularity of the infarcted segment:[45] Atelectasis may also contribute to this hypervascularity.

5. Organization: Eccentric or concentric plaque, web, or stenosis.

6. Recanalization with opacification of a new channel.

7. Pruning and attenuation of the branches: This is also a late sequela of pulmonary embolization.

If the AP arteriogram does not demonstrate an embolus, oblique arteriograms must be obtained. For the latter, segmental magnification arteriography guided by the V/Q scan provides the greatest accuracy.[44] Contrast injection into a lobar or segmental artery is essential for improving arterial opacification and diagnostic accuracy. Both the pigtail and the Grollman catheters can usually be advanced deep into the left or right pulmonary arteries to provide preferential opacification of the segmental arteries. Alternatively, a multiple hole multipurpose or balloon catheter can be used for selective arteriography.

PITFALLS IN DIAGNOSIS (Figs. 20–24 and 20–25; see also Fig. 20–19).

1. Streaming artifacts: Layering of contrast medium and inflow of unopacified blood often give rise to an artifact that simulates an embolus. However, evaluation of several films shows that the appearance of the artifact changes. In the presence of a thrombus, the proximal vessel is completely opacified (see Fig. 20–17C). In inflow artifacts, serial

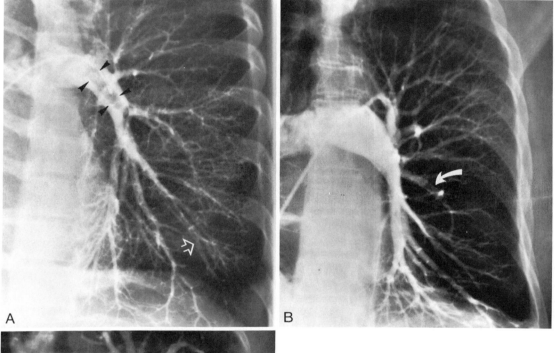

**Figure 20–17.** Pulmonary embolus presenting as intraluminal defect. *A,* LAO left pulmonary arteriogram shows a nonobstructing embolus (*arrowheads*). There is another embolus in a segmental branch (*open arrow*). *B,* LAO left pulmonary arteriogram from another patient shows an embolus in a segmental branch (*arrow*), *C,* Left posterior oblique pulmonary arteriogram from the same patient shown in *B.* The embolus is defined more clearly (*arrow*).

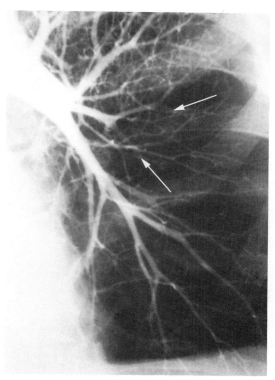

*Figure 20–18.* Pulmonary embolus causing an abrupt cut-off. LAO left pulmonary arteriogram shows abrupt termination of several branches (*arrows*). The lower lobe vessels are attenuated and fewer branches are opacified. Oligemia of the lower lobe is partly due to the presence of a large bulla.

films show inflow of unopacified blood into the proximal pulmonary arteries during the preceding systole, which then leads to poor opacification of some distal branches and simulates thromboemboli.

2. Overlapping or parallel vessels: These can occasionally simulate an embolus (Fig. 20–24).

3. Hypoperfusion in the left middle lung field: On the parenchymal phase of the arteriogram, a relatively hypovascular zone is frequently observed in the mid-portion of the left lung field. This is unrelated to embolic disease and is due to the anatomy of the left lung.

4. Vascular crowding: Atelectasis may be present in the absence of pulmonary emboli (Fig. 20–25).

## Nonangiographic Methods for Detection of Pulmonary Emboli

Other methods that have been or may be used for the detection of pulmonary emboli are computed tomography, magnetic resonance, and angioscopy.[46, 47] However, at the present stage of development, the sensitivity of these methods and the capability of resolving emboli in subsegmental vessels are far less than those of selective magnification arteriography.

## MISCELLANEOUS DISEASES

### Aneurysms

Most aneurysms of the pulmonary arteries are acquired (eg, mycotic, traumatic, or due to an arteritis or connective tissue disorder).[48] Mycotic aneurysms occur in patients with necrotizing pneumonias, chronic tuberculosis (Rasmussen's aneurysm), or following septic emboli (eg, sepsis, intravenous drug abuse)[48, 49] (Fig. 20–26). In connective tissue disorders (eg, Marfan's syndrome), there is dilatation of the main pulmonary artery and the proximal left and right pulmonary arteries. Aneurysms of the peripheral branches are not characteristic of this disorder. Dilatation of the central pulmonary arteries is also present in untreated atrial septal defects and pulmonary hypertension. Congenital peripheral pulmonary artery aneurysms are seen in association with arteriovenous malformations and sequestration.[5]

### Arteriovenous Malformations

Pulmonary arteriovenous malformation (AVM) may occur as an isolated abnormality or in association with hereditary hemorrhagic telangiectasia (Rendu-Osler-Weber syndrome). The pulmonary AVMs are multiple in approximately one third of patients, and 70% of the lesions are found in the lower lobes, often close to the surface of the lungs.[50] Up to 60% of patients with pulmonary AVMs may have hereditary hemorrhagic telangiectasia.[50] Conversely, 15% of patients with hereditary hemorrhagic telangiectasia have pulmonary AVMs.[51] The true incidence is probably much higher, however, since the smaller lesions may not be detectable without computed tomography of the chest or pulmonary arteriography. Occasionally, diffuse pulmonary telangiectasia may be present.[52, 53] In patients with the hereditary form, 40 to 50% have telangiectatic lesions of the skin, mucous membranes, and parenchymal and hollow organs.[54] The malformation is present from birth and is manifested gradu-

*Text continued on page 608*

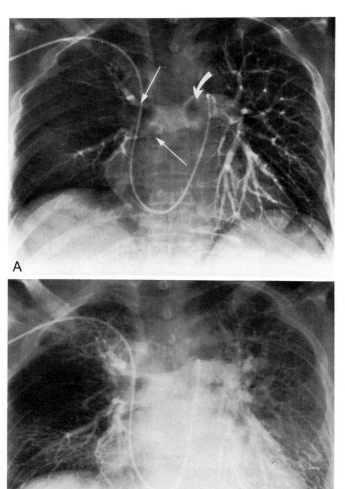

*Figure 20–19.* Large pulmonary embolus with wedge-shaped oligemia. *A,* Early arterial phase of main pulmonary arteriogram shows a large saddle embolus in the right pulmonary artery (*straight arrows*). Inflow of unopacified blood into the main pulmonary artery simulates an embolus (*curved arrow*). *B,* Later film from the same arteriogram shows a wedge-shaped oligemic area in the midportion of the right lung field (compare with the left lung). In addition, the main pulmonary artery is opacified. *Note:* Main pulmonary arteriograms are no longer performed for thromboembolic disease because of poorer resolution of smaller branches.

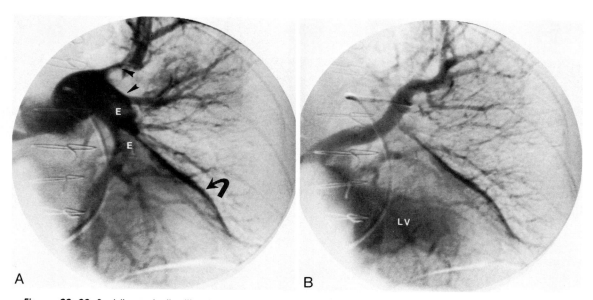

A   B

*Figure 20–20.* Saddle emboli with absent venous drainage. *A,* Left pulmonary arteriogram using DSA shows multiple emboli in the upper and lower lobe arteries (arrowheads and E). Curved arrow points to subtraction artifact caused by cardiac motion. *B,* Venous phase from same study shows no opacification of the main left inferior pulmonary vein. LV = left ventricle.

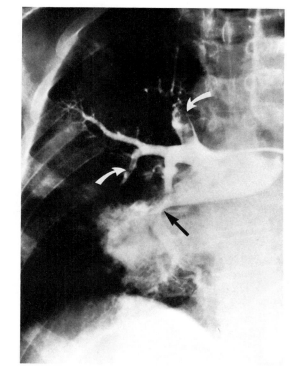

*Figure 20–21.* Multiple pulmonary emboli. Right pulmonary arteriogram in a patient with mycosis fungoides shows multiple emboli (*arrows*).

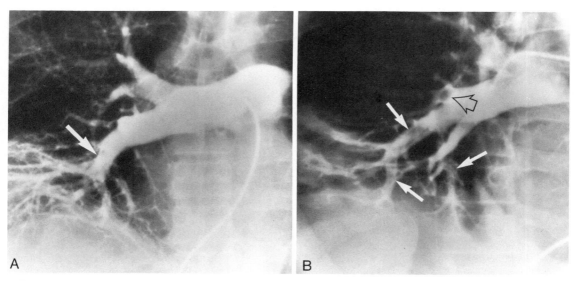

**Figure 20–22.** Value of oblique arteriography for detection of emboli. *A,* AP right pulmonary arteriogram shows a suspicious area at the base (*arrow*). There is a segmental parenchymal consolidation and hyperemia. *B,* Right anterior oblique arteriogram delineates the emboli in the lower lobe branches (*arrows*).

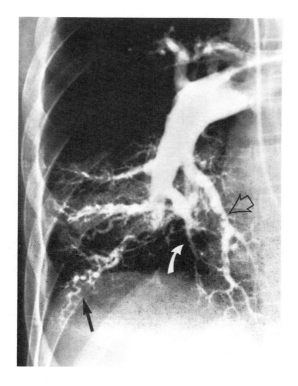

**Figure 20–23.** Chronic arterial abnormalities of the right lower lobe vessels due to pulmonary embolization. Several large vessels are occluded. Other branches show increased tortuosity (*black arrow*), attenuation (*curved arrow*), and stenosis (*open arrow*).

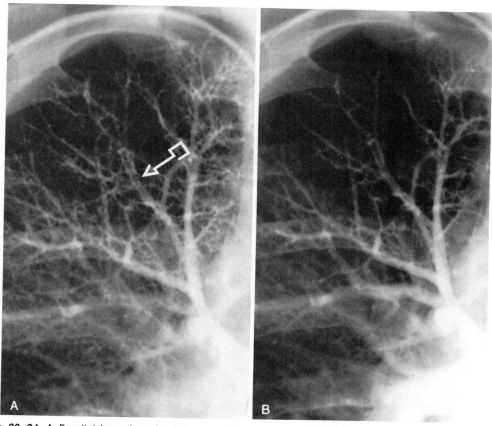

*Figure 20–24.* *A,* Parallel branches simulating a pulmonary embolus (*arrow*). *B,* Earlier frame from the same arteriogram shows two separate vessels.

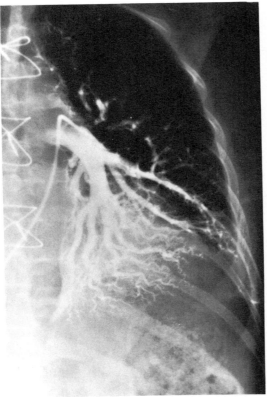

*Figure 20–25.* Left pulmonary arteriogram shows left lower lobe arterial crowding due to atelectasis.

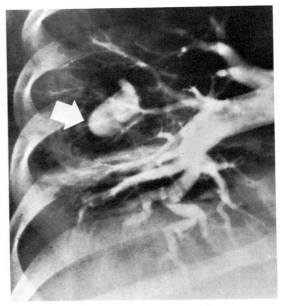

*Figure 20–26.* Mycotic pulmonary artery aneurysm (*arrow*) in a patient with necrotizing pneumonia.

ally as the abnormal vessels are subjected to higher pulmonary artery pressures.

The majority of patients (56%) with pulmonary AVMs are asymptomatic, and symptoms can generally be correlated with the size and number of AVMs.[50] A single AVM of less than 2 cm is usually asymptomatic. The most frequent symptoms and physical findings, in descending order of frequency, are dyspnea, cyanosis, clubbing of digits, and hemoptysis. Other manifestations are cerebrovascular accidents (hemorrhagic or embolic, the latter due to a paradoxical embolus) and brain abscesses. A right to left shunt is present with polycythemia and low arterial $pO_2$. Often a bruit can be heard over larger lesions.

On the chest radiograph, the AVMs appear as oval or round lobulated masses. A feeding artery and draining vein can frequently be identified. The angiographic appearance permits identification of two different types (Figs. 20–27 and 20–28):

1. Simple type: This occurs in 80% of pul-

monary AVMs and is characterized by a direct artery to vein communication. The venous limb is dilated, giving rise to a fusiform or saccular venous aneurysm. Ninety-five per cent of such AVMs involve the pulmonary arteries, whereas in the remainder the blood supply comes from a systemic artery.[50] Paradoxical embolization occurs in this type of AVM.

2. Complex type: This type occurs in 20% of pulmonary AVMs and is characterized by one or more feeding arteries and prominent draining veins. An interposed network of

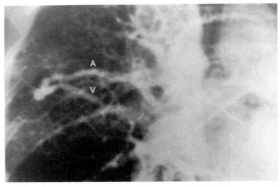

*Figure 20–27.* Simple pulmonary AVM. Close-up of right pulmonary arteriogram shows a simple upper lobe AVM. A = artery; V = vein.

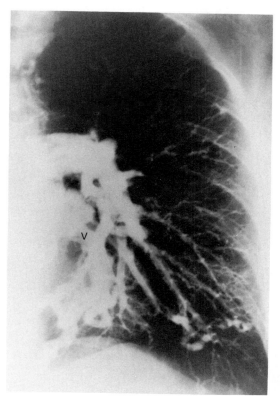

*Figure 20–28.* Complex pulmonary AVM. Left pulmonary arteriogram shows a large complex AVM in the lower lobe. In addition, there are several smaller simple AVMs. V = vein.

tortuous, dilated vascular channels is present between the arteries and veins.

Acquired pulmonary arteriovenous fistulae may be due to schistosomiasis, ruptured aneurysm, trauma, infection, or hepatogenic pulmonary angiodysplasia.[49, 55]

## Coarctation

Coarctation of the pulmonary arteries is a rare anomaly. It may affect a single artery or multiple vessels may be involved, and it may be proximal or distal in location (Fig. 20–29). On histological examination, the stenoses are due to fibrous proliferation of the intima. Pulmonary coarctation is frequently associated with pulmonary hypertension. The following are some of the modes of presentation[5, 56–58]:

1. Sporadic: This is an isolated abnormality with multiple central or peripheral pulmonary artery coarctations.

2. Congenital: This may be associated with other congenital cardiovascular abnormalities

(60% of cases).[56] The associated abnormalities include pulmonary valve stenosis, atrial and ventricular septal defects, patent ductus arteriosus, and aortic stenosis.

3. Familial: In this type, there is coarctation of the central pulmonary arteries and supravalvar aortic stenosis.

4. Post-rubella syndrome: Both the central and the peripheral pulmonary arteries are involved.

5. In association with idiopathic hypercalcemia.

## Chronic Inflammatory Diseases and Sepsis

In chronic inflammatory processes (eg, tuberculosis, bronchiectasis, sarcoidosis complicated by aspergillosis), there is hypertrophy of the bronchial and intercostal arteries. In addition, enlarged transpleural and transdiaphragmatic arterial channels are present. Mycotic pulmonary artery aneurysms (Ras-

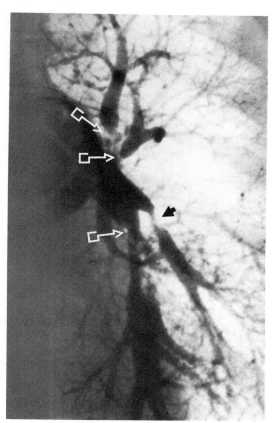

*Figure 20–29.* Coarctations of the pulmonary arteries. Left pulmonary arteriogram shows multiple stenoses of the proximal branches (*arrows*).

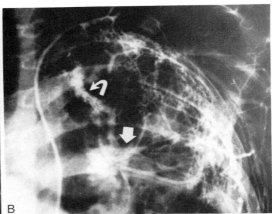

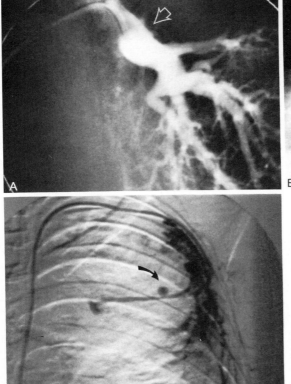

*Figure 20–30.* Pulmonary sarcoidosis with chronic left upper lobe infection. *A,* Digital subtraction left pulmonary arteriogram. There is occlusion of the left upper lobe arteries (*arrow*). *B,* Late film from left subclavian arteriogram shows numerous transpleural collaterals with opacification of the left pulmonary arteries (*straight arrow*). Markedly enlarged vasa vasorum are also opacified (*curved arrow*). *C,* Arteriogram of the lateral thoracic artery shows a mycotic aneurysm of the anterior intercostal artery (*arrow*).

mussen's aneurysms) may develop as a result of the inflammatory process. Aneurysm rupture leads to hemorrhage and rarely to formation of an arteriovenous fistula.[49] Mycotic aneurysms may also develop in the intercostal arteries and can be a source of hemorrhage (Fig. 20–30). In hepatogenic pulmonary angiodysplasia, multiple small arteriovenous shunts are present in patients with chronic hepatic cirrhosis.[55]

Microscopic arteriovenous shunts are present in the normal lungs.[59] In patients with sepsis, pulmonary arteriovenous shunting is observed in the absence of an abnormal arteriovenous communication (Fig. 20–31). Such arteriovenous shunting may also be present in some patients with pneumonia. Atelectasis is usually associated with delayed opacification and emptying of the affected vessels.

## Foreign Body Embolization

Sheared off catheter fragments and central venous lines usually lodge within the right atrium or ventricle.[60] Whereas longer fragments may remain in the vena cava, small catheter fragments may end up in the pulmonary arteries. Obstruction of a pulmonary artery branch with superimposed thrombosis will be demonstrated on arteriography performed prior to percutaneous retrieval (Fig. 20–32).

## Sequestration

**Intralobar Sequestration.** This is a congenital malformation consisting of a nonfunctional segment of lung enclosed within the visceral pleura. It is found most frequently in the posterior basal segment of the lower lobes. In two thirds of patients, intralobar sequestration occurs on the left side.[61] Typically, it is discovered in children and young adults and only occasionally in infants.[62]

Arterial supply to the sequestered lobe is from a systemic vessel and venous return to the left atrium, giving rise to a left to left shunt (Fig. 20–33). In some patients, venous return may be to the right atrium. Occasion-

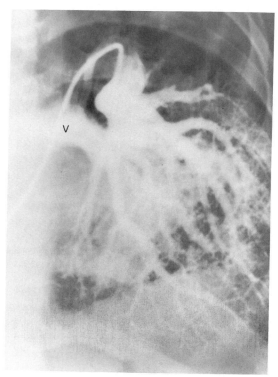

*Figure 20–31.* Pulmonary arteriovenous shunting in sepsis. Left pulmonary arteriogram shows early opacification of the left pulmonary vein (V).

2. Anomalous systemic arterial supply to the lower lobe from below the diaphragm.

3. Venous return to the pulmonary vein or left or right atrium.

4. Anomalies of the systemic veins.

5. A defect in the right hemidiaphragm with herniation of the liver.

On arteriography, the systemic artery drapes the lower lobe without penetrating it. In sequestration, the anomalous vessel penetrates and divides within the abnormal pulmonary tissue.

## Trauma

Pulmonary arteriography is very rarely indicated for the evaluation of acute chest trauma. In most cases, the injury affects the lungs or major airways. In severe blunt trauma, aortic injury is the major concern. Rarely, blunt or penetrating trauma may lead to formation of an aneurysm of a pulmonary artery.[67]

## Tumors

Pulmonary arteriography is used for preoperative evaluation of the resectability of certain mediastinal and perihilar neoplasms.[68] It is performed in conjunction with superior venacavography and azygos venography and is complementary to mediastinoscopy and computed tomography.

The two main indications for pulmonary arteriography are (1) determination of resectability of a mediastinal or hilar neoplasm in the absence of distant metastases, and (2) preoperative measurement of pulmonary artery pressure as a guide and prognostic indicator for pneumonectomy (ie, whether the patient can tolerate a pneumonectomy).

For the assessment of resectability, a main (or left or right) pulmonary arteriogram is obtained. The venous phase is also evaluated for obstruction of pulmonary veins. Demonstration of encasement or occlusion of the main pulmonary artery, proximal left or right pulmonary arteries, intrapericardial pulmonary veins, SVC, or innominate, azygos, or hemiazygos veins provides evidence of nonresectability (Fig. 20–34; also see Chapter 13, Fig. 13–4A). However, a neoplasm may be found to be unresectable in the absence of angiographically demonstrable major vessel involvement in 46% of patients.[68] Encasement or obstruction of the pulmonary arteries, simulating neoplastic encasement, is also

ally, the shunt is very large, leading to congestive heart failure.[62] Commonly, the feeding artery originates from the descending thoracic aorta, less frequently from the abdominal aorta or its branches, and occasionally from intercostal arteries.[61, 63] Histologically, these arteries are of the elastic type, similar to the pulmonary arteries.[63]

**Extralobar Sequestration.** This is also a congenital abnormality but differs from the intralobar type in that it is contained within its own visceral pleura.[64] It also occurs more frequently on the left side (89%), close to the hemidiaphragm. The blood supply is also from a systemic source (most commonly the thoracic aorta), but venous drainage is into a systemic vein (usually the IVC or azygos or hemiazygos system).[65] The diagnosis of sequestration can be made relatively easily by aortography. Selective arteriography of the abnormal vessel is usually not necessary.

**Pseudosequestration.** This is also a congenital abnormality in which the following findings have been described[66]:

1. Hypoplasia of the right lower lobe with a normal bronchial tree.

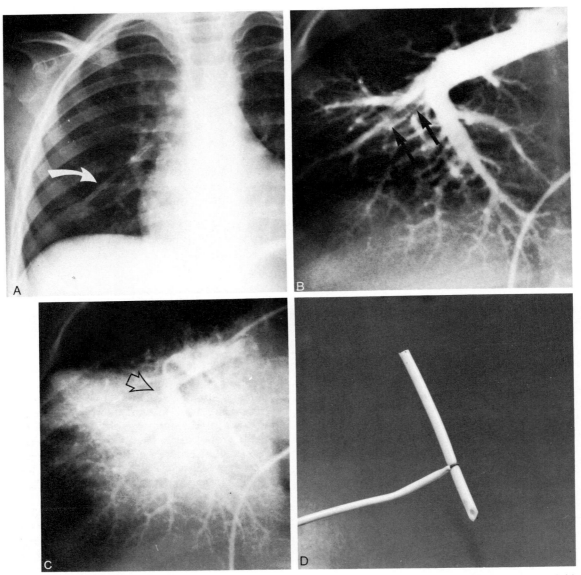

*Figure 20–32.* Foreign body. *A,* PA chest radiograph of a 2 year old girl shows a catheter fragment in the right lower lobe (*arrow*). *B,* Right lower lobe pulmonary arteriogram shows a thrombus surrounding the catheter fragment (*arrows*). *C,* Late film from the same study shows no opacification of the affected vessel (*open arrow*) and oligemia of the affected lung segment. *D,* Catheter fragment after percutaneous retrieval.

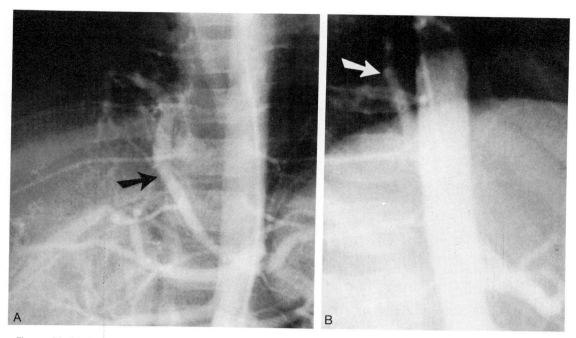

**Figure 20–33.** Pulmonary sequestration. AP (*A*) and lateral (*B*) lower thoracic aortogram shows an anomalous vessel (*arrow*) supplying the sequestered segment.

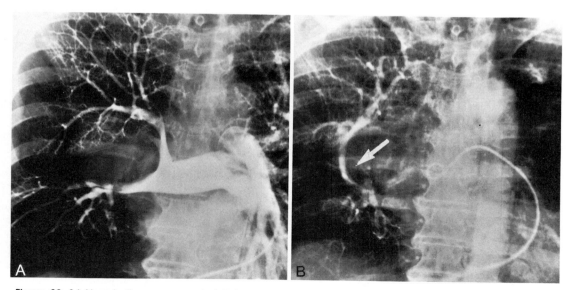

**Figure 20–34.** Neoplastic encasement. *A,* Pulmonary arteriogram shows encasement of right pulmonary artery branches by a hilar tumor. *B,* Venous phase from the same arteriogram shows displacement and encasement of the superior pulmonary vein (*arrow*).

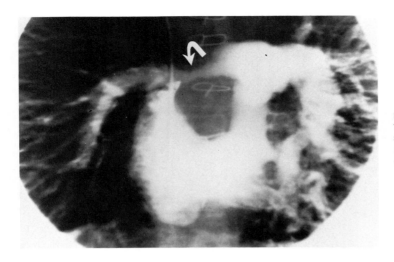

*Figure 20–35.* Intravenous DSA of the pulmonary arteries shows stenosis of the right pulmonary artery due to non-specific granulomatous inflammation (*arrow*). In addition, the left pulmonary artery is ectatic.

observed in benign granulomatous diseases[69] (Fig. 20–35).

For patients in whom pulmonary functional abnormalities have been detected by noninvasive testing, a balloon catheter is placed in the pulmonary artery to the abnormal (tumor containing) lung. The balloon is inflated. Pulmonary artery pressure is measured proximal to the balloon occlusion. This can be done through another catheter placed in the opposite pulmonary artery or via a double or triple lumen occlusion balloon catheter.

A wide range of post-occlusion pressure elevations are observed.[70] This does not appear to correlate with the presence or absence of pulmonary artery hypertension prior to balloon occlusion. In general, elevation of the mean post-occlusion pulmonary artery pressure to above 26 mm Hg indicates a higher risk for postoperative cardiopulmonary complications.[70] Elevation of the mean pulmonary artery pressure above 35 mm Hg or systemic hypoxemia ($pO_2 < 45$ mm Hg) indicates that a pneumonectomy is not feasible.

## REFERENCES

1. Boijsen E, Kozuka T: Angiographic demonstration of systemic arterial supply in abnormal pulmonary circulation. AJR 106:70–80, 1969.
2. Bessolo RJ, Maddison FE: Scimitar syndrome. Report of a case with unusual variations. AJR 103:572–576, 1968.
3. Kleinman PK: Pleural telangiectasia and absence of a pulmonary artery. Radiology 132:281–284, 1979.
4. Kirkpatrick SE, Girod DA, King H: Aortic origin of the right pulmonary artery. Surgical repair without a graft. Circulation 36:777–782, 1967.
5. Ellis K, Seaman WB, Griffiths SP, et al: Some congenital anomalies of the pulmonary arteries. Semin Roentgenol 2:325–341, 1967.
6. Flisak ME, Chandrasekar AJ, Marsan RE, et al: Systemic arterialization of lung without sequestration. AJR 138:751–753, 1982.
7. Capitanio MA, Ramos R, Kirkpatrick JA: Pulmonary sling. Roentgen observations. AJR 112:28–34, 1971.
8. Mills SR, Jackson DC, Older RA, et al: The incidence, etiologies and avoidance of complications of pulmonary angiography in a large series. Radiology 136:295–299, 1980.
9. Almen T, Aspelin P, Levin B: Effect of ionic and nonionic contrast medium on aortic and pulmonary arterial pressure. An angiocardiographic study in rabbits. Invest Radiol 10:519–525, 1975.
10. Ferris EJ, Athanasoulis CA, Clapp PR: Inferior vena cavography correlated with pulmonary angiography. Chest 59:651–653, 1971.
11. Grollman JH Jr, Gypes MT, Helmer E: Transfemoral selective bilateral pulmonary arteriography with a pulmonary artery seeking catheter. Radiology 96:202–204, 1970.
12. Greene R, O'Connell RS, Snow R, et al: Bedside balloon occlusion pulmonary angiography in acute respiratory failure: Correlation with magnification post mortem injections and pathological findings (Abstract). Am Rev Resp Dis 121:143, 1980.
13. Bynum LJ, Wilson JE III, Christensen EE, et al: Radiographic techniques for balloon occlusion pulmonary angiography. Radiology 133:518–528, 1979.
14. Baker DV Jr, Warren R, Homans J, et al: Pulmonary embolism. Evaluation of a policy for prophylaxis and therapy. N Engl J Med 242:923–928, 1950.
15. Sasahara AA, Sharma GVRK, Barsamian EM, et al: Pulmonary thromboembolism. Diagnosis and treatment. JAMA 249:2945–2950, 1983.
16. Vollmar F, Rüdiger K-D: Statistische Untersuchungen zur Häufigkeit von Lungenembolien und hämorrhagischen Lungeninfarkten im Obduktionsgut. Zbl Allg Path 115:138–144, 1972.
17. Freiman DG, Suyemoto J, Wessler S: Frequency of pulmonary thromboembolism in man. N Engl J Med 272:1278–1280, 1965.
18. Coon WW: The spectrum of pulmonary embolism. Twenty years later. Arch Surg 111:398–402, 1976.
19. Menzoian JO, Sequiera JC, Doyle JE, et al: The

therapeutic and clinical course of deep vein thrombosis. Am J Surg 146:581–585, 1983.

20. Moreno-Cabral R, Kistner RL, Nordyke RA: Importance of calf vein thrombophlebitis. Surgery 80:735–742, 1976.

21. Tow DE, Wagner HN Jr: Recovery of pulmonary arterial blood flow in patients with pulmonary embolism. N Engl J Med 276:1053–1059, 1967.

22. Sautter RD, Fletcher FW, Emanuel DA, et al: Complete resolution of massive pulmonary thromboembolism. JAMA 189:948–949, 1964.

23. Könn G, Schejbal V: Pathologie der Lungenarterienembolie. Med Klin 69:167–174, 1974.

24. Bordt J, Müller K-M: Lungendurchblutung bei Lungenarterienembolien ohne Lungeninfarkt. Fortschr Roentgenstr 126:87–89, 1977.

25. Lapp H: Über die Sperrarterien der Lunge und der Anastomosen zwischen den A. bronchiales und A. pulmonales, Über ihrer Bedeutung insbesondere für die Entstehung des hämorrhagischen Infarktes. Frankfurter Z Path 62:537–550, 1951.

26. Mathur VS, Dalen JE, Evans H, et al: Pulmonary angiography one to seven days after experimental pulmonary embolism. Invest Radiol 2:304–312, 1967.

27. Fred HL, Axelrad AA, Lewis JM, et al: Rapid resolution of pulmonary thromboemboli in man. JAMA 196:121–123, 1966.

28. Barritt DW, Jordan SC: Anticoagulant drugs in the treatment of pulmonary embolism. A controlled trial. Lancet 1:1309–1312, 1960.

29. Alpert JS, Smith R, Carlson J, et al: Mortality in patients treated for pulmonary embolism. JAMA 236:1477–1480, 1976.

30. Gorham LW: A study of pulmonary embolism. Part II. The mechanism of death; based on a clinicopathological investigation of 100 cases of massive and 285 cases of minor embolism of the pulmonary artery. Arch Intern Med 108:189–207, 1961.

31. Adams JT, McEvoy RK, DeWeese JA: Primary deep venous thrombosis of the upper extremity. Arch Surg 91:29–42, 1965.

32. Smith GT, Dammin GJ, Dexter L: Postmortem arteriographic studies of the human lung in pulmonary embolization. JAMA 188:143–151, 1964.

33. Sasahara AA, Barsamian EM, Cella G, et al: Acute pulmonary embolism. Part I. Diagnosis. Vasc Diagn Therap 29–60, 1981.

34. McIntyre KM, Sasahara AA: The hemodynamic responses to pulmonary embolism in patients without prior cardiopulmonary disease. Am J Cardiol 28:288–294, 1971.

35. Moses DC, Silver TM, Bookstein JJ: The complementary roles of chest radiography, lung scanning, and selective pulmonary angiography in the diagnosis of pulmonary embolism. Circulation 49:179–188, 1974.

36. Gilday DL, Poulose KP, DeLand FH: Accuracy of detection of pulmonary embolism by lung scanning correlated with pulmonary angiography. AJR 115:732–738, 1972.

37. Bookstein JJ, Feigin DS, Seo KW, et al: Diagnosis of pulmonary embolism. Experimental evaluation of the accuracy of scintigraphically guided pulmonary arteriography. Radiology 136:15–23, 1980.

38. Hull RD, Hirsh J, Carter CJ, et al: Pulmonary angiography, ventilation lung scanning, and venography for suspected pulmonary embolism and abnormal perfusion lung scan. Ann Intern Med 98:891–899, 1983.

39. Robinson AE, Puckett CL, Green JD, et al: In vivo demonstration of small airway bronchoconstriction following pulmonary embolism. Radiology 109:283–286, 1973.

40. Robin ED: Overdiagnosis and overtreatment of pulmonary embolism: The emperor may have no clothes. Ann Intern Med 87:775–781, 1977.

41. Cavaluzzi JA, Alderson PO, White RI: Pulmonary embolism with unilateral lung scan defects and matching infiltrates. J Assoc Can Radiol 30:162–164, 1979.

42. McIntyre KM, Sasahara AA: Hemodynamic alterations related to extent of lung scan perfusion defect in pulmonary embolism. J Nucl Med 12:166–170, 1971.

43. Bossart PJ, Sniderman KW, Beinart C, et al: Pulmonary arteriography: The importance of multiple projections. Cardiovasc Intervent Radiol 5:105–107, 1982.

44. Novelline RA, Baltarowich OH, Athanasoulis CA, et al: The clinical course of patients with suspected pulmonary embolism and a negative pulmonary arteriogram. Radiology 126:561–567, 1978.

45. Bookstein JJ: Segmental arteriography in pulmonary embolism. Radiology 93:1007–1012, 1969.

46. Shure D, Moser KM, Harrel JH II, et al: Identification of pulmonary emboli in the dog: Comparison of angioscopy and perfusion scanning. Circulation 64:618–621, 1981.

47. Moore EH, Gamsu G, Webb WR, et al: Pulmonary embolus: Detection and followup using magnetic resonance. Radiology 153:471–472, 1984.

48. Boyd LJ, McGavack TH: Aneurysm of the pulmonary artery. A review of the literature and report of two new cases. Am Heart J 18:562–578, 1939.

49. Lundell C, Finck E: Arteriovenous fistulas originating from Rasmussen aneurysms. AJR 140:687–688, 1983.

50. Dines DE, Arms RA, Bernatz PE, et al: Pulmonary arteriovenous fistulas. Mayo Clin Proc 49:460–465, 1974.

51. Hodgson CH, Burchell HB, Good A, et al: Hereditary hemorrhagic telangiectasia and pulmonary arteriovenous fistula. Survey of a large family. N Engl J Med 261:626–636, 1959.

52. Sagel SS, Greenspan RH: Minute pulmonary arteriovenous fistulas demonstrated by magnification pulmonary arteriography. Radiology 97:529–530, 1970.

53. Hales MRL: Multiple small arteriovenous fistulae of the lungs. Am J Pathol 32:927–943, 1956.

54. Sloan RD, Cooley RN: Congenital pulmonary arteriovenous aneurysm. AJR 70:183–210, 1953.

55. Oh KS, Bender TM, Bowen A, et al: Plain radiographic, nuclear medicine and angiographic observations of hepatogenic pulmonary angiodysplasia. Pediatr Radiol 13:111–115, 1983.

56. Gay BB, Franch RH, Shuford WH, et al: The roentgenologic features of single and multiple coarctations of the pulmonary artery and branches. AJR 90:599–613, 1963.

57. Arvidsson H, Karnell J, Moeller T: Multiple stenosis of the pulmonary arteries associated with pulmonary hypertension, diagnosed by selective angiocardiography. Acta Radiol 44:209–216, 1955.

58. Orell SR, Karnell J, Wahlgren F: Malformation and multiple stenoses of the pulmonary arteries with pulmonary hypertension. Acta Radiol 54:449–459, 1960.

59. Tobin CE: Arteriovenous shunts in the peripheral pulmonary circulation in the human lung. Thorax 21:197–204, 1966.

60. Kadir S, Athanasoulis CA: Percutaneous retrieval of intravascular foreign bodies. *In* Athanasoulis CA, et al (eds.): Interventional Radiology, Philadelphia, WB Saunders Company, 1982, pp 379–390.

61. Turk LN III, Lindskog GE: The importance of angiographic diagnosis in intralobar pulmonary sequestration. J Thorac Cardiovasc Surg 41:299–305, 1961.

62. White JJ, Donahoo JS, Ostrow PT, et al: Cardiovascular and respiratory manifestations of pulmonary sequestration in childhood. Ann Thorac Surg 18:286–294, 1974.

63. Ferris EJ, Smith PL, Mirza FH, et al: Intralobar pulmonary sequestration: value of aortography and pulmonary arteriography. Cardiovasc Intervent Radiol 4:17–23, 1981.

64. Weir JA: Congenital anomalies of the lung. Ann Intern Med 52:330–348, 1960.

65. Ranniger K, Valvassori GE: Angiographic diagnosis of intralobar pulmonary sequestration. AJR 92:540–546, 1964.

66. Macpherson RI, Whytehead L: Pseudosequestration. J Can Assoc Radiol 28:17–25, 1977.

67. Symbas PN, Scott HW Jr: Traumatic aneurysm of the pulmonary artery. J Thorac Cardiovasc Surg 45:645–649, 1963.

68. Benfield JR, Bonney H, Crummy AB, et al: Azygograms and pulmonary arteriograms in bronchogenic carcinoma. Arch Surg 99:406–409, 1969.

69. Hietala S-O, Stinnett RG, Faunce HF III, et al: Pulmonary artery narrowing in sarcoidosis. JAMA 237:572–573, 1977.

70. Rams JJ, Harrison RW, Fry WA, et al: Operative pulmonary artery pressure measurements as a guide to postoperative management and prognosis following pneumonectomy. Dis Chest 41:85–90, 1962.

# THE LYMPHATIC SYSTEM

## Lymphography

The main purposes of this chapter are to describe the technique of lymphography and familiarize the reader with basic lymphographic abnormalities. Detailed review of the subject can be found in references 1 and 2.

Although lymphography has largely been replaced by computed tomography (CT) for the evaluation of lymphadenopathy, it nevertheless plays an important role in the evaluation of patients with a negative CT examination. The main advantage of lymphography over CT is that it permits assessment of the internal architecture of lymph nodes. Furthermore, abnormal lymph nodes can be biopsied percutaneously, thus avoiding a more invasive procedure.

Preliminary studies with magnetic resonance imaging indicate that this may provide an additional imaging modality for the evaluation of enlarged lymph nodes.[3]

Lymphoscintigraphy now plays an increasingly important role in the evaluation of patients with lymphedema. With the availability of safe, nonionic, water-soluble contrast agents that can also be injected intraparenchymally,[4] contrast lymphangiography may regain importance as a diagnostic modality, since it permits evaluation of the morphology of both the lymph channels and the lymph nodes.

## ANATOMY

Endothelial-lined lymphatic capillaries begin in the soft tissues and join to form larger lymphatic channels. These drain through regional lymph nodes into the central lymphatics. Larger lymph vessels have a structure similar to that of veins, ie, an intima, media, adventitia, and valves. The last are responsible for the beaded appearance on lymphography. Communications exist between the blood-containing vascular system and the lymphatics in the lymph nodes and via the thoracic duct.

Lymph nodes are encapsulated structures consisting of collections of lymphoid cells contained within a network of reticular fibers and connective tissue. The reticular fibers form the sinus system of the lymph nodes (Figs. 21–1 and 21–2).

**Lymphatic System of the Upper Extremities.** A deep and a superficial lymphatic system are present and both drain into the axillary lymph nodes. The latter are comprised of five groups: anterior, posterior, lateral, central, and apical.[5] The deep lymph channels follow the blood vessels and drain primarily into the lateral group of axillary nodes. The superficial lymph vessels consist of a medial and a lateral group.

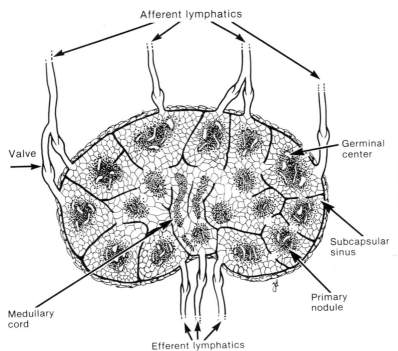

*Figure 21–1.* Sketch showing histological anatomy of a normal lymph node. Medullary cord = medullary lymph follicle; primary nodule = cortical lymph follicle.

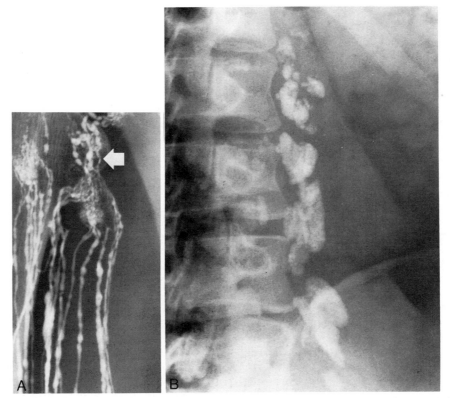

*Figure 21–2.* Lymphographic appearance of normal lymph nodes. *A,* Channel phase. Arrow points to efferent channels. Beaded appearance is due to valves in the narrow segments. *B,* Nodal phase.

**Lymphatic System of the Lower Extremities** (Fig. 21–3). The lower extremities also have a deep (subfascial) and a superficial system. The deep system consists of three groups of lymph vessels—anterior, fibular, and posterior—that accompany the main veins of the calf.[5, 6] The posterior group is the largest. Unlike the vessels of the superficial system, these vessels do not bifurcate, ie, the number of channels does not increase as they course centrally.[6] On the way to the inguinal region, the deep lymphatics pass through the popliteal nodes. Under normal conditions, no communications are observed between the deep and the superficial systems.[7]

The superficial lymphatics are divided into an anterior and a posterior group. The anterior group is further subdivided into a lateral and a medial group. The medial anterior lymphatics are larger and greater in number than the lateral anterior lymphatics. They accompany the greater saphenous vein and are opacified by cannulation of a medially located lymph channel at the foot. The lateral anterior lymphatics are opacified by injecting a laterally located lymph channel at the foot. These cross over to the medial side midway over the calf. Both systems continue centrally along the medial aspect of the thigh and bifurcate, ie, increase in number to 12 to 15 channels, before reaching the inguinal nodes.

The posterior group of superficial lymphatics is smaller in size and fewer in number. These lymphatics are opacified by injecting contrast medium in a lymph channel behind the lateral malleolus. They drain into the popliteal nodes, which are four to five in number, and continue along the deep femoral vessels.[8]

The inguinal nodes are located below the inguinal ligament and consist of a deep and a superficial group. The former are two to three in number, are usually large, and lie closer to the inguinal ligament. The superficial nodes are subdivided into a superior and an inferior group. Nodes of the superior group (9 to 12 in number) lie closer to the inguinal ligament and drain the perineal region. They are less frequently opacified on pedal lymphography. Nodes of the inferior group lie closer to the femoral canal.

**Lymphatic System of the Pelvis and Retroperitoneum** (Figs. 21–3 to 21–5). In the pelvis, the lymph channels and nodes accompany the major vessels and are named after them. In the external iliac region, three lymphatic chains are present: lateral, middle, and medial. The medial chain contains the largest number of vessels and lies medial to the external iliac vein. The middle and lateral chains are smaller, and the former is often not opacified on lymphography.

The node of Rosenmueller is located medial to the femoral vein (Fig. 21–5). The obturator node is the middle node of the medial external iliac chain.[9]

The internal iliac lymphatics, with 8 to 10 lymph nodes, are located along the branches of the internal iliac vessels. These communicate with the medial common iliac chain and drain the pelvic organs and muscles. They are infrequently opacified on pedal lymphography.

The external iliac lymphatics continue as the common iliac chains along the common iliac artery. The lateral chain lies posterolateral to the common iliac artery. The medial chain is located posteromedial to the vessels. The middle chain may be anteriorly or posteriorly located. Knowledge of these locations is important when attempting percutaneous lymph node biopsy.

The iliac lymphatics continue into the abdomen along the aorta as left and right paraaortic trunks and the mid-aortic chain. The paraaortic channels do not extend beyond the lateral margins of the lumbar transverse processes, with the exception of an occasional vessel that may deviate laterally for a short distance. On the lateral projection, they remain within 3 cm of the anterior surface of the vertebral bodies. Cross filling occurs frequently and is usually at the lower lumbar level. Tributaries to the paraaortic lymphatics come from the lumbar, gonadal, renal, adrenal, and abdominal wall lymphatics.

**Cisterna Chyli and Thoracic Duct** (Fig. 21–6). The aortic trunks terminate in the cisterna chyli, which is located at L1–L2. The cisterna is a saccular dilatation of the lymph vessels that also receives the mesenteric/abdominal visceral lymphatics. In many individuals, only one of the aortic chains reaches the cisterna. In some individuals, a true cisterna does not form, and instead there are multiple interconnected saccular dilatations.

From the cisterna chyli, the thoracic duct continues towards the neck. It is between 1 and 3 mm in diameter in its mid-portion, but the proximal and terminal portions are wider (up to 5 to 7 mm). Occasionally, the thoracic duct is partially duplicated, or it may divide

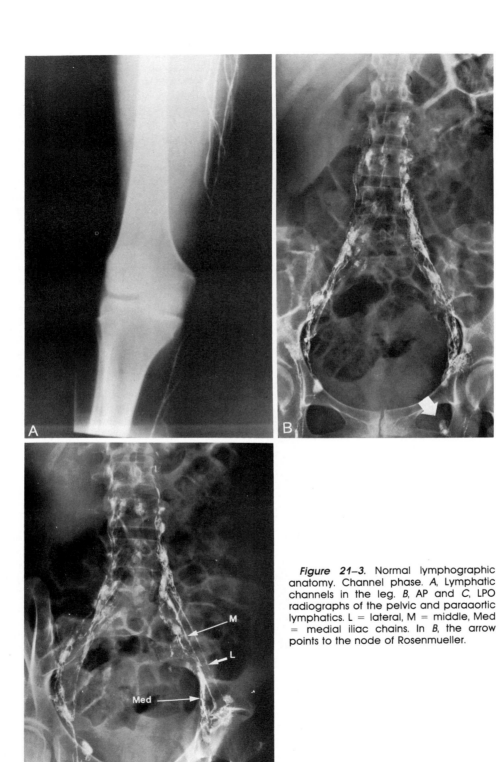

*Figure 21–3.* Normal lymphographic anatomy. Channel phase. *A*, Lymphatic channels in the leg. *B*, AP and *C*, LPO radiographs of the pelvic and paraaortic lymphatics. L = lateral, M = middle, Med = medial iliac chains. In *B*, the arrow points to the node of Rosenmueller.

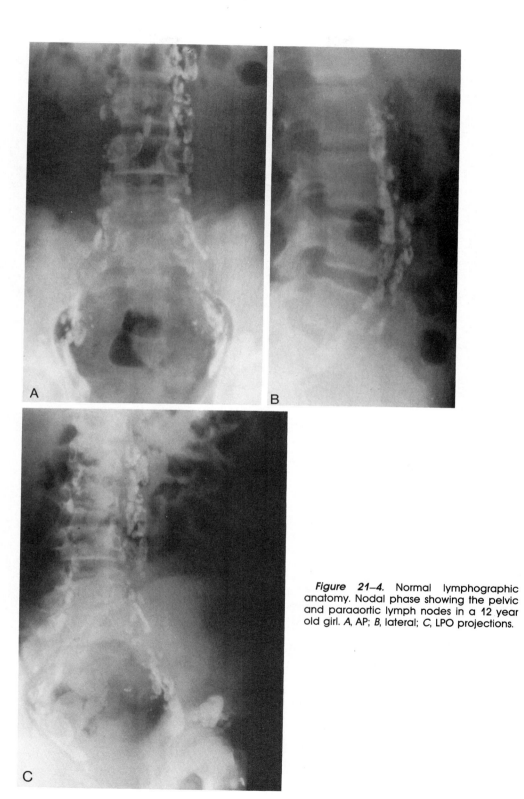

*Figure 21–4.* Normal lymphographic anatomy. Nodal phase showing the pelvic and paraaortic lymph nodes in a 12 year old girl. *A,* AP; *B,* lateral; *C,* LPO projections.

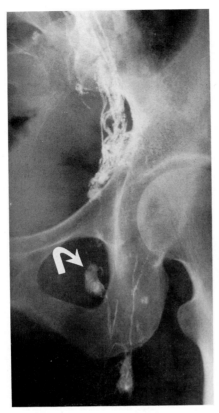

*Figure 21–5.* Node of Rosenmueller (*curved arrow*).

into several branches before entering the venous system.

The thoracic duct lies between the azygos vein and the aorta, ie, to the right of the latter. At the level of the fifth thoracic vertebra, it crosses over to the left and terminates at the venous angle formed by the left subclavian and internal jugular veins. It carries the lymph from the entire body, with the exception of the dome of the liver and right chest, neck, and arm. The latter are drained by the right lymphatic duct, which empties into the right venous angle.[5]

**Lymphatic Drainage from the Pelvis and Genital Organs.** Lymphatic drainage from the testis is along the spermatic cord to lymph nodes located at the terminal portion of the testicular vein and the paraaortic nodes (L1–L2 on the left and L1–L3 on the right).[10] The former are usually not demonstrated by pedal lymphography but are opacified by testicular lymphography. In addition, some drainage occurs to the external iliac nodes. Lymphatic drainage from the epididymis goes to the superficial inguinal nodes. Lym-

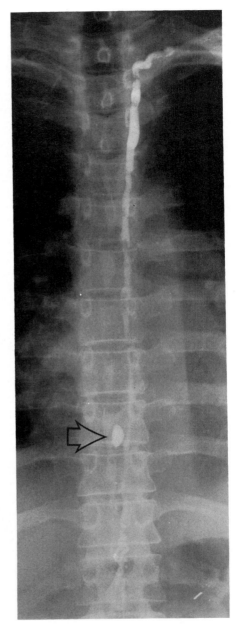

*Figure 21–6.* Normal thoracic duct. Open arrow points to myelographic contrast medium.

phatic drainage from the prostate goes to the internal iliac and presacral lymph nodes, with the exception of the posterior prostatic surface, which drains into the external iliac nodes.[5]

Lymphatic drainage from the female genitalia is as follows[5]:

1. Ovary: Along ovarian vessels to the paraaortic nodes and to the iliac nodes.

2. Cervix/lower uterus: External and internal iliac and sacral nodes.
3. Fundus/upper uterus: External iliac and paraaortic nodes.
4. Vagina
   a. Upper: Internal and external iliac nodes.
   b. Mid: Internal iliac nodes.
   c. Lower vagina and external genitalia: superficial inguinal nodes.

Lymphatic drainage from the urinary bladder occurs mainly to the external iliac and occasionally to the internal or common iliac lymph nodes.

## TECHNIQUE FOR LYMPHOGRAPHY

Lymphography is usually performed as an outpatient procedure. As for other angiographic studies, the patient is instructed to abstain from eating for at least 8 hours before the lymphogram. Clear liquids and medication are permitted. Premedication is usually not required, unless the patient is anxious.

The instruments required for lymphography are listed in Table 21–1. Several blue dyes have been used for opacification of

#### TABLE 21–1. Materials for Lymphography

1% lidocaine
Blue dye
Ethiodol, two vials (Savage Laboratories, Missouri City, Texas)
Hot plate with bowl of water to heat Ethiodol
Injector, Harvard apparatus (Bard Medsystems, Division of CR Bard Inc, North Reading, Massachusetts)
Sterile gauze and towels
Two packs of Steri-Strips (3M, Surgical Products Division, St Paul, Minnesota)
One pair sterile stockings
Two 30 gauge lymphography sets (BD & Company, Rutherford, New Jersey)
One bowl with bacteriostatic water or normal saline (50 ml)
Two Kelly clamps
Two Halsted clamps
Two curved mosquito clamps
One suture scissors
One fine forceps without teeth
One forceps with teeth
One blade handle with No. 15 blade
One needle holder
One 10 ml three ring syringe for lidocaine
Two 10 ml disposable syringes for Ethiodol
Three tuberculin syringes
One 20 ml disposable syringe
Two 25 gauge needles
One pack 4–0 silk ties
One pack 4–0 Dermalon on cutting needle

lymphatic channels, including methylene blue and patent blue violet. We currently use isosulfan blue (Lymphazurin 1%, Hirsch Industries, Cherry Hill, New Jersey 08034). Ten per cent of this dye is excreted through the urine, while the remainder is excreted through the biliary tract. Urinary excretion leads to discoloration of the urine for 2 to 3 days. The preparation for intracutaneous injection is as follows: 0.5 ml of a 1% lidocaine solution added to 0.5 ml of isosulfan blue in a tuberculin syringe. We have not observed precipitation of this mixture.

The contrast medium used for lymphography is Ethiodol (iodinated ethyl esters of fatty acids of poppyseed oil, Savage Laboratories, Missouri City, Texas). The iodine content is 37%. Ninety per cent is retained by the lymph nodes and the remainder enters the pulmonary bed, mainly via the thoracic duct. In individuals with normal pulmonary function, this goes unnoticed. However, in patients with compromised pulmonary function, this may cause dyspnea and decreased $pO_2$ as a result of a decrease in the pulmonary diffusion capacity. In some patients, infusion of Ethiodol is associated with a transient low-grade temperature elevation.

In patients with obstruction of the paraaortic lymphatics, Ethiodol may enter the mesenteric lymphatics.[11] Paraaortic lymphatic obstruction associated with IVC obstruction predisposes to hepatic embolization via lympho-portal communications.[12]

The sites for blue dye injection are as follows:

Cervical lymphography: Behind the ears.

Arm: Dorsum of the hand, between the fingers.

Leg (superficial): Between the toes.

Leg (deep): Abductor hallucis muscle,[6] sole of the foot.[7]

The lymph channels are visualized through the skin as blue streaks. In dark-skinned individuals, it may not be possible to see these channels transcutaneously. In individuals with dermal backflow due to lymphatic obstruction, the dermal lymphatic capillaries are opacified.

**Preparation and Cannulation** (Figs. 21–7 to 21–13).

1. The skin between the first and second and the third and fourth toes is cleaned with alcohol, and 0.5 ml of blue dye mixed with lidocaine is injected intracutaneously in each location (Fig. 21–7). The patient is instructed to flex and extend the toes for 3 to 5 minutes

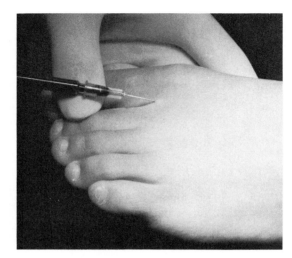

*Figure 21–7.* Intradermal injection of blue dye using a 25 gauge needle.

*Figure 21–8.* Sterile stocking with oval window.

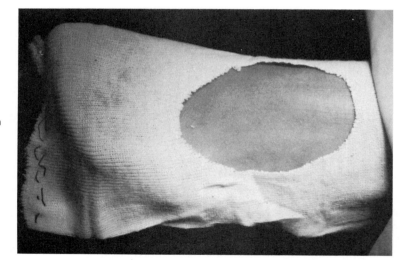

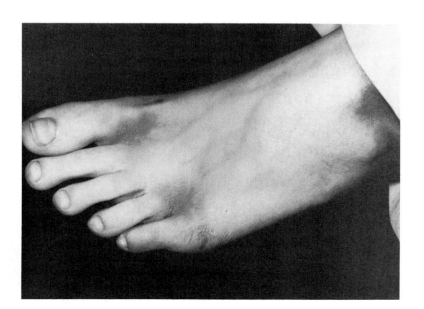

*Figure 21–9.* Transcutaneous appearance of lymph vessels.

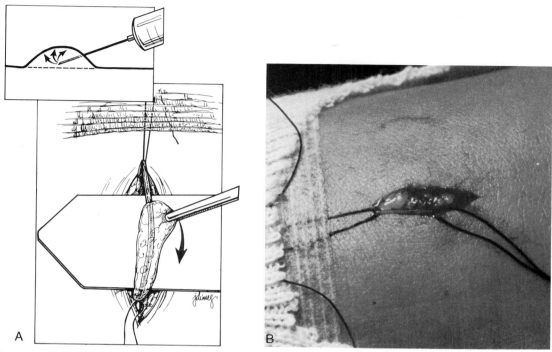

**Figure 21–10.** Technique for preparation of a lymph vessel. *A*, Subcutaneous injection of local anesthetic (*inset*) and removal of perilymphatic tissue. *B*, Lymph vessel after preparation for cannulation.

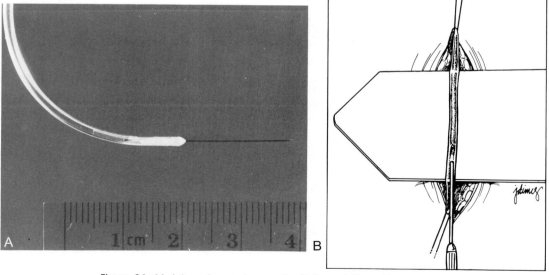

**Figure 21–11.** *A*, Lymphography needle. *B*, Cannulation of lymph vessel.

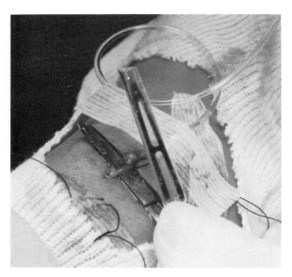

*Figure 21–12.* Hair clip method for stabilization. Note that the proximal tip has been cut off to facilitate unimpeded flow of contrast medium.

in order to facilitate lymphatic uptake and transportation of the dye.

2. The feet, to the ankles, are washed with soap and water and dried.

3. Hair, if present on the dorsum of the feet, is shaved.

4. The feet are prepped with povidone-iodine (Betadine) or another antimicrobial skin preparation and air dried. Sterile stockings are then placed over the feet, and an oval-shaped window is cut out to expose the working area (Fig. 21–8).

5. Lymphatic channels are located over the dorsum of the foot (Fig. 21–9). Lymphatic filling can be enhanced by massaging the area injected with the blue dye. Lidocaine, 1%, without epinephrine is injected generously into the subcutaneous tissues around the transcutaneously visualized lymphatics (Fig. 21–10). A lymphatic channel may not be visualized in dark-skinned individuals. In this case and in individuals in whom a blue dye cannot be used, lidocaine is injected into the subcutaneous tissues over the base of the second metatarsal bone. Injection of a large volume (5 to 10 ml) of lidocaine serves a twofold purpose: (1) it provides durable local anesthesia and (2) the imbibition of the perilymphatic tissue with lidocaine facilitates the process of preparation, ie, removal of fat and other perilymphatic tissues. In addition, lidocaine may have an antispasmodic effect on the lymph channels themselves.

6. A longitudinal incision (2 to 3 cm) is made parallel to the lymph vessels, and the subcutaneous tissues are dissected bluntly.

7. A curved mosquito clamp is passed under a suitable lymph vessel to isolate it. A narrow piece of waxed paper, approximately 1 cm × 3 cm (from the Steri-Strip), or cardboard (from the lymphography needle packing) is placed under the lymph vessel (Fig. 21–10A). In addition, a 4–0 silk tie is placed at each end of the exposed vessel.

8. A pair of fine forceps (without teeth) are used to remove the perilymphatic tissues. These must be removed completely in order to permit successful cannulation.

9. A slight tension is applied to the proximal tie (towards the ankle), and the tie is taped to the skin with a Steri-Strip. This obstructs the vessel temporarily, permitting it to be distended. The silk tie closer to the toes is used to apply tension at the time of cannulation.

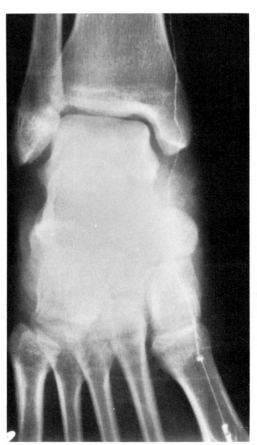

*Figure 21–13.* Radiograph obtained to confirm intralymphatic injection of Ethiodol shows a normal lymph channel.

10. A tuberculin syringe containing normal saline is attached to the lymphography needle (Fig. 21–11). For cannulation, the needle is held almost parallel to the lymph vessel. After the needle tip is inserted into the lymph vessel, some saline is injected. If the tip is intraluminal, this will distend the lymph vessel. Once the lymph vessel is distended, the needle tip is advanced further into it. The needle is secured in place with a Steri-Strip, and tension on the proximal tie is released to permit unobstructed flow of contrast medium. The tubing from the lymphography needle is also taped to the skin and then attached to the injector. The patient is instructed not to flex or extend the toes for the duration of the infusion. It is not necessary to place a tie around the needle unless there is leakage of contrast medium as a result of multiple attempted punctures. An alternative technique for securing the needle is the use of a hair clip (Fig. 21–12).

11. Contrast medium is injected via a constant infusion pump at 0.10 to 0.15 ml per minute for a total of 5 to 7 ml per leg or 4 to 5 ml per arm.

After about 1 minute, intralymphatic infusion is confirmed by fluoroscopy or a radiograph (Fig. 21–13). A single leg infusion opacifies the ipsilateral iliac lymphatic system, but because of cross filling, bilateral paraaortic lymph nodes are usually opacified.

Most patients experience cramplike calf pain as the contrast medium ascends into the calf. Occasionally, this is responsible for extremity motion, which can dislodge the needle. We have been successful in preventing this pain in over 90% of patients by injection of 0.5 ml of lidocaine into the lymph vessel immediately before contrast infusion (Howes V and Kadir S, unpublished data).

Upon completion of the infusion, the incision is rinsed with saline and cleaned with hydrogen peroxide. The skin is sutured and an antimicrobial ointment is applied. The following radiographs are obtained immediately thereafter and at 24 hours:

1. Pelvis: AP, lateral, both obliques, and an angled view (prone, 25° tube angulation towards the feet).

2. Lumbosacral spine: AP, lateral, and obliques.

3. Chest: PA, lateral.

The angled view is particularly helpful, as it separates the iliac nodes. The skin sutures are removed in 7 to 10 days.

**Lymphography Without Blue Dyes.** Lymphography can also be performed without blue dyes if there is a known allergy to the dyes. Lymph channels are thin walled and glisten, whereas veins have thicker walls and increase in opacity if blood flow is augmented by massaging the distal foot. When attempting lymphography without the aid of blue dyes, the presence of intralymphatic Ethiodol must be confirmed soon after infusion is begun. Alternatively, fluorescein may be used to locate the lymph vessels.[13]

## NORMAL AND ABNORMAL LYMPH NODES

For the interpretation of the lymphangiogram, both the channel and the nodal phases must be evaluated. The former is important for evaluation of small metastatic foci and lymphatic obstruction. The lymph nodes must be evaluated for size, number, contour, and internal architecture.

Under normal circumstances, the contrast medium is cleared from the lymph vessels within 3 to 4 hours. Stasis, ie, slower emptying, is occasionally observed in normal older individuals. However, in most cases, it is indicative of lymphatic obstruction. Extravasation of contrast medium into the perilymphatic tissues occurs with the use of very fast infusion rates. It also occurs in patients with lymphatic obstruction.

The lymphographic appearance of lymph nodes depends upon the degree of opacification and the histology. The larger lymph nodes are oval shaped and are oriented along the long axis of the vessel they accompany. Smaller lymph nodes are round in configuration. Normal lymph nodes do not exceed a diameter of 2.6 cm.[14] Often several smaller lymph nodes may be clustered together and may thus simulate an abnormality (multiple filling defects). Radiographs obtained in different projections help to delineate the nodes and exclude any abnormality.

Lymphographic contrast material is located within the sinuses. Lymph follicles do not take up contrast medium and thus appear as small black dots, giving the normal lymph node a fine, homogeneous, granular appearance (see Figs. 21–2 and 21–4). Normal lymph nodes are sharply outlined and the appearance is uniform for the entire group. On the nodal phase, the hilus of the lymph node appears as a round or cleftlike filling defect. The channel phase shows efferent lymphatic channels emanating from this region.

The size and number of the lymph nodes may vary in normal individuals. In general, the fewer the lymph nodes, the larger their size and vice versa.[15] Centrally located lymph nodes are usually smaller, whereas the more peripheral ones, eg, inguinal, are the largest.

As the lymph follicles enlarge, they demonstrate a coarse granularity. With further enlargement there is less contrast medium uptake and the lymph node appears foamy. Replacement of the normal nodal lymphatic tissue by tumor, granuloma, or scar tissue appears as a filling defect on the lymphangiogram. In animal experiments, intranodal deposits as small as 3 mm could be detected by lymphography.[16]

## Benign Diseases of the Lymph Nodes

The benign nodal abnormalities described below may simulate malignancy and are the most frequent causes for misinterpretation of lymphograms.[15, 17-19]

**Follicular Hyperplasia.** The lymph node is enlarged, with enlargement of the follicles and lymph channels. The node may appear hyperdense as a result of increased accumulation of contrast medium in the dilated sinuses, or it may have a coarse granular or even foamy appearance. Usually, the architecture is normal, but occasionally a single filling defect, similar to a metastatic deposit, may be found. Follicular hyperplasia is observed in systemic inflammatory diseases (eg, viral infections, toxoplasmosis, gamma globulinopathies, sarcoidosis, psoriasis, and rheumatoid arthritis).[15, 17, 18, 20, 21] It may also occur as a focal abnormality, especially in the inguinal area.

**Reactive (Sinus) Hyperplasia** (Figs. 21–14 and 21–15). The lymphographic changes in reactive hyperplasia can be indistinguishable from those of follicular hyperplasia. The lymph nodes are also enlarged and can have a coarse granular or foamy appearance.

Reactive hyperplasia is essentially a tumor-induced inflammatory response in regional lymph nodes, but may also be generalized. The former is seen in lymph nodes located more central to those affected by metastatic disease or in regional lymph nodes following surgery. The generalized form is observed in systemic diseases such as lymphoma, leuke-

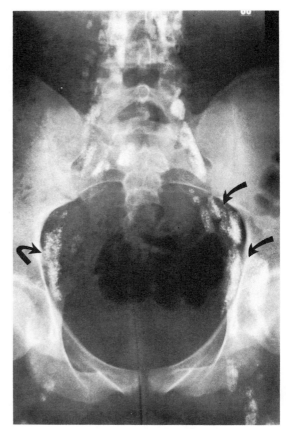

**Figure 21–14.** Reactive hyperplasia (biopsy proven) of the pelvic nodes (*arrows*) in a young homosexual man with nodular sclerosing Hodgkin's lymphoma.

mias, collagen diseases, lymphadenopathy syndrome, and certain immune disorders.[17, 18] When generalized, reactive hyperplasia may be difficult to differentiate from lymphoma. A similar lymphographic picture is also found in hydantoin-induced and angioimmunoblastic lymphadenopathy.[22, 23]

**Fibrolipomatosis** (Fig. 21–16). Fibrotic change with fatty replacement of the lymph nodes occurs as a result of the normal aging process. It develops most frequently in the cervical, axillary, and inguinal lymph nodes and occasionally in the iliac nodes. The central portion of the lymph node is replaced, leaving a rim of lymphatic tissue. In the channel phase, a few attenuated lymphatics may be seen traversing the node.

**Radiation Changes.** Radiation causes atrophy of the lymph nodes and fibrosis with a decrease in the number of lymphatics. On lymphography, the nodal architecture is distorted with inhomogeneous filling.

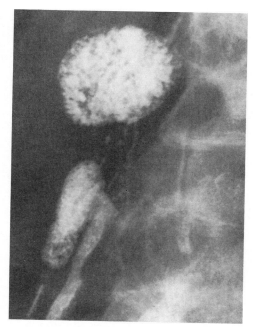

*Figure 21–15.* Reactive hyperplasia in a 51 year old woman with epidermoid carcinoma of the cervix. The right paraaortic lymph node is enlarged and globular. The sinuses are enlarged and droplets of Ethiodol contained in the sinuses give the node a hyperdense appearance.

## Malignant Diseases of the Lymph Nodes

**Lymphomas.** The accuracy of lymphography for detection of lymphoma is about 95%.

It is higher for Hodgkin's disease than for other types of lymphoma;[24] in a patient with a negative lymphogram, the likelihood of Hodgkin's disease is only 2%. However, lymphography may underestimate the extent of disease in a significant number of patients.[25]

Several patterns of nodal involvement are observed (Figs. 21–17 to 21–20):

1. Most frequently, the nodes are enlarged, increased in number, and have a foamy, lacey architecture. The outer margins are usually preserved. Often, the enlarged node becomes globular and the marginal sinus is prominent.[14]

2. Nodular, punched-out defects, both marginal and centrally located, are observed in the nodular type of lymphomas. The involved nodes are generally enlarged, but the uninvolved section may have a normal architecture.

3. No nodal abnormality may be demonstrated if the disease is still in the microscopic stage.

4. Total lymphatic obstruction due to complete nodal replacement may be seen.

5. In patients treated by radiation, reactive hyperplasia of nodes excluded from the radiation field may be observed.[26]

**Metastases.** Several patterns of lymph node involvement are also observed in metastatic disease. Metastases usually involve the regional lymph nodes but may extend centrally. Microscopic nodal metastases may be present in a significant number of patients

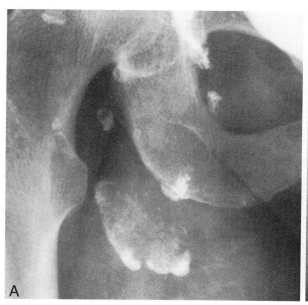

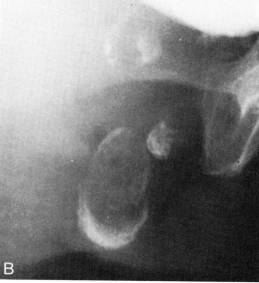

*Figure 21–16.* Fibrolipomatosis. *A,* AP projection. *B,* LPO projection.

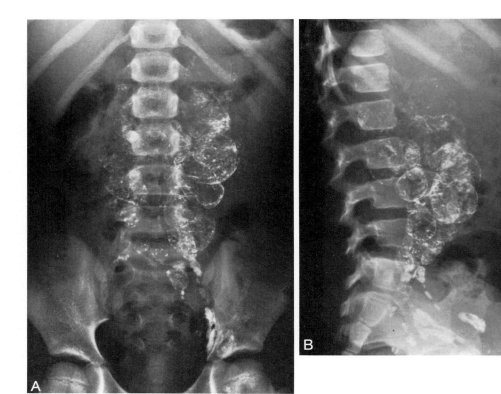

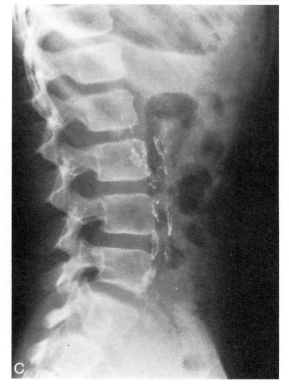

*Figure 21–17.* Hodgkin's disease. *A* and *B,* AP and lateral lymphogram shows massively enlarged globular lymph nodes. Dense droplets of contrast medium (punctate) are present in the dilated sinuses. Note that bilateral paraaortic lymph nodes have been opacified from a left leg lymphangiogram. *C,* Lateral film after treatment shows a dramatic reduction in the size of the nodes.

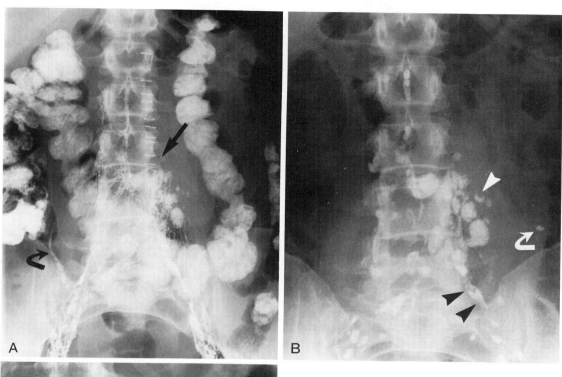

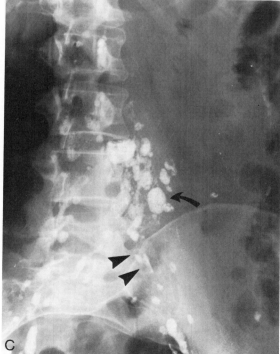

**Figure 21–18.** Nodular sclerosing Hodgkin's lymphoma in a 46 year old woman. *A,* Channel phase shows obstruction of the left paraaortic channels due to tumorous nodes (*straight arrow*). There is deviation of channels and a collateral is opacified (*curved arrow*). Contrast medium in the colon is from a preceding CT examination. *B* and *C,* Nodal phase. Multiple displaced and abnormal nodes are present. Nodular defects (*arrowheads*) and reactive hyperplasia (*black curved arrow*) are seen. Curved white arrow points to mesenteric lymph node.

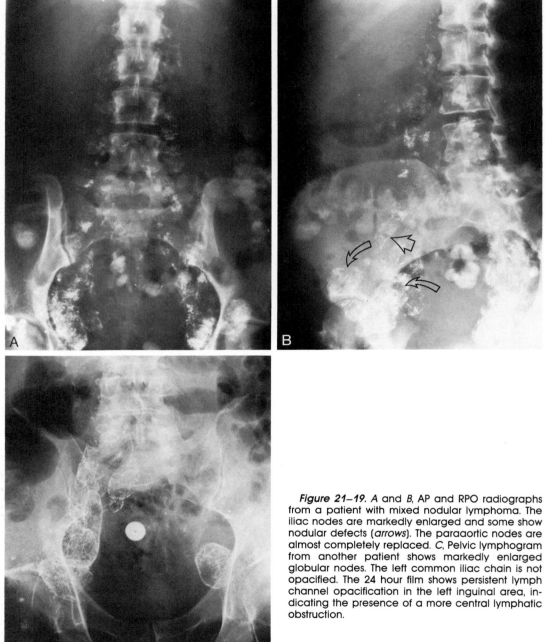

*Figure 21–19.* A and B, AP and RPO radiographs from a patient with mixed nodular lymphoma. The iliac nodes are markedly enlarged and some show nodular defects (*arrows*). The paraaortic nodes are almost completely replaced. *C,* Pelvic lymphogram from another patient shows markedly enlarged globular nodes. The left common iliac chain is not opacified. The 24 hour film shows persistent lymph channel opacification in the left inguinal area, indicating the presence of a more central lymphatic obstruction.

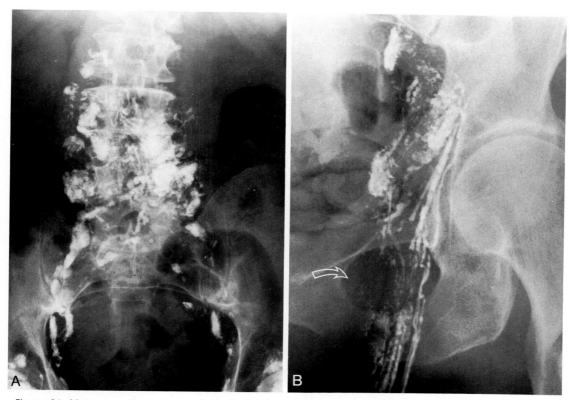

**Figure 21-20.** Large cell lymphoma. *A,* Markedly abnormal nodes are seen in the paraaortic chain along with stasis of contrast medium in the lymphatics. Several nodes in the left iliac chain are not opacified. *B,* Channel phase shows lymphatics bypassing node replaced by tumor (*arrow*).

with normal nodal architecture on lymphography.[27, 28]

The accuracy of lymphography for detection of metastases from testicular tumors is only 76%.[29] It does not reflect the true extent of disease because of inability of pedal lymphography to opacify the regional lymph nodes located at the junction of the testicular and renal veins. In ovarian tumor metastases, the iliac and paraaortic lymph nodes are involved, and the overall accuracy of lymphography is 91.7%.[27] The majority of false-negative interpretations are due to the presence of microscopic metastases. In comparison, the overall accuracy of CT for detecting lymph node metastases from pelvic malignancies has been reported at 77%.[30]

1. Smaller metastases involve a portion of the node and are often eccentric (Fig. 21-21). The remainder of the node may have a coarse granular appearance or normal architecture. The lymph nodes appear punched out or moth-eaten and may be normal in size or enlarged. Similar defects may be observed in the normal hilus and in fatty replacement. In

the latter, efferent lymph vessels are seen during the channel phase. In metastatic disease, there is absence of such vessels in the region of the defect and a segment of the marginal sinus does not opacify. Granulomatous infection, eg, sarcoidosis and tuberculosis, may also simulate metastatic disease.[17, 21]

2. Nonopacification of nodes completely replaced by tumor (Fig. 21-22): In such cases, displaced or obstructed (demonstrating contrast stasis) lymph vessels and collateral channels may be visualized. Occasionally, this is also observed in benign conditions eg, sarcoidosis.[21] In some cases, a rim of nodal tissue is seen (ghost node). In benign conditions (fatty replacement, follicular hyperplasia), the rim is usually complete (but may appear incomplete in one or the other projection, when not seen in profile) (see Fig. 21-16).

3. In seminoma metastasis, the lymph nodes are enlarged and foamy and may resemble lymphoma.

4. There may be diffuse nodal enlargement

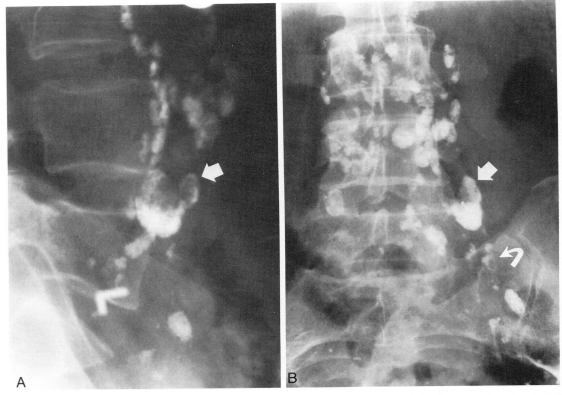

*Figure 21–21.* Metastatic vaginal carcinoma. *A,* lateral and *B,* AP views show nodal enlargement and metastatic deposits (*arrows*). A smaller node containing a central metastasis is also seen (*curved arrow*). On the AP view, a 22 gauge biopsy needle is seen in the node (*straight arrow*). Several paraaortic nodes show reactive hyperplasia.

without lymphographic abnormality.[17] Histological examination demonstrates microscopic metastatic foci.

5. Obstruction and displacement of lymphatic channels with opacification of collaterals.

6. Skip lesions may be present, eg, in carcinoma of the cervix.

PITFALLS IN DIFFERENTIAL DIAGNOSIS. Nonneoplastic stimuli may lead to a variety of abnormalities in the lymph nodes that may simulate malignancy. Reactive changes in the lymph nodes are the most frequent source of error in the interpretation of lymphangiograms in patients with lymphoma.[18, 19] The inguinal lymph nodes are frequently abnormal as a result of inflammatory disease and fibrofatty proliferation and should therefore be evaluated only if they serve as a regional drainage center.

1. Enlarged lymph nodes with normal architecture: This is observed in normal individuals and in patients with systemic infection and occasionally in microscopic metastatic involvement.

2. Normal-sized lymph node with marginal defect: This may be a normal finding (hilus defect or incomplete filling of a normal node) or due to an infection, granuloma, metastasis, or lymphoma.[17] Rarely, follicular hyperplasia may cause such a defect.

3. Enlarged nodes with coarse granularity or foaminess: This can be due to reactive or follicular hyperplasia, lymphoma, sarcoidosis, metastasis (seminoma), angioimmunoblastic lymphadenopathy, or hydantoin-induced lymphadenopathy.[17, 21-23]

4. Nonvisualization of lymph nodes: This may occur in normal lymph nodes or indicate complete replacement by a neoplastic process. In the latter, stasis and deviated channels are observed.

5. Persistent opacification of lymphatic channels on 24 hour films: In the absence of other nodal abnormalities, this finding is nonspecific and is observed in normal older

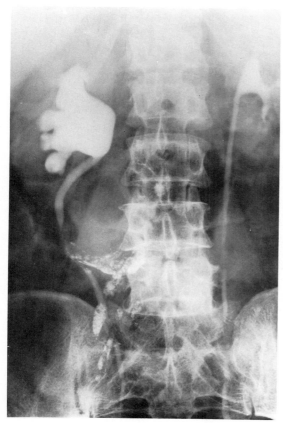

*Figure 21–22.* Metastatic adenoepidermoid carcinoma of the cervix. There is marked nodal enlargement with partial obstruction of the right ureter. The nodes completely replaced by tumor do not opacify.

individuals.[14] When seen in association with other abnormalities, it is indicative of the presence of retroperitoneal disease.

## LYMPHEDEMA AND THE CHYLOUS SYNDROMES

### Lymphedema

**Primary Lymphedema.** Lymphedema (primary or secondary) is the result of an imbalance between the formation and transportation of lymphatic fluid. Primary lymphedema is the result of a developmental anomaly that may manifest at birth or during the neonatal period (congenital lymphedema), during adolescence (lymphedema praecox), or in adulthood (lymphedema tarda). The underlying abnormality is aplasia or hypoplasia (decrease in number and caliber) of the superfi-

cial lymphatics.[31, 32] The deep system is unaffected. The anatomical abnormality is usually bilateral, although the clinical manifestation is frequently unilateral.[33]

There is dermal backflow of the intracutaneously injected blue dye. The lymphangiogram (Fig. 21–23) shows decrease in the number and caliber of lymph vessels (eg, one to two vessels in the calf and one to four in the thigh), filling of collaterals, and dermal lymphatics with delayed emptying. The dermal lymphatics may be dilated and tortuous. Hyperplasia (ectasia) of the lymph channels is observed in 10 to 15% of cases.[1] Extravasation of contrast medium is seen as a result of increased permeability of the defective lymph channels.[32] In uncomplicated cases, there is no lymphatic obstruction.[33]

**Secondary Lymphedema** (Fig. 21–24). This type is more common than the primary variety. The most common cause is malignant obstruction. Other causes are benign tumors, radiation fibrosis, postoperative states, infection, parasites (filariasis), trauma, and thrombophlebitis.[6, 33, 34] Lymphangiograms performed early in the course of obstruction (in patients without infection or filariasis) demonstrate normal lymphatic anatomy of the distal extremity. However, there is stasis of the contrast medium and extravasation as a result of the increased intralymphatic pressure. In the chronic stages, alterations in the distal lymph channels may make the lymphangiographic picture indistinguishable from that of primary lymphedema.[33] In filariasis, blind-ending lymph channels are seen.[34]

**Lymphangiectasis/Lymphangioma** (Fig. 21–25). In the extremities, lymphangiectasis (lymphatic hyperplasia) manifests as tortuous ectatic, valveless vessels similar to varicose veins.[32] It is usually a congenital abnormality but may also develop following trauma and chronic destruction (see Fig. 21–24).[35] In the abdomen, it leads to chylous ascites, and in the chest it is responsible for chylothorax and chylopericardium.[36, 37] Intestinal lymphangiectasis is associated with protein-losing enteropathy. On the lymphangiogram, the contrast medium enters the intestinal lymphatics and may extravasate into the intestinal lumen.[38]

Lymphangioma is a rare benign congenital lesion of the lymph vessels. Three types are identified: simple (capillary), cavernous, and cystic lymphangioma (cystic hygroma).[36]

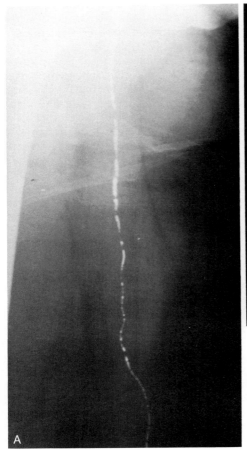

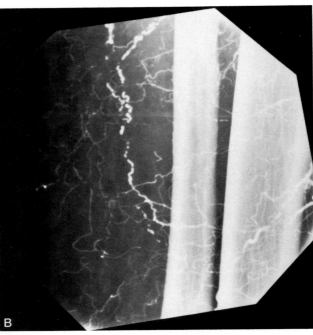

*Figure 21–23.* Primary lymphedema. *A,* Lymphedema prae-cox. There is hypoplasia of the lymphatics with opacification of a single channel (compare with Fig. 21–2). *B,* Lymphedema tarda. Spot film shows opacification of dermal lymphatics.

Lymphangiomas may occur as solitary lesions or may be multiple and affect multiple organs, including bone.

**Lymphovenous Communication and Lymphocele.** Lymphovenous communications are observed in chronic obstruction, after operation or trauma, or in association with neoplasms. Such communications may occur at any level after trauma or operation. In neoplastic obstruction, they are usually found in the retroperitoneum (eg, lympho-portal).

Most lymphoceles occur after radical lymph node dissection, most frequently for pelvic malignancy. They are also observed after renal transplantation, vascular reconstructive surgery, and trauma. Rarely, a lymphocele may occur as a complication of chemotherapy.[39]

### The Chylous Syndromes

The underlying abnormality in nontraumatic chylous effusion is incompetence of the lymph vessel valves.[1] This may be due to a congenital lymphatic abnormality, lymphatic obstruction (malignant, infectious), or venous obstruction.

**Chylous Ascites.** In adults, congenital chylous ascites is rare (1% of cases).[40] It is most frequently acquired as a result of an inflammatory process (35%), tumor (30%), idiopathic causes (23%), or trauma, which is often minor (11%). In children, congenital abnormalities are the most frequent etiology (39%). Other causes are inflammatory processes (15%), trauma (12%), and tumor (3%).[40] The etiology is undetermined in one third of patients. Rupture of a dilated, obstructed lymphatic or a laceration leads to a fistulous communication with the peritoneal cavity with accumulation of chylous ascites.

**Chylothorax.** The most frequent cause of chylothorax is a neoplasm.[41] Other causes are inflammatory diseases, trauma (blunt, penetrating, operative, or associated with subclavian venous catheter insertion), and idiopathic processes. In the neonate, the etiology

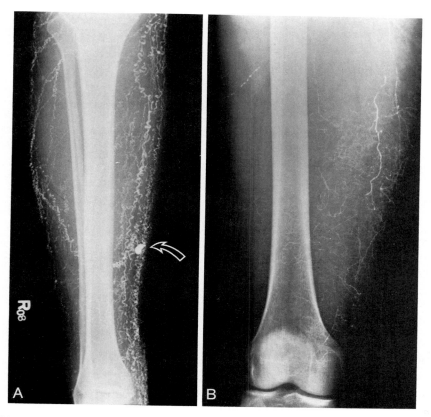

**Figure 21–24.** Secondary lymphedema. *A*, Patient with lymphoma. Markedly tortuous, dilated dermal lymph vessels (lymphatic varices) are opacified. A small lymphatic cyst is present (*arrow*). *B*, Posttraumatic lymphedema. A network of fine dermal lymph vessels is opacified. The normal superficial lymphatic vessels are not seen.

is often elusive. In older children it is often due to a congenital lymphatic abnormality[36] (Fig. 21–25*B*).

**Chyluria.** This occurs as a result of a fistulous communication between the lymphatic system and the urinary tract. It is observed as a complication of filariasis,[42] or may occur in association with malignant obstruction or chronic infection (eg, tuberculosis) and trauma. We have observed chyluria in one patient following embolization of a large renal cell carcinoma.

In patients with chylous syndromes, lymphangiography is used to diagnose the etiology of the obstruction and to localize the site of obstruction. Injection of a colored dye into the lymph vessel preoperatively can be used for intraoperative localization of the site of leakage.

## PATIENT SELECTION AND COMPLICATIONS OF LYMPHOGRAPHY

Ethiodol lymphography is contraindicated in patients with contrast allergy, severe dysp-

nea, chronic pulmonary obstructive disease, or right to left intracardiac or pulmonary shunts.

Pulmonary embolization of Ethiodol occurs in 55% of patients[43] (Fig. 21–26). However, in a large review, clinically significant pulmonary complications were observed in only 0.4% of patients.[44] They are more likely to occur in patients with lymphatic obstruction and may be more severe with infusion of larger volumes of Ethiodol.[43] In individuals with normal pulmonary function, pulmonary embolization of Ethiodol remains unnoticed. In patients with chronic obstructive pulmonary disease or dyspnea, such embolization may compromise pulmonary function, resulting in severe dyspnea and decrease in $pO_2$. If lymphography must be performed in such individuals, a single extremity is studied at one time and the volume of contrast medium is reduced to 4 to 5 ml per lower extremity. Another potentially serious but fortunately rare complication is chemical pneumonitis.

Serious complications are very infrequent.

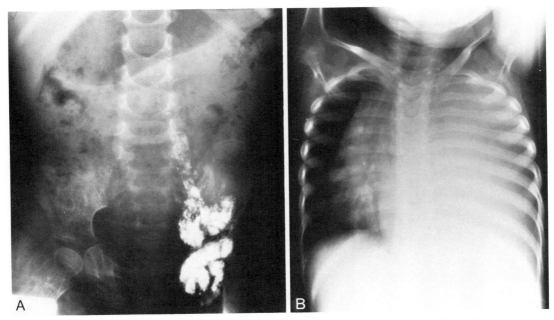

*Figure 21–25.* Lymphangioma. *A,* Left leg lymphogram shows a large lymphangioma in the left groin and pelvis. *B,* Chest radiograph from the same child shows a left-sided chylothorax.

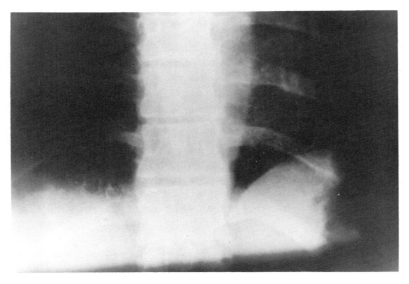

*Figure 21–26.* Asymptomatic pulmonary embolization of Ethiodol. Close-up view shows the contrast medium in pulmonary artery branches in the paraspinal region bilaterally.

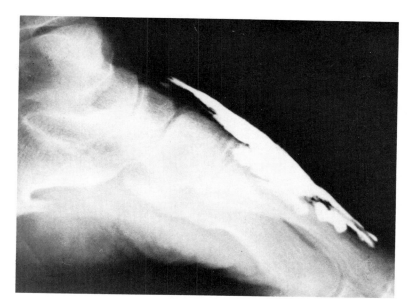

*Figure 21–27.* Subcutaneous-paralymphatic infusion of Ethiodol.

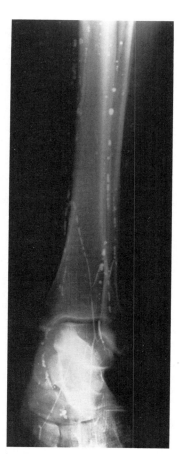

*Figure 21–28.* Inadvertent intravenous infusion of Ethiodol. The contrast medium shows the typical droplet configuration of intravenous contrast. In addition, the branching pattern and location of the opacified vessels is characteristic for veins.

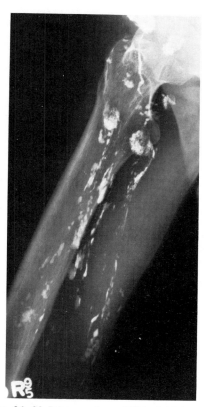

*Figure 21–29.* Extravasation of Ethiodol into the perilymphatic space.

The mortality associated with the procedure is 0.01%.[44] Potential complications are allergy to the blue dye or Ethiodol, inadvertent venous or paralymphatic infusion, and wound infection (Figs. 21–27 and 21–28). Careful fluoroscopic or radiographic monitoring within 1 to 2 minutes of starting the infusion will detect intravenous or paralymphatic infusion before any significant volume of Ethiodol is infused. Paralymphatic infusion of a small volume of Ethiodol is usually without sequelae.

Extravasation of contrast medium into the perilymphatic spaces is most frequently a consequence of a rapid infusion (Fig. 21–29). It also occurs in lymphatic obstruction.

## REFERENCES

1. Viamonte M Jr, Rüttimann A (eds): Atlas of Lymphography. Stuttgart, New York, Georg Thieme Verlag, 1980.
2. Clouse ME, Wallace S (eds): Lymphatic Imaging: Lymphography, Computed Tomography and Scintigraphy. 2nd ed. Baltimore, The Williams & Wilkins Company, 1985.
3. Dooms GC, Hricak H, Crooks LE, et al: Magnetic resonance imaging of the lymph nodes: Comparison with CT. Radiology 153:719–723, 1984.
4. Siefert HM, Mützel W, Schöbel C, et al: Iotasul, a water soluble contrast agent for direct and indirect lymphography. Results and preclinical investigations. Lymphology 13:150–157, 1980.
5. Warwick R, Williams PL: Gray's Anatomy. 35th Brit Edit. Philadelphia, WB Saunders Company, 1973, pp 727–744.
6. Vitek J, Kaspar Z: The radiology of the deep lymphatic system of the leg. Br J Radiol 46:120–124, 1973.
7. Larson DL, Lewis SR: Deep lymphatic system of the lower extremity. Am J Surg 113:217–220, 1967.
8. Malek P, Kolc J, Belan A: Lymphography of the deep lymphatic system of the thigh. Acta Radiol 51:422–428, 1959.
9. Herman PG, Benninghoff DL, Nelson JH, et al: Roentgen anatomy of the ilio-pelvic-aortic lymphatic system. Radiology 80:182–193, 1963.
10. Chiappa S, Uslenghi C, Bonadonna G, et al: Combined testicular and foot lymphangiography in testicular carcinomas. Surg Gynecol Obstet 123:10–14, 1966.
11. Mihara K, Koga K, Tsurudome H, et al: Extravasation of contrast medium into the gastrointestinal tract following lymphangiography: report of 2 cases. Gastrointest Radiol 6:239–242, 1981.
12. Lechner G, Riedl P, Zechner O: Zum Mechanismus der Kontrastmitteldarstellung der Leber nach Lymphographie. Fortschr Roentgenstr 125:355–357, 1976.
13. Doss LL, Alyea JL, Waggoner CM, et al: Fluorescein-aided isolation of lymphatic vessels for lymphangiography. AJR 134:603–604, 1980.
14. Takahashi M, Abrams HL: The accuracy of lymphangiographic diagnosis in malignant lymphoma. Radiology 89:448–460, 1967.
15. Greening RR, Wallace S: Further observations in lymphangiography. Radiol Clin North Am 1:157–173, 1963.
16. Fischer HW, Zimmerman GR: Roentgenographic visualization of lymph nodes and lymphatic channels. AJR 81:517–534, 1959.
17. Viamonte M Jr, Altman D, Parks R, et al: Radiologic-pathologic correlation in the interpretation of lymphangioadenograms. Radiology 80:903–916, 1963.
18. Parker BR, Blank N, Castellino RA: Lymphographic appearance of benign conditions simulating lymphoma. Radiology 111:267–274, 1974.
19. Castellino RA, Billingham M, Dorfman RF: Lymphographic accuracy in Hodgkin's disease and malignant lymphoma with a note on the "reactive" lymph node as a cause of most false-positive lymphograms. Invest Radiol 9:155–165, 1974.
20. Miyaji H, Nakagawa E, Sugimoto H: Lymphography in toxoplasmosis. A case report. Lymphology 13:59–61, 1980.
21. Lohkamp F, Hiness R: Extrathorakale Sarkoidose der retroperitonealen Lymphknoten und der Milz mit Aszites. Fortschr Roentgenstr 125:358–361, 1976.
22. Sayoc AS, Howland WJ: Lymphangiographic findings of Mesantoin-induced pseudolymphoma. Radiology 111:579–580, 1974.
23. Cunningham JJ, Jackson DV Jr: Lymphographic and echographic findings in angioimmunoblastic lymphadenopathy. Arch Intern Med 137:1693–1695, 1977.
24. Marglin S, Castellino R: Lymphographic accuracy in 632 consecutive, previously untreated cases of Hodgkin disease and non-Hodgkin lymphoma. Radiology 140:351–353, 1981.
25. Schaner EG, Head GL, Doppman JL, et al: Computed tomography in the diagnosis, staging, and management of abdominal lymphoma. J Comput Tomogr 1:176–180, 1977.
26. Castellino R: Observations on "reactive (follicular) hyperplasia" as encountered in repeat lymphography in the lymphomas. Cancer 34:2042–2050, 1974.
27. Musumeci R, De Palo G, Kenda R, et al: Retroperitoneal metastases from ovarian carcinoma: reassessment of 365 patients studied by lymphography. AJR 134:449–452, 1980.
28. Castellino RA: The role of lymphography in "apparently localized" prostatic carcinoma. Lymphology 8:16–20, 1975.
29. Zaunbauer W, Kunz R, Leuppi R: Die diagnostische Zuverlässigkeit der Lymphographie bei Patienten mit malignen Hodentumoren. Fortschr Roentgenstr 126:335–338, 1977.
30. Walsh JW, Amendola MA, Konerding KF, et al: Computed tomographic detection of pelvic and inguinal lymph-node metastases from primary and recurrent pelvic malignant disease. Radiology 137:157–166, 1980.
31. Fonkalsrud EW, Coulson WF: Management of congenital lymphedema in infants and children. Ann Surg 177:280–285, 1973.
32. Craig O: Primary lymphedema and lymphatica porosa. Radiology 92:1216–1222, 1969.
33. Buonocore E, Young JR: Lymphangiographic evaluation of lymphedema and lymphatic flow. AJR 95:751–765, 1965.
34. Cohen LB, Nelson G, Wood AM, et al: Lymphangiography in filaria lymphoedema and elephantiasis. Am J Trop Med Hyg 10:843–848, 1961.
35. Pirschel J, Hagemann H: Posttraumatische Lymphangiektasie. Fortschr Roentgenstr 127:592–593, 1977.
36. Fonkalsrud EW: Surgical management of congenital

malformations of the lymphatic system. Am J Surg 128:152–159, 1974.

37. Gallant TE, Hunziker RJ, Gibson TC: Primary chylopericardium: The role of lymphangiography. AJR 129:1043–1045, 1977.

38. Gold RH, Youker JE: Idiopathic intestinal lymphangiectasis (primary protein-losing enteropathy). Lymphographic verification of enteric and peritoneal leakage of chyle. Radiology 109:315–316, 1973.

39. Jones WB, Rhamy RK, Faber RB, et al: Lymphocele. A complication of cancer chemotherapy. JAMA 239:1419–1420, 1978.

40. Vasko JS, Tapper RI: The surgical significance of chylous ascitis. Arch Surg 95:355–368, 1967.

41. Roy PH, Carr DT, Payne WS: The problem of chylothorax. Mayo Clin Proc 42:457–467, 1967.

42. Koehler PR, Chiang T-C, Lin C-T, et al: Lymphography in chyluria. AJR 102:455–465, 1968.

43. Bron KM, Baum S, Abrams HL: Oil embolism in lymphangiography. Incidence, manifestations, and mechanisms. Radiology 80:194–202, 1963.

44. Hessel SJ, Adams DF, Abrams HL: Complications of angiography. Radiology 138:273–281, 1981.

# THE BILIARY SYSTEM

## SEVEN

## Cholangiography

### ANATOMY

The hepatic ducts have a lobar and a segmental distribution (Figs. 22–1 and 22–2). The right hepatic duct is formed by the anterior and posterior segmental ducts. Occasionally, these segmental ducts join the left or common hepatic duct separately. The left hepatic duct is formed by medial and lateral segmental ducts. Either a single medial segmental duct or several smaller ducts join the lateral segmental ducts to form the left hepatic duct. The lateral segment is drained by two major ducts: an anterior-superior duct and a larger posterior-inferior duct. The left hepatic duct is usually longer and slightly wider in its central portion than the right hepatic duct. Bile ducts from the caudate lobe drain into either the left or the right hepatic ducts.

The common hepatic duct is formed at the porta hepatis by the junction of the left and right hepatic ducts. The distal 1.5 to 2 cm of each of these ducts lies outside the liver parenchyma. The common hepatic duct may vary in length from 1 to 5 cm. It is closely related to the hepatic artery, which lies to the left of it, and to the portal vein, which runs posteriorly and to the left. It is joined by the cystic duct from the right side to form the common bile duct (CBD).

The CBD drains into the duodenum at the papilla of Vater. It is joined by the pancreatic duct at the ampulla. The ampullary sphincter (of Oddi) is a thickened circular muscle around the distal CBD, pancreatic duct, and

ampulla. On cholangiography, the diameter of the normal unobstructed CBD is between 6 and 8 mm. It may appear larger if there is distention following injection of contrast medium or atony after administration of medication.

### Variant Anatomy

Several variants of biliary anatomy have been described.[1, 2] In fact, such variant anatomy is observed in 47% of individuals undergoing biliary surgery.[2] Most variants (other than variations in length and anomalous junction of the cystic duct) are accessory ducts, which account for 38% of such anomalies. Failure to recognize such anatomical variants is a major cause of operative complications, leading to accidental ligation, bile fistula, and stricture formation.

### CHOLANGIOGRAPHY

Percutaneous transhepatic cholangiography (PTC) alone as a diagnostic procedure is being performed less frequently, primarily because of the improved diagnostic accuracy of computed body tomography and abdominal ultrasonography. In addition, endoscopic retrograde cholangiopancreatography (ERCP) has become readily available.

PTC is usually performed in conjunction with percutaneous transhepatic biliary drainage (PBD). Only 5% of patients referred to us for evaluation and treatment of biliary

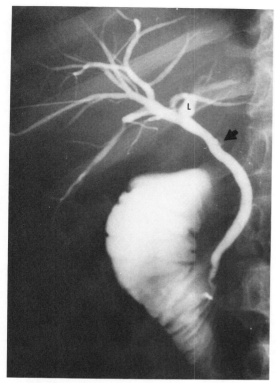

**Figure 22–1.** Normal PTC through a 22 gauge needle. L = left hepatic duct. Arrow points to cystic duct.

disease do not require PBD catheters. Although the following discussion will focus primarily upon PTC, it must be kept in mind that patients with biliary obstruction require PBD as part of their management.

## Indications and Contraindications for PTC

The main indications for PTC are:

1. Differentiation between obstructive and nonobstructive jaundice, ie, surgical versus nonsurgical jaundice in patients with marginally abnormal liver function tests.

2. Demonstration of site of obstruction.

3. Determination of the etiology of the obstruction.

4. Delineation of biliary anatomy prior to operation.

5. Establishment of PBD as a preoperative measure, for palliation, for access to the biliary tract for interventional procedures (eg, stricture dilation, stone retrieval), and management of biliary sepsis.

6. Evaluation of functional disturbances (eg, post-cholecystectomy syndrome, papil-

lary stenosis), and bilio-intestinal anastomosis.

Fever and sepsis due to cholangitis are not contraindications for PTC followed by PBD, because biliary drainage for relief of obstruction and biliary diversion in patients with postoperative complications are therapeutic.[3-5] The presence of a small or moderate amount of ascites is a relative contraindication. However, PTC may be performed if significant benefit is anticipated from the procedure. Abnormal blood clotting parameters and severe ascites are contraindications for PTC.

PTC can be performed safely if the prothrombin time and partial thromboplastin time are not prolonged by more than 25% of the control values and if platelets are normal. Alternatively, fresh frozen plasma and platelets are given at the time of the procedure.

### Pre-cholangiogram Workup

Most patients referred for PTC have completed an extensive workup for the differentiation of the type of jaundice and determination of the site of obstruction. Such a workup includes liver function tests, abdominal ultrasonography, computed body tomography (CT), and, in some cases, ERCP. Although clinical assessment can differentiate between obstructive and nonobstructive jaundice in 75 to 80% of cases,[6] liver function tests may be normal in some patients with biliary obstruction.[7, 8]

Both ultrasonography and CT are used for demonstration of ductal dilatation and identification of the site and etiology of obstruction. Under optimal conditions, ductal dilatation may be demonstrated by ultrasound in as many as 90% of cases. An accuracy of 97% (for level) and 94% (for etiology) of the obstruction is reported for systematic evaluation with CT.[9, 10]

Although both these examinations are highly accurate in complete obstruction with dilated ducts, partial obstruction with nondilated ducts may not be recognized by these studies.[7, 8, 11] Since the intra- and extrahepatic ducts may remain nondilated during the early phases of biliary obstruction, demonstration of normal caliber ducts is not a reliable criterion for excluding obstructive jaundice. On the other hand, demonstration of biliary dilatation by these studies, even in the absence of jaundice, is highly suggestive of the presence of a partially obstructing or

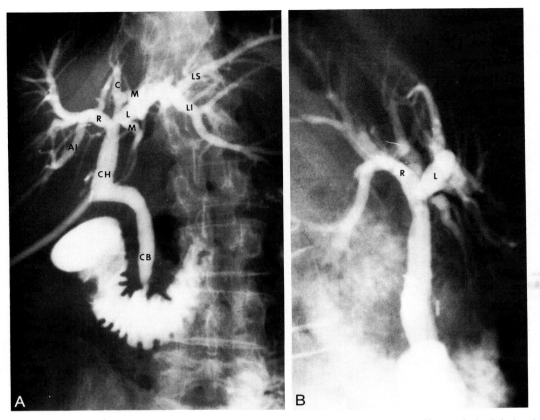

**Figure 22–2.** AP (*A*) and lateral (*B*) T-tube cholangiograms showing normal anatomy. AI = anterior-inferior right hepatic duct; C = caudate lobe duct; CB = choledochus; CH = common hepatic duct; L = left hepatic duct; LI = lateral inferior and LS = lateral superior left lobe ducts; M = medial segment ducts; R = right hepatic duct. *Note*: The course of the common hepatic duct is deviated as a result of surgical placement of a T-tube.

nonobstructing lesion.[12] Occasionally, dilatation of the extrahepatic ducts is seen in the absence of disease.[13]

ERCP is successful in identifying the site and cause of obstruction in between 70 and 90% of cases.[6, 14] In experienced hands, this procedure is not only highly successful but also safe, with only a 2 to 3% complication rate and 0.1 to 0.2% mortality.[14] In some patients, radionuclide hepatobiliary imaging may provide a sensitive method for the detection of early or partial biliary obstruction.[15]

In patients with complete biliary obstruction, PTC is successful in 100% of cases. In those with nondilated ducts, the success rate is about 85%. The additional advantage of PTC is that therapeutic PBD is available immediately. Biliary drainage has also become available in conjunction with ERCP.

Properly performed PTC with or without PBD is the only reliable technique that provides the most accurate delineation of intra- and extrahepatic biliary anatomy. In patients with marginally abnormal liver function tests and nonobstructed ducts on CT and ultrasonography, PTC should be performed to exclude a partially obstructing lesion. Other authors also support the view that PTC is preferable to ERCP for the evaluation of obstructive jaundice.[16]

Table 22–1 lists the most frequent causes of obstructive jaundice. Partial ductal obstruction or jaundice in the absence of CT or ultrasonographically demonstrable bile duct abnormality is seen in metastatic disease, biliary strictures, calculi, and sclerosing cholangitis. Other rare causes of benign biliary obstruction are aberrant hepatic vessels[17] and parasitic disease.[18]

### Premedication

Intramuscular injections of a sedative and an analgesic are given before the procedure (see Chapter 4). All patients must receive intravenous antibiotic coverage. Two or three

**TABLE 22–1. Major Causes of Obstructive Jaundice**

| Lesion | Incidence (%) | |
|---|---|---|
| | Smith* | JHH† |
| Malignancy* | 24 | |
| Pancreatic carcinoma | 18 | 32 |
| Ampullary/duodenal carcinoma | | 4 |
| Metastatic disease | 2 | 9 |
| Cholangiocarcinoma | 3 | 20 |
| Benign disease: | 76 | |
| Traumatic stricture/operative complications | 44 | 10 |
| Calculi | 21 | 8 |
| Pancreatitis | 8 | |
| Sclerosing cholangitis | 1 | 7 |
| Miscellaneous: | | |
| Benign and malignant causes | | 10 |

*3527 operatively treated patients
†350 patients treated with PBD, between 1978 and 1984 at The Johns Hopkins Hospital.

antibiotics are used in combination: gentamicin or tobramycin, a cephalosporin, and ampicillin. If only two antibiotics are given, ampicillin may be omitted. Aminoglycosides should not be used in patients with compromised renal function. Unless indicated for some other reasons (eg, sepsis, fever), the first dose of the antibiotic is administered 1 hour before the study. This provides maximal blood levels at the time of PTC. This practice, together with minimization of catheter manipulation in patients with a history of cholangitis and avoidance of overinjection into obstructed ducts, has virtually eliminated episodes of sepsis.

Antibiotic coverage is continued for at least 24 hours after PTC or until satisfactory PBD is established and the patient is afebrile. Systemic antibiotic therapy does not influence the bacterial composition of bile in an obstructed system, but does provide protection from systemic complications. The incidence of infected bile is particularly high in patients with partial obstruction and calculi.

During PTC and PBD, all patients should have EKG monitoring. An intravenous line must be placed (preferably in the left arm) for emergency medication and additional analgesics. Morphine should not be used as premedication in patients being evaluated for functional disturbances of the papilla.

## Approach

PTC can be performed via an anterior or a lateral approach. The anterior approach for PTC of the right hepatic ducts has been used by some authors, but has failed to gain popularity.[19, 20] With this method, the PTC needle is inserted at a 45° angle from the body surface, via the subcostal region, in the mid-clavicular line. The disadvantages of this approach are increased radiation to the operator's hands and a somewhat higher risk of bilio-vascular fistula formation.

The lateral approach is used most frequently for PTC of both the right and the left ducts. PTC of the left ducts can also be performed via the subxiphoid approach with or without ultrasound guidance.

## Puncture Site

Fixed anatomical landmarks (intercostal space, spine) are notoriously unreliable. The liver must be entered below the right costophrenic sulcus. To determine its position, excursion of the right hemidiaphragm is observed in maximal inspiration. In general, the sulcus extends 1 to 2 cm below the costophrenic angle as visualized on fluoroscopy. Thus, the skin entry site should be at least one or, if feasible and especially for PBD, two intercostal spaces below the costophrenic angle, in the anterior to mid-axillary line. A metal clamp is placed on the skin surface to mark the anticipated puncture site as the diaphragmatic excursion is evaluated.

The needle puncture is made in the mid or lower half of the intercostal space. An attempt should be made to stay away from the rib periosteum, as this is extremely sensitive. In addition, if a duct is entered that is suitable for placement of a PBD catheter (over a 0.018 inch wire), proximity to the rib is undesirable because the PBD catheter often leads to chronic periosteal irritation and occasionally to osteomyelitis.

The proximal duodenum has been used as a relatively reliable landmark for localization of the liver hilus.[21] In most patients, the junction of the left and right hepatic ducts is located several centimeters above it. The duodenum can be opacified with oral contrast medium or localized by placement of a nasogastric tube. We have not found it necessary to intubate or opacify the duodenum for successful PTC.

## Puncture

Local anesthetic is infiltrated at the anticipated skin entry site with a 25 gauge needle. For deeper injection, a 22 gauge needle is used. The patient is instructed to stop breathing in mid-respiration, and the needle is advanced to the liver capsule while continuously injecting the anesthetic. A small skin incision is made, and the subcutaneous tissues are spread apart with a mosquito clamp.

A 22 gauge skinny (Chiba) needle is inserted through the skin. The patient is instructed to stop breathing in mid-respiration, and the needle is advanced into the liver in a single, continuous, gentle thrust (Fig. 22–3). If the patient resumes respiration prematurely (induced by pain), the needle must not be inserted any farther (to prevent damage to ducts or blood vessels). The needle is advanced only when the patient is not breathing. The depth of needle insertion is determined by liver size, angle of insertion, and the bile ducts that need to be opacified (left or right). For the right-sided ducts, the needle tip is advanced to 1 to 2 cm from the vertebral spine or 2 to 3 cm from the dome of the liver. If a left duct puncture is to be performed, the anterior axillary line is chosen for needle insertion, and the needle tip is advanced past the midline.

Once the needle is in place, the patient is instructed to resume shallow respirations. The stylet is removed, and a connecting tubing with a 10 ml syringe containing 60% contrast medium is attached to the hub. Contrast medium is injected continuously as the needle is withdrawn slowly and the tip is observed by fluoroscopy. Multiple blood vessels are often entered. These are recognized by the following criteria (Fig. 22–4):

1. Prompt washout occurs after contrast injection is stopped.

2. The hepatic vein flow is towards the right atrium, and often several parallel channels are opacified.

3. The portal vein flow is towards the liver periphery, and a hepatic parenchymal stain is seen. Injection into a hepatic artery branch gives a similar picture.

In addition, dilated lymphatic channels and the cisterna chyli may be opacified (Fig. 22–5). This is usually an indication of the presence of biliary obstruction or parenchymal disease.

As a bile duct is entered, the dense contrast is seen entering its branches. The duct is recognized easily by the typical branching pattern and persistence of dense contrast even when the injection is stopped (see section on Pitfalls in Diagnosis). Contrast flow is towards the liver hilus. If there is any doubt concerning the fluoroscopic impression, a spot film should be obtained before continuing to inject contrast medium.

If no bile duct is entered, the needle is withdrawn to the liver periphery and the stylet is reinserted. The needle tip should not exit from the liver substance, but should remain at least 1 to 3 cm from the liver surface. A single puncture hole in the liver capsule is desirable. Multiple holes predispose to leakage of bile and blood into the peritoneal cavity.

Generally, the first needle pass is directed towards the dome of the liver. The angle for each subsequent needle pass is adjusted by about 10° (towards the porta), and the needle is reinserted during suspended respiration (see Fig. 22–3). If multiple portal vein branches are entered, the needle course should be adjusted anteriorly by about 10°.

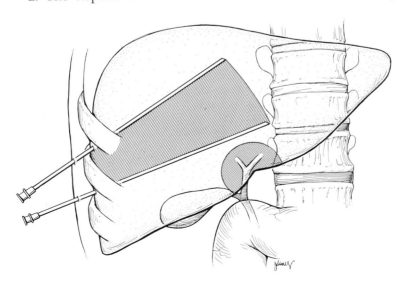

**Figure 22–3.** Technique for PTC of the right hepatic ducts. The fan-shaped shaded area between the two PTC needles represents the zone most likely to yield successful duct puncture. Puncture of the extrahepatic segments of the left and right hepatic ducts (*dotted area*) must be avoided.

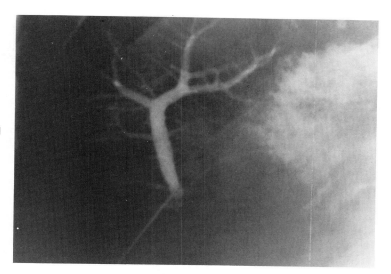

*Figure 22–4.* Appearance of a portal vein branch on PTC.

The procedure is repeated until a bile duct is entered or until 10 to 15 passes have been made.

However, if after 8 to 10 passes the needle insertion site is to be changed, ie, another intercostal space is to be used for PTC, the first needle is withdrawn to the liver periphery and left in place until the study is completed. In this way, leakage of bile and blood will be avoided.

Once a duct is entered, 10 to 20 ml of contrast medium is injected slowly to opacify the system. In nonobstructed ducts, this usually provides satisfactory opacification. In an obstructed biliary system, it is frequently not possible to opacify the distal extrahepatic ducts without a tilt table or injection of a larger volume of contrast medium. In such cases, therapeutic PBD should be performed to decompress the ducts. Once a larger catheter is inserted and some bile is removed, the distal ducts can be opacified to evaluate the site of obstruction. In this way, overinjection of contrast medium and sepsis are avoided.

Tilting or turning the patient (upright for the CBD; left posterior oblique or left lateral decubitus for the left hepatic ducts) may be necessary to facilitate opacification of some segments. We have found that altering the patient's position frequently results in dislodgment of the needle tip. Thus, if these

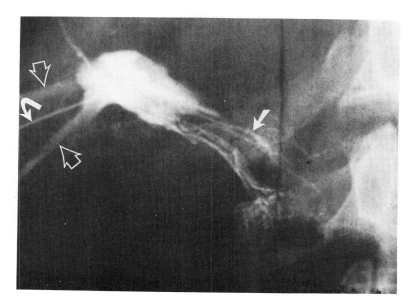

*Figure 22–5.* Opacification of liver lymphatics (*straight arrow*) during PTC. Dense intraparenchymal deposition of contrast medium is present. Several dilated bile ducts are opacified (*open arrows*). The lymphatic drainage is towards the cisterna chyli. Curved arrow points to PTC needle.

maneuvers are used, contrast injection should be monitored fluoroscopically. In addition, all the necessary radiographs of the ducts opacified in the supine position should be obtained prior to tilting or turning the patient. If there is partial or complete obstruction and PBD is performed, these maneuvers are not necessary since a complete cholangiogram can be obtained through the thin-walled Teflon sheath of the PBD needle.

A drainage catheter can be inserted through the 22 gauge needle puncture site if an appropriate right hepatic duct has been entered. A 0.018 inch coat hanger wire is inserted through the 22 gauge needle and is torqued into the common duct. The needle is removed, and the thin-walled Teflon sheath from the PBD needle is inserted over the 0.018 inch wire. The wire is replaced by a 0.038 inch torque wire, which is used to advance the Teflon sheath into the bowel or the distal duct. A PBD catheter is then inserted over a Lunderquist exchange wire.

For PBD, the shortest, most direct route between the liver surface and the bile ducts is generally desirable, ie, perpendicular to the long axis of the body. For PTC, a craniad angulation from a low intercostal space puncture can also be used, especially in large livers. A very low position, however, may predispose to inadvertent puncture of the gallbladder.

A sheath needle has been used for a one-step approach to PTC and PBD. The advantage of this approach is that only a single puncture is necessary for both PTC and PBD. The main disadvantage is that the duct that is entered must be utilized for catheter insertion; ie, selection of a more suitable duct is not possible unless a second puncture is made. Although this is a larger needle, bile leakage is not a problem as long as the system is decompressed. Catheter removal may be associated with significant bleeding. If only PTC is performed with the sheath needle, the tract can be embolized at the time of sheath removal. Alternatively, the catheter can be removed gradually over 2 to 4 hours to permit thrombosis of the tract.

Left hepatic duct puncture is usually necessary if these ducts do not opacify from the right (ie, are isolated as a result of stricture or tumor). Occasionally, a severely stenosed left hepatic duct will occlude completely after a right PBD catheter is inserted (see Fig. 22–35). Once the catheter is in place, the location of the left hepatic ducts can usually be predicted from the cholangiogram. A skinny needle is used for PTC of the left ducts via the subxiphoid approach (Fig. 22–6). We have not found it necessary to use ultrasound guidance for PTC or PBD of the left ducts.

### Films

Radiographs (14 × 14 inch or 105 mm spot films if a large field image intensifier is available) are obtained in the supine and left and right posterior oblique (~ 25 to 30°) positions. In addition, spot films of the pertinent areas

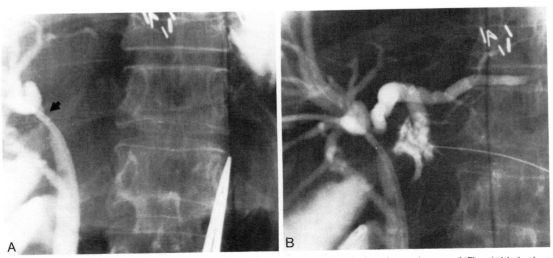

*Figure 22–6.* Subxiphoid approach for left duct PTC in a patient with cholangiocarcinoma. *A,* The right ducts are opacified through a PBD catheter and the site of obstruction is identified (*arrow*). A metal clamp is placed at the skin entry site for left duct puncture. *B,* The 22 gauge needle is advanced and contrast injection opacifies the occluded left hepatic ducts.

(eg, calculi, obstructing tumor) are obtained. The distal CBD and sphincter should be evaluated for functional disturbances and the presence of strictures or stenoses. Spot films should be used to document the sphincter in the relaxed phase, if necessary after intravenous injection of glucagon.

## Post-PTC Care

Specific care of the patient is not necessary after uncomplicated PTC. Bed rest is prescribed for 3 to 4 hours. During this period, vital signs are monitored and the abdomen is checked for tenderness and guarding. Antibiotic coverage is continued for 24 hours in uncomplicated cases.

## Biliary Pressure Measurement and Pharmacocholangiography

Contrary to some opinions, accurate intraductal pressures cannot be obtained consistently with a 22 gauge needle unless a dilated or central duct is entered. In the smaller peripheral ducts, the bevel is often partially extraductal (Fig. 22–7). Although contrast medium enters the duct freely, accurate pressure reading is not possible. Similarly, we have often found it difficult to aspirate bile through the 22 gauge needle. Accurate pressures can be measured through the thin-walled sheath of the PBD needle. The normal intraductal pressure is less than 20 cm $H_2O$. Intraductal pressures may be elevated in patients premedicated with morphine.

Pharmacocholangiography is indicated for differentiation between fixed anatomical and

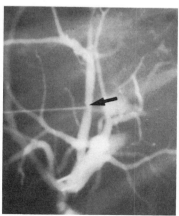

*Figure 22–7.* Close-up of 22 gauge needle entry site into right hepatic duct shows partially extraductal location of the bevel (*arrow*).

functional stenoses of the distal common duct. In addition, glucagon relaxation of the sphincter can be used as an aid for transpapillary expulsion of smaller calculi (less than 6 mm in maximal diameter).[22] The dosage is 1 mg glucagon, which is injected intravenously.

## Failed Cholangiogram

The main reasons for a failed cholangiogram are an inadequate number of needle passes, fast needle withdrawal, or intermittent injections of contrast medium. In addition, if subcapsular or significant intraparenchymal (extraductal) contrast medium has accumulated, contrast entering the biliary tree on a subsequent needle pass may be obscured and remain unrecognized. If such a situation exists, the procedure should be terminated and attempted again the following day.

If a biliary radicle has not been entered after 8 to 10 passes, the needle entry site should be changed and subsequent passes made through a different intercostal space. With this approach, our success rate for PTC in patients with nonobstructed ducts and in those with sclerosing cholangitis has exceeded 90%.

## Complications of PTC

The incidence and severity of pain during PTC are proportional to the number of needle passes. Pain is located in the right upper quadrant, subxiphoid, or substernal region or is referred to the shoulder. Occasionally, the pain is severe. With an increasing number of needle passes, the requirement for analgesia also increases. Extravasation of large amounts of contrast medium into the liver parenchyma or injection into the subcapsular space is very painful. If the procedure is prolonged, some patients become restless and uncooperative, and despite administration of large doses of analgesics, it may be difficult to continue the study. At this point, it is wise to terminate the study and reattempt PTC the following day.

Serious complications are reported in 3 to 6% of patients undergoing PTC (Table 22–2).[23, 24] Routine antibiotic coverage, decompression of obstructed ducts, and use of the skinny needle have decreased the incidence of serious complications at our institution.

**TABLE 22–2.** Major Complications of PTC

|  | PTC | |
| --- | --- | --- |
|  | Ref. 24* | Ref. 23* |
| Number of procedures | 905 | 2745 |
| Major complications (%): | 5.4 |  |
| Emergency operation | 2.8 |  |
| Sepsis | 3.1 | 1.6 |
| Bile leakage/peritonitis | 2.6 | 0.8 |
| Hemorrhage | 0.4 | 0.2 |
| Death | 0.1 | 0.1 |

*Review of published reports.

Fever and chills are due to bacteremia. Vasovagal reactions occur occasionally and are easily managed with intravenous atropine (0.6 to 0.8 mg). PTC with the skinny needle is rarely associated with significant bleeding, although intrahepatic hematomas and transient arterioportal fistulae[25] and traumatic aneurysms of hepatic artery branches have been observed. Persistent hemobilia is usually associated with the insertion of the larger PBD catheters or operatively placed Silastic stents (see Chapter 15, Figs. 15–34 and 15–35).

Bile leakage and peritonitis have been reported after skinny needle cholangiography.[26] Bile peritonitis is an infrequent but potentially lethal complication. Asymptomatic bile leakage occurs much more frequently. Bilious pleural effusion results from a high puncture in which the needle has traversed the pleural space. Rarely, it may also be due to transdiaphragmatic transportation of intraperitoneal fluid. Acute renal failure may occur if large volumes of contrast medium are used or in patients with compromised renal function.[27]

Inadvertent puncture of the gallbladder can occur if a low hepatic puncture is made. If there is no obstruction of the cystic or distal ducts, bile is aspirated and the needle removed. If the cystic duct is obstructed, insertion of a drainage catheter may be necessary. This is not required if the gallbladder communicates with the common duct and the latter is decompressed through a PBD catheter.

PITFALLS IN DIAGNOSIS

1. Periductal injection of contrast medium (Fig. 22–8): A partially extraductal position of the 22 gauge needle may result in intra- and periductal contrast injection. This can simulate ductal dilatation on fluoroscopy. The distinction is made by evaluation of the spot films, which demonstrate indistinct margins with periductal injection, whereas intraductal

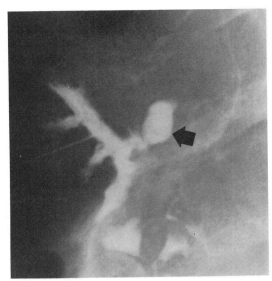

**Figure 22–8.** Periductal injection of contrast medium simulating intraductal opacification. Spot film demonstrates a fuzzy outline of the extraductal contrast medium. Intraductal contrast medium is also present and has a smooth outline (*arrow*).

contrast medium has a smooth outline in the absence of mural abnormality.

2. Portal vein opacification simulating a bile duct (Fig. 22–9): Stasis of contrast medium in severe portal hypertension may simulate a bile duct on fluoroscopy. Although blood returns on aspiration, this is often considered the result of a traumatic puncture. Again, spot films should be obtained to assess the situation.

3. Compression artefacts (Fig. 22–10): As the normal hepatic artery crosses the common hepatic duct, it may cause extrinsic compression that can be misinterpreted as a tumor or calculus.[28] This defect may be eccentric or bandlike or may appear concentric as a result of bilateral compression.

## CONGENITAL ABNORMALITIES

### Caroli's Disease/Congenital Hepatic Fibrosis

Congenital cystic dilatation (or communicating cavernous ectasia) of the hepatic ducts is an autosomal recessive disorder that is often associated with renal abnormalities of varying severity (tubular ectasia, medullary sponge kidney, multiple cysts); rarely, a choledochal cyst may also be present.[29-31] Dilatation of the bile ducts results from an abnormality in the connective tissues of these ducts.[32]

Although the exact etiology remains unclear, clinical observations and animal exper-

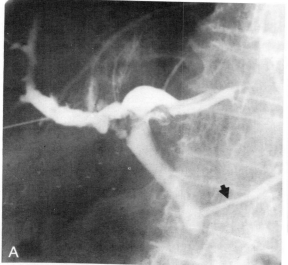

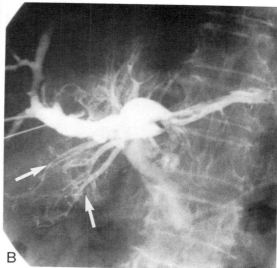

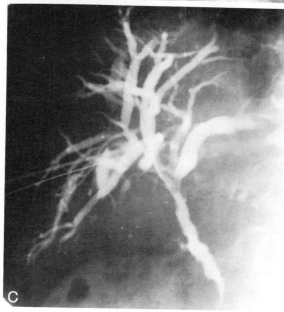

*Figure 22–9.* Stasis of contrast medium in the portal vein simulating intraductal contrast medium in a patient with cholangiocarcinoma. *A,* There is dense opacification of intrahepatic branches and faint opacification of the main portal vein. Opacification of the coronary vein (*arrow*) can be mistaken for the pancreatic duct on fluoroscopy. *B,* Repeat contrast injection through a 5 Fr sheath shows diffuse thrombosis of smaller portal vein branches (*arrows*) causing severe portal hypertension. *C,* Cholangiogram through the PBD needle sheath.

iments have shown that epithelial-lined cysts, identical to those found in Caroli's disease, develop after hepatic infarction following occlusion of the hepatic capillary bed.[33, 34] Thus, it is postulated that the etiology of Caroli's disease may lie in neonatal hepatic artery occlusion.[33] In our own experience in patients with hepatic artery embolization, no such cysts were observed despite embolization with Ivalon microspheres and Gelfoam powder, both of which are also capillary occluding agents. However, this microvascular infarction theory may explain the development of peripheral bile duct cysts in patients with congenital hepatic fibrosis.

Caroli's disease may manifest with or without periportal hepatic fibrosis. Although some authors consider these to be extreme manifestations of the same disease, others believe they represent separate entities.[29, 30, 32, 35] In the type without hepatic fibrosis, the clinical history is characterized by recurrent cholangitis and the formation of calculi. In Caroli's disease with hepatic fibrosis, there are proliferative changes in the small biliary ducts and periportal fibrosis, leading to portal hypertension. Calculi and cholangitis are usually absent.

Both sexes are affected with equal frequency, and the onset of symptoms is usually in the second to third decade of life and occasionally during infancy.[29, 30] Typical symptoms are recurrent episodes of cramplike abdominal pain and fever due to cholan-

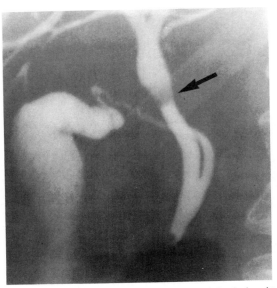

**Figure 22–10.** Bandlike compression defect due to right hepatic artery (*arrow*). Note anomalously low and left-sided insertion of the cystic duct and a pseudocalculus at the sphincter.

gitis and obstructing biliary calculi. These may be complicated by liver abscesses and septicemia, both of which are the most frequent causes of death.

**Cholangiography.** This is indicated to confirm the diagnosis, determine the etiology of biliary obstruction, and delineate the anatomy. In addition, PBD can be performed for relief of obstruction.

The cholangiogram is quite characteristic (Fig. 22–11). There is segmental dilatation of the intrahepatic ducts throughout the liver. Ectasia of the extrahepatic ducts is also frequently present.[32] In addition, hepatic abscesses and biliary calculi may be demonstrated. The dilated segments can be quite large and difficult to opacify on PTC. In patients on long-term biliary drainage, a decrease in the size of these ducts is observed, indicating that their size is related to the degree and duration of obstruction.

In congenital hepatic fibrosis, there is cystic dilatation of the peripheral biliary ducts that may assume significant proportions and thus simulate Caroli's disease.[32] On histological examination, proliferative changes are present in these ducts, in addition to severe periportal fibrosis. In polycystic disease of the liver, the cysts are lined by columnar epithelium, contain serous fluid, and do not communicate with the bile ducts. Such cysts may occasionally be responsible for obstructive jaundice.[36]

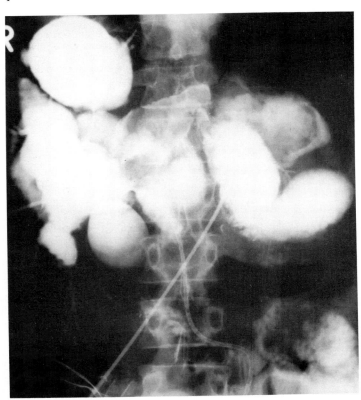

**Figure 22–11.** Caroli's disease. There is marked saccular and cylindrical dilatation of the intrahepatic ducts. Bilateral PBD catheters have been inserted.

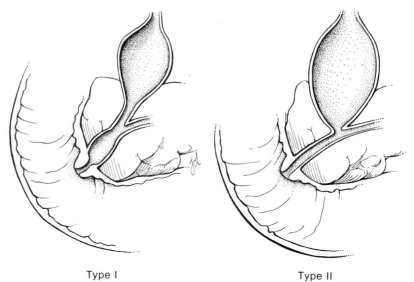

*Figure 22–12.* Choledochal cysts. Diagrammatic representation of the anomalous CBD–pancreatic duct junction.

Type I                    Type II

## Choledochal Cyst

This is also an uncommon congenital abnormality leading to biliary ectasia. Both extra- and intrahepatic ducts are affected in 73% of patients.[37] In the remainder, only the extrahepatic ducts are affected. Abnormality of the intrahepatic ducts is unilateral in 42% of patients and involves the left lobe exclusively.[37] In the remainder, both lobes are affected. Dilatation of the intrahepatic ducts may be due to the congenital abnormality or secondary to a stenosis of the common hepatic duct, which is observed in 16% of patients.

The ectasia of the CBD is most frequently cystic but may be cylindrical or a combination of the two types. It may be segmental or diffuse, or multiple cystic dilatations may be present.[38]

The development of choledochal cysts is most likely related to an anomalous junction of the CBD and pancreatic duct that gives rise to an abnormally long common channel.[39, 40] Two types are recognized (Figs. 22–12 to 22–14): In the first type (Kimura Type I), the pancreatic duct enters the proximal or mid CBD; in the second type (Kimura Type II), the CBD drains into the pancreatic duct.[39] In the Type I abnormality, ductal dilatation is mild and symptoms are not severe. In the Type II abnormality, ductal dilatation is usually pronounced and symptoms are severe and appear at a younger age. This abnormal

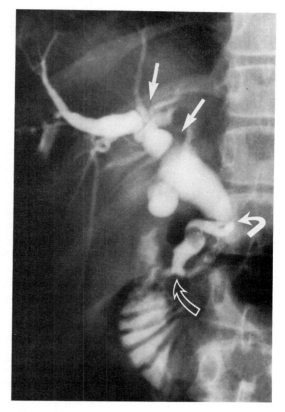

*Figure 22–13.* Type II choledochal cyst with congenital strictures of the CBD (*curved arrow*), the common hepatic duct, and at the junction of the left and right hepatic ducts (*straight arrows*). Open arrow points to anomalous junction of the CBD and the pancreatic duct. A distal CBD calculus is present.

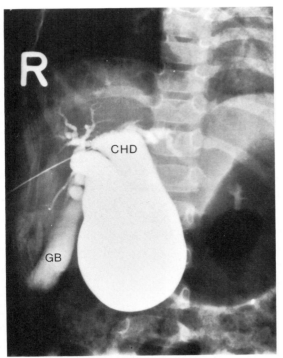

**Figure 22–14.** Choledochal cyst. 5 year old girl with massive saccular ductal ectasia. CHD = common hepatic duct; GB = gallbladder.

union, along with an absent ductal sphincter mechanism, permits free reflux of pancreatic enzymes into the CBD, resulting in cholangitis and ectasia. The higher intrapancreatic ductal pressure prevents reflux of bile into the pancreatic duct.[40]

Clinically, choledochal cysts manifest with recurrent abdominal pain (> 75% of patients) and recurrent jaundice (about 50% of patients) and less frequently with an intermittently palpable mass. Females are affected more often than males (3:1 ratio).[41] Onset of symptoms may vary from childhood to the seventh decade of life, but most patients are 20 years old or younger. Choledochal cysts may be complicated by cholangiocarcinoma in about 3% of patients, and calculus formation is reported in 8%.[38, 41, 42]

**Cholangiography.** Choledochal cysts can be diagnosed by ultrasonography.[43] Cholangiography is indicated for the definition of the intra- and extrahepatic anatomy and for the preoperative assessment of the CBD–pancreatic duct junction.

The cholangiogram shows ectasia of the common hepatic and common bile ducts (Figs. 22–13 and 22–14). These can be mas-

sively dilated, and despite the injection of a large volume of contrast medium, the distal portion of the CBD may not be opacified. Some dilatation of the intrahepatic ducts is also present.

## Choledochocele

This is a rare congenital abnormality that represents a herniation of the CBD into the duodenum. On cholangiography, the appearance of the distal CBD is similar to that of a ureterocele. A smooth saclike or clublike dilatation of the intramural segment of the CBD is seen.

Choledochoceles may remain asymptomatic or manifest with intermittent colicky abdominal pain and occasionally with jaundice or pancreatitis. They are readily demonstrated on cholangiography. On upper gastrointestinal barium studies, a smooth mass is observed in the region of the papilla. Barium does not enter the choledochocele from the duodenum.

Two different types are recognized[44] (Figs. 22–15 and 22–16):

1. Cystic dilatation of the distal CBD that involves the papilla of Vater: The sac drains into the duodenum via an opening that is located eccentrically, close to its neck.

2. Thin-necked, diverticulum-like outpouching of the distal CBD: This drains into the duodenum via the normally situated opening.

## INFLAMMATORY DISEASES

### Bacteriology of Biliary Obstruction

Bacteria are not found in the normal, unobstructed biliary system. However, gallbladder bile samples obtained intraoperatively during biliary surgery grew bacteria in 22% of patients with biliary disease in one series.[45] Choledochal bile cultures were negative despite the presence of calculi or obstruction.

Seeding of the biliary tract with enteric organisms occurs in obstruction. The incidence of bacterial seeding is significantly higher in patients with incomplete or partial obstruction (64%) than in those with complete obstruction (10%).[46] In addition, the incidence of infected bile is twice as high in jaundiced patients with calculi as in those with malignant obstruction.[47] However, despite heavy bacterial seeding, some patients

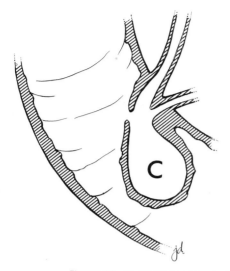 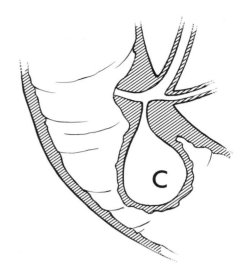

**Figure 22–15.** Choledochocele (C). Diagrammatic representation of the different types.

may not develop clinical symptoms of cholangitis.

We found positive bile cultures in 29% of patients undergoing PBD. The most frequent organisms were *E. coli* (21%), *Klebsiella* (21%); enterococci (18%), and *Proteus* species (15%). Several days or weeks after PBD, bacterial cultures were positive in 97% of patients and revealed predominantly enterococci and less

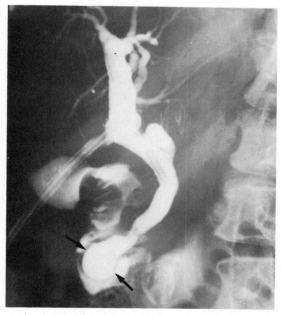

**Figure 22–16.** T-tube cholangiogram shows a choledochocele (*arrows*). Courtesy of Dr Francis J. Scholz. (From Scholz FJ et al: Radiology 118:25–28, 1976. Used with permission.)

frequently *Serratia, E. coli,* and *Klebsiella.* In other reports, the incidence of infected bile in patients with obstructive jaundice has been between 25% (elective operation) and 94% (emergency operation), and *E. coli* was found to be the most frequent pathogen.[46, 47]

Bacterial seeding occurs in 80% of patients with bilioenteric anastomoses, but symptoms of cholangitis are present in fewer than 50% of these patients.[46]

## Bacteremia: Mechanisms of Bacterial Dissemination

Blood cultures obtained at the time of septicemia in patients with acute cholangitis grow the same organisms as those cultured from the bile. This is also true for cultures obtained in patients with cholangiography-induced septicemia. In either case, a transient increase in intraductal pressure is the triggering mechanism.[48, 49] The clinical picture is characterized by chills and fever and occasionally by shock. The last may also be induced by endotoxins.[50] There are several potential mechanisms by which bacteria enter the blood stream:

1. Biliovenous pathway: Direct communication is said to exist between the terminal bile ducts and the vascular system at the sinusoidal level.[51, 52] In animal studies, biliovenous reflux is observed when the intraductal pressure exceeds the secretory biliary pressure.[53]

2. Biliolymphatic pathway: In animal studies, bacteria have been recovered from the

lymphatic ducts after minimal increases in intraductal pressure above the normal ductal pressure.[48] A larger increase resulted in biliovenous reflux. The lymphatic pathway may play a greater role in patients with chronic disease or obstruction. In such patients, it is not uncommon to opacify dilated lymphatic channels during PTC (see Fig. 22–5). It is also our impression that this is the most likely mechanism of delayed septicemia occurring after the procedure is completed.

3. Iatrogenic biliovenous or biliolymphatic communications: Mucosal laceration commonly occurs during PTC and guide wire manipulation for the placement of PBD catheters. In addition, the venous system is entered frequently and a transient direct iatrogenic communication is established. In the presence of such iatrogenic communications, transient increases in intraductal pressure, associated with the injection of contrast medium, are responsible for biliovenous or biliolymphatic reflux and bacteremia. This mechanism may also be responsible for bacteremia occurring during operation.

4. The mechanism for the development of septicemia following cholangiography through indwelling drainage catheters is most likely a result of biliovenous reflux. Digital subtraction studies performed during cholangiography demonstrate an intense hepatic parenchymal stain. This is similar to the hepatogram seen during hepatic arteriography and is indicative of retrograde sinusoidal filling (Fig. 22–17) (unpublished data).

## Cholangitis

Acute cholangitis is usually the result of infection proximal to an obstruction in the biliary system. The most frequent cause of obstruction is benign disease, ie, stricture (36%), calculi (30%).[54] Other less frequent causes are sclerosing cholangitis, obstructed drainage catheters, and neoplasms. The last are a less frequent cause of acute cholangitis, because the incidence of infected bile proximal to a malignant occlusion is low.[46]

Clinically, cholangitis is characterized by recurrent episodes of sepsis (fever, chills, elevated white blood cell count). Interestingly, over 75% of patients with cholangitis have had biliary surgery. The classic Charcot's triad (fever and chills, jaundice, and right upper quadrant pain) is present in only 70% of patients.[54] The intensity of symptoms or the magnitude of alteration of the laboratory values does not always correlate with severity of the disease. Bile cultures are positive in over 90% of patients, and 50% of these patients have two or more organisms per culture.[54] *E. coli* is the most frequently cultured organism, followed by *Klebsiella, Pseudomonas,* and enterococci. The overall mortality rate is high (13 to 16%), even with treatment.[54, 55]

In acute suppurative cholangitis, which accounts for 14% of cases of acute cholangitis, there is occlusion or near occlusion of the biliary tree, which contains purulent material under pressure.[54-56] The most frequent causes of biliary obstruction in acute suppurative

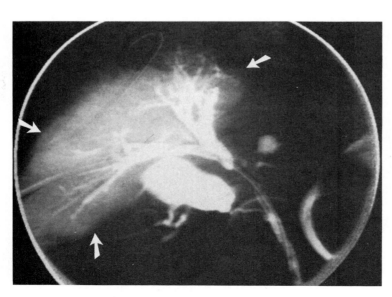

*Figure 22–17.* Hepatic parenchymal staining on cholangiography, demonstrated by digital subtraction (*arrows*). The contrast medium was injected through the percutaneously placed drainage catheter and did not result in cholangitis.

cholangitis are calculi and malignancy.[54-56] Symptoms are usually more severe than those of nonsuppurative cholangitis. If there is complete obstruction of the CBD, shock, lethargy, mental confusion, and coma occur in over half the patients. Acute suppurative cholangitis has a very high mortality (between 40 and 60%) despite operative treatment.[55, 56] If untreated, it is usually fatal.

**Cholangiography.** PTC is indicated for determining the location and etiology of the obstruction. This must be followed by therapeutic PBD for relief of the obstruction. In addition, bile can be obtained for culture. Catheter manipulation should be minimized in order to avoid sepsis and septic shock.

The inflammatory changes in acute cholangitis do not demonstrate specific cholangiographic findings but may include edema, mural irregularity, demonstration of food particles, etc. The appearance of the obstructing lesions is described in the sections dealing with the different diseases.

## Pancreatitis

PTC is rarely indicated in patients with acute pancreatitis unless there is evidence for an obstruction (tumor, stone). When PTC is performed during an acute episode, narrowing or abrupt occlusion of the distal CBD may be seen as a result of the edema and enlargement of the pancreatic head. As the swelling subsides, a stricture from previous episodes of pancreatitis, tumor, or calculus may be demonstrated.

In patients with chronic pancreatitis, the cholangiogram shows relatively typical abnormalities. However, such cholangiographic findings are occasionally present in patients with cysts, abscesses, or carcinoma of the head of the pancreas. In addition, the clinical picture may be confusing, as some patients with chronic pancreatitis present with jaundice and others may have painless pancreatitis.[57]

**Cholangiography** (Fig. 22–18). The main features are narrowing and displacement of the CBD.

1. The narrowing is usually long and gently tapered, involving the entire CBD, but may exclude the ampullary segment. It can also be short and abruptly tapered and may involve the mid CBD only. The ducts proximal to it are dilated.

2. The mucosal surface is usually smooth but can be irregular and thus simulate a neoplasm.

3. Displacement or distortion of the distal CBD occurs as a result of the edema and fibrosis, and thus the stage of the disease can be correlated with the cholangiographic abnormality.[58] Initially, there is loss of the normal curvature of the distal CBD. In advanced disease, the distal CBD is displaced medially and assumes a reversed C configuration. Less frequently, it is displaced laterally. There may be reflux of contrast medium into a dilated pancreatic duct. However, such reflux alone is not evidence for the presence of pancreatitis.[58]

## Sclerosing Cholangitis

The etiology of this disease is unknown. It may occur as an isolated abnormality or in association with inflammatory bowel disease. Histologically, it is a chronic obliterative, fibrotic, inflammatory process (pericholangitis) that affects both the intra- and the extrahepatic ducts. Seventy per cent of the patients are males and two thirds are less than 45 years old.[59]

Clinically, there is a gradual onset of symptoms, and the actual diagnosis may not be made for a considerable period of time. Symptoms include fatigability, pruritus, abdominal pain, and intermittent jaundice. The last is the most frequent initial symptom. Fever is the presenting symptom in one third of patients and occurs most frequently in patients with previous biliary tract surgery.[60] Occasionally, the full clinical picture of acute cholangitis may be present and is usually indicative of a complication (eg, calculi, severe obstruction, or carcinoma). Laboratory data indicate cholestasis. Fourteen per cent of patients have chronic or recurrent pancreatitis and 53% have undergone previous biliary surgery.[60]

The disease is progressive over many years, leading to biliary cirrhosis and portal hypertension and occasionally to development of biliary carcinoma. Varices frequently develop at the ileostomy stoma in patients with inflammatory bowel disease and at the insertion site of surgically placed Silastic stents.

The development of carcinoma is heralded by the detection of a polypoid mass, progressive dilatation, or progressive stricture formation on serial cholangiograms.

The inflammatory bowel disease most frequently associated with sclerosing cholangitis is ulcerative colitis and is observed in 66% of patients.[61] Occasionally, the bowel disease

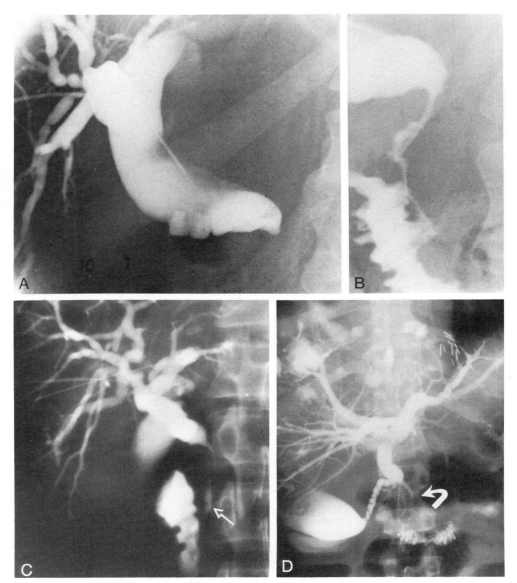

*Figure 22–18.* Pancreatitis. *A,* The common hepatic duct is dilated and horizontally oriented and ends in a nipple-like configuration. *B,* Contrast injection into obstructed segment shows an irregular, edematous CBD and duodenal mucosa. *C,* Cholangiogram from another patient shows a concentrically tapered stenosis of the mid-CBD. The distal CBD (*arrow*) is normal. *D,* Cholangiogram from a different patient shows a reversed C-shaped, smoothly tapered CBD stenosis (*curved arrow*) and multiple intrahepatic abscesses.

may predate the clinical manifestation of sclerosing cholangitis. The natural history and cholangiographic appearance of sclerosing cholangitis in patients with or without associated inflammatory bowel disease remain the same.[59, 61]

**Cholangiography.** Cholangiography is indicated for diagnosis, detection of complications, and, more recently, for preoperative stenting (ie, prior to resection of extrahepatic ducts and hepaticojejunostomy with place-

ment of Silastic stents) and percutaneous balloon dilatation.[62] Preoperatively placed PBD catheters are extremely helpful for intraoperative localization of the CBD and are also used to guide the placement of transhepatic Silastic stents after resection of the diseased extrahepatic ducts.

Multifocal short or long strictures are observed on cholangiography. Both the intra- and the extrahepatic ducts are involved in 68 to 89% patients, and the cholangiographic appearance of the disease in these two location may be different.[60, 63] The intrahepatic ducts are the sole location of the disease in 3 to 10% of patients, and the extrahepatic ducts in only 3% of patients.[60, 63] The areas affected most severely are the distal left and right hepatic and proximal common hepatic ducts.[60] On cholangiography, the main findings in intrahepatic disease include[61, 63] (Figs. 22–19 to 22–21):

1. Skip lesions with mild to moderate focal stenoses, especially at the bifurcations, without intervening areas of dilatation (ie, uninvolved duct segments are of normal caliber).

2. Severe long stenoses, especially at duct bifurcations, giving rise to a threadlike lumen: The segments between the stenoses may be of normal caliber or slightly dilated.

3. Focal circumferential stenoses with alternating segments of dilatation, leading to a beaded appearance: This is not a common cholangiographic appearance (Fig. 22–20).

4. Fine serrations of the intrahepatic ducts, representing early or mild changes: These are seen on close examination.

5. Diffuse obstruction of the smaller peripheral ducts: Only the central ducts are opacified, resulting in a "pruned tree" appearance. We have noted that nonvisualization of peripheral ducts is often due to incomplete opacification. Thus, poor ductal filling alone is an unreliable criterion for the severity or progression of disease.

The extrahepatic ducts may also show several patterns (Figs. 22–22 to 22–24):

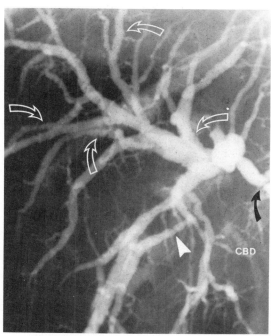

**Figure 22–20.** Sclerosing cholangitis. Early cholangiographic changes are seen in the right intrahepatic ducts. There is a fine mucosal serration (*curved open arrows*) of several ducts. In addition, there is mild beading and focal stricture of the right (*arrowhead*) and left hepatic ducts (*curved black arrow*). The common hepatic duct is severely strictured. CBD = common bile duct.

1. Smooth or irregular stenoses and threadlike ducts.

2. Skip lesions giving rise to a beaded appearance or several segmental stenoses.

3. Segmental or diffuse mural abnormality without stenosis: This can be in the form of fine, brushlike serrations, a coarse, nodular thickening (cobblestone appearance), or

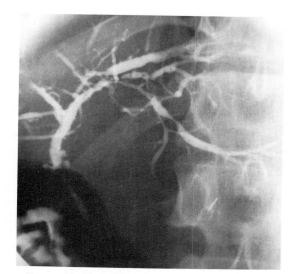

**Figure 22–19.** Sclerosing cholangitis. Multiple skip lesions without dilatation of intervening segments are present.

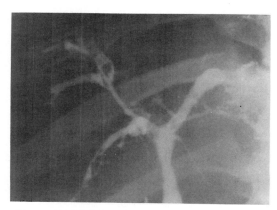

**Figure 22–21.** Sclerosing cholangitis. "Pruned tree" appearance of the intrahepatic ducts is seen. There is ectasia of the left hepatic duct.

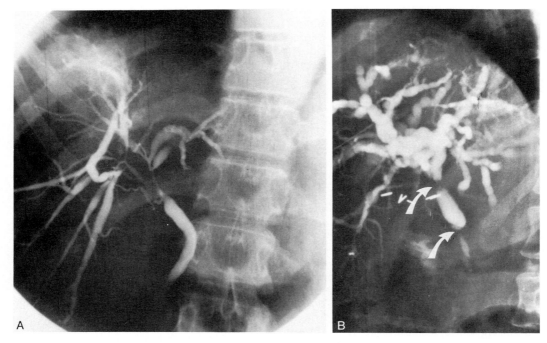

**Figure 22–22.** Sclerosing cholangitis: *A,* There are threadlike stenoses of the distal left, the right, and the common hepatic ducts. The intrahepatic ducts are slightly dilated. *B,* Stenoses of the common hepatic and common bile ducts (*arrows*) with dilatation of the intrahepatic ducts and uninvolved segment of the common hepatic duct.

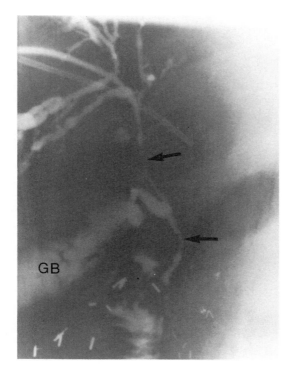

**Figure 22–23.** Sclerosing cholangitis. There is diffuse narrowing of the common hepatic and common bile ducts (*arrows*). Skip lesions are seen in the left hepatic ducts and beading is present on the right. GB = gallbladder.

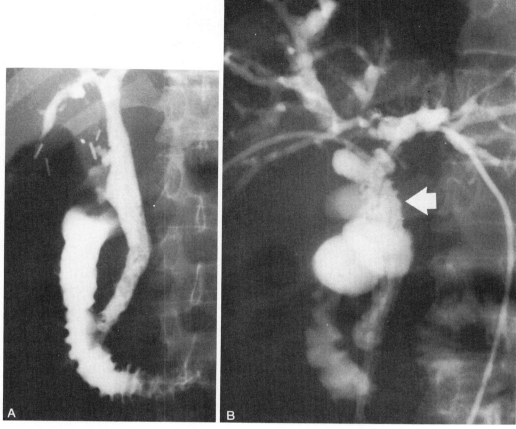

*Figure 22–24.* Sclerosing cholangitis. *A*, Ectasia of the extrahepatic ducts. The CBD has a cobblestone appearance. *B*, Ectasia of the intra- and extrahepatic ducts. There are multiple sacculations in these ducts. Arrow points to the sacculations in the common hepatic duct.

small sacculations.[61, 63] Although fine serrations and diverticula may be characteristic for sclerosing cholangitis, focal nodularity can also be seen in neoplasms.

4. Ductal ectasia with mural irregularity: This occurs infrequently.

Unlike other causes of biliary obstruction, in sclerosing cholangitis there may be no dilatation of the bile ducts proximal to a stricture, because the pericholangitis and fibrosis render the ducts nondistensible. However, the disease may spare the intrahepatic ducts, leading to their dilatation, and may thus simulate other types of strictures (neoplastic, iatrogenic).

PITFALLS IN DIAGNOSIS

1. Nondilated intrahepatic ducts with strictures of the extrahepatic ducts: This may be indistinguishable from diffuse hepatic metastases and cholangiocarcinoma (see Fig. 22–46). Other causes for a similar cholangio-graphic appearance are hepatic cirrhosis, polycystic liver disease, lymphoma, and incomplete ductal opacification.

2. Segmental stricture of the extrahepatic ducts (see Figs. 22–22, 22–33A, 22–35, and 22–37): The differential diagnosis includes cholangiocarcinoma versus sclerosing cholangitis versus benign postoperative stricture. Occasionally, differentiation between these is difficult on the basis of the cholangiographic picture alone. The clinical history may not be helpful, as many of these patients have had biliary surgery, and ulcerative colitis occurs with equal frequency in patients with sclerosing cholangitis and those with cholangiocarcinoma. The presence of skip lesions and nondistensibility of the ducts proximal to the obstruction helps to identify patients with sclerosing cholangitis. A history of intra- or postoperative complications helps identify patients more likely to have

benign postoperative strictures. Multicentric cholangiocarcinoma does occur (see Figs. 22–35 and 22–37), but multiple iatrogenic strictures of the extrahepatic ducts are distinctly unusual in patients who have not been treated by chemotherapy or arterial embolization.

3. Beading of duct segments is not characteristic for sclerosing cholangitis. It is observed in other types of biliary obstruction (see Fig. 22–37).

**Iatrogenic Sclerosing Cholangitis.** Iatrogenic bile duct stenoses simulating sclerosing cholangitis have been observed in patients treated by hepatic arterial infusion of 5-fluorodeoxyuridine (5-FUDR)[63a] and following embolization with capillary occluding agents.[63b]

## NON-NEOPLASTIC CAUSES OF OBSTRUCTIVE JAUNDICE

Some of the non-neoplastic causes of obstructive jaundice have been discussed in the section dealing with inflammatory diseases. Other causes will be discussed in the section on biliary trauma.

### Calculi

The principal components of biliary calculi are cholesterol, calcium bilirubinate, and calcium carbonate. Only a small percentage of stones are truly "pure." The majority (about 90%) of calculi encountered in the United States are predominantly cholesterol containing, and the remainder are pigment stones. Cholesterol calculi are amenable to chemical dissolution with chenodeoxycholic and ursodeoxycholic acid. Most calculi have a complex structure with a protein-pigment nucleus containing calcium bilirubinate.[64] The pathogenesis of biliary calculi is discussed in reference 65.

Cholelithiasis occurs more frequently in women (ratio of 2–4:1), and its incidence increases with age and parity. Common duct stones occur in 15% of patients with cholecystolithiasis. Retained common duct stones are observed in about 4% of patients undergoing cholecystectomy for cholelithiasis. Most common duct stones originate in the gallbladder, and as many as 20% of calculi, usually less than 6 mm, pass spontaneously into the duodenum. Larger stones cause obstructive jaundice, cholangitis, and pancreatitis (if the pancreatic duct is obstructed). Predisposing factors for common

duct stones are hemolytic diseases, Caroli's disease, and benign or malignant strictures.

The amount of calcium within a calculus determines its radiopacity. Pure cholesterol calculi are radiolucent and most mixed stones are radiopaque. Approximately 15% of calculi have sufficient calcium to permit detection on plain radiographs of the abdomen. Contrast cholangiography is the most accurate method for the detection of calculi in the extrahepatic ducts. Ultrasonography and CT, although accurate in a large number of patients, are unreliable if the stones are small or radiolucent.[66] ERCP is used for both diagnosis and retrieval of CBD calculi. In addition, choledochoscopy is now used for retrieval of retained calculi.

**Cholangiography** (Figs. 22–25 and 22–26). PTC is performed in patients with obstructive jaundice and when ERCP fails. On cholangiography, the calculi are usually well outlined. They are easily differentiated from tumors by demonstration of mobility. Very rarely, an inflammatory fibrous reaction may lead to fixation of the calculus to the CBD wall, thereby simulating a tumor. Similarly, an impacted calculus may be difficult to differentiate from an ampullary tumor. Large, lucent calculi are easily identified during cholangiography with undiluted (60%) contrast medium, but may be obscured if diluted contrast medium is used. On the other hand, partially calcified and small calculi are frequently obscured by dense contrast medium. Thus, cholangiographic evaluation for calculi must be performed with both undiluted (60%) and diluted (approximately 20%) contrast medium.

### Mirizzi Syndrome

This syndrome is characterized by extrinsic right-sided compression of the common hepatic duct by a large gallstone impacted in the cystic duct or gallbladder neck. This is frequently associated with the formation of a fistula between the gallbladder and the common duct.[67] In most cases, the diagnosis can be established by ultrasonography, but preoperative confirmation and definition of biliary anatomy require PTC.[68] Extrinsic compression of the common hepatic duct by lymphadenopathy or neoplasm (gallbladder, common duct, or rarely, pancreatic) may simulate this syndrome on cholangiography.

### Pseudocalculus

A bandlike impression upon the common hepatic duct may be due to extrinsic compression by the right hepatic artery[28] (see Fig. 22–

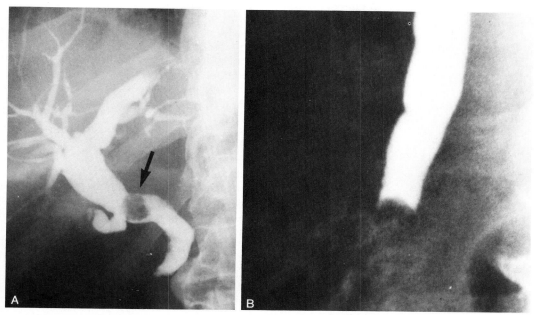

**Figure 22–25.** Common duct calculi. *A,* There is a large lucent calculus in the proximal CBD (*arrow*). The distal CBD is tapered and occluded by pancreatic carcinoma. *B,* Impacted distal CBD calculus.

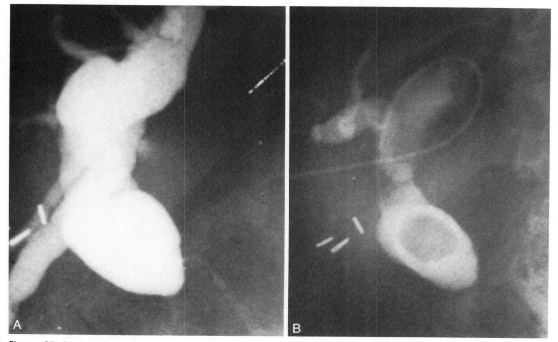

**Figure 22–26.** Partially calcified calculus obscured by dense contrast. *A,* Cholangiogram using undiluted (60%) contrast medium. A calculus is not seen. *B,* Repeat cholangiogram after injection of approximately 20% contrast medium shows the large CBD calculus.

10). Occasionally, this compression defect may simulate a calculus.[69] Oblique views confirm the extrinsic nature of the defect.

A pseudocalculus is frequently observed at the papilla[70] (Fig. 22–27; see also Fig. 22–10). It can be differentiated from a true calculus by observing the relaxation phase of the sphincter. Intravenous glucagon may be necessary to obtain sphincter relaxation. More proximally, inflow of bile from the cystic duct can also simulate a calculus or polyp (Fig. 22–28).

## Strictures

The most frequent cause of benign biliary strictures is operative trauma. Less frequent causes are chronic pancreatitis, perforated duodenal ulcer, erosion by calculi, abscesses, and external trauma. Iatrogenic benign biliary strictures have also been observed following hepatic artery embolization and infusion of chemotherapeutic agents.[63a, 63b, 70a] Congenital strictures occur in patients with chole-

dochal cysts (see Fig. 22–13). In one large series, a benign traumatic stricture was the cause of surgical jaundice in 44% of patients.[71] In 99% of these patients, the stricture resulted from operative trauma. In our own experience, 7% of the first 350 patients who underwent PBD had benign biliary strictures, and all of these strictures were postoperative.

Strictures are observed more frequently in women, because of a higher incidence of biliary surgery in such patients. Operative ductal trauma is recognized intraoperatively in only half the patients.[72] In the remainder, it manifests in the immediate postoperative period as increased and prolonged bile leakage from drains, cholangitis, and occasionally jaundice and abscess formation. Late manifestations (months or years later) are recurrent cholangitis and jaundice. Untreated, the stricture leads to progressive jaundice, cholangitis, sepsis, and the formation of liver abscesses proximal to the obstruction.

Postoperative strictures are caused by focal ischemia and fibrosis. They are most com-

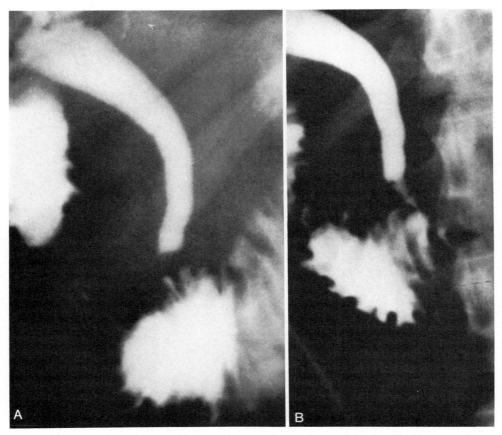

*Figure 22–27.* Pseudo-calculus. *A,* Abrupt termination of the CBD due to contraction of the sphincter, simulating a distal calculus. *B,* Later film showing the sphincter in the relaxed phase.

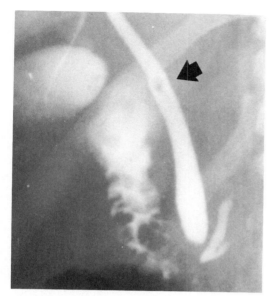

*Figure 22–28.* Inflow of unopacified bile into CBD simulating a polyp or calculus (*arrow*).

monly located in the common hepatic duct and less frequently in the CBD or intrahepatic ducts. Anastomotic strictures are observed at bilioenteric anastomoses. Calculi are observed proximal to strictures in approximately one third of these patients.

In some patients with postoperative bile leakage and infection, temporary biliary diversion through the PBD catheter (ie, external drainage of bile for several days) permits healing of the traumatized segment. If diversion is instituted early in the postoperative period (before infection sets in), it is conceivable that stricture formation may be avoided.

**Cholangiography.** This is indicated for establishing a diagnosis and for preoperative decompression. In many patients, the strictures can be managed by percutaneous transhepatic balloon dilatation or the insertion of large-diameter stents.[73] In addition, the calculi can be retrieved percutaneously.

The cholangiographic findings are shown in Figures 22–29 and 22–30. Postoperative strictures are usually short and cause a relatively abrupt change in the caliber of the duct. They are usually eccentric and have angulated or rounded margins. Longer strictures, especially those with a changing caliber, should arouse suspicion of an underlying malignancy (see Fig. 22–33). The ducts proximal to the stricture are dilated and intrahepatic abscesses may be present. If the laceration has not sealed, extravasation of contrast medium is observed.

PITFALLS IN DIAGNOSIS

1. Distal CBD strictures must be differentiated from functional disturbances (eg, benign papillary stenosis) with the aid of glucagon.

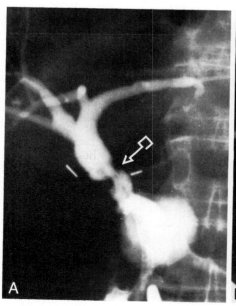
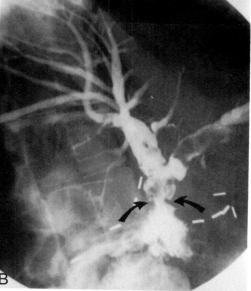

*Figure 22–29.* Benign biliary strictures. *A,* Proximal common bile duct stricture (*arrow*) caused by operative trauma during cholecystectomy. *B,* Anastomotic stricture. There is a short, angulated stenosis at the anastomosis (*arrows*). Multiple calculi are present in the proximal ducts. (*A,* From Gallagher DJ et al: Radiology 156:625–629, 1985. Used with permission.)

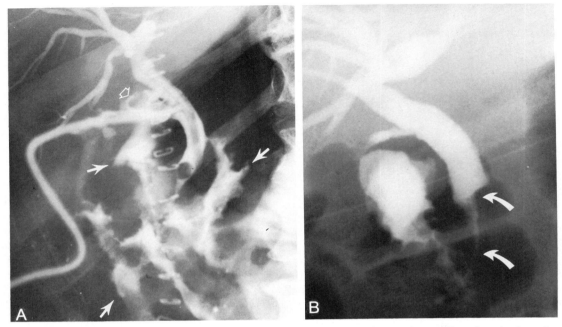

**Figure 22–30.** Traumatic postoperative stricture. *A*, T-tube cholangiogram shows extravasation of contrast medium into a paraduodenal abscess (*closed arrows*). Calculi are present in the distal CBD and the cystic duct remnant (*open arrow*). *B*, Repeat cholangiogram several weeks later (after PBD and percutaneous retrieval of calculi) shows the distal CBD stricture (*arrows*). (*A* from Kadir S et al: AJR 138:25–29, 1982. Used with permission.)

2. Benign inflammatory strictures (due to chronic pancreatitis) or iatrogenic strictures must be differentiated from malignant strictures due to carcinoma of the CBD, pancreas, or ampulla. Benign strictures, including those occurring at anastomoses, are usually short. Long strictures, especially those with central extension (even though they may be smooth), are highly suggestive of tumor (see Figs. 22–33 and 22–42C).

## TRAUMA

Blunt abdominal trauma may result in injury to the intra- or extrahepatic bile ducts. Laceration of intrahepatic ducts with extravasation of bile may lead to the development of post-traumatic bile cysts of the liver.[74, 75] These may manifest clinically, several days or years after the acute injury, as jaundice or hepatic abscess secondary to biliary obstruction. Blunt trauma to the extrahepatic ducts may lead to laceration with bile leakage, choledochoduodenal fistula, or complete transection. Late sequelae of such injury are benign strictures.

Penetrating injury to the intrahepatic ducts frequently results in hemobilia (usually as a result of hepatic artery to bile duct fistula and occasionally portal vein to bile duct fistula). Extravasation of bile from an extrahepatic ductal injury can cause bile peritonitis, which is associated with a high mortality.

The most frequent type of iatrogenic injury to the bile ducts is operative trauma.[71] Such injury is recognized intraoperatively in only 50% of patients.[72] In the immediate postoperative period, increasing jaundice is observed if the common hepatic duct or CBD has been ligated or clipped accidentally. Laceration or transection manifests as increased and prolonged bile leakage and abscess formation. Late sequelae are bile duct strictures (see also earlier section on Strictures).

Iatrogenic bile duct injury is also observed in patients undergoing PTC and PBD. Perforation of the extrahepatic ducts following catheter and guide wire manipulation is rare. This is usually inconsequential and heals spontaneously if the patient is placed on external biliary drainage. Failure to decompress the biliary system may lead to biloma and abscess formation.

Severe, nonremitting hemobilia following PBD is observed in 2 to 3% of patients. This is most frequently due to a false aneurysm of the hepatic artery (see Chapter 15, Fig.

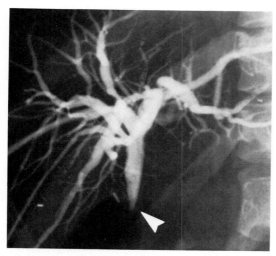

*Figure 22–31.* Inadvertent ligation of the distal common hepatic duct. Cholangiogram through a multiple hole straight catheter placed at the occlusion (*arrowhead*).

15–34). Hepatic arteriography is diagnostic, and transcatheter embolization is the treatment of choice.

**Cholangiography** (Figs. 22–30 and 22–31). Cholangiography is indicated in patients who have excessive bile leakage or increasing jaundice following blunt, penetrating, or iatrogenic bile duct injury. Patients with hemobilia require hepatic arteriography.

In patients with inadvertent ligation of the common hepatic duct or CBD, the dilated duct ends blindly. In such patients, a multiple hole straight drainage catheter should be wedged into the occluded segment prior to surgery. The catheter serves as a marker for intraoperative localization of the obstructed duct.

If the bile duct has been lacerated or transected, contrast medium may accumulate in a cavity. In such patients, decompression of the intrahepatic ducts and temporary biliary diversion via PBD catheters facilitate healing of the traumatized segments. Subsequently, operative reconstruction of the bile ducts may be performed electively, or the strictures may be dilated percutaneously.[3, 4, 73]

## TUMORS

### Benign Tumors

Since benign tumors of the bile ducts are rarely symptomatic, they are diagnosed in-

frequently during life, and thus only a few have been reported.[76-78] Adenoma is the most common lesion and may be cystic or papillary. Other tumors include polyps, papilloma, leiomyoma, fibroma, granular cell myoblastoma, and neurinoma.[76] The most frequent location of these tumors is the CBD.[78] The most frequent symptom is jaundice, which is often intermittent. Other symptoms include pain, cholangitis, weight loss, and hemobilia.

Cystadenoma is an infrequent benign biliary tumor. It causes intermittent jaundice and occurs more frequently in women. Cystadenoma arises in the intrahepatic ducts in 85% of patients and is commonly located on the right side.[79] The diagnosis can be made by ultrasonographic demonstration of a thick-walled, multiloculated cystic mass.[80] The cysts are lined with biliary epithelium but do not communicate with the biliary system. Percutaneous cyst aspiration and contrast opacification can be used to aid in the differential diagnosis.[81]

**Cholangiography** (Fig. 22–32). Unless an intraluminal mass is demonstrated, the cholangiographic features are not specific. Such findings can be observed in other lesions, including other cysts (eg, echinococcal), malignant tumors, hematoma, metastases, Mir-

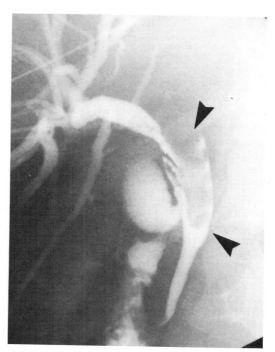

*Figure 22–32.* Intraductal cystadenoma (*arrowheads*).

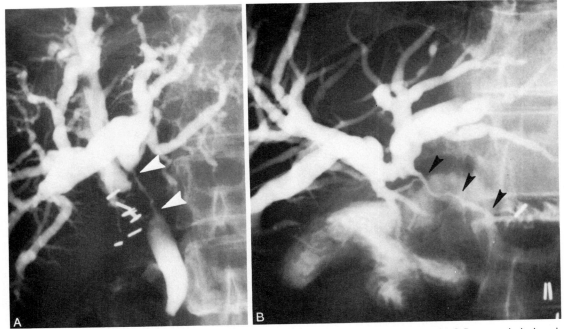

*Figure 22–33.* A, Cholangiocarcinoma arising in the common hepatic duct (*arrowheads*). B, Recurrent cholangio-carcinoma at the hepatico-jejunostomy anastomosis (*arrowheads*). Note that the strictured segments have an irregular lumen.

izzi syndrome, and abscesses and show compression of the duct with proximal dilatation.

## Malignant Tumors

### Cholangiocarcinoma

The incidence of cholangiocarcinoma at autopsy is less than 0.5%.[82] The most common type (found in over two thirds of patients) is a well-differentiated adenocarcinoma. Other malignant neoplasms include anaplastic adenocarcinoma, cystadenocarcinoma, squamous cell carcinoma, and leiomyosarcoma. The tumor may occur as a nodular mass 2 to 5 cm in diameter (most frequent type), stricture, papillary mass, or diffusely infiltrating lesion. It may be confined to the duct wall and thus escape detection at surgery,[82-84] in which case it appears as a stricture on cholangiography. The diffusely infiltrating (sclerosing) type is responsible for inciting an intense fibrotic reaction. Without the aid of cholangiography, this type of tumor may be confused with a benign stricture (eg, due to sclerosing cholangitis), since only ductal thickening is palpable at operation.[83, 84]

The most frequent locations are the distal left and right and the common hepatic ducts (more than 50% of cases). The junction of the left and right hepatic ducts is involved in 20.5 to 45.5% of cases, the CBD in 33 to 40.5% of cases.[84, 85] The tumor arises in the cystic duct in 6% of cases.[82] Occasionally, a single major intrahepatic duct is affected. Such patients may not have jaundice, but cholangitis and formation of a hepatic abscess can occur proximal to the occlusion. More frequently, the affected lobe atrophies. Rarely, the cholangiocarcinoma may calcify and can thus be mistaken for an obstructing calculus.

The mode of spread is through local extension along the ducts or into the liver substance. In the former, there is progressive occlusion of the segmental ducts. Common hepatic duct tumors may invade and occlude the hepatic artery and portal vein, thus making them unresectable. Metastases to the regional lymph nodes or omentum are observed in 15% of cases.[86] Local recurrence after resection is observed more frequently (Fig. 22–33B). Because of the absence of a large mass and the infiltrating nature, cholangiocarcinoma frequently escapes detection by CT.

**Clinical Considerations.** The most common symptom is a gradual onset of fluctuating, painless jaundice. Other symptoms are weight loss, fatigability, and intermittent epigastric pain due to ductal obstruction. Ten per cent of patients have cholangitis, and occasionally cholecystitis or hemobilia may be the initial symptom.[83, 84]

Cholangiocarcinoma occurs more commonly in men, with a peak incidence in the sixth and seventh decades of life, but has also been observed in patients in their twenties.[82] Between 30 and 50% of patients have a history of calculi, and many patients have previously undergone cholecystectomy and common duct exploration.[82, 86, 87] Ten per cent of patients also have a history of other malignancies, whereas a few have ulcerative colitis or have undergone surgery for choledochal cysts.[84]

Less than 20% of lesions are resectable, owing to the presence of local spread or metastases.[85] Death is most frequently due to liver failure as a result of obstructive jaundice and repeated cholangitis, sepsis, or hepatic abscesses and rarely is due to widespread metastases. The treatment of choice of localized lesions is resection with hepaticojejunostomy and long-term stenting with operatively placed Silastic transhepatic stents.[87] The 5 year survival for patients with all forms of tumor is 30%.[88] In patients with inoperable lesions, transcatheter irradiation with iridium-192 seeds may provide relief of the obstruction.[89]

**Cholangiography.** Cholangiography remains the only reliable method for establishing the diagnosis of cholangiocarcinoma. PTC is performed for diagnosis and drainage catheters are inserted for decompression. Most patients require bilateral PBD catheters. In addition, in patients with resectable tumors, preoperative placement of left and right hepatic catheters in the duodenum aids in intraoperative localization of the CBD and decreases the operating time considerably.[62]

The cholangiographic appearance of cholangiocarcinoma depends upon its location and histopathological characteristics. In almost all cases, the extrahepatic ducts are involved. Typically, the tumor is located in the common hepatic duct, with extension into the liver along the left and right hepatic ducts. As the tumor extends centripetally, multiple smaller and larger ducts are occluded and isolated from the main ductal system. Thus, it is not unusual to enter an isolated ductal system on PTC. Three main types of cholangiographic abnormalities are observed (Figs. 22–33 to 22–39):

1. Focal narrowing: A short or long (3 to 4 cm) concentric stricture is seen. Occasionally, the short stricture may appear as an "apple core" type annular constriction. Longer strictures may be smooth or have a nodular appearance. Short strictures are observed in any location, ie, from the junction of the left and right hepatic ducts to the distal CBD. Proximal common hepatic duct lesions often extend into the main lobar ducts. The ducts proximal to the stricture are dilated, whereas the distal ducts are of normal caliber. If the tumor is located in the distal CBD, it can be difficult to differentiate from an ampullary or pancreatic carcinoma and occasionally from a benign stricture due to chronic pancreatitis.

2. Diffuse narrowing: This may involve all the extrahepatic ducts or a large segment thereof and may extend into the intrahepatic ducts. An identical picture may be seen in patients with sclerosing cholangitis and occasionally in patients with metastatic disease (see Fig. 22–46).

3. Exophytic, intraductal tumor mass.

In our experience, the first type is seen most frequently. Failure to opacify all the intrahepatic ducts on cholangiography is indicative of intrahepatic extension and isola-

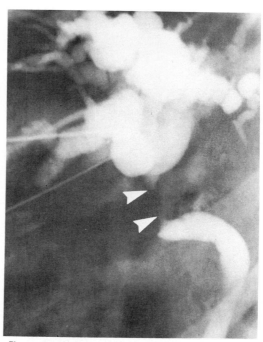

**Figure 22–34.** Cholangiocarcinoma. There is an "apple core" lesion of the common hepatic duct (*arrowheads*).

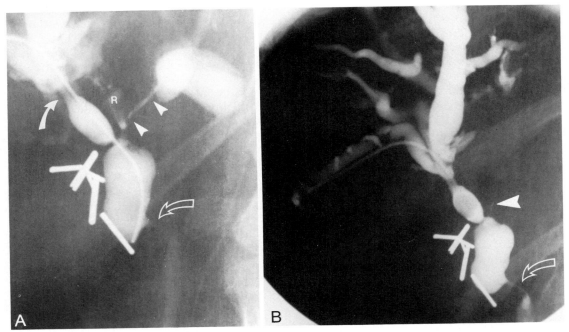

*Figure 22–35.* Multicentric cholangiocarcinoma. *A,* There is anomalous drainage of a right hepatic duct (R) into the left hepatic duct. The junction of the left and right hepatic ducts is severely strictured with extension of the tumor into the left hepatic duct (*arrowheads*). Focal strictures of the right hepatic duct (*solid arrow*) and the CBD (*open arrow*) are also present. The uninvolved segments (skip areas) are dilated. *B,* Cholangiogram following insertion of a catheter. The stricture of the CBD is more clearly defined (*curved arrow*). The left hepatic duct is no longer opacified (*arrowhead*) because of edema resulting from the guide wire manipulation.

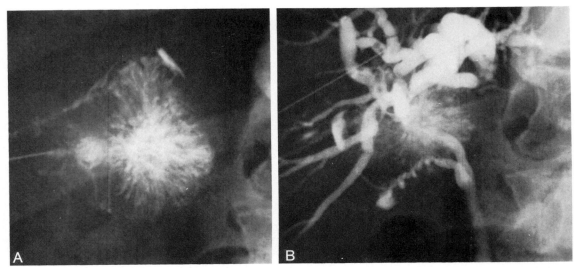

*Figure 22–36.* Cholangiocarcinoma. *A,* Inadvertent contrast injection into the tumor during PTC demonstrates a starburst pattern. *B,* Subsequent PTC shows both severe narrowing of the common hepatic duct due to the mass and dilatation of the intrahepatic ducts.

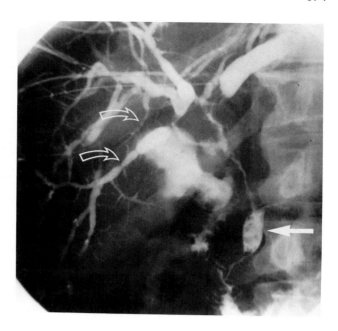

**Figure 22–37.** Cholangiocarcinoma of the common hepatic duct and CBD with a skip area in the mid-CBD (*solid arrow*). The tumor also extends into the left and right hepatic ducts. There is beading of the right hepatic ducts (*curved arrows*).

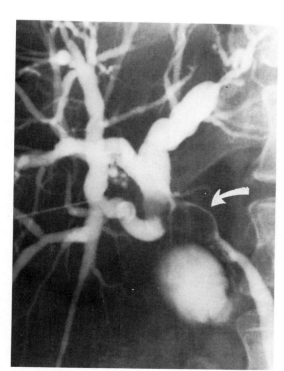

**Figure 22–38.** Cholangiocarcinoma appearing as an intraluminal mass in the common hepatic duct (*arrow*).

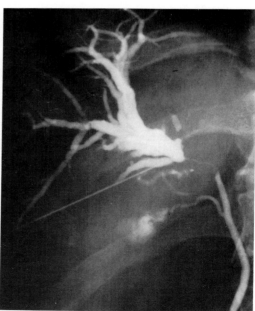

**Figure 22–39.** Cholangiocarcinoma arising at the junction of the left and right hepatic ducts (Klatskin's tumor). The left ductal system has been isolated and does not opacify.

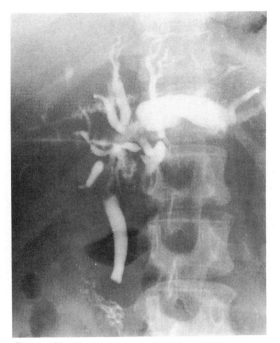

*Figure 22–40.* Carcinoma of the gallbladder with invasion into the liver. There is isolation of multiple segmental and lobar ducts. Most of the right hepatic ducts are isolated and not opacified.

tion of segmental ducts. In such patients, PTC of the remaining segments is performed after insertion of PBD catheters in the ducts that are opacified. In most patients, two catheters, ie, for the right and left hepatic ducts, provide satisfactory drainage. Occasionally, two PBD catheters are needed to drain the right lobe.

PITFALLS IN DIAGNOSIS

These are the same as the pitfalls for the diagnosis of sclerosing cholangitis and have been discussed earlier.

### Carcinoma of the Gallbladder

This is the most common biliary cancer and is 9 times more common than extrahepatic bile duct cancers.[88] It occurs more often in women, and the peak incidence is in the sixth and seventh decades of life. Frequently, it is an incidental finding at cholecystectomy for cholelithiasis. Although 80% of patients with gallbladder carcinoma have cholelithiasis, only a few patients with cholelithiasis have carcinoma of the gallbladder.

At the time of diagnosis, 77% of tumors have either regional or distant metastases.[88] The most common pathway of spread is via the lymphatics, but spread may be vascular, neural, intraductal, intraperitoneal, or via di-

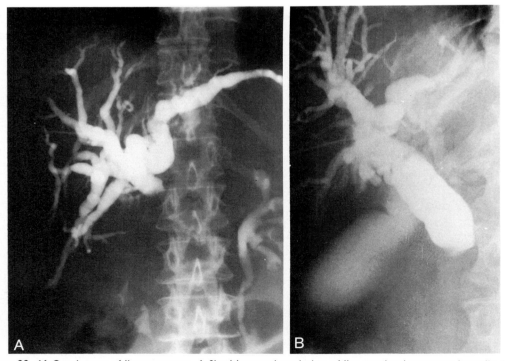

*Figure 22–41.* Carcinoma of the pancreas. *A,* Short tapered occlusion of the proximal common hepatic duct. *B,* Occlusion of the distal CBD with a nipple-like termination.

rect extension.[90] Symptoms may mimic benign gallbladder disease (eg, acute or chronic cholecystitis). Pain is present in 76% and jaundice in 38% of patients.[91]

**Cholangiography.** Transhepatic cholangiography and PBD are performed for evaluation of the extent of intrahepatic involvement and relief of obstructive jaundice. The cholangiogram may show obstruction of the common hepatic duct, and occasionally a tumor mass is demonstrated. Frequently, there is multifocal obstruction with isolation of several intrahepatic ducts (Fig. 22–40). Intraductal spread of tumor may also occur and is more common with the papillary type.[90]

## Carcinoma of the Pancreas and Ampulla

Carcinoma of the pancreas is the most frequent cause of malignant biliary obstruction. Tumors of the body and tail are less likely to produce obstructive jaundice. Pancreatic carcinoma is the fourth most frequent cause of death from malignancy and has a dismal prognosis, with less than 10% 1 year survival. Most patients are in the sixth decade or older, and 75% present with obstructive jaundice.

Malignant tumors of the ampulla are found in 0.096% of autopsies.[92] They are responsible for obstruction of the extrahepatic ducts in

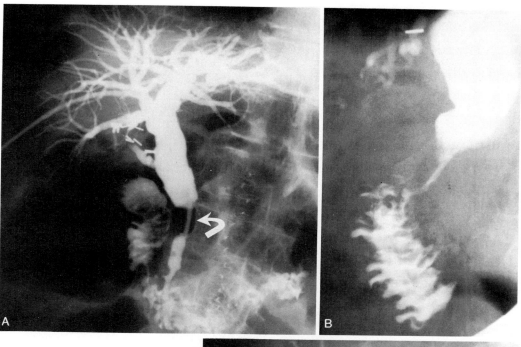

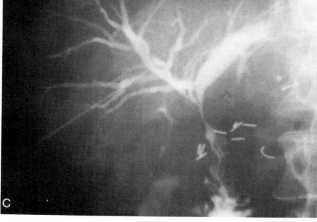

*Figure 22–42.* Carcinoma of the pancreas. *A,* Short segmental occlusion of the mid-CBD (*arrow*). A PBD catheter has been inserted. *B,* "Rat tail" stricture of the distal CBD. *C,* Smooth stricture of the distal left and right hepatic and common hepatic ducts and hepatico-jejunostomy due to recurrent carcinoma.

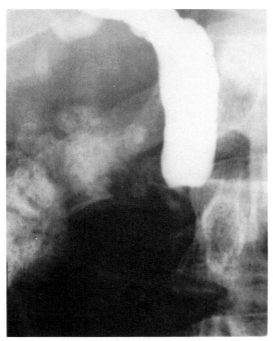

*Figure 22–43.* Ampullary carcinoma. There is an abrupt occlusion of the distal CBD with a meniscus. Compare with Figure 22–25*B*.

8% of patients.[93] The diagnosis can usually be established by endoscopy and endoscopic biopsy.

**Cholangiography.** Cholangiography is rarely indicated for establishing the diagnosis of pancreatic carcinoma but is performed together with palliative PBD and for the subsequent placement of an endoprosthesis. Similarly, in patients with ampullary or duodenal carcinoma, PTC and PBD are indicated for preoperative biliary decompression. In patients in whom ERCP fails (ie, the papilla cannot be cannulated), PTC is necessary to delineate anatomy, determine the extent of the lesion, and differentiate the lesion from an obstructing, impacted calculus. In addition, PBD is performed for the relief of jaundice.

In patients with carcinoma of the pancreatic head, one or more of the following cholangiographic findings are observed (Figs. 22–41 and 22–42):

1. Concentric narrowing and obstruction of the mid and distal CBD with pronounced dilatation of the proximal ducts: The encased segment either is severely stenosed with a

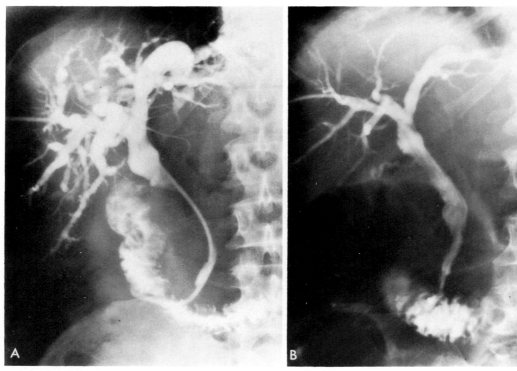

*Figure 22–44. A,* Extrahepatic biliary obstruction due to lymphoma. *B,* Cholangiogram after treatment shows return of the duct to normal size. (From Kadir S et al: Selected Techniques in Interventional Radiology. Philadelphia, WB Saunders, 1982.)

tapered (eg, "rat tail") appearance or it ends in a nipple-like occlusion.

2. Alteration in the course of the common hepatic duct and CBD due to the mass: The course of the more proximal extrahepatic ducts is altered as a result of the dilatation. There is often a relatively abrupt angulation between the dilated proximal duct and the encased segments. Frequently, the dilated proximal duct assumes a horizontal (transverse) position. This is not specific for carcinoma of the pancreas, as it is also observed in patients with ampullary tumors and pancreatitis (see Fig. 22–18). In addition, horizontally oriented extrahepatic ducts are observed in about 5% of normal individuals.

3. Occasionally, the tumor may metastasize to the portal nodes or infiltrate along the ducts, causing proximal strictures (Fig. 22–42C).

In ampullary tumors, the cholangiogram shows a nodular mass or a meniscus (Fig. 22–43). Occasionally, a stricture is present. Calculi may form proximal to the obstruction.

## Lymphoma

Extrahepatic biliary obstruction can also be caused by lymphoma. The cholangiogram shows diffuse narrowing of the extrahepatic ducts and dilatation of the intrahepatic ducts. Following successful therapy, the extrahepatic ducts regain normal diameter (Fig. 22–44).

## Metastases

Jaundice in patients with diffuse hepatic metastases is due to obstruction of the intrahepatic ducts. Such metastases are diagnosed by CT, and PTC is usually not indicated. Obstruction of the extrahepatic ducts by metastatic disease most frequently involves the porta hepatis. The most common primary tumors are stomach, pancreatic, lung, breast, and colonic carcinoma. Direct spread of pancreatic or gallbladder carcinoma or lymphangitic spread of stomach and ovarian carcinoma can also be responsible for obstruction.

**Cholangiography.** PTC is indicated to determine the location of the obstruction and for percutaneous drainage. In some patients, transductal biopsy can provide material for establishing a diagnosis. Three different cholangiographic patterns are observed (Figs. 22–45 to 22–47; see also Fig. 22–40):

1. Extrinsic compression: Periportal metastases may cause compression of the ducts with proximal dilatation. Intrahepatic metas-

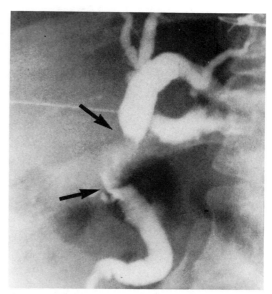

**Figure 22–45.** Metastasis to the common hepatic duct from carcinoma of the colon (*arrows*) leading to complete occlusion of several right hepatic ducts.

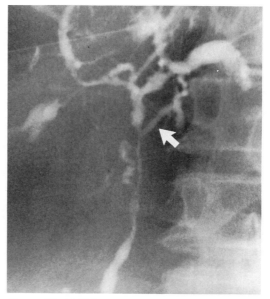

**Figure 22–46.** Diffuse intra- and extrahepatic metastases. There is diffuse narrowing of the common hepatic and proximal common bile ducts. The right hepatic ducts are not dilated (with the exception of a few segments), despite the severity of obstruction. There is some dilatation of the left hepatic duct. An anomalous left hepatic duct drains directly into the common hepatic duct (*arrow*). This cholangiographic appearance is indistinguishable from that of sclerosing cholangitis or cholangiocarcinoma.

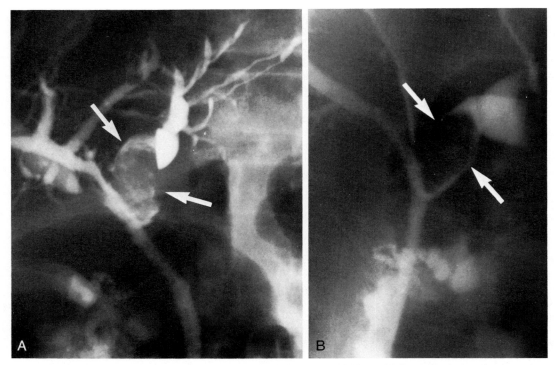

**Figure 22–47.** Intraductal metastasis from carcinoma of the colon. AP (*A*) and lateral (*B*) cholangiograms show a mass in the left hepatic duct (*arrows*).

tases also cause compression, but ductal dilatation is often absent or only segmental.

2. Strictures or stenoses: Focal or diffuse strictures may be observed. These are due to metastasis to the duct or ductal invasion. The mucosal outline may be smooth or irregular. Diffuse involvement of the extrahepatic ducts can simulate sclerosing cholangitis or cholangiocarcinoma. Proximal ductal dilatation is absent in the presence of intrahepatic metastases. Occasionally, an "apple core" type lesion is present.

3. Intraductal metastases with segmental ductal obstruction: Intraductal growth is also observed in hepatoma (see Chapter 15, Fig. 15–53).

## REFERENCES

1. Braasch JW: Congenital anomalies of the gallbladder and bile ducts. Surg Clin North Am 38:627–630, 1958.
2. Hayes MA, Goldenberg IS, Bishop CC: The developmental basis for bile duct anomalies. Surg Gynecol Obstet 107:447–456, 1958.
3. Kadir S, Baassiri A, Barth KH, et al: Percutaneous biliary drainage in the management of biliary sepsis. AJR 138:25–29, 1982.
4. Zuidema GD, Cameron JL, Sitzmann JV, et al: Percutaneous transhepatic management of complex biliary problems. Ann Surg 197:584–593, 1983.
5. Kaufman SL, Kadir S, Mitchell S, et al: Percutaneous transhepatic biliary drainage for bile leaks and fistulas. AJR 144:1055–1058, 1985.
6. Conn HO: AGA Workshop. Diagnostic techniques in hepatobiliary disease. Gastroenterology, 75:1175–1177, 1978.
7. Beinart C, Efremidis S, Cohen B, et al: Obstruction without dilation. Importance in evaluating jaundice. JAMA 245:353–356, 1981.
8. Muhletaler CA, Gerlock AJ, Fleischer AC, et al: Diagnosis of obstructive jaundice with nondilated bile ducts. AJR 134:1149–1152, 1980.
9. Pedrosa CS, Casanova R, Rodriguez R: Computed tomography in obstructive jaundice. I. The level of obstruction. Radiology 139:627–634, 1981.
10. Pedrosa CS, Casanova R, Lezana AH, et al: Computed tomography in obstructive jaundice. II. The cause of obstruction. Radiology 139:635–645, 1981.
11. Greenwald RA, Pereiras R Jr, Morris SJ, et al: Jaundice, choledocholithiasis and a nondilated common duct. JAMA 240:1983–1984, 1978.
12. Weinstein DP, Weinstein BJ, Brodmerkel GJ: Ultrasonography of biliary tract dilatation without jaundice. AJR 132:729–734, 1979.
13. Gross BH, Harter LP, Gore RM, et al: Ultrasonic evaluation of common bile duct stones. Prospective comparison with endoscopic retrograde cholangiopancreatography. Radiology 146:471–474, 1983.
14. Cotton PB: Progress report, ERCP. Gut 18:316–341, 1977.

15. Zeman RK, Lee C, Jaffe MH, et al: Hepatobiliary scintigraphy and sonography in early biliary obstruction. Radiology 153:793–798, 1984.

16. Elias E, Hamlyn AN, Jain S, et al: A randomized trial of percutaneous transhepatic cholangiography versus endoscopic retrograde cholangiography for bile duct visualization in cholestasis. Gut 16:831, 1975.

17. Luttwack EM, Schwartz A: Jaundice due to obstruction of the common duct by aberrant artery: Demonstration of celiac anomaly by translumbar aortography and simultaneous choledochogram. Ann Surg 153:134–137, 1961.

18. Sullivan WG, Koep LJ: Common bile duct obstruction and cholangiohepatitis in clonorchiasis. JAMA 243:2060–2061, 1980.

19. Flemma RJ, Capp MP, Shingleton WW: Percutaneous transhepatic cholangiography. Arch Surg 90:5–10, 1965.

20. Kittredge RD, Finby N: Percutaneous transhepatic cholangiography. AJR 101:592–604, 1967.

21. Ohto M, Ono T, Tsuchiya Y, et al: Cholangiography and Pancreatography. Baltimore, University Park Press, 1978.

22. Latshaw RF, Kadir S, Witt WS, et al: Glucagon induced choledochal sphincter relaxation: Aid for expulsion of impacted calculi into the duodenum. AJR 137:614–616, 1981.

23. Ariyama J: Percutaneous transhepatic cholangiography. In Margulis AR, Burhenne HJ (eds): Alimentary Tract Radiology. St. Louis, The CV Mosby Company, 1983 pp 2229–2241.

24. Kreek MJ, Balint JA: "Skinny needle" cholangiography—results of a pilot study of a voluntary prospective method for gathering risk data on new procedures. Gastroenterology 78:598–604, 1980.

25. Hellekant C: Vascular complications following needle puncture of the liver. Clinical Angiography. Acta Radiol Diagn 17:209–222, 1976.

26. Juhler GL, Conroy RM, Fuelleman RW: Bile leakage following percutaneous transhepatic cholangiography with the Chiba needle. Arch Surg 112:954–958, 1977.

27. Gregory MC: Acute renal failure after percutaneous cholangiography. Arch Intern Med 144:1288–1289, 1984.

28. Watanabe H, Matsumoto T, Maekawa T: Filling defects at the hepatic hilum due to compression by the right hepatic artery in cholangiography. Gastrointest Radiol 7:263–267, 1982.

29. Caroli J, Couinaud C, Soupault R, et al: Une affection nouvelle, sans doute congénitale, des voies biliares. La dilatation kystique unilobaire des canaux hépatiques. Semaine Hop Paris 14:136–142, 1958.

30. Mujahed Z, Glenn F, Evans JA: Communicating cavernous ectasia of the intrahepatic ducts (Caroli's disease). AJR 113:21–26, 1971.

31. Gots RE, Zuidema GD: Dilatation of the intrahepatic biliary ducts in a patient with a choledochal cyst. Am J Surg 119:726–728, 1970.

32. Faust H, Gyr K: Zur Diagnostik kongenitaler zystischer Gallengangsdilatationen im Zusammenhang mit neuen therapeutischen Möglichkeiten. Fortschr Roentgenstr 126:209–212, 1977.

33. Doppman JL, Dunnick NR, Girton M, et al: Bile duct cysts secondary to liver infarcts: Report of a case and experimental production by small vessel hepatic artery occlusion. Radiology 130:1–5, 1979.

34. Peterson IM, Neumann CH: Focal hepatic infarction with bile lake formation. AJR 142:1155–1156, 1984.

35. Unite I, Maitem A, Bagnasco FM, et al: Congenital hepatic fibrosis associated with renal tubular ectasia. A report of 3 cases. Radiology 109:565–570, 1973.

36. Erguen H, Wolf BH, Hissong SL: Obstructive jaundice caused by polycystic liver disease. Radiology 136:435–436, 1980.

37. Todani T, Watanabe Y, Fujii T, et al: Congenital choledochal cyst with intrahepatic involvement. Arch Surg 119:1038–1043, 1984.

38. Todani T, Watanabe Y, Narusue M, et al: Congenital bile duct cysts. Classification, operative procedures, and review of 37 cases including cancer arising from a choledochal cyst. Am J Surg 134:263–269, 1977.

39. Kimura K, Ohto M, Ono T, et al: Congenital cystic dilatation of the common bile duct: relationship to anomalous pancreaticobiliary ductal union. AJR 128:571–577, 1977.

40. Babbitt DP, Starshak RJ, Clemett AR: Choledochal cyst: a concept of etiology. AJR 119:57–62, 1973.

41. Yamaguchi M: Congenital choledochal cyst. Analysis of 1433 patients in the Japanese literature. Am J Surg 140:653–657, 1980.

42. Flanigan DP: Biliary carcinoma associated with biliary cysts. Cancer 40:880–883, 1977.

43. Kangarloo H, Sarti DA, Sample WF, et al: Ultrasonic spectrum of choledochal cysts in children. Pediatr Radiol 9:15–18, 1980.

44. Scholz FJ, Carrera GF, Larsen CR: The choledochocele: Correlation of radiological, clinical and pathological findings. Radiology 118:25–28, 1976.

45. Lou SMA, Mandal AK, Alexander JL, et al: Bacteriology of the human biliary tract and the duodenum. Arch Surg 112:965–967, 1977.

46. Flemma RJ, Flint LM, Osterhout S, et al: Bacteriologic studies of biliary tract infection. Ann Surg 166:563–572, 1967.

47. Kreighley MRB, Drysdale RB, Quoraishi AH, et al: Antibiotic treatment of biliary sepsis. Surg Clin North Am 55:1379–1390, 1975.

48. Huang T, Bass JA, Williams RD, et al: The significance of biliary pressure in cholangitis. Arch Surg 98:629–632, 1969.

49. Mixer HW, Rigler LG, Gonzalez-Oddone MV: Experimental studies on biliary regurgitation during cholangiography. Gastroenterology 9:64–80, 1947.

50. Kreighley MRB, Wilson G, Kelley JP: Fatal endotoxic shock of biliary tract origin complicating transhepatic cholangiography. Br Med J 3:147–148, 1973.

51. Rouiller C: Les canalicules biliares. Acta Anat 26:94–109, 1956.

52. Edlund Y, Hanzon V: Demonstration of the close relationship between bile capillaries and sinusoid walls. Acta Anat 17:105–111, 1953.

53. Jacobsson B, Kjellander J, Rosengren B: Cholangiovenous reflux. An experimental study. Acta Chir Scand 123:316–321, 1962.

54. Boey JH, Way LW: Acute cholangitis. Ann Surg 191:264–270, 1980.

55. Dow RW, Lindenauer SM: Acute obstructive suppurative cholangitis. Ann Surg 169:272–276, 1969.

56. Reynolds BM, Dargan EL: Acute obstructive cholangitis. A distinct clinical syndrome. Ann Surg 150:299–303, 1959.

57. Goulston SJM, Gallagher ND: Chronic painless pancreatitis. Gut 3:252–254, 1962.

58. Sacks MD, Partington PF: Cholangiographic diagnosis of pancreatitis. Radiology 76:32–38, 1956.

59. LaRusso NF, Wiesner RH, Ludwig J, et al: Primary sclerosing cholangitis. N Engl J Med 310:899–903, 1984.

60. Cameron JL, Gayler BW, Sanfey H, et al: Sclerosing cholangitis. Anatomical distribution of obstructive lesions. Ann Surg 200:54–60, 1984.

61. McCarty RL, LaRusso NF, Wiesner RH, et al: Primary sclerosing cholangitis: Findings on cholangiography and pancreatography. Radiology 149:39–44, 1983.

62. Kadir S, Cameron JL: Unpublished data.

63. Li-Yeng C, Goldberg HI: Sclerosing cholangitis: Broad spectrum of radiographic features. Gastrointest Radiol 9:39–47, 1984.

63a. Botet JF, Watson RC, Kemeny N, et al: Cholangitis complicating intraarterial chemotherapy in liver metastasis. Radiology 156:335–337, 1985.

63b. Doppman JL, Girton ME: Bile duct scarring following ethanol embolization of the hepatic artery: An experimental study in monkeys. Radiology 152:621–626, 1984.

64. Been JM, Bills PM, Lewis D: Microstructure of gallstones. Gastroenterology 76:548–555, 1979.

65. Weisberg HF: Pathogenesis of gallstones. Ann Clin Lab Sci 14:243–251, 1984.

66. Suzuki M, Takashima T, Funaki H, et al: CT diagnosis of common bile duct stone. Gastrointest Radiol 8:327–331, 1983.

67. Cornud F, Grenier P, Belghiti J, et al: Mirizzi syndrome and biliobiliary fistulas: Roentgenologic appearance. Gastrointest Radiol 6:265–268, 1981.

68. Cruz FO, Barriga P, Tocornal J, et al: Radiology of the Mirizzi syndrome: Diagnostic importance of the transhepatic cholangiogram. Gastrointest Radiol 8:249–253, 1983.

69. Baer JW, Abiri M: Right hepatic artery as a cause of pseudocalculus in the biliary tree. Gastrointest Radiol 7:269–273, 1982.

70. Mujahed Z, Evans JA: Pseudocalculus defect in cholangiography. AJR 116:337–341, 1972.

71. Marlow LS: Obstructions of the bile duct. Br J Surg 66:69–79, 1979.

70a. Makuuchi M, Sukigara M, Mori T, et al: Bile duct necrosis: Complication of transcatheter hepatic embolization. Radiology 156:331–334, 1985.

72. Way LW, Dunphy JE: Biliary stricture. Am J Surg 124:287–295, 1972.

73. Gallagher DJ, Kadir S, Kaufman SL, et al: Percutaneous management of benign postoperative biliary strictures. Radiology 156:625–629, 1985.

74. Tucker JK, Everett WG, Smith JM: Roux loop drainage for post-traumatic biliary cyst. Br Med J 2:22, 1975.

75. Levin DC, Watson RC, Sos TA, et al: Angiography in blunt hepatic trauma. AJR 119:95–101, 1973.

76. Chu PT: Benign neoplasms of the extrahepatic biliary ducts. Review of the literature and report of a case of fibroma. Arch Pathol 50:84–97, 1950.

77. Hossack KF, Herron JJ: Benign tumours of the common bile duct: Report of a case and review of the literature. Aust NZ J Surg 42:22–26, 1972.

78. Dowdy GS Jr, Olin WG Jr, Shelton EL Jr, et al: Benign tumors of the extrahepatic bile ducts. Arch Surg 85:503–513, 1962.

79. Ishak KG, Willis GW, Cummins SD, et al: Biliary cystadenoma and cystadenocarcinoma. Report of 14 cases and review of the literature. Cancer 39:322–338, 1977.

80. Nagorney DM, LeSage GD, Carboneau JW, et al: Cystadenoma of the proximal common hepatic duct: The use of abdominal ultrasonography and transhepatic cholangiography in diagnosis. Mayo Clin Proc 59:118–121, 1984.

81. Frick MP, Feinberg SB: Biliary cystadenoma. AJR 139:393–395, 1982.

82. Sako K, Seitzinger GL, Garside E: Carcinoma of the extrahepatic bile ducts. Review of the literature and report of 6 cases. Surgery 41:416–437, 1957.

83. Braasch JW: Carcinoma of the bile duct. Surg Clin North Am 53:1217–1227, 1973.

84. Lees CD, Zapolanski A, Cooperman AM, et al: Carcinoma of the bile ducts. Surg Gynecol Obstet 151:193–198, 1980.

85. Broe PJ, Cameron JL: The management of proximal biliary tract tumors. Adv Surg 15:47–91, 1981.

86. Ross AP, Braasch JW, Warren KW: Carcinoma of the proximal bile ducts. Surg Gynecol Obstet 136:923–928, 1973.

87. Cameron JL, Broe PJ, Zuidema GD: Proximal bile duct tumors. Surgical management with Silastic transhepatic biliary stents. Ann Surg 196:412–419, 1982.

88. Krain LS: Gallbladder and extrahepatic bile duct carcinoma. Analysis of 1808 cases. Geriatrics 27:111–117, 1972.

89. Conroy RM, Shahbazian AA, Edwards KC, et al: A new method for treating carcinomatous biliary obstruction with intracatheter radium. Cancer 49:1321–1327, 1982.

90. Fahim RB, McDonald JR, Richards JC, et al: Carcinoma of the gallbladder: a study of its modes of spread. Ann Surg 156:114–124, 1962.

91. Piehler JM, Crichlow RW: Primary carcinoma of the gallbladder. Surg Gynecol Obstet 147:929–942, 1978.

92. Lieber MM, Stewart HL, Lund H: Carcinoma of the periampullary portion of the duodenum. Ann Surg 109:383–429, 1939.

93. Ransom HK: Carcinoma of the pancreas and extrahepatic bile ducts. Am J Surg 40:264–281, 1938.

# COMPLICATIONS

## EIGHT

## Complications of Angiography

Complications associated with angiography must be evaluated in light of the patient's overall condition. A comparison of patients undergoing angiography and a similar group whose procedure was scheduled but later canceled showed similarity in the number and onset of serious complications.[1] Another study of complications associated with renal angiography revealed that patients with underlying renal abnormalities were at a much higher risk for post-angiography complications.[2] These studies and other unpublished clinical observations indicate that many of the major complications observed in patients undergoing diagnostic angiography are related to the severity of their underlying illnesses and may not be avoidable despite the most meticulous technique.

### CONTRAST REACTIONS

Contrast reactions are observed in about 3% of patients undergoing arteriography or venography.[3] Although minor contrast reactions tend to recur after renewed exposure to contrast medium, major, life-threatening reactions do not.[4] However, with a few exceptions, it is difficult to predict which patient will have a reaction. In individuals with a past history of a contrast reaction, the incidence of another such reaction is three and one half times that of the normal population.[4] Similarly, the incidence of bronchospasm following exposure to contrast medium is three and one half times higher in patients with asthma.

Major nonfatal contrast reactions occur in 0.14% of patients undergoing arteriography and 0.09% of patients having venography.[3] A fatal reaction occurs more frequently after venography than after arteriography (0.02% versus 0.004%). Laryngeal edema following intraarterial contrast injection occurs in less than 0.06% of patients.[5, 6]

Many of the "reactions" reported by patients are not true contrast reactions. A precise description of the incident should be obtained, and if there is any doubt, the patient should be premedicated. Our approach for patients with previous contrast reactions has been as follows:

1. Minor reactions (urticaria): Premedicate with antihistamines: outpatients—25 to 50 mg of diphenhydramine (Benadryl) IV as soon as intravenous access has been established (*before the procedure!*); inpatients—50 mg of Benadryl PO the evening before the study and repeat dose IM together with other premedication.

2. Moderate reactions (eg, bronchospasm): Premedicate with antihistamine as for minor reactions and, in addition, add 100 mg of hydrocortisone every 6 hours for at least three doses. The third dose is given together with the premedication for angiography.

3. Severe reactions (laryngospasm, anaphylaxis, shock, cardiopulmonary arrest): First, reassess the indications for angiography. Then explore the possibility of using noniodinated contrast media (eg, carbon dioxide for pelvis and lower extremity DSA), radionuclide studies, or other noninvasive procedures (eg, real time ultrasonography for demonstration of deep venous thrombosis).

Although a second severe contrast reaction occurs infrequently,[4] we recommend that appropriate precautionary measures be taken. Our approach has been as follows:

1. Antihistamine and hydrocortisone prep similar to that used for moderately severe reactions. The effectiveness of Benadryl can be enhanced by using an $H_2$ receptor antagonist, ie, cimetidine (Tagamet).[7a] The latter has also been used for the treatment of an allergic reaction not responsive to steroids and Benadryl.[7b]

2. Anesthesia standby, ie, anesthesiologist and equipment available in the angiography room during the procedure.

Although the protective value (from repeat contrast reactions) of steroid and antihistamine medication has been questioned by some,[4] our experience with many patients undergoing multiple repeat contrast examinations has provided unquestionable evidence that minor and moderate contrast reactions (urticaria, bronchospasm) can be avoided by such premedication (in combination with appropriate sedation). On the other hand, steroids have been shown to be of little help in preventing contrast toxicity.[7] Table 23–1 lists the treatment of the different types of contrast reactions.

## RENAL COMPLICATIONS OF ANGIOGRAPHY

Contrast-induced renal failure is defined as an increase in the serum creatinine level by at least 20% or 0.3 mg/dl in the post-angiography period.[2] Factors that predispose to contrast-induced renal complications include preexisting renal diseases, marginal or abnormal renal function, diabetes mellitus, myeloma, hyperuricemia, proteinuria, dehydration, and advanced age (> 55 years).[2, 8, 9] Additional factors are the volume of contrast medium used and the administration of concomitant medication, eg, nephrotoxic antibiotics.

**TABLE 23–1.** Treatment of Contrast Reactions

| Reaction | Treatment |
|---|---|
| Urticaria | 25–50 mg of Benadryl IV |
| Bronchospasm | 0.2–0.5 mg of epinephrine subcutaneously* <br> 25–50 mg of Benadryl IV <br> (100 to 1000 mg of hydrocortisone IV)† |
| Laryngospasm/ laryngeal edema | 0.2–0.4 mg of epinephrine diluted in 10 ml of normal saline (slow IV injection) <br> 100 to 1000 mg of hydrocortisone <br> (25 to 50 mg Benadryl IV and 300 mg cimetidine‡ in 100 ml D5W infused over 15 to 20 minutes) <br> Intubation§ |
| Cardiopulmonary arrest/shock | Cardiopulmonary resuscitation |

*Alternatively, 0.2 to 0.4 mg diluted in 10 ml of normal saline for slow IV injection.

†In severe bronchospasm.

‡Cimetidine is used in conjunction with Benadryl in patients not responding to epinephrine and hydrocortisone.

§If the other treatment is unsuccessful.

Patients undergoing multiple contrast studies are also at increased risk for such complications. These patients are a frequently overlooked group. Because of cost containment policies, multiple contrast studies may be scheduled within a short period of time in an inadequately hydrated patient, eg, scheduling of CT and percutaneous transhepatic cholangiography with biliary drainage. In the latter study, large volumes of contrast medium may be injected intravenously into the hepatic or portal vein branches. In addition, such patients are often on nephrotoxic antibiotics.

In most patients, contrast-induced renal failure is transient, with recovery occurring over several days or weeks. Some of these patients may require dialysis for correction of electrolyte imbalance.

Renal complications can be avoided by careful screening and identification of the

**TABLE 23–2.** Complications (%) of Percutaneous Arteriography*

| Type of Complication | Approach | | |
|---|---|---|---|
| | Femoral | Axillary | Translumbar |
| Puncture site complications: | | | |
| Hematoma | 0.26 | 0.68 | 0.53 |
| Occlusion/thrombosis | 0.14 | 0.76 | 0 |
| False aneurysm | 0.05 | 0.22 | 0.05 |
| Arteriovenous fistula | 0.01 | 0.22 | 0 |
| Death | 0.03 | 0.09 | 0.05 |

*Adapted from Hessel SJ et al: Radiology 138:273–281, 1981.

high-risk group. Following identification of such patients, the feasibility of other studies that do not require contrast medium must be considered. If angiography is performed, the following measures are recommended:

1. Order overnight hydration: 100 to 125 ml/hour. This may not be possible in patients with marginal cardiac reserve.

2. Use DSA, if applicable, for the evaluation of vascular abnormalities.

3. Use carbon dioxide as the contrast agent for infrarenal arterial studies.

4. Perform a limited examination, eg, a staged procedure.

## COMPLICATIONS RELATED TO CATHETERIZATION

In a survey of a large number of procedures, the overall complication rates for percutaneous arteriography were as follows: femoral, 1.73%; axillary, 3.29%; translumbar, 2.89%.[5] Table 23–2 lists the incidence and type of puncture site complications. In another review of 1762 percutaneous axillary artery catheterizations, the overall incidence of complications was 2.1%, with only 0.5% serious complications.[10] Fatal complications are reported in 0.03 to 0.06% of patients undergoing angiography.[5, 11]

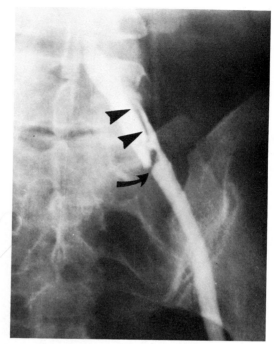

**Figure 23–1.** Dissection without occlusion. Left common iliac arteriogram shows a focal dissection (*arrowheads*). This occurred during an attempt at traversing the eccentric stenosis (*curved arrow*).

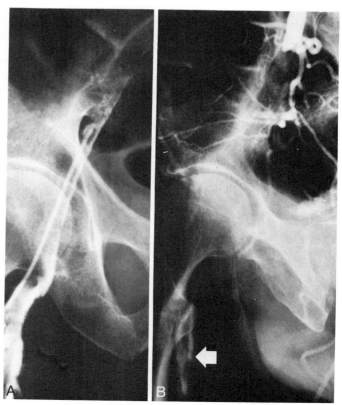

**Figure 23–2.** Dissection with occlusion during forced insertion of a guide wire. *A,* Contrast injection shows intramural position of the arterial catheter. *B,* Oblique common iliac arteriogram via the contralateral approach shows complete occlusion of the external iliac and common femoral arteries. Arrow points to residual extravasated contrast medium in the right groin (from the injection shown in *A.*)

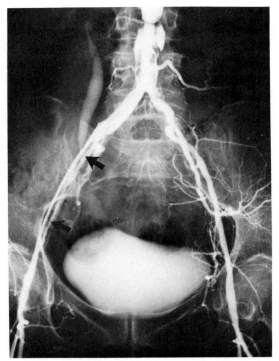

*Figure 23–3.* Severe atherosclerosis of the distal aorta and right external iliac artery simulating arterial dissection. Note the well-defined, smooth edges of the plaque in the external iliac artery (*arrows*).

The higher complication rate associated with axillary artery catheterization observed in one survey[5] may have been related to inexperience with the technique (only 3.87% of cases reviewed were performed via the axillary approach) or may reflect severity of the occlusive disease. In addition, it was not specified whether a true axillary or a high brachial puncture was performed. In our experience, the high brachial puncture is associated with a much greater incidence of serious complications.

Hematoma is the most frequent complication of percutaneous catheterization. The majority of hematomas are due to improper or inadequate compression or multiple catheter exchanges. If the latter is anticipated, an arterial sheath should be used to reduce intimal traumatization and leakage of blood. In the groin, a hematoma may also be due to a high common femoral or external iliac artery puncture.[12]

Arterial dissection is a potentially serious complication that may be associated with thrombosis. This is usually due to forced insertion of a guide wire or advancement of a nonpigtail catheter without the aid of a

guide wire in a severely diseased vessel (Figs. 23–1 and 23–2). Severe atherosclerosis may occasionally simulate arterial dissection (Fig. 23–3).

## Complications of Translumbar Aortography

Serious complications related to translumbar aortography are infrequent and are reported in only 0.58% of cases.[5]

Retroperitoneal hemorrhage, which is usually minor, occurs in almost all patients.[13] The sheath needle and the soft-tipped, high torque wire used by us has provided an added measure of safety, making this technique a very attractive alternative to the femoral approach in many patients with diminished femoral pulses.

Complications observed with this technique include contrast extravasation, intramural contrast injection, dissection, and inadvertent cannulation of aortic branches (Figs. 23–4 to 23–6). The majority of such complications have occurred with the older method, ie, without the sheath needle. When

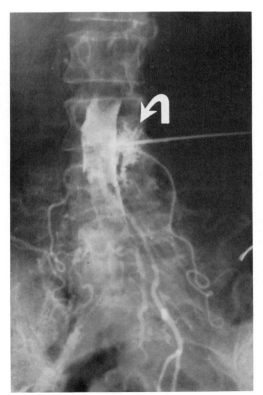

*Figure 23–4.* Complication of TLA. The contrast injection is partially extraluminal (*arrow*) and partially intramural.

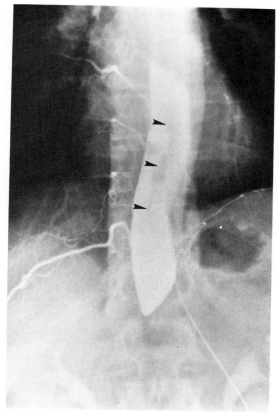

*Figure 23–5.* Complication of TLA. Retrograde aortic dissection due to forceful insertion of guide wire and sheath. Contrast medium has been injected into the false lumen. Arrowheads point to the intimal flap. The dissection was no longer seen on a subsequent aortogram performed via the axillary approach.

used properly, the currently employed method, using the sheath needle and soft-tipped, high torque J guide wires, is remarkably safe.

## Complications of Selective Catheterization

The most frequent complications of selective catheterization are arterial dissection due to guide wire or catheter trauma and subintimal injection of contrast medium. Such complications are reported in 2% of catheterizations.[6] Intramural contrast injection is recognized by persistent dense opacification at the catheter tip. This usually persists after contrast medium has washed out from the remainder of the vessel (Fig. 23–7). In severe trauma, the vessel may occlude as the result of a flap created by intimal disruption (Fig. 23–8). Guide wire or catheter trauma predisposes to the development of stenoses and false aneurysms.[6, 14] Contrast extravasation also occurs as a result of an excessively forceful injection or overinjection into small vessels (Figs. 23–9 and 23–10).

## Thromboembolism

Thromboembolic occlusion of the distal vascular bed is reported in 0.4 to 0.6% of arterial catheterizations.[6, 15] The most frequent sources of the thromboemboli are the arterial puncture site and distal catheter

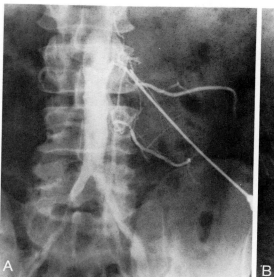

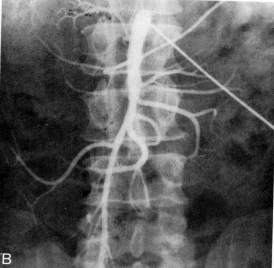

*Figure 23–6.* Inadvertent cannulation of aortic branches. *A,* TLA needle tip lies in a lumbar artery. *B,* TLA needle tip is in the superior mesenteric artery.

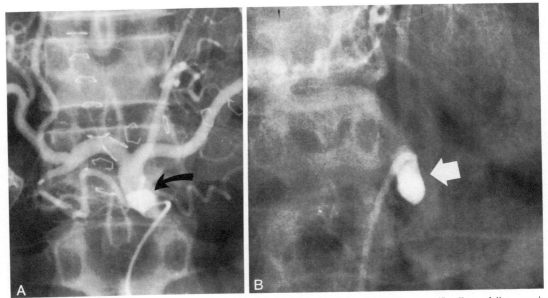

**Figure 23–7.** Subintimal injection of contrast medium. *A,* Early film shows dense opacification of the proximal celiac artery (*arrow*). *B,* Late film from a celiac arteriogram in another patient after the intraluminal contrast medium has washed out. Arrow points to the intramurally injected contrast medium in the proximal celiac artery. The catheter tip is against the arterial wall. *Note:* This complication can be avoided by using a catheter with side holes.

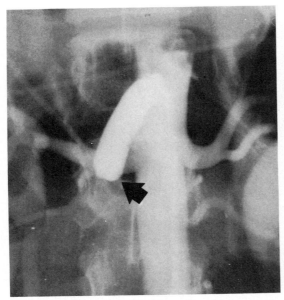

**Figure 23–8.** Arterial dissection with subintimal contrast injection. Superior mesenteric arteriogram shows occlusion of the proximal superior mesenteric artery (*arrow*).

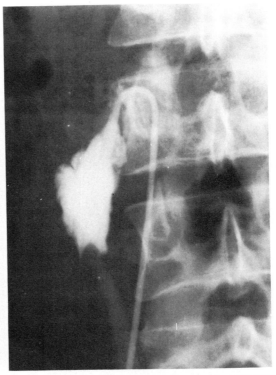

**Figure 23–9.** Contrast extravasation due to a forceful injection through an end hole catheter with the tip against the wall. This occurred during an attempt at catheterization of the right testicular vein.

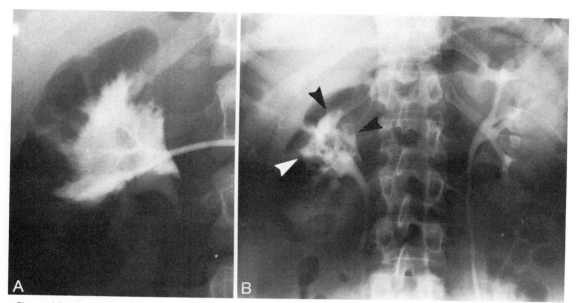

*Figure 23–10.* Contrast extravasation due to overinjection of a small vessel. *A,* Arteriogram of an accessory renal artery shows a dense parenchymal stain. *B,* Abdominal radiograph obtained approximately 1 hour later also shows the extravasation (*arrowheads*).

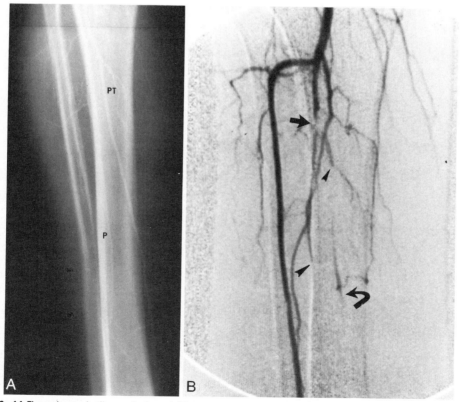

*Figure 23–11.* Thromboembolic occlusion. *A,* Right leg arteriogram in a patient who was evaluated for peripheral vascular disease shows patent posterior tibial (PT) and peroneal (P) arteries. *B,* Intraarterial DSA performed several days later shows a thrombus in the posterior tibial–peroneal trunk (*arrow*) and occlusion of these arteries distally (*arrowheads*). Further distally, the posterior tibial artery is reconstituted via collaterals (*curved arrow*).

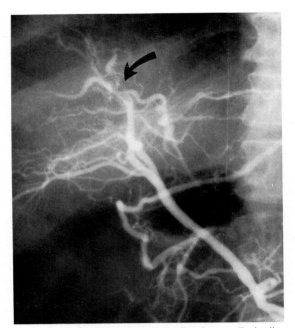

*Figure 23–12.* Thromboembolization from catheter tip. Arteriogram of the replaced right hepatic artery shows a thrombus in the intrahepatic branches (*arrow*).

(Figs. 23–11 and 23–12). Small thrombi are occasionally observed at the arterial puncture site (see Chapter 3, Fig. 3–45). Such thrombi develop as a result of intimal trauma from needle puncture or catheter insertion. Larger thrombi may be superimposed upon arterial spasm or atherosclerotic stenosis, thus leading to occlusion. Upon catheter removal, a thrombus may embolize distally (Fig. 23–11; see also Fig. 23–14). In the leg, most thrombi lodge in the popliteal artery or in the proximal segments of its branches.

Clotted catheters may be a source for peripheral embolization and should be removed without further manipulation. The technique for exchange of such catheters is described in Chapter 3, Figure 3–54.

Most distal emboli are clinically silent and are usually discovered incidentally. If there is suspicion of distal embolization, the following should be evaluated: skin temperature and color, distal pulses (if necessary with the aid of the Doppler flow probe), and systolic ankle pressure measurements. Significantly diminished skin temperature (in comparison with the opposite extremity) or livid or mottled discoloration with absent distal pulses is indicative of limb-threatening embolization.

The Doppler-derived ankle systolic pressure is a sensitive indicator for detection of smaller emboli. A decrease in systolic pressure of greater than 20 mm Hg over the pre-arteriographic value is indicative of embolic occlusion[16]

Whereas smaller emboli lyse spontaneously and often remain clinically silent, larger emboli can be retrieved percutaneously or lysed by intraarterial infusion of thrombolytic agents (Figs. 23–13 and 23–14).[17]

Cholesterol embolization is a rare complication of angiography.[18] It has been observed after atraumatic catheterization of the abdominal aorta. If the source of cholesterol emboli lies above the mesenteric vessels, bowel and renal infarctions occur. Renal damage is usu-

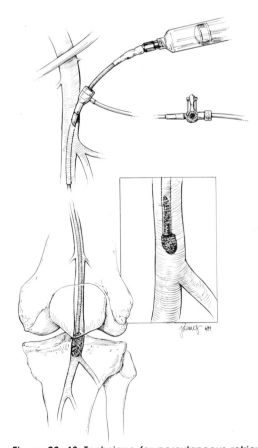

*Figure 23–13.* Technique for percutaneous retrieval of thromboemboli. An 8 to 9 Fr nontapered catheter is inserted through an arterial sheath. When the catheter tip is in contact with the thrombus, suction is applied with a 50 ml Luer-Lok plastic syringe. The catheter is withdrawn slowly and removed through the sheath, while maintaining suction. Several attempts may be necessary before the thrombus is removed.

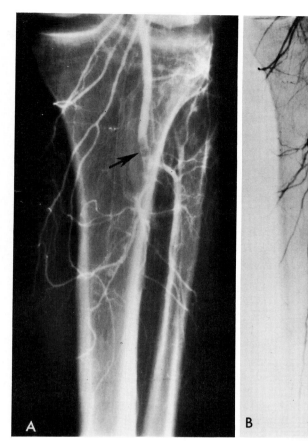

**Figure 23–14.** Thrombolytic therapy for distal thromboemboli. *A*, Arteriogram obtained 4 hours after diagnostic arteriography to evaluate a cold, pulseless extremity shows a thromus in the popliteal artery (*arrow*). *B*, Arteriogram after intraarterial streptokinase (60,000 Units over 30 minutes) shows complete lysis. (From Kadir S et al: Selected Techniques in Interventional Radiology. Philadelphia, WB Saunders, 1982.)

ally permanent. The clinical manifestations of cholesterol embolization were discussed in Chapter 11.

## Vascular Spasm

A diminished arterial pulse or occlusion at the puncture site can also be due to intramural injection of the local anesthetic (see Chapter 3, Fig. 3–1). Absence of a pulse at the arterial puncture site following catheter removal is not always due to thrombosis. For example, diminished pulses caused by arterial spasm are frequently observed in children. Follow-up examination after several hours reveals restoration of distal pulses as the spasm resolves.

The etiology of the spasm is mechanical injury to the intima, eg, the use of a large catheter (large relative to the diameter of the arterial lumen). If the pulse does not return within 6 to 8 hours or if there is deterioration of the peripheral circulation, a repeat arteriogram may be indicated to determine the etiology and location of the obstruction. In children, systemic heparinization for the duration of the catheterization has almost eliminated thrombotic occlusion of the femoral vessels.

Arterial spasm is also observed during catheterization of smaller vessels, especially in the extremities and in younger individuals (Fig. 23–15). Such spasm may be responsible (in part) for the higher incidence of complications associated with a high brachial artery puncture. Spasm also occurs in the venous system and is also induced by guide wire or catheter manipulation.

In both the arterial and the venous systems, spasm is recognized by (1) inability to move the catheter or (2) resistance to catheter movement. The latter can be very painful. Such vascular spasm usually resolves spontaneously within a few minutes. During this period, the catheter should be attached to a continuous flush (heparinized solution of 5% dextrose). If the spasm involves an artery, an attempt should be made to withdraw the catheter as soon as possible.

Spasm is most severe in the extremity

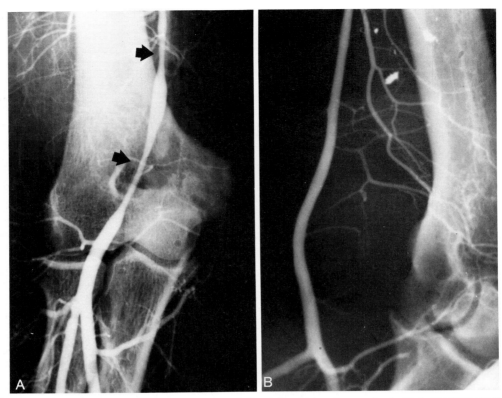

***Figure 23–15.*** Catheter-induced arterial spasm simulating intimal injury in a patient with bullet injury to the arm. *A,* Brachial arteriogram shows two areas of arterial spasm (*arrows*). *B,* Repeat arteriogram several minutes later shows a normal lumen. The oblique view also demonstrates a hematoma with anterior displacement of the brachial artery.

arteries. If it persists, a bolus of heparin (3000 to 5000 U) is given, and a vasodilator is injected in an attempt to relieve the spasm and to maintain the distal circulation (reserpine, 0.5 to 1.0 mg, or tolazoline [Priscoline], 25 mg intraarterially). Focal spasm at the femoral artery puncture site may be treated with periarterial injection of 5 to 10 ml of lidocaine (Xylocaine).

## PYROGENIC REACTIONS

Pyrogenic reactions (fever up to 103° F, shaking chills, and hypotension) are observed in 0.03% of catheterizations.[19] The onset of symptoms is usually 1½ to 3 hours after catheterization and may occur towards the end of the procedure or after the patient is returned to the floor. The symptoms may last up to 24 hours. Blood cultures do not grow bacteria, but there is leukocytosis with a shift towards the left.

This reaction is caused by fever-producing substances called pyrogens. These are heat-stable, water-soluble substances consisting of large polysaccharide molecules that are most frequently derived from gram-negative bacteria.[20] The most frequent sources of contamination are sterilized reusable catheters, stopcocks, etc. A similar reaction is occasionally seen in association with intravascular injection of contrast medium.

## SYNCOPE

Syncope, or a "vaso-vagal reaction," is caused by an inadequate venous return due to gravitational intravascular pooling of blood. This occurs as a result of vagal overstimulation. Clinically, it is manifested as bradycardia, arterial hypotension, and a low central venous pressure. Management involves:

1. Elevation of the legs to augment venous return.

2. Pushing intravenous fluids (with the exception of patients with marginal cardiac compensation or congestive heart failure).

3. If the above measures are not successful, injection of 0.6 to 0.8 mg of atropine intravenously.

## REFERENCES

1. Baum S, Stein GN, Kuroda KK: Complications of "no arteriography." Radiology 86:835–838, 1966.
2. Cochran ST, Wong WS, Roe DJ: Predicting angiography-induced acute renal function impairment: clinical risk model. AJR 141:1027–1033, 1983.
3. Shehadi WH, Toniolo G: Adverse reactions to contrast media. A report from the Committee on Safety of Contrast Media of the International Society of Radiology. Radiology 137:299–302, 1980.
4. Shehadi WH: Contrast media adverse reactions: Occurrence, recurrence, and distribution patterns. Radiology 143:11–17, 1982.
5. Hessel SJ, Adams DF, Abrams HL: Complications of angiography. Radiology 138:273–281, 1981.
6. Sigstedt B, Lunderquist A: Complications of angiographic examinations. AJR 130:455–460, 1978.
7. Lalli AF, Greenstreet R: Reactions to contrast media: Testing the CNS hypothesis. Radiology 138:47–49, 1981.
7a. Black JW, Duncan WAM, Durant CJ, et al: Definition and antagonism of histamine $H_2$ receptors. Nature 236:385–390, 1972.
7b. Myers G, Bloom FL: Cimetidine (Tagamet) combined with steroids and $H_1$ antihistamines for the prevention of serious radiographic contrast material reactions. Cath. Cardiovasc. Diagn. 7:65–69, 1981.
8. Diaz-Buxo JA, Wagoner RD, Hattery RR, et al: Acute renal failure after excretory urography in diabetic patients. Ann Intern Med 83:155–158, 1975.
9. Byrd L, Sherman RL: Radiocontrast-induced acute renal failure: A clinical and pathophysiologic review. Medicine 58:270–279, 1979.
10. Molnar W, Paul DJ: Complications of axillary arteriotomies. An analysis of 1762 consecutive studies. Radiology 104:269–276, 1972.
11. Lang EK: A survey of the complications of percutaneous retrograde arteriography. Seldinger technic. Radiology 81:257–263, 1963.
12. Kaufman JL: Pelvic hemorrhage after percutaneous femoral angiography. AJR 143:335–336, 1984.
13. Amendola MA, Tisnado J, Fields WR, et al: Evaluation of retroperitoneal hemorrhage by computed tomography before and after translumbar aortography. Radiology 133:401–404, 1979.
14. Long JA Jr, Krudy A, Dunnick NR, et al: False aneurysm formation following arteriographic intimal dissection. Serial studies in 2 patients. Radiology 135:323–326, 1980.
15. Jacobsson B, Paulin S, Schlossman D: Thromboembolism of leg following percutaneous catheterization of femoral artery for angiography. Acta Radiol 8:97–108, 1969.
16. Barnes RW, Slaymaker EE, Hahn FJY: Thromboembolic complications of angiography for peripheral arterial disease: Prospective assessment by Doppler ultrasound. Radiology 122:459–461, 1977.
17. Sniderman KW, Bodner L, Saddekni S, et al: Percutaneous embolectomy by transcatheter aspiration. Radiology 150:357–361, 1984.
18. Lonni YG, Matsumoto KK, Lecky JW: Postaortographic cholesterol (atheromatous) embolization. Radiology 93:63–65, 1969.
19. Swan HJC: Infections, inflammation, and allergic reactions. Cooperative study on cardiac catheterization. Circulation 37(Suppl III)49–51, 1968.
20. Bennett IL Jr, Beeson PB: The properties and biological effects of bacterial pyrogens. Medicine 29:365–400, 1950.

# Index

Page numbers in *italics* refer to illustrations; t following a page number indicates a table.

691

# ABBREVIATIONS

**AAI:** ankle arm index
**ACTH:** adrenocorticotropic hormone
**AP:** anteroposterior
**APUD:** amine precursor uptake and decarboxylation

**BUN:** blood urea nitrogen (normal 10–25 mg/dl)

**CBD:** common bile duct
**cP:** centipoise
**CSP:** corrected sinusoidal pressure
**CT:** computed tomography

**DSA:** digital subtraction angiography

**ERCP:** endoscopic retrograde cholangiopancreatography

**FMD:** fibromuscular dysplasia
**FNH:** focal nodular hyperplasia
**FUDR:** 5-fluorodeoxyuridine

**GDA:** gastroduodenal artery

**HWP:** hepatic vein wedge pressure

**IMA:** inferior mesenteric artery
**IVC:** inferior vena cava

**LAO:** left anterior oblique
**LGA:** left gastric artery
**LHA:** left hepatic artery
**LLT:** long length taper (guide wire with 15 cm flexible end)
**LPO:** left posterior oblique
**LT:** long taper (guide wire with 10 cm flexible end)

**MEN:** multiple endocrine neoplasia
**MRI:** magnetic resonance imaging

**PBD:** percutaneous (transhepatic) biliary drainage
**PCW:** pulmonary capillary wedge pressure
**PTC:** percutaneous transhepatic cholangiography

**RAD:** right anterior oblique
**RPD:** right posterior oblique

**SLE:** systemic lupus erythematosus
**SMA:** superior mesenteric artery
**SVC:** superior vena cava

**TDW:** tip deflecting wire
**TLA:** translumbar aortography

**VMA:** vanillylmandelic acid
**V/Q:** ventilation-perfusion lung scan